Pharmacology: In Vivo Imaging

Pharmacology: In Vivo Imaging

Editor: Felix Jackson

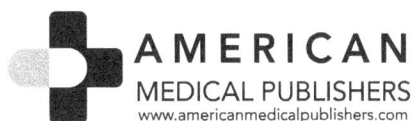

AMERICAN
MEDICAL PUBLISHERS
www.americanmedicalpublishers.com

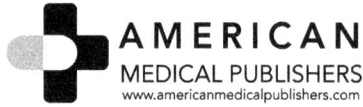

AMERICAN
MEDICAL PUBLISHERS
www.americanmedicalpublishers.com

Cataloging-in-Publication Data

Pharmacology : in vivo imaging / edited by Felix Jackson.
    p. cm.
Includes bibliographical references and index.
ISBN 978-1-63927-556-4
1. Pharmacology. 2. Diagnostic imaging. 3. Drugs. 4. Pharmacy. I. Jackson, Felix.
RM301 .P43 2022
615--dc23

American Medical Publishers,
41 Flatbush Avenue,
1st Floor, New York,
NY 11217, USA

ISBN 978-1-63927-556-4 (Hardback)

Contents

Permissions

List of Contributors

Index

Preface

Every book is initially just a concept; it takes months of research and hard work to give it the final shape in which the readers receive it. In its early stages, this book also went through rigorous reviewing. The notable contributions made by experts from across the globe were first molded into patterned chapters and then arranged in a sensibly sequential manner to bring out the best results.

Pharmacology is a branch of medicine which is associated with the study of drug action. A drug can be characterized as any man-made, natural, or endogenous molecule. These drugs can have a biochemical or physiological effect over the cell, tissue, organ, or organism. In vivo imaging or preclinical imaging refers to the visualization of living animals for research purposes, such as drug development and cancer research. Imaging modalities are used in identifying changes, either at the organ, tissue, cell, or molecular level. The imaging systems can be characterized into morphological/anatomical and molecular imaging techniques. The aim of this book is to present researches that have transformed this discipline and aided its advancement. It contains some path-breaking studies in the field of pharmacology and in vivo imaging. The book is appropriate for students seeking detailed information in this area as well as for the experts.

It has been my immense pleasure to be a part of this project and to contribute my years of learning in such a meaningful form. I would like to take this opportunity to thank all the people who have been associated with the completion of this book at any step.

Editor

Serial Measurements of Splanchnic Vein Diameters in Rats using High-Frequency Ultrasound

Bridget M. Seitz[1], Teresa Krieger-Burke[2], Gregory D. Fink[1] and Stephanie W. Watts[1]*

[1] Department of Pharmacology and Toxicology, Michigan State University, East Lansing, MI, USA, [2] In Vivo Facility, Michigan State University, East Lansing, MI, USA

Edited by:
Nicolau Beckmann,
Novartis Institutes for BioMedical
Research, Switzerland

Reviewed by:
Nadezhda A. German,
Texas Tech University Health
Sciences Center, USA
Craig J. Goergen,
Purdue University, USA

*Correspondence:
Stephanie W. Watts
wattss@msu.edu

The purpose of this study was to investigate serial ultrasound imaging in rats as a fully non-invasive method to (1) quantify the diameters of splanchnic veins in real time as an indirect surrogate for the capacitance function of those veins, and (2) assess the effects of drugs on venous dimensions. A 21 MHz probe was used on anesthetized male Sprague–Dawley rats to collect images containing the portal vein (PV), superior mesenteric vein (SMV), abdominal inferior vena cava (IVC), and splenic vein (SpV; used as a landmark in timed studies) and the abdominal aorta (AA). Stable landmarks were established that allowed reproducible quantification of cross-sectional diameters within an animal. The average diameters of vessels measured every 5 min over 45 min remained within $0.75 \pm 0.15\%$ (PV), $0.2 \pm 0.09\%$ (SMV), $0.5 \pm 0.12\%$ (IVC), and $0.38 \pm 0.06\%$ (AA) of baseline (PV: 2.0 ± 0.12 mm; SMV: 1.7 ± 0.04 mm; IVC: 3.2 ± 0.1 mm; AA: 2.3 ± 0.14 mm). The maximal effects of the vasodilator sodium nitroprusside (SNP; 2 mg/kg, i.v. bolus) on venous diameters were determined 5 min post SNP bolus; the diameters of all noted veins were significantly increased by SNP, while mean arterial pressure (MAP) decreased 29 ± 4 mmHg. By contrast, administration of the venoconstrictor sarafotoxin (S6c; 5 ng/kg, i.v. bolus) significantly decreased PV and SpV, but not IVC, SMV, or AA, diameters 5 min post S6c bolus; MAP increased by 6 ± 2 mmHg. In order to determine if resting splanchnic vein diameters were stable over much longer periods of time, vessel diameters were measured every 2 weeks for 8 weeks. Measurements were found to be highly reproducible within animals over this time period. Finally, to evaluate the utility of vein imaging in a chronic condition, images were acquired from 4-week deoxycorticosterone acetate salt (DOCA-salt) hypertensive and normotensive (SHAM) control rats. All vessel diameters increased from baseline while MAP increased (67 ± 4 mmHg) in DOCA-salt rats compared to SHAM at 4 weeks after pellet implantation. Vessel diameters remained unchanged in SHAM animals. Together, these results support serial ultrasound imaging as a non-invasive, reliable technique able to measure acute and chronic changes in the diameter of splanchnic veins in intact rats.

Keywords: ultrasound, serial imaging, splanchnic veins, venous capacitance, venous diameter$_5$, cardiovascular diseases

INTRODUCTION

Dysregulation of venous capacitance (venous volume at a given transmural pressure) is proposed to contribute to the etiology of heart failure, arterial hypertension, hepatic cirrhosis, pre-eclampsia, postural hypotension and shock (Safar and London, 1987; Reilly et al., 2001; Stewart et al., 2004; Aardenburg et al., 2005; Li et al., 2008; Burchell et al., 2013). Splanchnic veins, located within the abdominal region, represent the largest blood volume reservoir within the human body (Gelman, 2009), and also exhibit the largest degree of active capacitance response of all venous beds in the body (Tyberg, 2002). Therefore, they play an important role in the regulation of the circulation by affecting cardiac preload, and thus, cardiac output and blood pressure. Early methods to study splanchnic venous capacitance and its regulation were highly invasive and could only be readily applied in experimental animals (Brooksby and Donald, 1971). Later approaches that were applicable to humans included examining the distribution of blood-sequestered radionuclides (Schmitt et al., 2002), impedance plethysmography (Leunissen et al., 1993), and direct imaging of the large veins (Stewart and Montgomery, 2004). For example, ultrasonographic assessment of the dimensions of large veins [particularly the inferior vena cava (IVC)] has been used to estimate venous capacitance as a measure of intravascular volume status in patients with septic shock (Schefold et al., 2010) and in patients on hemodialysis (Brennan et al., 2006).

Recent advancements in ultrasound technology include the development of high-frequency transducers (up to 70 MHz for rodent imaging). The associated enhanced signal processing at rapid frame rates (132 frames/second), with superior resolution[1], enables quality ultrasound imaging in small animals (Deshpande et al., 2010; Stuart et al., 2011). The specific probe used in this study, the 21 MHz MS250 probe, has a resolution of 75 μM axial by 165 μm lateral[2]. Importantly, rapid real-time imaging allows longitudinal measurements of the structure and function of small structures without significant impact on the animal or its physiology.

While the current literature highlights many uses of high-frequency ultrasound in rodent cardiovascular models (Coatney, 2001; Slama et al., 2003; Chen et al., 2012), imaging of the abdominal veins has not been widely described in animal research. While many rat splanchnic veins can be readily visualized using ultrasound (Knipp et al., 2003), there is no report of a technique that observes several major splanchnic vessels (both veins and arteries) at once with repeated measures of the same location along a specific splanchnic vessel. The ability to re-locate and measure a precise section along a vessel is critical to allow the continuous evaluation of diameter changes of that vessel during pharmacological interventions, or in chronic pathological states. We have therefore developed a technique for serial ultrasound imaging and measurement of

the splanchnic vessel diameters in the anesthetized rat with the goal of providing a reproducible, longitudinal, and non-invasive index of the capacitance function of these vessels. Validation of this technique included determining if imaging could reliably detect acute changes (seconds to minutes) in splanchnic vein diameters caused by venoactive drugs. Another focus was testing whether imaging could detect stable changes in the diameter of splanchnic veins in chronic conditions such as hypertension. Finally, this work was essential in developing a tool that would allow interrogation of the role of the venous circulation in drug-induced blood pressure changes. Specifically, our laboratories are dedicated to understanding how serotonin (5-HT, 5-hydroxytryptamine) lowers blood pressure chronically (Diaz et al., 2008). In vitro work on isolated splanchnic veins strongly supports the ability of 5-HT to cause direct venodilation but not arterial dilation (Watts et al., 2015). As such, a validated mechanism by which to investigate in vivo venous diameter would allow us to connect in vitro and in vivo studies, a powerful approach when investigating cause and effect. This work suggests the feasibility of using serial ultrasound imaging to investigate venous function in rodents.

MATERIALS AND METHODS

Animals

MSU Institutional Animal Care and Use Committee approved all protocols used in this study. Male Sprague–Dawley rats at 6-weeks of age (300–350 g; Charles River Laboratories,) were used in all experiments. Rats were housed in a temperature–controlled room (22°C) with 12-h light/dark cycles and given standard chow and distilled water ad libitum.

Ultrasound Imaging

All animals were anesthetized using isoflurane (1.5–2.5% in oxygen, titrated to maintain stable heart rate (HR), respiration rate, and body temperature). The upper abdomen was shaved and depilatory cream (Nair^{TM}) applied below the xiphoid process. Animals were positioned supine on a heated platform [Vevo 2100 Imaging Station (integrated rail system); Visualsonics, Toronto, Canada], as shown in **Figure** . Coupling gel was applied to all four paws and the paws were taped to conductive pads on the platform to allow continuous collection of HR, respiratory rate, body temperature, and electrocardiograms (ECGs) during ultrasound image collection. Body temperature was monitored continuously, via a rectal probe, and maintained at 37°C throughout the experiment using the heated table and when necessary, a supplemental heat lamp. Warmed ultrasound gel was applied to the abdominal skin, just below the xiphoid process to couple the transducer (21 MHz probe; Visualsonics MS250) for imaging. The transducer head was locked in the adjustable arm of the Vevo mechanical rail-system to allow accurate hands-free transducer positioning during image collection. The height of the transducer was set to apply minimal pressure to the abdomen while still allowing adequate views of the abdominal vessels of interest. Once the transducer was positioned, the x–y knobs of the platform were used to move the transducer small increments in

[1]http://www.visualsonics.com/products/vevo-2100

[2]www.visualsonics.com/customer/docs/product_info_vevo2100/Vevo_2100-Transducers_v2.8.pdf

A

C

B

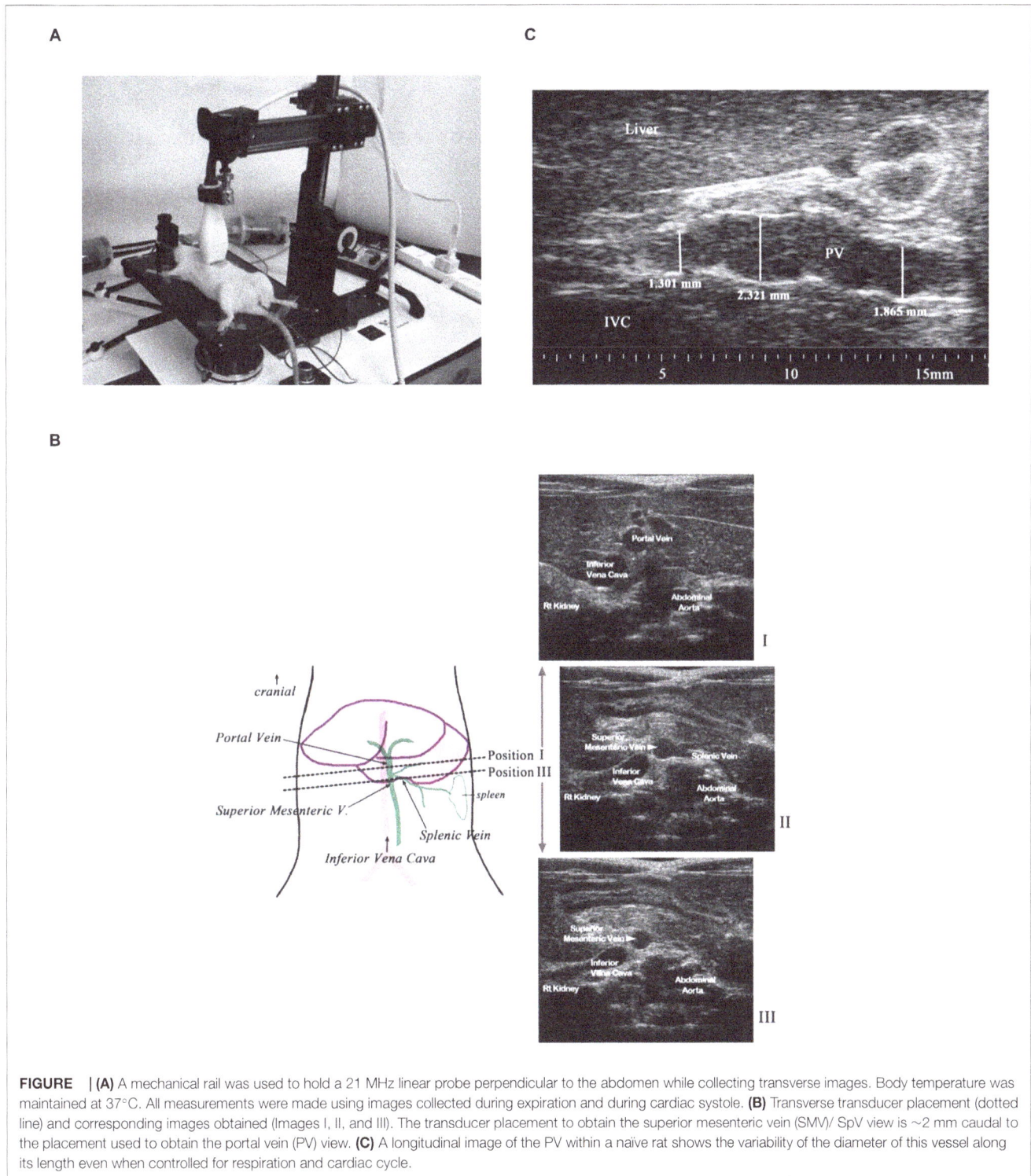

FIGURE | **(A)** A mechanical rail was used to hold a 21 MHz linear probe perpendicular to the abdomen while collecting transverse images. Body temperature was maintained at 37°C. All measurements were made using images collected during expiration and during cardiac systole. **(B)** Transverse transducer placement (dotted line) and corresponding images obtained (Images I, II, and III). The transducer placement to obtain the superior mesenteric vein (SMV)/ SpV view is ~2 mm caudal to the placement used to obtain the portal vein (PV) view. **(C)** A longitudinal image of the PV within a naïve rat shows the variability of the diameter of this vessel along its length even when controlled for respiration and cardiac cycle.

the cranial and caudal directions to display the major abdominal vessels significant to this study: abdominal aorta (AA), IVC, and portal vein (PV) in the same view. Transverse B-mode images were collected at 25 frames per second in two locations, as seen in **Figure** . In Image I, we focused on a transverse view at the level of the PV exiting the liver, which provides simultaneous cross-sectional images of the AA, IVC, and PV; these structures are labeled as such. Image II displays the splenic vein (SpV), the established landmark for locating the noted veins. Finally, image III provides a transverse view ~2 mm caudal to Image I, at a level just below the branching of the SpV (shown in image II), and shows the structures of the superior mesenteric vein

(SMV), SpV, and IVC. **Figure**   shows a longitudinal image of the PV (as it exits the liver) during systole and expiration. All ultrasound images were saved as cine loops for subsequent measurement and analyses of vessel diameters. This technique was used to collect baseline and post dose images during drug interventions. Ultrasound recordings from individual rats during chronic studies were collected at the same time each day and feeding schedule remained consistent throughout the studies. We assumed venous pressure remained stable during each of these interventions and cardiac function did not change, except in DOCA animals. The AA was used as a control abdominal blood vessel for which minimal dynamic changes in measureable diameter were expected.

Ultrasound Image Analysis

All vessel diameter measurements were made by the same ultrasonographer with considerable experience in the use of the Vevo Imaging system. Cine loops of the images were viewed on a desktop station using Vevo LAB 1.7.1 software (Visualsonic, Toronto, Canada). All vessel diameters were measured using image frames from periods of cardiac systole and during expiration. Both vertical and horizontal diameters (vessel height and vessel width) of vessel cross-sections were measured and then averaged to obtain final values from each time point.

Time Course Studies

We performed two time course studies: (1) images were collected for three animals every 5 min over the course of 45 min (acute); (2) images were collected for five animals every 2 weeks over the course of 8 weeks (chronic).

Blood Pressure Monitoring

Rats used in the sodium nitroprusside (SNP) and sarafotoxin experiments were anesthetized with isoflurane (2% in oxygen) and a femoral arterial catheter was implanted for blood pressure monitoring. The catheter was placed through a 1–1.5 cm incision in the left inguinal area into the left femoral artery immediately prior to ultrasound imaging. The tip of the catheter was advanced to the AA and the catheter was attached to a transducer connected to a data acquisition system (Powerlab, ADinstruments) to record mean arterial pressure (MAP) and HR during imaging. Rats remained anesthetized throughout catheter placement and subsequent imaging.

Vasodilation Study- Sodium Nitroprusside (SNP)

After 3 min of baseline recordings of abdominal vessel images and blood pressure, each animal received a 2 mg/kg bolus (0.3 mL, tail vein) of SNP (5054, Sigma Chemical CO., St Louis, MO, USA). Ultrasound images were collected every minute over 30 min with 30 min being the time at which MAP returned to near baseline values. Data were collected at 5 min post-bolus, the point at which the MAP had reach nadir while vessel diameters initial achieved near maximum dilation during the 30 min of the experiment. These maximum changes were reported graphically. MAP was measured continuously via a femoral arterial catheter connected

to data acquisition software on an ADInstruments Powerlab (Chart 7.0, Colorado Springs, CO, USA). The SpV was not used as an endpoint in this particular study, but solely as a landmark. Seven animals were used in this study.

Vasoconstriction Study- Sarafotoxin (S6c)

After 3 min of baseline recordings of abdominal vessel images and blood pressure, each animal received a 5 ng/kg bolus (0.3 mL, tail vein) of S6c (88-9-35, American Peptide, Sunnyvale, CA, USA). Ultrasound images were collected every minute over 15 min at which time all imaged vessels and MAP had returned back to baseline values. Data was graphed at 5 min' post-bolus, the point of maximum vessel diameter change. MAP was measured continuously via a femoral arterial catheter connected to data acquisition software on an ADInstruments Powerlab (Chart 7.0, Colorado Springs, CO, USA). The SpV was not used as an endpoint in this particular study, but solely as a landmark. Five animals were used in this study.

Deoxycorticosterone Acetate-Salt Study (DOCA-Salt)

All rats used during the DOCA-salt study underwent a left uninephrectomy. A DOCA pellet was implanted subcutaneously in half of the rats to deliver the drug at a dose of 200 mg/kg. The other rats underwent a SHAM pellet surgery (SHAM group). All rats were switched from distilled drinking water, to water containing 1% NaCl plus 0.2% KCl for 4 weeks. All rats were imaged at baseline (prior to any intervention), and again 4 weeks after surgery/pellet implantation. Systolic arterial pressure was measured 4 weeks after surgery in conscious rats via the tail cuff method (Malkoff, 2005; Kent Scientific Corp, CODA 6); this was the only time blood pressure was measured. There were four animals in each group: DOCA-salt and SHAM.

Data Analysis

Values were either expressed as mean ± SEM of the number of animals in the experiment, or a percent change from baseline. The baseline was determined by 3 min of image collection, prior to injection or during the 1st day of imaging prior to treatment. Statistical analyses were performed using paired two-tailed t-tests when comparing vessel images to baseline values. A repeated measures ANOVA were performed when comparing vessel diameter values at different time points in timed studies. (GraphPad Prism 6). In all cases, a p-value of <0.05 was considered significant.

RESULTS

Ultrasound Transducer Placement

The splanchnic vein diameters varied considerably along the length of those vessels within the same rat as shown in **Figure** and it was therefore imperative that a landmark be identified to allow repeated placement of the transducer at the exact location along a particular vein. Preliminary work suggested the SpV could be used as a landmark to locate and differentiate the PV and the SMV as shown in **Figure**   , image II. Because it was important to visualize the branching of the SpV off the parent vessels and to include multiple vessels of interest within the same view, a transverse positioning of the ultrasound transducer as seen in **Figure**   was determined to provide the optimal views for measurements of the PV, SMV, SpV, IVC, and AA diameters. In addition, the use of high-frequency ultrasound allowed the collection of images throughout the cardiac and respiratory cycles despite the rapid heart and respiratory rates of rats. Data could be generated from vessels during systole and exhalation specifically.

Acute Time Course Study

Vessel diameters measured every 5 min in anesthetized rats were unchanged with no statistical difference from baseline diameters through at least 45 min as seen in **Figure** . The diameters remained within $0.75 \pm 0.15\%$ (PV), $0.2 \pm 0.09\%$ (SMV), $0.5 \pm 0.12\%$ (IVC), and $0.38 \pm 0.06\%$ (AA) of baseline measurement for each noted vessel. The SpV was not imaged in this particular study.

Acute Pharmacologic Intervention Studies

The venodilator SNP and the venoconstrictor S6c were used in separate experiments to investigate the ability of our imaging method to detect acute drug-induced changes in venous diameter. A single iv bolus of SNP at 2 mg/kg caused significant peak increases in PV, SMV, SpV, and IVC diameters by 5 min post drug administration as seen in **Figures**   ; (PV: $34.70 \pm 2.2\%$, SMV: $28 \pm 4.1\%$, SpV: $39.3 \pm 4.7\%$, and IVC: $6.6 \pm 4.8\%$ change from baseline). Actual diameters of vessels at baseline are reported in the foundation of each bar. In contrast, there was little change in the diameter of the AA to SNP despite MAP being significantly reduced by 29 ± 4 mmHg. In separate rats, a single 5 ng/kg iv bolus of S6c caused a peak decrease in the diameters of the SMV ($11.9 \pm 2.0\%$), PV ($20.5 \pm 1.6\%$), and SpV ($13.5 \pm 2\%$) 5 min after injection, while MAP increased 6 ± 2 mmHg as shown in **Figures**   . The percent change

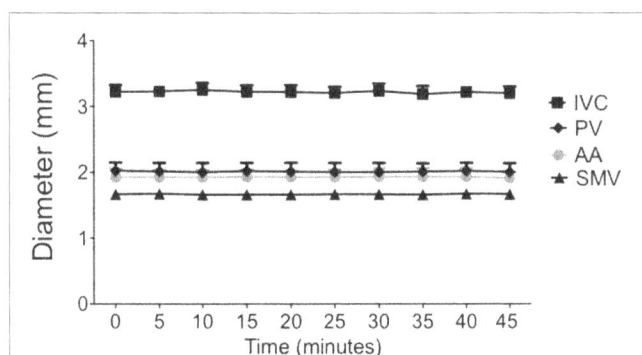

FIGURE | Under isoflurane anesthesia, animals were imaged every 5 min over 45 min to determine the stability and consistency of each vessel diameter. Points on the graph represent vessel diameters (means ± SEM of three animals).

from baseline in vein diameter for both PV and SMV in the presence of S6c were statistically significant (p-value of <0.05) with SMV (p-value 0.067) and MAP (p-value 0.105) close to significance. The SMV image was not included in **Figure** since SMV did not show a statistical significance in the presence of sarafotoxin. There was little change in the diameters of the IVC or AA. Baseline diameters are reported in the foundation of each bar.

In addition, the arterial catheter which was placed in the femoral artery to measure MAP, during each acute pharmacologic intervention study, had no significant affect on the diameter of the PV, SMV, or AA when compared to similar imaged vessels without an arterial catheter (data not shown). There was a modest reduction in the IVC diameter of animals with (3.13 ± 0.11 mm) and without an arterial catheter (3.34 ± 0.05 mm; $p < 0.05$). These differences could possibly be attributed to the larger variability in the diameter size of the IVC, or be a response to occlusion of the femoral artery during catheter insertion. It is important to note, measurements were always compared to baseline, as our focus was on change from baseline rather than actual diameter changes.

Chronic Time Course Study

In a longitudinal imaging study, we evaluated the stability of the splanchnic veins and AA diameters measurements within an animal when acquired every 2 weeks, over 8 weeks. Vascular diameters measured using our imaging technique were extremely stable over 8 weeks, showing the average of the percent changes from baseline at 8 weeks to be within $2.0 \pm 0.5\%$ (PV), $0.95 \pm 0.2\%$ (SMV), $11.7 \pm 8\%$ (IVC), and $0.9 \pm 0.6\%$ (AA), as shown in **Figure** . The SpV was not imaged in this particular study. There was no statistical difference between the time points of the imaged vessels. These findings support the ability to consistently relocate a specific cross-section of abdominal vessel of interest over multiple imaging sessions spanning many weeks within an individual animal. Interestingly, vessel diameters remained stable despite a steady body weight gain (200 g) over the course of the experiment (**Figure**   ). All animals used in these studies were mature rats (10–12 weeks of age at the start of each experiment) with stable body lengths, however.

Deoxycorticosterone Acetate-Salt Study (DOCA-Salt)

We applied our imaging method to an experimental model of hypertension, DOCA-salt hypertension, in which we have previously demonstrated abnormalities of venous capacitance regulation (Fink et al., 2000). The current experiment involved ultrasound imaging of splanchnic vessels at baseline and again after 4-weeks of established DOCA-salt hypertension. While vascular diameters were similar in the two groups of rats at baseline prior to treatment (less than a 4% difference in any vessel diameters between groups prior to treatment), we observed an overall increase in the vessel diameters of DOCA-salt treated animals compared with vehicle controls at 4 weeks of treatment as quantified and imaged in **Figures**   . Diameters increased significantly from baseline in the DOCA-salt treated group,

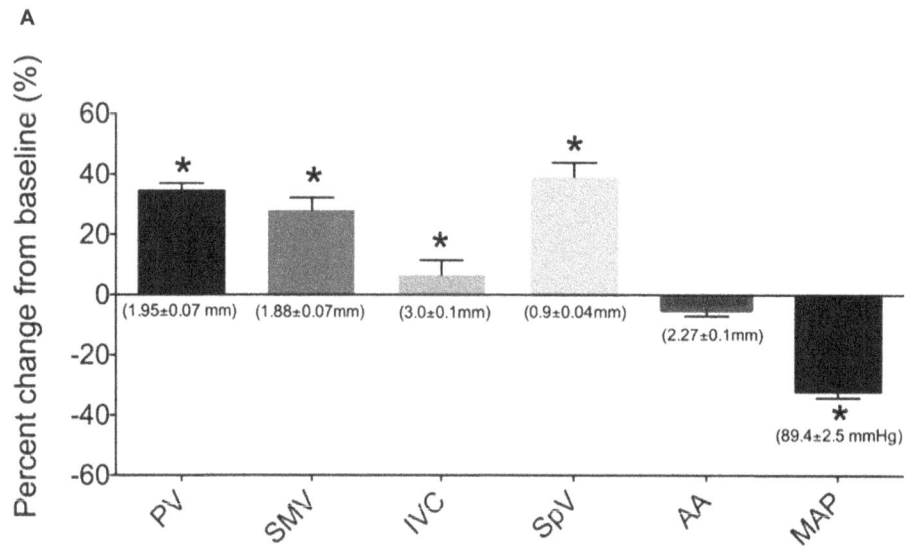

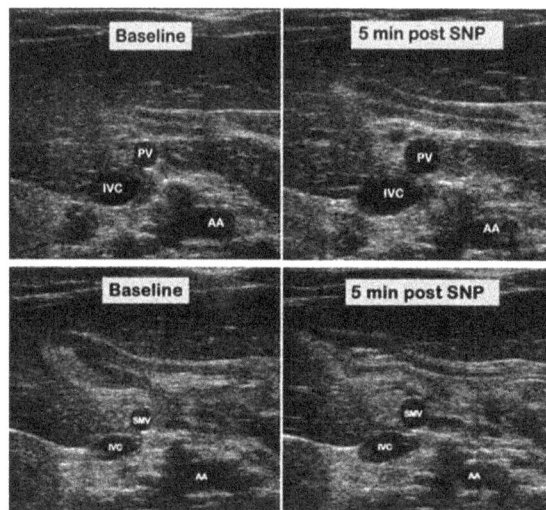

FIGURE | **(A)** Percent change from baseline (baseline measured 3 min prior to drug treatment) of vessel diameters and MAP at 5 min post SNP i.v bolus. Bars represent means ± SEM of seven animals. Asterisks depicts statistically different from baseline, $P < 0.05$. **(B)** Images of PV, IVC, SMV, and AA at baseline and 5 min post SNP. Baseline diameters of vessels are shown in the foundation of each bar.

$32.3 \pm 4.6\%$ (PV), $30.8 \pm 6.7\%$ (SMV), $20.6 \pm 6.4\%$ (IVC), $44.3 \pm 4\%$ (SpV), but not in the AA $16.2 \pm 6.9\%$ of the DOCA-salt treated group or vehicle group, $0.1 \pm 0.4\%$ (PV), $0.7 \pm 2.1\%$ (SMV), $-6.8 \pm 4.7\%$ (IVC), $0.7 \pm 11.5\%$ (SpV), and $0.9 \pm 1.4\%$ (AA). Tail-cuff blood pressure was 67 ± 4 mmHg higher in DOCA-salt versus SHAM rats.

DISCUSSION

The goal of the present study was to develop and validate a non-invasive imaging method to make reliable and reproducible serial measurements of splanchnic vein diameters in anesthetized rats as an aid to understanding the role of vascular capacitance

in cardiovascular regulation. We investigated several different vein segments (PV, SMV, IVC, and SpV) because multiple veins contribute to splanchnic vascular capacitance function, and each segment is unique in terms of structure and contractile regulation (Schmitt et al., 2002). Our approach to this goal featured the use of: high frequency ultrasound; an adjustable arm and mechanical rail-system to allow for accurate, stable, hands-free transducer positioning during image collection; identification of reliable anatomical landmarks to facilitate reproducible transducer location; and the measurement of vessels during systole and expiration only (as cardiac and respiratory cycles strongly influence the dimensions of the compliant abdominal veins). The PV, SMV, and SpV all showed marked changes when rats were infused with either S6c or SNP, while the IVC remained

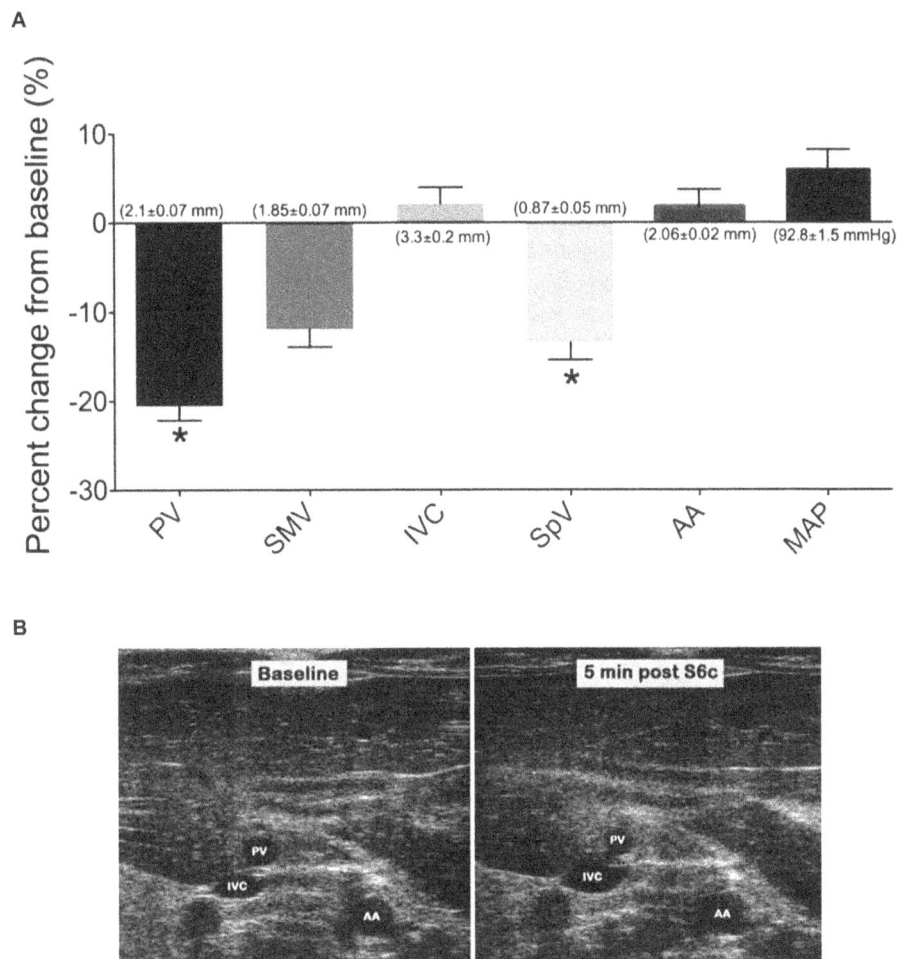

FIGURE | (A) Graph represents the percent change from baseline (measured 3 min prior to drug treatment) of vessel diameters and MAP at 5 min post S6c i.v bolus. Bars represent means ± SEM of five animals. Asterisks depicts statistically difference from baseline, $P < 0.05$. **(B)** Images of PV, IVC, and AA at baseline and 5 min post S6c. Baseline diameters of vessels are shown in the foundation of each bar.

relatively stable. This may occur because the effectors of S6c and SNP are differently functional in these compared veins (e.g., is the amount of ET_B receptors different, is the expression of guanylate cyclase different, respectively?). Alternatively, diameter changes to the PV, SMV, and SpV may lead to compensatory changes in the IVC that mask effects that might be seen in an isolated IVC. The varying responses of specific vessels *in vivo* highlight the importance of simultaneous and collective diameter measurements.

Our initial study showed that use of this approach produced quite stable measurement of vessel diameters over 45 min in anesthetized, temperature-controlled rats. The stability of the vessel diameters over this time period, in the absence of any intervention, allowed us to conduct subsequent experiments to examine the acute effects of venoactive drugs on splanchnic vessel diameters. Administration of the venodilator SNP and the venoconstrictor S6c resulted in anticipated increases and decreases in splanchnic venous diameters, respectively. These two compounds were chosen because of their relative venoselectivity.

This difference in reactivity highlights one of the many differences between veins and arteries, including veins possessing lower smooth muscle content and exposure to lower levels of cyclic strain (Sung et al., 2007). In isolated rat veins and arteries, S6c causes a venoconstriction but not an arterial constriction (Tykocki et al., 2009). This was the best tool we had available that would permit relatively selective venoconstriction and, used with SNP as a recognized vasodilator, demonstrates that we could observe and quantify both venous constriction and dilation. It is important to note that we did not measure pressure within the abdominal veins during image acquisition; therefore firm conclusions cannot be drawn about whether the observed diameter changes were primarily passive or active in nature. However, in a previous study (Schwarzacher et al., 1992) in rabbits that reported changes in the diameter of the abdominal vena cava in response to venoactive drugs, only very small alterations in venous pressure were observed. Thus the diameter changes we observed were likely due to active alterations in venous smooth muscle tone.

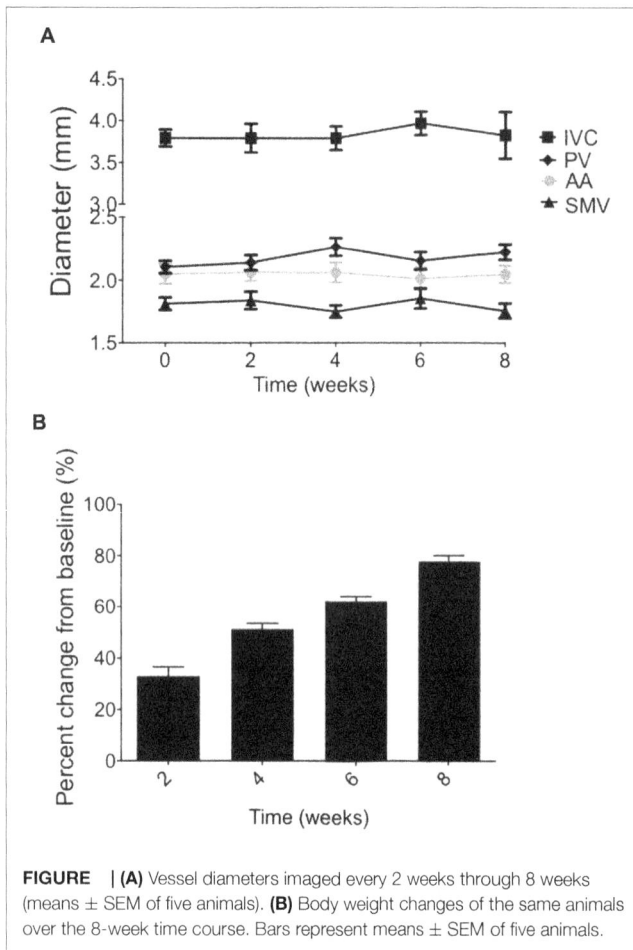

FIGURE | (A) Vessel diameters imaged every 2 weeks through 8 weeks (means ± SEM of five animals). (B) Body weight changes of the same animals over the 8-week time course. Bars represent means ± SEM of five animals.

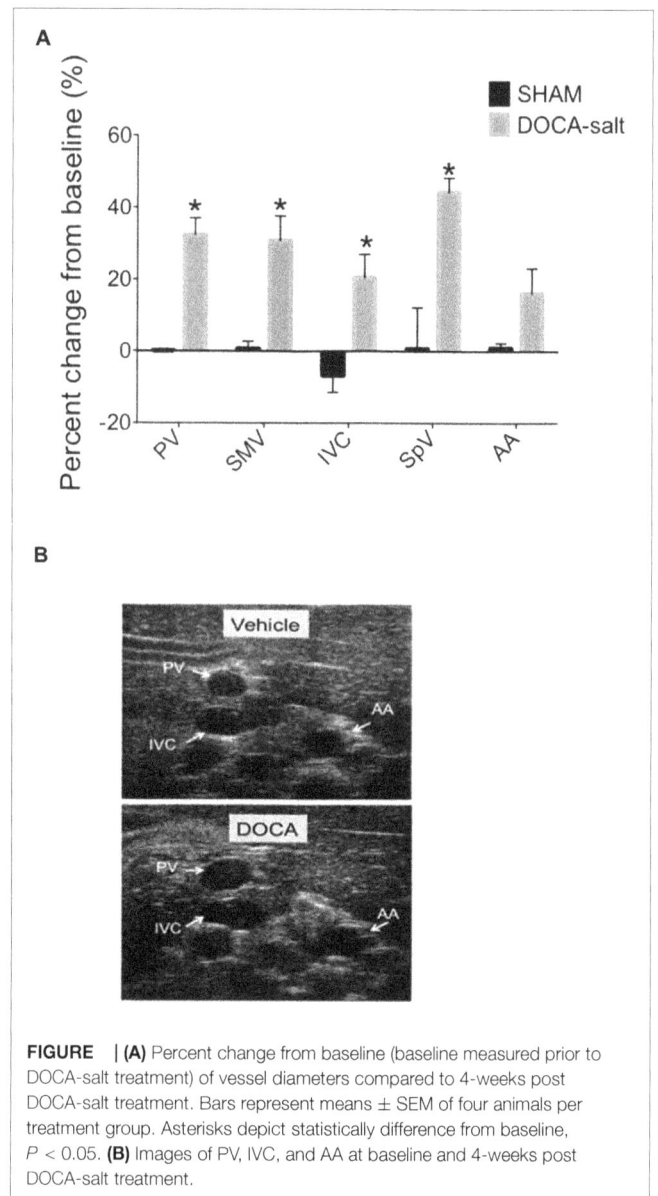

FIGURE | (A) Percent change from baseline (baseline measured prior to DOCA-salt treatment) of vessel diameters compared to 4-weeks post DOCA-salt treatment. Bars represent means ± SEM of four animals per treatment group. Asterisks depict statistically difference from baseline, $P < 0.05$. (B) Images of PV, IVC, and AA at baseline and 4-weeks post DOCA-salt treatment.

In order to validate this imaging technique for use in more chronic longitudinal studies, in a further experiment we investigated the stability of the splanchnic vein and AA diameters within an animal when acquired every 2 weeks over an 8 weeks period. The key to this approach was the ability to accurately relocate a specific cross-section of the splanchnic vessel of interest. The consistency of vessel diameter measurements observed in this chronic time course study indicates that these vessels can serve as their own control in experiments examining the potential impact of interventions on long-term changes in vascular diameter. Therefore, we applied our imaging technique to study splanchnic venous diameters in an experimental model of chronic hypertension, i.e., DOCA-salt hypertension. The results showed a significantly increased diameter of all the splanchnic veins in DOCA-salt rats, whereas no increases were observed in SHAM rats. We have previously reported increased venoconstriction in conscious DOCA-salt rats (Fink et al., 2000) so anticipated that we would observe reduced splanchnic venous diameters in these animals. However, venomotor tone in splanchnic veins is primarily controlled by sympathetic activity, and isoflurane anesthesia is known to dramatically reduce sympathetic activity (Bencze et al., 2013). So the increases in venous diameters we observed in DOCA-salt rats under anesthesia are likely due to passive effects (unopposed

by sympathetic venoconstriction) of the volume expansion and cardiac hypertrophy that occur in chronic DOCA-salt rats (Kobrin et al., 1990; Titze et al., 2006). This experiment highlights the complexities of evaluating moment-to-moment regulation of venous diameter; and indicates the desirability of using multiple, and minimally invasive, approaches to that evaluation. Nevertheless, the results support the ability of our vein imaging technique to detect chronic, physiologically significant changes in venous diameter in intact (albeit anesthetized) rats.

There are some additional limitations to the current study that deserve mention. First, we only studied a relatively small number of male Sprague–Dawley rats between 6 and 20 weeks of age. Venous diameters measured by ultrasound vary by age and sex in humans (Kutty et al., 2014; Gui et al., 2015) and are likely to do so in rats as well. Likewise, it is quite possible that the approach described here may need to be modified if applied to other strains of rats, to female rats, or to sexually immature or old rats. Second, although we found that weight gain of ∼200 g (∼80% increase) did not significantly affect the diameters of any abdominal vein, studies in humans suggests that venous diameter correlates modestly with body surface area and height (Gui et al., 2015). Third, all animals were imaged only in one spatial plane, i.e., supine. It is possible that altering the posture of the rat would result in different findings for splanchnic vein diameters. Four, since each vessel of interest courses a distinct 3-dimensional plane, it is acknowledged that the combined image may not represent exact perpendicular views of all three vessels at the same time. However, obtaining a single images depicting all three vessels makes possible the evaluation of simultaneous changes to these various vessel sizes that is not possible with constant repositioning of the transducer over each separate vessel. This includes the important ability of being able to directly compare and contrast arterial vs. venous responses. Finally, a relevant consideration for any measurement technique is the time and effort required to master it (Bowra et al., 2015) but since all values here were obtained by a single highly experienced rodent ultrasonographer, we cannot comment on how long it would take for a novice to achieve the kind of stable, reproducible measurements we report.

CONCLUSION

Although, ultrasound imaging the abdominal vessels, particularly the PV and IVC, is not novel in experimental research or clinical settings, investigation of diameter change in multiple splanchnic vessels is novel as they relate to venous capacitance. There is no current publication that measures vein diameters

in the splanchnic vasculature, a highly capacitive and compliant region important in blood pressure regulation. We anticipate that this technique will be useful in a number of different ways. The goal of the present study was to lay the foundation for repeatable measures, and illustration of changes in one model in which alterations in venous function have been suggested (e.g., the DOCA-salt model). Once we, and hopefully others, accept this type of approach than we can begin to interrogate disease models that would benefit from investigate of the venous circulation. These include other models of experimental and genetic hypertension, hyperlipidemia, obesity and heart failure.

AUTHOR CONTRIBUTIONS

SW devised original idea, helped with data analysis, draft revisions, read the final version of the manuscript and worked on this revision. This work was funded by a grant of which she is PI. BS planned and performed experiments, analyzed data and was in charge of pulling this manuscript together (including making figures, etc). She contributed significantly to this revision. TK-B planned and performed experiments, analyzed data, and prepared figures, commented on revisions and final drafts. She contributed significantly to this revision. GF helped with ideas, analysis, experimental planning, working on drafts, and read the final version. He contributed significantly to this revision.

FUNDING

This work was supported by NIH HL107495 (SW) and P01HL070687 (SW and GF).

REFERENCES

Aardenburg, R., Spaanderman, M. E., Courtar, D. A., Van Eijndhoven, H. W., De Leeuw, P. W., and Peeters, L. L. (2005). A subnormal plasma volume in formerly preeclamptic women is associated with a low venous capacitance. *J. Soc. Gynecol. Investig.* 12, 107–111. doi: 10.1016/j.jsgi.2004.09.002

Bencze, M., Behuliak, M., and Zicha, J. (2013). The impact of four different classes of anesthetics on the mechanisms of blood pressure regulation in normotensive and spontaneously hypertensive rats. *Physiol. Res.* 62, 471–478.

Bowra, J., Uwagboe, V., Goudie, A., Reid, C., and Gillett, M. (2015). Interrater agreement between expert and novice in measuring inferior vena cava diameter and collapsibility index. *Emerg. Med. Australas.* 27, 295–299. doi: 10.1111/1742-6723.12417

Brennan, J. M., Ronan, A., Goonewardena, S., Blair, J. E., Hammes, M., Shah, D., et al. (2006). Handcarried ultrasound measurement of the inferior vena cava for assessment of intravascular volume status in the outpatient hemodialysis clinic. *Clin. J. Am. Soc. Nephrol.* 1, 749–753. doi: 10.2215/CJN.00310106

Brooksby, G. A., and Donald, D. E. (1971). Dynamic changes in splanchnic blood flow and blood volume in dogs during activation of sympathetic nerves. *Circ. Res.* 29, 227–238. doi: 10.1161/01.RES.29.3.227

Burchell, A. E., Sobotka, P. A., and Hart, E. C. (2013). Chemohypersensitivity and autonomic modulation of venous capacitance in the pathophysiology of acute decompensated heart failure. *Curr. Heart Fail. Rep.* 10, 139–146. doi: 10.1007/s11897-013-0135-y

Chen, J. Y., Chen, H. L., Wu, S. H., Tsai, T. C., Lin, M. F., Yen, C. C., et al. (2012). Application of high-frequency ultrasound for the detection of surgical anatomy in the rodent abdomen. *Vet. J.* 191, 246–252. doi: 10.1016/j.tvjl.2010.12.024

Coatney, R. W. (2001). Ultrasound imaging: principles and applications in rodent research. *ILAR J.* 42, 233–247. doi: 10.1093/ilar.42.3.233

Deshpande, N., Needles, A., and Willmann, J. K. (2010). Molecular ultrasound imaging: current status and future directions. *Clin. Radiol.* 65, 567–581. doi: 10.1016/j.crad.2010.02.013

Diaz, J., Ni, W., Thompson, J., King, A., Fink, G. D., and Watts, S. W. (2008). 5-Hydroxytryptamine lowers blood pressure in normotensive and hypertensive rats. *J. Pharmacol. Exp. Ther.* 325, 1031–1038. doi: 10.1124/jpet.108.136226

Fink, G. D., Johnson, R. J., and Galligan, J. J. (2000). Mechanisms of increased venous smooth muscle tone in desoxycorticosterone acetate-salt hypertension. *Hypertension* 35, 464–469. doi: 10.1161/01.HYP.35.1.464

Gelman, S. (2009). Venous function and central venous pressure. *Anesthesiology* 108, 735–748. doi: 10.1097/ALN.0b013e3181672607

Gui, J., Guo, J., Nong, F., Jiang, D., Xu, A., Yang, F., et al. (2015). Impact of individual characteristics on sonographic IVC diameter and the IVC diameter/aorta diameter index. *Am. J. Emerg. Med.* 33, 1602–1605. doi: 10.1016/j.ajem.2015.06.047

Knipp, B. S., Ailawadi, G., Sullivan, V. V., Roelofs, K. J., Henke, P. K., Stanley, J. C., et al. (2003). Ultrasound measurement of aortic diameters in rodent models of aneurysm disease. *J. Surg. Res.* 112, 97–101. doi: 10.1016/S0022-4804(03)00114-8

Kobrin, I., Eimerl, J., Mekler, J., and Ben-Ishay, D. (1990). Cardiac hypertrophy developing during DOCA-salt treatment is dissociated from systemic and regional hemodynamics. *Am. J. Hypertens.* 3, 136–139.

Kutty, S., Li, L., Hasan, R., Peng, Q., Rangamani, S., and Danford, D. A. (2014). Systemic venous diameters, collapsibility indices, and right atrial measurements in normal pediatric subjects. *J. Am. Soc. Echocardiogr.* 27, 155–162. doi: 10.1016/j.echo.2013.09.002

Leunissen, K. M., Kouw, P., Kooman, J. P., Cheriex, E. C., deVries, P. M., Donker, A. J., et al. (1993). New techniques to determine fluid status in hemodialyzed patients. *Kidney Int. Suppl.* 41, 50–56.

Li, Y., Liu, H., Gaskari, S. A., Tyberg, J. V., and Lee, S. S. (2008). Altered mesenteric venous capacitance and volume pooling in cirrhotic rats are mediated by nitric oxide. *Am. J. Physiol. Gastrointest. Liver Physiol.* 295, G252–G259. doi: 10.1152/ajpgi.00436.2007

Malkoff, J. (2005). Non-invasive blood pressure for mice and rats. *Animal Lab News*, 1–3.

Reilly, P. M., Wilkins, K. B., Fuh, K. C., Haglund, U., and Bulkley, G. B. (2001). The mesenteric hemodynamic response to circulatory shock: an overview. *Shock* 15, 329–343. doi: 10.1097/00024382-200115050-00001

Safar, M. E., and London, G. (1987). Arterial and venous compliance in sustained essential hypertension. *Hypertension* 10, 133–139. doi: 10.1161/01.HYP.10.2.133

Schefold, J. C., Storm, C., Bercker, S., Pschowski, R., Oppert, M., Krüger, A., et al. (2010). Inferior vena cava diameter correlates with invasive hemodynamic measures in mechanically ventilated intensive care unit patients with sepsis. *J. Emerg. Med.* 38, 632–637. doi: 10.1016/j.jemermed.2007.11.027

Schmitt, M., Blackman, D. J., Middleton, G. W., Cockcroft, J. R., and Frenneaux, M. P., (2002). Assessment of venous capacitance. Radionuclide plethysmography: methodology and research applications. *Br. J. Clin. Pharmacol.* 54, 565–576. doi: 10.1046/j.1365-2125.2002.t01-7-01689.x

Schwarzacher, S., Weidinger, F., Schemper, M., and Raberger, G., (1992). Blockade of endothelium-derived relaxing factor synthesis with NG-nitro-L-arginine methyl ester leads to enhanced venous reactivity in vivo. *Eur. J. Pharmacol.* 229, 253–258. doi: 10.1016/0014-2999(92)90563-J

Slama, M., Susic, D., Varagic, J., Ahn, J., and Frohlich, E. D., (2003). Echocardiographic measurements of cardiac output in rats. *Am. J. Physiol. Heart Circ. Physiol.* 284, H691–H697. doi: 10.1152/ajpheart.00653.2002

Stewart, J. M., McLeod, K. J., Sanyal, S., Herzberg, G., and Montgomery, L. D. (2004). Relation of postural vasovagal syncope to splanchnic hypervolemia in adolescents. *Circulation* 110, 2575–2581. doi: 10.1161/01.CIR.0000145543.88293.21

Stewart, J. M., and Montgomery, L. D. (2004). Regional blood volume and peripheral blood flow in postural tachycardia syndrome. *Am. J. Physiol. Heart Circ. Physiol.* 287, H1319–H1327. doi: 10.1152/ajpheart.00086.2004

Stuart, F., Hossack, J., and Adamson, S. L. (2011). Micro-ultra sound for preclinical imaging. *Interface Focus* 1, 576–601. doi: 10.1098/rsfs.2011.0037

Sung, H. J., Yee, A., Eskin, S. G., and McIntire, L. V. (2007). Cyclic strain and motion control produce opposite oxidative responses in two human endothelial cell types. *Am. J. Physiol. Cell Physiol.* 293, C87–C94. doi: 10.1152/ajpcell.00585.2006

Titze, J., Luft, F. C., Bauer, K., Dietsch, P., Lang, R., Veelken, R., et al. (2006). Extrarenal Na+ balance, volume, and blood pressure homeostasis in intact and ovariectomized deoxycorticosterone-acetate salt rats. *Hypertension* 47, 1101–1107. doi: 10.1161/01.HYP.0000221039.17735.1a

Tyberg, J. (2002). How changes in venous capacitance modulate cardiac output. *Eur. J. Physiol.* 445, 10–17. doi: 10.1007/s00424-002-0922-x

Tykocki, N. R., Gariepy, C. E., and Watts, S. W. (2009). Endothelin ET(B) receptors in arteries and veins: multiple actions in the vein. *J. Pharmacol. Exp. Ther.* 329, 875–881. doi: 10.1124/jpet.108.145953

Watts, S. W., Darios, E. S., Seitz, B. M., and Thomspon, J. M. (2015). 5-HT is a potent relaxant in rat superior mesenteric veins. *Pharmacol. Res. Perspect.* 3:e00103. doi: 10.1002/prp2.103

Conflict of Interest Statement: The authors declare that the research was conducted in the absence of any commercial or financial relationships that could be construed as a potential conflict of interest.

2

Drug Development in Alzheimer's Disease: The Contribution of PET and SPECT

Lieven D. Declercq[1], Rik Vandenberghe[2], Koen Van Laere[3], Alfons Verbruggen[1] and Guy Bormans[1]*

[1] *Laboratory for Radiopharmacy, Department of Pharmaceutical and Pharmacological Sciences, KU Leuven, Leuven, Belgium,* [2] *Laboratory for Cognitive Neurology, Department of Neurosciences, KU Leuven, Leuven, Belgium,* [3] *Nuclear Medicine and Molecular Imaging, Department of Imaging and Pathology, KU Leuven, Leuven, Belgium*

Edited by:
Albert D. Windhorst,
VU University Medical Center,
Netherlands

Reviewed by:
Bashir M. Rezk,
Southern University at New Orleans,
USA
Carmen Gil,
Centro de Investigaciones Biologicas
(CIB–CSIC), Spain

*Correspondence:
Guy Bormans
guy.bormans@pharm.kuleuven.be

Clinical trials aiming to develop disease-altering drugs for Alzheimer's disease (AD), a neurodegenerative disorder with devastating consequences, are failing at an alarming rate. Poorly defined inclusion-and outcome criteria, due to a limited amount of objective biomarkers, is one of the major concerns. Non-invasive molecular imaging techniques, positron emission tomography and single photon emission (computed) tomography (PET and SPE(C)T), allow visualization and quantification of a wide variety of (patho)physiological processes and allow early (differential) diagnosis in many disorders. PET and SPECT have the ability to provide biomarkers that permit spatial assessment of pathophysiological molecular changes and therefore objectively evaluate and follow up therapeutic response, especially in the brain. A number of specific PET/SPECT biomarkers used in support of emerging clinical therapies in AD are discussed in this review.

Keywords: Alzheimer's disease, PET, SPECT, drug development, biomarkers

INTRODUCTION

The worldwide prevalence of AD is estimated at 35 million, a number expected to quadruple by 2050, due to the increasing lifespan of the world population (Brookmeyer et al., 2007). With an unfavorable prognosis and a life expectancy of approximately 8–10 years, AD is becoming one of the most costly diseases for society (Thies and Bleiler, 2013). In spite of increasing knowledge

Abbreviations: 5-HT, 5-hydroxytryptamine; 5-HTRs, 5-HT receptors; 5-HTT, 5-HT transporter; α-APP, α-amyloid precursor protein; Aβ, amyloid beta; ACh, acetylcholine; AChE, acetylcholinesterase; AD, Alzheimer's disease; ADAS-cog, Alzheimer's disease assessment scale-cognitive subscale; ALA, α-lipoic acid; APP, amyloid precursor protein; BACE1, β-site APP-cleaving enzyme 1; BBB, blood–brain barrier; BPSD, behavioral and psychological symptoms of dementia; BZDs, benzodiazepines; CBD, corticobasal degeneration; ChAT, choline acetyltransferase; CIBIC+, clinician's interview-based impression of change; CNS, central nervous system; CSF, cerebrospinal fluid; CT, computerized tomography; CTI, clinical trial identifier; D_1R, dopamine$_1$-like receptors; DA, dopamine; DAT, dopamine transporter; DLB, dementia with Lewy bodies; ECT, EudraCT-number; EMA, European medicines agency; FDA, food and drug administration; FTD, frontal temporal dementia; GABA, gamma-amino butyric acid; GSK, glycogen synthase kinase; HCs, healthy controls; mAChR, muscarinic acetylcholine receptor; MAPT, microtubule-associated protein tau gene; MCI, mild cognitive impairment; MMSE, mini-mental state examination; MOAs, monoamine oxidases; MRI, magnetic resonance imaging; nAChRs, nicotinic acetylcholine receptors; NFTs, neurofibrillary tangles; PBR, peripheral benzodiazepine receptor; PET, positron emission tomography; P-gp, permeability glycoprotein; PHFs, paired helical filaments; PSP, progressive supranuclear palsy; p-tau, phosphorylated tau; rCBF, regional cerebral blood flow; SERT, 5-HT reuptake transporter; SP, senile plaques; SPE(C)T, single photon emission (computed) tomography; TSPO, translocator protein; VDAC, voltage dependent anion channel.

about the genetics, epidemiology, and histopathological features of AD there is, at this moment, only symptomatic treatment available. However, already at early clinical signs, intrinsic disease progression has developed for a long time; patients rapidly decline and develop irrevocable brain damage (Masters et al., 2006; Romano and Buratti, 2013). Therefore, there is a great need for efficient treatment that should be initiated in a very early phase of the disease. Strict definite diagnosis can still only be made post-mortem, on the basis of two pathological hallmarks: SP and NFTs (Hyman et al., 2012), although use of biomarkers is strongly advocated in research guidelines (Dubois et al., 2014). More than 90% of clinical trials aiming to intervene at the causative pathological elements have failed to produce disease altering effects. A major concern hereby is the lack of objective biomarkers assisting in the evaluation of inclusion- and outcome criteria of participating patients, as many participants turned out to be misdiagnosed, particularly in the early AD disease stages (Jack et al., 2010; Barthel et al., 2015; James et al., 2015). Currently five biomarkers for AD have been used for evaluation of disease and monitoring of disease progression (Jack et al., 2010): CSF levels of $A\beta_{42}$, CSF levels of total tau and p-tau$_{181}$ and p-tau$_{231}$, structural imaging (CT and MRI) and functional imaging (PET with [^{18}F]FDG). Elevated levels of CSF tau and reduced levels of CSF $A\beta$ allow the prediction of, respectively, the NFT load and the SP deposits (Ahmed et al., 2014; de Souza et al., 2014; Wurtman, 2015). Therefore, these CSF levels appear to be useful biomarkers in the diagnosis of AD (Wallin et al., 2006; Weiner et al., 2015). Nonetheless, CSF sampling requires an invasive lumbar puncture, quantification of CSF levels is hampered by interlaboratory variability and CSF values do not provide regional information on tau- and $A\beta$ deposits. The regional concentration of tau- and $A\beta$ deposits is however essential for a differential diagnosis of AD, especially among the different tauopathies (Hampel and Teipel, 2004; Gozes et al., 2009; Hampel et al., 2010). Structural volume measurement can be used to measure regional cerebral atrophy. Although not highly specific for AD due to overlap with 'normal' aging, the degree of atrophy follows neuropathological progression in AD and severity of volume loss correlates well with disease progression (Masters et al., 2006; Jack et al., 2010). Regarding the biomarkers that can be visualized and quantified by the molecular imaging techniques PET and SPECT, there are three important applications to be considered, that could contribute to successful drug development in clinical trials. The first one is the ability of PET and SPECT to provide quantitative and spatial *in vivo* assessment of, for example, the amyloid- and tau burden in AD patients. By doing so, inclusion and exclusion criteria in clinical trials can be verified more objectively than what was possible now with the previous biomarkers. Indeed, the use of specific radiotracers, for various targets, may provide accurate differential diagnosis (even at early AD stages) and true confirmation of the availability of the drug target, which allows physicians to reliably select patients for clinical trials to evaluate novel AD therapeutics (Barthel et al., 2015). Another important role for these molecular imaging techniques is the assessment and quantitative follow-up of drugs aiming to intervene at the specific molecular pathophysiological processes.

Using highly selective PET- or SPECT radioligands, the true biological effect of novel clinical candidates can be established and true quantitative assessment is possible (Barthel et al., 2015). Thirdly, molecular imaging can be applied to measure the dose-related occupancy of specific targets caused by drugs under test, which allows the characterization of the optimal therapeutic window and thus a more effective design of subsequent clinical drug trials (Broich et al., 1998; Passchier et al., 2002). Although PET is able to provide a much higher spatial resolution and dynamic scanning with higher temporal resolution and better quantification than SPECT, SPECT cameras are more widely available and cheaper than PET cameras. Both the availability and the economical aspect are important to consider when performing large multi-center clinical trials (Rahmim and Zaidi, 2008).

The most frequently used PET radiopharmaceutical is 2-[^{18}F]fluoro-2-deoxy-D-glucose ([^{18}F]FDG, **Figure**), a glucose derivative which allows measurement of brain glucose metabolism directly related with viability of brain tissue in AD (Barthel et al., 2015). This commercially available compound, with various clinical applications, has been well established in routine clinical practice, but also in the recruitment and follow-up of the majority of AD clinical trials which use PET as biomarker technique (Barthel et al., 2015). Indeed, several AD clinical trials are currently recruiting and following up patients with [^{18}F]FDG (CTI: NCT02593318, NCT01561053, and NCT02560753). Although FDG-PET is able to provide information about regional glucose metabolism, which can aid in the detection and prognosis of MCI for further progression to AD, there is a great need for PET- and SPECT radiopharmaceuticals which deliver more target-specific information of a variety of (patho)physiological processes that are happening in AD. In this review we will therefore focus on some of the major molecular pathophysiological changes known to occur in AD, along with emerging pharmacological treatment approaches. Furthermore, specific attention will be attributed to the role that PET- and SPECT biomarkers (can) play during these clinical trials.

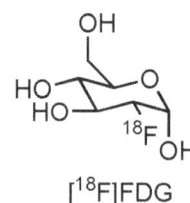

FIGURE | Structure of [^{18}F]FDG.

CHOLINERGIC HYPOTHESIS

Acetylcholinesterase

The cholinergic hypothesis states that a decreased cholinergic neurotransmission, caused by a degeneration of cholinergic neurons in the basal forebrain, leads to several cognitive and functional conditions, associated with the symptoms of AD (Davies and Maloney, 1976; Bartus et al., 1982). Furthermore, the disruption of AChE seems to be associated with NFT- and Aβ deposits (Tavitian et al., 1993).

Acetylcholine, a neurotransmitter synthesized presynaptically by ChAT, is released in the synaptic cavity, where it is able to interact with nicotinic and muscarinic cholinergic receptors on pre- and postsynaptic membranes. Synaptic transmission is eventually stopped by the hydrolysis of ACh by AChE (Lleo et al., 2006). Both ChAT and AChE expression is reduced in cortical regions of AD patients (Davies and Maloney, 1976; Coyle et al., 1983; Vogels et al., 1990).

Inhibition of AChE was the first approach to treat AD, and this led to the FDA approval of eventually four AChE inhibitors: galantamine, rivastigmine, donepezil, and tacrine, though the latter one was largely discontinued due to hepatotoxicity issues (Wu et al., 2010). All inhibitors showed however only mild symptomatic improvement in patients with mild to moderate AD (Burns et al., 1999; Rosler et al., 1999; Farlow et al., 2000; Greenberg et al., 2000; Raskind et al., 2000; Tariot et al., 2000; Wilcock et al., 2000; Winblad et al., 2001). Several new agents are currently under development (Aprahamian et al., 2013), two of which have been evaluated in clinical trials: phenserine (Winblad et al., 2010; Darreh-Shori et al., 2014) and huperzine A (Rafii et al., 2011). Phenserine, structurally related to rivastigmine, showed a prolonged, but mild inhibition of AChE in AD patients. Researchers suggested an add-on therapy with donepezil to improve the clinical efficacy of this class of agents. Low dosage of huperzine A, a reversible AChE inhibitor, showed no significant improvement on the ADAS-cog [the primary cognitive outcome measure in mild to moderate AD patients (259)], in a phase II trial in mild to moderate AD patients. Higher dosage and a long term evaluation were suggested by the authors. A phase III trial (CTI:NCT01282619) using sustained-release huperzine A is currently ongoing (Ghezzi et al., 2013).

Visualization of the cholinergic system could be done by using radiolabeled ACh analogs or inhibitors of AChE (Tavitian et al., 1993; Irie et al., 1994; Iyo et al., 1997; Kilbourn et al., 1996). Both pathways have been pursued by researchers, but at present only two carbon-11 labeled compounds have been clinically evaluated on AD patients: [11C]MP4A and [11C]MP4P, two N-[11C]methylpiperidine esters (acetate and propionate, **Figure**). Moreover, both compounds were used to evaluate the effect of donepezil or rivastigmine in AD patients. Scans

with [11C]MP4A or [11C]MP4P, taken before and after treatment with donepezil or rivastigmine, showed significant (up to 40%) cerebral cortical or frontal cortical inhibition of the AChE activity. Modest symptomatic improvement was recorded for all AD patients during these trials (Kuhl et al., 2000; Shinotoh et al., 2001; Kaasinen et al., 2002). These studies show the usefulness of both tracers for therapeutic monitoring of AChE inhibitors, as well as the possibility to evaluate newly developed drugs that target AChE (Shinotoh et al., 2004). Nonetheless, carbon-11 labeled compounds have the limitation that an on-site cyclotron is needed, which limits their widespread use. The lack of significant cognitive improvement and the fact that the cholinergic deficit is not an early event in the development of AD (Gilmor et al., 1999), has challenged the cholinergic hypothesis (Francis et al., 1999; Bartus, 2000; Terry and Buccafusco, 2003; Contestabile, 2011). Nevertheless, two decades after FDA approval of tacrine, AChE inhibitors remain (out of necessity) the mainstay for the current symptomatic treatment of AD.

Muscarinic ACh Receptor

The presynaptic cholinergic signal is transmitted through the release of the neurotransmitter ACh, which can interact with both muscarinic and nicotinic ACh receptors (the latter one discussed in the next section). The pre-and postsynaptic muscarinic ACh receptor (mAChR) is a plasmamembrane, GTP binding protein coupled receptor, of which five subtypes exist (M_1-M_5) (Bonner et al., 1987; Peralta et al., 1987; Bonner, 1989). Due to the involvement in several neurological and psychiatric disorders, this target has been the topic of many research papers during the past few decades (Palacios et al., 1990; Tandon et al., 1991; Maziere, 1995). A comprehensive autoradiography study using tritium labeled compounds on the distribution of M_1-M_4 muscarinic receptors of histopathological diagnosed AD patients by Rodríguez-Puertas et al. (1997) showed that the decrease of M_1 muscarinic receptors followed the general pattern of neurodegeneration as recorded in the Braak stages (Braak and Braak, 1991), while the M_2 muscarinic receptor displayed significant reduction in the hippocampal area (up to 64%) and a significant increase in the striatum (up to 468% in the putamen), although this increase was not confirmed by other research groups (Eckelman, 2002). The density of M_{3-4} receptors on the other hand, was not altered compared to their density in brains of HCs. Interestingly, several research groups demonstrated that the stimulation of the M_1- and M_3 muscarinic receptors lead to an increase of the neuroprotective non-amyloidogenic pathway (formation of α-APP) (Buxbaum et al., 1992; Nitsch et al., 1992). Stimulation of these receptors could thus provide means for a decrease in Aβ production, a hypothesis which was confirmed in several studies (Wolf et al., 1995; Savonenko et al., 2005; Tsang et al., 2006). Little is known about the M_5 muscarinic receptor, the latest receptor to be cloned (Bonner et al., 1988; Liao et al., 1989), although some research groups have demonstrated possible involvement in regulation of the cerebral blood flow and DA release (Yamada et al., 2001).

A number of clinical trials have been carried out to examine the potential role of mAChR agonists/antagonists on the clinical

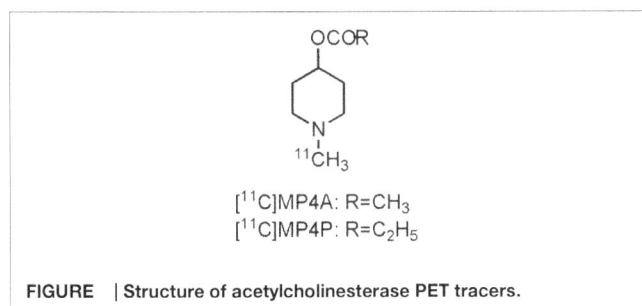

OCOR

N

$^{11}CH_3$

[11C]MP4A: R=CH₃
[11C]MP4P: R=C₂H₅

FIGURE | Structure of acetylcholinesterase PET tracers.

symptoms of AD patients. In the group of the selective M_1 agonists, talsaclidine showed a significant decrease (up to 27% compared to placebo) in the Aβ-CSF levels in a randomized, double-blind, placebo controlled trial on AD patients with a MMSE score between 12 and 26. Results should, however, be interpreted with some caution, as suggested by the researchers, since assessment of the amyloid burden in AD patients by CSF has some flaws as biomarker, furthermore there was no mention on any cognitive improvement alongside the drop in Aβ CSF levels (Hock et al., 2000). Yet, another M_1 selective agonist, cevimeline (AF102B), an FDA approved drug for the treatment of dry mouth in Sjögren's syndrome, did show cognitive improvement in the ADAS-cog and word recognition scales in a single-blind-placebo-controlled parallel group study with patients with probable AD (Fisher et al., 1996). Dual selectivity for both the M_1- and M_2-receptor on the other hand, as it is the case for RS-86, showed no consistent cognitive improvement in a double-blind, placebo-controlled trial on mild to moderate AD patients (Bruno et al., 1986). Palacios et al. (1986) hypothesized that RS-86' failure could be due to the concomitant stimulation of the M_1- and M_2 receptor, where stimulation of M_2 might inhibit the effects of the M_1 receptor. On the other hand, milameline, a partial agonist for all five muscarinic receptor subtypes, demonstrated an effect on the rCBF in the frontal and subcortical regions of AD patients as part of an 'add-on study' during a Phase III clinical trial of this drug. AD participants were evaluated with SPECT, using the cerebral blood flow tracer ^{99m}Tc-exametazime (^{99m}Tc-HMPAO), during the performance of two cognitive tasks. Although a modest increase (of 26%) of rCBF was demonstrated, the authors suggested that there may be neuropsychopharmacological effects associated with the intake of milameline during the performance of cognitive demanding tasks (Trollor et al., 2006). And finally, in a large-scale clinical trial, xanomeline, a M_1- and M_4-receptor agonist and M_5 receptor antagonist (Grant and El-Fakahany, 2005), was evaluated in a randomized, double-blind, placebo-controlled trial on mild to moderate AD patients. Significant cognitive improvement was hereby shown in the ADAS-cog (drug vs. placebo; $p \leq 0.05$), and the CIBIC+ scale (drug vs. placebo; $p \leq 0.02$), demonstrating that a muscarinic receptor agonist can ameliorate cognitive symptoms in AD patients (Bodick et al., 1997).

Only one imaging agent, with affinity for the M_1- and M_4 muscarinic receptor (Piggott et al., 2002), has been clinically evaluated on AD patients thus far, namely $[^{123}I]$I-quinuclidinyl benzilate ((R,R) $[^{123}I]$I-QNB) (**Figure**). Eighteen mild to moderate AD patients and their age-matched HCs were evaluated with $[^{123}I]$I-QNB. Significantly reduced uptake ($p \leq 0.001$) was noted in the frontal rectal gyrus, right parahippocampal gyrus, left hippocampus, and regions of the left temporal lobe, compared to the HCs (Pakrasi et al., 2007). Nevertheless, conflicting results have been reported by other research groups with this tracer (Holman et al., 1985; Weinberger et al., 1991; Wyper et al., 1993; Kemp et al., 2003), although the sample sizes in these other studies were smaller. In another study, $[^{123}I]$I-QNB was used as a biomarker to evaluate the density of the mAChR on 20 patients receiving the AChE inhibitor

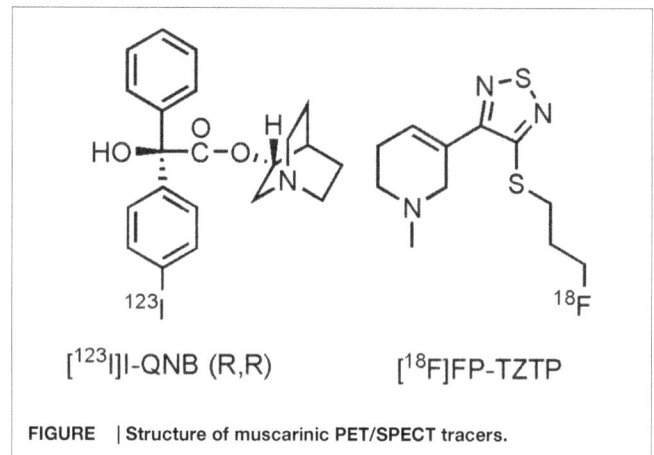

FIGURE | Structure of muscarinic PET/SPECT tracers.

donepezil (Brown et al., 2003). No distinction could be made between donepezil responders and non-responders, furthermore no positive correlation was found between $[^{123}I]$I-QNB scans and the extent of cognitive improvement on the ADAS-cog scale, apart from the insular cortex, were an inverse correlation was found. Researchers suggest that response to donepezil may thus be greater in patients with clear cholinergic deficits. Several efforts have been made to develop carbon-11 and fluorine-18 labeled tracers for muscarinergic receptors (Farde et al., 1996; Eckelman, 2001; Xie et al., 2004). A clinical trial in the US with 3-(3-(3-([^{18}F]fluoropropyl)thio)-1,2,5-thiadiazol-4-yl)-1,2,5,6-tetrahydro-1-methylpyridine ($[^{18}F]$FP-TZTP) (Ravasi et al., 2012; **Figure**), which binds to the M_2 receptor, on AD patients has been completed (CTI: NCT00001917), but results are yet to be published. Lastly, recruitment for a study with HCs and AD patients using an M_4 positive allosteric modulator $[^{11}C]$MK-6884 (structure not yet available), will soon start (CTI: NCT02621606). Future PET- and SPECT compounds hold promise to evaluate inclusion- and outcome criteria with novel drugs targeting the muscarinic receptor, as well as to establish therapeutic windows via dose-occupancy studies.

Nicotinic ACh Receptor

nAChRs are ionotropic receptors, part of the ligand-gated ion channel superfamily (Cooper and Millar, 1997; Castelan et al., 2008; Criado et al., 2011; Valles and Barrantes, 2012). They consist of a hetero-or homopentameric structure, assembled from 17 possible subunits: α_{1-10}, β_{1-4}, γ, δ, and ε (Karlin, 2002; Gotti and Clementi, 2004). The main subtypes of the nAChRs in the human CNS are, however, α_7, $\alpha_4\beta_2$, and $\alpha_3\beta_2$, although the latter one is not involved in the pathophysiology of AD (Wevers and Schroder, 1999; Pym et al., 2005). Reduction in nAChRs expression levels of several subtypes has indeed been revealed in regions with dense deposits of Aβ and NFTs (Pimlott et al., 2004; Oddo and Laferla, 2006; Buckingham et al., 2009). The α_7 nAChR is mainly expressed in the hippocampus, whereas the $\alpha_4\beta_2$ nAChR is homogenously expressed throughout brain (O'Brien et al., 2007; Valles and Barrantes, 2012). While loss of $\alpha_4\beta_2$ nAChR can cause memory deficits in AD patients

(Paterson and Nordberg, 2000; O'Brien et al., 2007; Kendziorra et al., 2011), a more complex relationship has been noted when evaluating the interaction between α_7 nAChR and Aβ in AD (Oddo and Laferla, 2006). Aβ can either interact as agonist or as antagonist of α_7 nAChR, depending on its concentration, where low concentrations may activate and high concentrations may inactivate α_7 nAChR (Dineley et al., 2002; Puzzo and Arancio, 2013; Sadigh-Eteghad et al., 2014). Observations in an AD transgenic mouse model overexpressing APP, presenilin-1, and tau (3xTg-ADmice) (Oddo et al., 2003; Billings et al., 2005; Kitazawa et al., 2005) were consistent with the aforementioned in vitro conclusions for human AD, demonstrating an age dependent reduction of α_7 nAChR, as higher Aβ may eventually block remaining α_7 nAChRs (Hernandez et al., 2010). For a more detailed discussion about the many different roles of nAChRs in AD, readers are referred to several reviews on the subject (Oddo and Laferla, 2006; Jurgensen and Ferreira, 2010; Vandenberghe et al., 2010).

Since nicotine can induce the release of presynaptic ACh and is involved in the modulation of many other neurotransmitters, such as GABA, DA, norepinephrine, and serotonin (Levin, 1992), several clinical studies have investigated the effect of nicotine on AD patients (Jones et al., 1992; Wilson et al., 1995; Snaedal et al., 1996; White and Levin, 1999). However, as mentioned in a review by Oddo and Laferla (2006), these trails failed to demonstrate any cognitive improvement in AD patients; only an increase in attention could be determined. Yet, clinical trials with two nAChR agonists did show cognitive improvement in mild to moderate AD patients (Potter et al., 1999; Deardorff et al., 2015). The first of them was encenicline (EVP-6124), a partial agonist of α_7 nAChR. This drug was well tolerated in Phase I and II trials, showing significant improvement in cognitive and functional domains (Deardorff et al., 2015). A currently ongoing Phase III trial involving mild to moderate AD patients, receiving or having already received AChE inhibitors, to assess the efficacy and tolerability of EVP-6124 (ECT: 2012-003209-92) in a large group of patients was halted due to severe gastrointestinal side-effects (Shugart, 2016). Another nAChR agonist, ABT-418, which has binding affinity for $\alpha_4\beta_2$, $\alpha_2\beta_2$, and $\alpha_3\beta_4$ (Potter et al., 1999), showed some cognitive improvement in the acquisition and retention of verbal information of patients with early AD (Mean MMSE score of 21.4). It is, however, unclear whether this compound will be further pursued in large clinical trials. Two other trials with nAChR agonists were less convincing; efficacy of ispronicline (TC-1734 or AZD-3480) a selective agonist of $\alpha_4\beta_2$ nAChR and $\alpha_2\beta_2$ nAChR (Gatto et al., 2004) was investigated in a large Phase IIb dose-finding study on mild to moderate AD patients (MMSE score: 12–26). Despite the fact that ispronicline caused significant improvement on patients with age-associated memory impairment (Dunbar et al., 2007, 2011), no significant improvement could be shown on the ADAS-cog scale in the latest Phase IIb study, although secondary outcome measurements did show some improvement (Frolich et al., 2011). Additional Phase II trials on mild to moderate AD patients were halted, since no superiority over donepezil could be demonstrated. Finally, in a Phase II trial on mild to moderate AD patients (MMSE score of 26–26 and 14–20, respectively), no cognitive improvement could

be observed with the $\alpha_4\beta_2$ nAChR selective agonist varenicline (Kim et al., 2014). Researchers concluded that the dosing regimen was not optimal and overall longer (than 6 weeks) trials may be needed to show cognitive improvement. In the light of these two failed clinical trials with $\alpha_4\beta_2$ nAChR agonists, another clarification could, however, be that the $\alpha_4\beta_2$ nAChR subtype may only play a minor role on cognitive processes in AD, and α_7 nAChR is therefore a more suitable target (Kim et al., 2014).

While nicotine was not really used as a therapeutic drug, as a carbon-11 labeled PET tracer it successfully showed reduction of nAChR in AD patients reflecting the loss of the nicotinic receptors during disease progression, in comparison with control subjects (Nordberg et al., 1990; Nordberg et al., 1995; Kadir et al., 2006). Additionally, a number of other clinical studies used [^{11}C]nicotine PET imaging (**Figure**), to assess the efficacy of the AChEIs tacrine and rivastigmine (Nordberg et al., 1992; Nordberg et al., 1997; Nordberg et al., 1998; Kadir et al., 2007). Significant increase in nAChR expression compared to baseline in several cortical areas could be demonstrated, after treatment with both tacrine and rivastigmine. [^{11}C]nicotine does, however, show high non-specific binding and rapid brain wash-out, making quantitative PET assessments of nAChR difficult. A few other PET radiotracers are currently under development for imaging of α_7 and $\alpha_4\beta_2$ nicotinic receptors (Toyohara et al., 2010; Meyer et al., 2014; Chalon et al., 2015); two structurally related compounds, one SPECT and one PET tracer, with affinity for the $\alpha_4\beta_2$ nicotinic receptor have already been evaluated on AD patients (O'Brien et al., 2007; Ellis et al., 2008; Sabri et al., 2008). Reduced tracer uptake was noted in AD patients in the frontal lobe, striatum, right medial temporal lobe and the pons after scans with-5-[^{123}I] iodo-3-[2(S)-2-azetidinylmethoxy]pyridine ([^{123}I]5IA-85350) (**Figure**), consistent with known reductions of the $\alpha_4\beta_2$ nicotinic receptor in AD (O'Brien et al., 2007). Its PET counterpart, 2-[^{18}F]fluoro-3-(2(S)-azetidinylmethoxy)pyridine (2-[^{18}F]FA-85380) (**Figure**), was able to demonstrate significant reduction (up to 75%) of the $\alpha_4\beta_2$ nicotinic receptor in MCI patients, which later on converted to AD (Sabri et al., 2008). In another study with 2-[^{18}F]FA-85380, the possible relationship between Aβ depositions and the reduction of the $\alpha_4\beta_2$ nicotinic receptor was studied by evaluating early to moderate AD patients (Okada et al., 2013). A negative correlation between the presence of Aβ in the medial frontal cortex and the nucleus basalis magnocellularis, as assessed by [^{11}C]Pittsburgh Compound B ([^{11}C]PiB, an Aβ tracer), and the binding of 2-[^{18}F]FA-85380 to the $\alpha_4\beta_2$ nicotinic receptor could be established. Both $\alpha_4\beta_2$ nicotinic receptor tracers suffer, however, from slow kinetics,

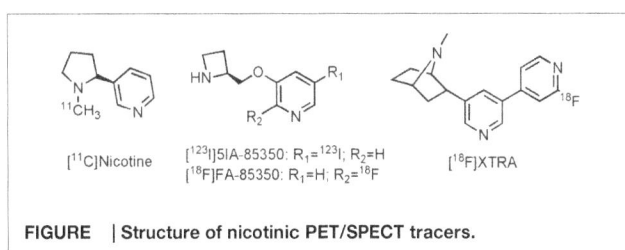

[^{11}C]Nicotine

[^{123}I]5IA-85350: R$_1$=^{123}I; R$_2$=H
[^{18}F]FA-85350: R$_1$=H; R$_2$=^{18}F

[^{18}F]XTRA

FIGURE | Structure of nicotinic PET/SPECT tracers.

leading to long scanning times, making routine application difficult (Meyer et al., 2014). Conversely, a novel $\alpha_4\beta_2$ nAChR tracer, 2-{5-[2-[^{18}F]fluoropyridin-4-yl]pyridin-3-yl}-7-methyl-7-azabicyclo[2.2.1]heptane ([^{18}F]XTRA) (Meyer et al., 2014) (**Figure**), showed much faster pharmacokinetics, which allow scanning within a reasonable time frame. Recruitment for a clinical trial with [^{18}F]XTRA on HCs, an AD or a MCI patient is currently ongoing (CTI:NCT01894646).

TAU HYPOTHESIS

As one of the pathological hallmarks in well over 20 neurodegenerative diseases (Lee et al., 2001), tau (*tubulin associated unit*), gained an increasing interest in the past few years, partly as a result of the large failure rate of clinical trials targeted toward the amyloid hypothesis (Barthel et al., 2015), but also due to recent availability of several tau specific PET ligands (Villemagne et al., 2015). As a member of the microtubule-associated protein (MAP) family, tau is mainly localized in the distal part of the neuronal axons (Binder et al., 1986). Consequently, the primary function of tau is stabilization and support of the microtubules (Weingarten et al., 1975). There are six different isoforms of tau, depending on alternative splicing of exon two, three, and ten of the MAPT. Localized on chromosome 17q32, this gene contains 16 exons (Neve et al., 1986). Exon two and three both encode a 29-aminoacid fragment at the N-terminal part of tau, yielding isoforms with none (0N), one (1N), or two inserts (2N). Exon ten on the other hand, encodes a 31-aminoacid fragment, which results in either three (3R) or four (4R) repeated binding domains at the C-terminus of the protein. The mature human brain contains thus six isoforms of tau: 0N3R, 1N3R, 2N3R, 0N4R, 1N4R, and 2N4R. Under normal conditions (and in AD) there is a 1:1 ratio of the 3R- and 4R isoforms, but this ratio somehow shifts in certain pathological conditions (Hong et al., 1998). The exact physiological role of these various isoforms remains to be elucidated, although 4R isoforms are better at promoting microtubuli assembly, and have greater binding affinity for microtubuli than the 3R isoforms (Goedert and Jakes, 1990; Butner and Kirschner, 1991). Under non-pathologic conditions, tau is a highly soluble protein with a limited secondary structure (Dunker et al., 2008), prone to several post-translational modifications. The most important one is phosphorylation on its serine and threonine residues, which modulates microtubule binding (Martin et al., 2011). Then again, in pathological conditions, such as AD, tau will become hyperphosphorylated, detaches from the microtubules and will self-aggregate into insoluble PHFs and NFTs, compromising neuronal cell function (Iqbal and Grundke-Iqbal, 2008). Different shapes and sizes of the aggregates can be found under diverse cognitive conditions, related to the presence of various isoforms, and post-translational modifications (Ballatore et al., 2007). In AD, the spreading of the tau pathology, which is thought to proceed in a prion-like manner (de Calignon et al., 2012), has been well-documented in the different Braak stages (Braak and Braak, 1991). Furthermore, several studies confirmed that this characteristic pattern of aggregated tau spread closely

correlates to the clinical symptoms of AD, as measured by the MMSE (Bancher et al., 1993, 1996; Duyckaerts et al., 1997; Grober et al., 1999). This makes tau an interesting target for drug development. Due to the complexity of aggregated tau as a drug target, several tau-associated approaches have been investigated.

Glycogen synthase kinase 3β, being the dominant isoform of three GSK-3 variants (Jaworski et al., 2011), is the main kinase responsible for the hyperphosphorylation of tau, and hence an important potential target for disease-modification (Maqbool et al., 2016). Diverse GSK-3 inhibitors were reported the last few years by many research groups (Noble et al., 2011; Berg et al., 2012; Maqbool et al., 2016). Lithium and valproate were the first compounds to be clinically evaluated, but due to inconsistent and overall disappointing results, they were largely discontinued (Noble et al., 2005; Hampel et al., 2009; Tariot and Aisen, 2009; Tariot et al., 2011). Several other GSK-3 inhibitors have, however, been pursued (Maqbool et al., 2016), two of which, tideglusib (NP0311212) and AZD1080, entered clinical trials (King et al., 2014; Lovestone et al., 2015). Development of AZD1080 was, however, halted in Phase I due to nephrotoxicity problems (Eldar-Finkelman and Martinez, 2011) and no clinical benefit was seen with tidelusib on patients with mild to moderate AD in Phase II clinical trials. Dose finding studies and longer trials are now required with the latter drug to examine its possible long term benefit (Lovestone et al., 2015). Another tau-associated approach is the inhibition of tau-aggregation (Bulic et al., 2009, 2010). The first of this class to be pushed in Phase II clinical trials, methylthioninium chloride (methylene blue, MTC), a phenothiazine derivative, was able to stabilize disease progression over a period of 50 weeks in mild and moderate AD patients (Wischik et al., 2015). The brain bioavailability of this charged drug remains, however, to be elucidated. The pro-drug of MTC, leuco-methylthioninium (TRx0237 or LMTX), with a superior pharmacological profile (Wischik et al., 2014) will now be evaluated in three parallel Phase III trials on mild to moderate AD patients and patients with FTD (CTI: NCT01689246, NCT01689233, and NCT01626378). And finally, an increasing interest toward tau immunotherapy has been noted, as means of removing tau aggregation by the patients' own immune system (Asuni et al., 2007). Two drugs of this kind, ACI-35 (ECT: 2015-000630-30) and AADvac1 (CTI: NCT02031198) are currently being evaluated in Phase I and II trials.

Despite the historical importance of tau as a pathological hallmark in AD (Graeber and Mehraein, 1999), only recently tau specific PET ligands have been developed. One of major issues during tau PET development is the lack of a representative tau-animal model, which may be explained by (ultra)structural differences between murine and humane tau (Duyckaerts et al., 2008). More than a few tracers are, however, currently being clinically evaluated. The first tau PET ligand to be reported was 2-(1-{6-[(2-[^{18}F]fluoroethyl)(methyl)amino]-2-naphthyl}ethylidene)malononitrile ([^{18}F]FDDNP) (**Figure**), although not specific for tau as such, high binding affinity was reported in several neurodegenerative diseases (Bresjanac et al., 2003; Small et al., 2006; Kepe et al., 2010; Nelson et al., 2011;

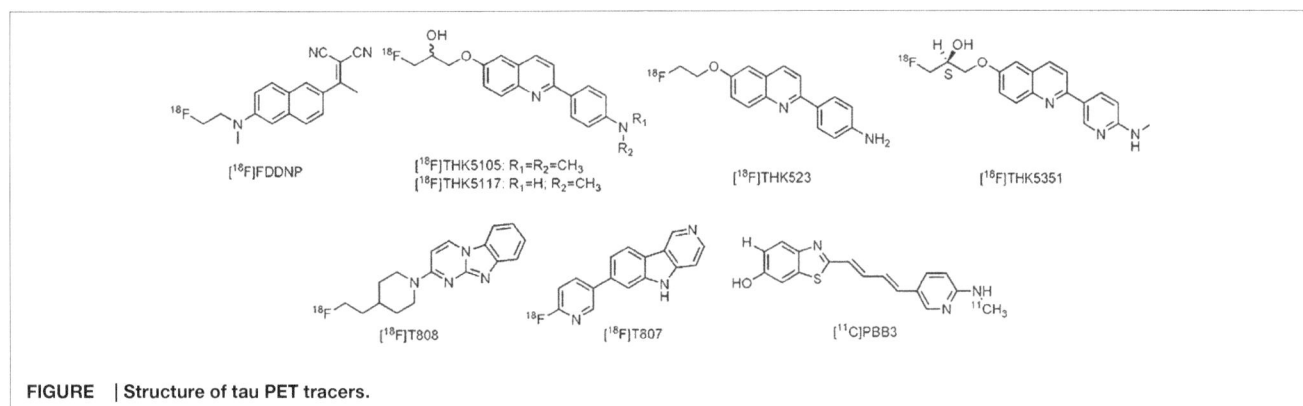

FIGURE | Structure of tau PET tracers.

Kepe et al., 2013; Small et al., 2013). Limited dynamic range of signal and relatively low affinity for tau, led to the development of novel tau directed ligands with similar structural moieties. Yet, the first real approach toward tau specific ligands was achieved by researchers of the Tohoku University in Japan with the development of 4-{6-[2-[^{18}F]fluoroethoxy]quinolin-2-yl} aniline ([^{18}F]THK523) (Fodero-Tavoletti et al., 2011) (**Figure**). While [^{18}F]THK523 was able to visualize the known pattern of tau distribution in AD patients, high white matter binding and unfavorable pharmacokinetics (Villemagne et al., 2014) led to the development of three novel 2-arylquinoline derivatives: 1-({2-[4-(dimethylamino)phenyl]quinolin-6-yl}oxy) -3-[^{18}F]fluoropropan-2-ol ([^{18}F]THK5105) (Okamura et al., 2014a), 1-[^{18}F]fluoro-3-({2-[4-(methylamino)phenyl]quinolin-6-yl}oxy)propan-2-ol ([^{18}F]THK5117) (Ishiki et al., 2015) and the optically pure (2S)-1-[^{18}F]fluoro-3-({2-[4-(methylamino) phenyl]quinolin-6-yl}oxy)propan-2-ol ([^{18}F]THK5351) (Harada et al., 2016) (**Figure**). All three compounds showed high binding in AD patients, with radiotracer retention in sites known for their tau deposition. Of these three compounds, [^{18}F]THK5351 showed superior pharmacokinetics, highest signal-to-noise ratio and the lowest white matter binding (Okamura et al., 2014b; Harada et al., 2016). Further clinical trials in Japan with [^{18}F]THK5351 are underway (UMIN-CTR: UMIN000013929 and UMIN000018496). Often considered by many research groups as the current benchmark in tau PET development, 11-{4-[2-[^{18}F]fluoroethyl]piperidin-1-yl}-1,8,10-triazatricyclo[7.4.0.0^{2,7}]trideca-2(7),3,5,8,10,12-hexaene ([^{18}F] T808 or [^{18}F]AV680), and 2-[^{18}F]fluoro-5-{5H-pyrido[4,3-b]indol-7-yl}pyridine ([^{18}F]T807 or [^{18}F]AV1451) (**Figure**) have high affinity and selectivity for tau over Aβ (Zhang et al., 2012; Xia et al., 2013; Shah and Catafau, 2014). A small first-in-man study with [^{18}F]T808 in eight AD patients (mean MMSE of 18) and their three age matched HCs, showed a rapid brain uptake and washout in HCs, and a tau pattern consistent with the Braak stages in the AD group (Chien et al., 2013). Interestingly, one of the AD patients who died a few weeks after his PET scan with [^{18}F]T808, showed close correlation with his histopathological staining (Dani et al., 2015). Nonetheless, substantial bone uptake was observed with this compound (Villemagne et al., 2015), which led to the development of [^{18}F]T807. In comparison to [^{18}F]T808,

[^{18}F]T807 has slower kinetics and a relatively lower affinity for tau, but [^{18}F]T807 does not show defluorination (Xia et al., 2013). Similar clinical findings as with [^{18}F]T808 were demonstrated with [^{18}F]T807 in a small first-in-man study on three HCs, in one patient with MCI (MMSE score of 26) and one severe AD patient (MMSE score of 7) in comparison with three HCs. Remarkably, the tracer retention was significantly lower in the patient with MCI, as compared to the patient with severe AD (Chien et al., 2012). A series of large clinical trials (ClinicalTrial.gov and EU Clinical Trials Register: search term: 'T807' OR 'AV1451' AND 'PET') is underway with [^{18}F]T807 to evaluate its applicability not only in AD, but also in several other tauopathies. Being thus far the only compound to be able to visualize tau (and possibly different isoforms) in AD, but also in PSP and CBD (Maruyama et al., 2013), 2-((1E, 3E)-4-(6-([^{11}C]methylamino)pyridin-3-yl)buta-1,3-dienyl)benzo[d]thiazol-6-ol ([^{11}C]PBB3) received a lot of interest (**Figure**). Clinical studies on AD patients and a CBD patient, as compared to HCs, showed increased tracer uptake, consistent with the Braak stages (for the AD case), and higher retention in the basal ganglia (for the CBD case). Stability issues and a challenging radiosynthesis might, however, limit its commercial use. Several other tau directed PET ligands from Roche, such as [^{11}C]RO6931643, [^{11}C]RO6924963, and [^{18}F]RO6958948 (structures not available) have been evaluated in a Phase I clinical trial, but data are yet to be published (CTI: NCT02187627) (Dani et al., 2015). Other clinical studies with [^{18}F]MK-6240, [^{18}F]MNI-798, and [^{18}F]MNI-815 (structures not available) on AD cases are currently recruiting patients (CTI: NCT02562989, NCT02640092, and NCT02531360). For a more detailed discussion about the current state of tau PET development, readers are referred to some excellent reviews on the subject (Okamura et al., 2014b; Zimmer et al., 2014; Dani et al., 2015). An important question that remains to be elucidated is for which isoforms these tau PET tracers have affinity; a question which may have major implications on the differential diagnosis of closely related neurodegenerative tauopathies. Nevertheless, the substantial progress that has been made in this field will make it possible to allow *in vivo* detection of tau in AD and thus the reassessment of inclusion- and outcome criteria of clinical trials aiming to intervene at tau-aggregates.

AMYLOID HYPOTHESIS

For many decades, the amyloid hypothesis has been the main pathological model of AD (Hardy and Higgins, 1992; Korczyn, 2008), accepted by most researchers, and only recently contested (Hardy, 2006). It postulates that extensive deposits of amyloid in the human brain are the central lesions in the development of AD, responsible for a neurotoxic cascade of events, which ultimately leads to dementia (Barage and Sonawane, 2015). Aβ peptides, the main component of SP (Gomez-Isla et al., 1997), are 39–43 amino acid residues, formed during the sequential cleavage of the transmembrane APP by β-secretase 1 (also called BACE1) (Haass, 2004), followed by the action of the γ-secretase (Selkoe, 2001). Under 'normal' conditions APP is cleaved in a non-amyloidogenic pathway by the action of initially α-secretase, forming α-sAPP, which may have a neuroprotective function (Pagani and Eckert, 2011). α-sAPP is then further cleaved by γ-secretase to eventually produce P3. The function of APP itself is unknown, although a possible role in the Cu-homeostasis has been proposed (Barnham et al., 2004). There are two main isoforms of Aβ: $A\beta_{40}$ and $A\beta_{42}$, the latter one being more prone to aggregation and regarded as the main neurotoxic species (Ballard et al., 2011). Once formed, Aβ species will undergo several characteristic changes, from small oligomers into larger fibrils, which eventually form diffuse and later neuritic plaques. These plaques frequently trigger astrocytosis, activation of microglial cells, cytokine release, and a multi-protein neuroinflammatory response (Barage and Sonawane, 2015). Just like the NFTs, amyloid depositions follow a specific pattern, as recorded by Braak and Braak (1991). In contrast to the NFTs, however, there is a poor correlation between the extent of these plaques and the degree of cognitive impairment (Nelson et al., 2012), furthermore non-demented individuals can heave substantial loads of Aβ deposition without revealing any clinical symptoms (Villemagne et al., 2008). Recently, several studies pointed toward Aβ oligomers, and not amyloid plaques, as the main toxic species in AD (Haass and Selkoe, 2007; Minati et al., 2009). For a more extensive discussion about the neuropathological role Aβ plays in AD, readers are referred to other reviews (Haass and Selkoe, 2007; Hardy, 2009; Barage and Sonawane, 2015).

Huge efforts have been undertaken to develop disease altering drugs that target the amyloid deposition, but unfortunately many failed during clinical trials (Barthel et al., 2015). Some of the most recent *ongoing* trials targeting the amyloid deposits are summarized in **Table** . Various therapeutic approaches are to be considered when targeting Aβ (Barage and Sonawane, 2015). We will discuss here the most important tactics, together with some of their constraints, as it is imperative to know why so many trials fail in this area. One of many methods applied, is the reduction of Aβ production through inhibition of β-and/or γ-secretase or activation of α-secretase (Cummings, 2008). Indeed, the therapeutic potential of BACE1 inhibitors has been demonstrated in BACE1 knockout mice, which produced significantly (15-fold) less Aβ (Luo et al., 2001; Roberds et al., 2001). Nonetheless, inhibition of BACE1 causes several problems, since BACE1 has been shown to have many physiological roles, which might lead to toxicity problems when using BACE1 inhibitors. Furthermore, BACE1 inhibitors need to be quite bulky, due to the relatively large active site and this can cause BBB passage issues (Ghezzi et al., 2013). Inhibition of the multimeric γ-secretase complex encounters similar problems as the use of BACE1 inhibitors,

TABLE | Ongoing clinical trials with drugs targeting the amyloid hypothesis (Han and Mook-Jung, 2014; Wischik et al., 2014; Apter et al., 2015).

Drug	Approach	Trial phase	CTI	PET biomarker*	EudraCT number
MK-8931	BACE1 inhibitor	3	NCT01953601	[18F]flutemetamol	2012-005542-38
		2/3	NCT01739348	[18F]flutemetamol	2011-003151-20
AZD3293	BACE1 inhibitor	2/3	NCT02245737	[18F]AV-45 / [18F]FDG	2014-002601-38
PF-03084014	γ-secretase inhibitor	2	NCT01981551	Not specified	/
NIC5-15	γ-secretase inhibitor	2	NCT01928420	Not specified	/
Bryostatin-1	α-secretase enhancer	2	NCT00606164	Not specified	/
		2	NCT02431468	Not specified	/
Solanezumab	Passive immunization	2/3	NCT01760005	[11C]PiB / [18F]FDG	2013-000307-17
		3	NCT01900665	[18F]AV-45	2013-001119-54
Gantenerumab	Passive immunization	3	NCT02051608	[18F]AV-45	2013-003390-95
		3	NCT01224106	Not specified	2010-019895-66
		2/3	NCT01760005	[11C]PiB / [18F]FDG	2013-000307-17
Crenezumab	Passive immunization	1	NCT02353598	[18F]AV-45	/
		2	NCT01998841	Not specified	/
		2	NCT01723826C	Not specified	2012-003242-33
BAN2401	Passive immunization	2	NCT01767311	Not specified	2012-002843-11
Gammagard	Passive immunization	2/3	NCT01561053	[18F]FDG	/
Aducanumab	Passive immunization	3	NCT02484547	Not specified	2015-000967-15
		3	NCT02477800	Not specified	2015-000966-72
		1	NCT02434718	Not specified	/

*C = Completed; PET biomarkers are either used as inclusion criteria and/or as outcome measure.

as γ-secretase has many other physiological roles as well, especially cleavage of the Notch receptor, necessary for growth and development (Yiannopoulou and Papageorgiou, 2013). Brain penetration seems to be an issue as well in this area (Imbimbo and Giardina, 2011). Increasing the α-secretase activity, and thus promoting the non-amyloidogenic pathway, is another way to reduce the Aβ load. Less is however known about the possible physiological consequences of such an upregulation (Barage and Sonawane, 2015). Another way of interfering with the Aβ load is by modulation of Aβ aggregation, as increasing evidence suggests that soluble oligomers, which act as intermediates for the formation of aggregates, are the most toxic species in AD disease (Dahlgren et al., 2002; Hoshi et al., 2003; Kayed et al., 2003). Yet, the most promising small molecules ultimately failed due to their (toxic) pharmacological profile (Santa-Maria et al., 2007; Rishton, 2008; Yiannopoulou and Papageorgiou, 2013). Several studies also showed the relationship of APP and Aβ with mitochondrial dysfunction in AD (Anandatheerthavarada et al., 2003; Lustbader et al., 2004; Caspersen et al., 2005); interaction of both proteins with mitochondrial matrix proteins, such as Aβ-binding alcohol dehydrogenase and adenosine triphosphate synthase subunit alpha, could directly lead to mitochondrial toxicity, and thus oxidative stress (Devi et al., 2006; Reddy and Beal, 2008). Numerous antioxidant agents have been described and evaluated in clinical trials with MCI- and AD patients, and several studies are still ongoing (Mecocci and Polidori, 2012; Polidori and Nelles, 2014). Conflicting results were, however, reported and overall small cognitive benefit was seen during these trials. Long-term trails are now warranted in order to establish clinical benefits in AD. Then again, several promising antioxidative compounds are currently being investigated (Qosa et al., 2015; Rigacci, 2015). Still, the primary action in targeting amyloid came from monoclonal antibodies. First discovered by Schenk et al. (1999) to be very effective in reducing the Aβ load in mice, the mechanism of action of amyloid immunotherapy remains, however, to be fully elucidated (Yiannopoulou and Papageorgiou, 2013). Nevertheless, only a small fraction (0.1% of the injected dose) of antibodies seems to be able to pass the BBB in humans (Banks et al., 2002). A higher fraction of antibodies in the brain may thus be needed to be therapeutically effective. This hurdle was the topic of two recently reported reviews (Lemere, 2013; Spencer and Masliah, 2014). Despite the low BBB's passage, one of the major concerns with immunotherapy is the development of serious side effects, for instance encephalitis (active immunization), microhemorrhages, or vasogenic edemas (passive immunization) (Orgogozo et al., 2003; Panza et al.,

2012). Another important factor to consider is the time of intervention in the AD state; immunotherapy is probably most efficacious in early disease states, when there is more function to preserve (Barthel et al., 2015). Efficient biomarkers, that can predict the conversion from MCI to AD, are therefore of utter importance. Using longitudinal PET biomarkers to assess and follow up the amyloid burden in clinical trials would indeed allow a more confident formulation of inclusion, but also outcome criteria (Barthel et al., 2015). Several amyloid PET tracers are currently being used for these purposes (see **Table**).

Although not FDA-approved, 2-{4-[[^{11}C]methylamino]phenyl}-1,3-benzothiazol-6-ol ([^{11}C]PiB) (**Figure**) has been used for many years as benchmark compound for *in vivo* imaging of the amyloid load in AD patients (Benadiba et al., 2012). Results of those trials have shown that clinically diagnosed AD cases have positive amyloid scans (Kemppainen et al., 2006; Jack et al., 2008, 2009; Lowe et al., 2009), and the ones that did not have positive scans, were most likely to be misdiagnosed (Rabinovici et al., 2007; Rabinovici et al., 2008). Furthermore, increased [^{11}C]PiB binding is able to predict the conversion of MCI to AD (Okello et al., 2009). [^{11}C]PiB has also been proven useful in the differential diagnosis of FTD and AD, as FTD patients typically have a normal [^{11}C]PiB uptake (Rowe et al., 2007; Engler et al., 2008). Interestingly, a close correlation has been noted with CSF Aβ levels (Tolboom et al., 2009; Weigand et al., 2011), firmly establishing [^{11}C]PiB as an Aβ biomarker. There are, however, a few limitations with [^{11}C]PiB as an amyloid biomarker; [^{11}C]PiB presumably binds to diffuse plaques and not to the more cognitive correlated neuritic plaques (Jack et al., 2013). Moreover, commercial use is excluded, due to the short half-life of carbon-11. Several attempts were thus undertaken to develop ^{18}F-labeled analogs (Koo and Byun, 2013). Three of them: 4-[(E)-2-[6-(2-{2-[2-[^{18}F]fluoroethoxy]ethoxy}ethoxy)pyridin-3-yl]ethenyl]-N-methylaniline ([^{18}F]florbetapir or [^{18}F]AV-45), 2-[3-[^{18}F]fluoro-4-(methylamino)phenyl]-1,3-benzothiazol-6-ol ([^{18}F]flutemetamol, [^{18}F]GE-067 or [^{18}F]AV-1) and 4-[(E)-2-[4-(2-{2-[2-[^{18}F]fluoroethoxy]ethoxy}ethoxy)phenyl]ethenyl]-N-methylaniline([^{18}F]florbetaben or [^{18}F]BAY 97-9172) (**Figure**) have already been approved by the FDA and the EMA for their binding to neuritic plaques. Another one, 2-[2-[^{18}F]fluoro-6-(methylamino)pyridin-3-yl]-1-benzofuran-6-ol ([^{18}F]AZD-4694 or [^{18}F]NAV4694) (**Figure**), is currently awaiting FDA-approval (Jack et al., 2013). Although all of the current ^{18}F-labeled compounds show significant increased uptake in AD patients as compared to HCs in clinical

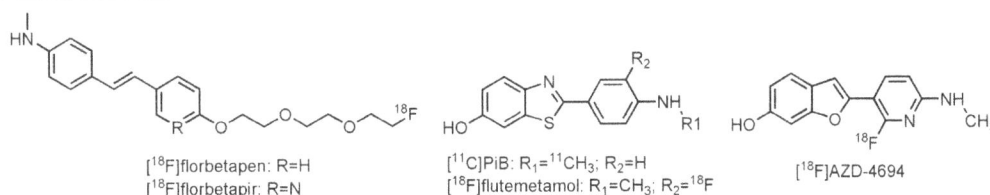

[^{18}F]florbetapen: R=H
[^{18}F]florbetapir: R=N

[^{11}C]PiB: R$_1$=^{11}CH$_3$; R$_2$=H
[^{18}F]flutemetamol: R$_1$=CH$_3$; R$_2$=^{18}F

[^{18}F]AZD-4694

FIGURE | Structure of Aβ PET tracers.

trials (Rowe et al., 2008, 2013; Barthel et al., 2011; Villemagne et al., 2011), they suffer from high non-specific white matter binding, as compared to [^{11}C]PiB (Benadiba et al., 2012; Rowe and Villemagne, 2013; Vandenberghe et al., 2013). Only [^{18}F]AZD-4694 has a white matter uptake similar to [^{11}C]PiB (Rowe et al., 2013). While a negative amyloid PET scan will exclude AD, a positive scan, on its own, is insuffient for the diagnosis of AD, as has been shown with [^{18}F]florbetapir in clinic (Yang et al., 2012). Furthermore, limited reimbursement of these recently approved compounds limits their use in clinical practice (Barthel et al., 2015). The use of amyloid PET may, however, reveal true AD cases. Moreover, the amyloid tracers are able to predict the conversion from MCI to AD, and this can considerably influence decision making in AD related clinical trials (Rowe and Villemagne, 2013).

GAMMA-AMINOBUTYRIC ACID RECEPTORS

The inhibitory GABA system in the CNS consists of three GABA receptor systems: $GABA_A$, $GABA_B$ and $GABA_C$ (Chebib and Johnston, 1999). Since $GABA_B$- and $GABA_C$ receptors have not been clinically evaluated in AD yet, focus will be toward the $GABA_A$ receptor. The $GABA_A$ receptor is a pentameric ligand gated ion channel, composed of a wide array of (possible) subunits: $\alpha_{1-6}, \beta_{1-3}, \gamma_{1-3}, \delta, \epsilon, \tau, \pi,$ and ρ_{1-3} (Mehta and Ticku, 1999). In order to be functional, the receptor seems to require the presence of at least one α- and one β-subunit. The most common composition is a pentamer composed of two α-, two β-, and one γ-subunit (Connolly et al., 1996). The GABA system plays an important role in AD, as it is one of the main culprits for the BPSD. Contributing to these BPSD, the GABA system is also known to modulate other neurotransmitters, such as serotonin, DA and ACh (Decker and McGaugh, 1991; Zorumski and Isenberg, 1991; Keverne, 1999). It has been a long standing, although contested (Lanctot et al., 2004), view that the GABA system undergoes little change during AD progression, due to dynamic plasticity of the system (Rissman et al., 2007). Recent findings suggest, however, otherwise and point to a severely altered GABAergic signaling in AD, with possible modulation of tau hyperphosphorylation (Lanctot et al., 2004; Limon et al., 2012; Nykanen et al., 2012). A more detailed discussion of the GABAsystem and its putative role in AD can be found in some extensive reviews (Marczynski, 1998; Lanctot et al., 2004; Rissman et al., 2007).

Benzodiazepines, which are allosteric modulators of the $GABA_A$ receptor (Hevers and Luddens, 1998), have long been used for the symptomatic treatment of anxiety and agitation in AD (Kirven and Montero, 1973; Covington, 1975; Sunderland et al., 1989; Zec and Burkett, 2008), nevertheless there is a need for randomized controlled trials to evaluate the true efficacy of these drugs in AD (Defrancesco et al., 2015). Caution is also to be advised with BZDs, as there are reports of rapid cognitive and functional decline in AD patients when taking these drugs for an extensive period of time (Zec and Burkett, 2008).

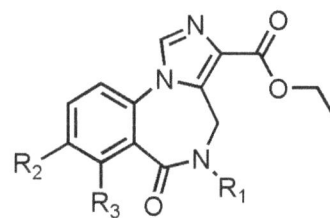

[^{11}C]flumazenil: $R_1=^{11}CH_3$; $R_2=F$; $R_3=H$
[^{123}I]iomazenil: $R_1=CH_3$; $R_2=H$; $R_3=^{123}I$

FIGURE | Structure of GABAergic PET/SPECT tracers.

There have been numerous endeavors to developed radiotracers for *in vivo* imaging of the $GABA_A$ receptors (Katsifis and Kassiou, 2004; Andersson and Halldin, 2013). Ethyl 12-fluoro-8-[^{11}C]methyl-9-oxo-2,4,8-triazatricyclo[8.4.0.0^{2,6}] tetradeca-1,3,5,10,12-pentaene-5-carboxylate ([^{11}C]flumazenil) (**Figure**), a $GABA_A$ antagonist with affinity for the α_{1-3} and α_5-subunit, is the most promising tracer thus far. Several clinical studies have been performed with [^{11}C]flumazenil (Savic et al., 1988; Heiss et al., 2004; Frankle et al., 2009, 2012; Andersson and Halldin, 2013), one of which was carried out on early AD patients (Mean MMSE: 21.2) to evaluate the $GABA_A$ receptor density. Researches demonstrated a marked decrease in [^{11}C]flumazenil binding, which correlated well with neuronal loss as evaluated by histopathological findings (Brun and Englund, 1981; Andersson and Halldin, 2013). The SPECT analog ethyl 11-[^{123}I]iodo-8-methyl-9-oxo-2,4,8-triazatricyclo[8.4.0.0^{2,6}]tetradeca-1,3,5,10,12-pentaene-5-carboxylate ([^{123}I]iomazenil) (**Figure**), showed significantly reduced uptake in the temporal, parietal end occipital cortex of moderate to severe AD patients (Soricelli et al., 1996; Fukuchi et al., 1997). In contrast to [^{11}C]flumazenil though, [^{123}I]iomazenil was not able to show significant changes in early AD patients (Pappata et al., 2010). Interestingly, in a direct PET-SPECT comparison study on healthy volunteers between [^{11}C]flumazenil and [^{123}I]iomazenil, the ^{123}I-labeled variant came out as the better candidate, due to a better fit in compartmental modeling with SPECT (Bremner et al., 1999). These radiopharmaceuticals not only hold promise to be used as inclusion- and outcome criteria for drugs combatting BPSD symptoms in AD, but they could also be used in dose-occupancy studies to assess the (sometimes small) therapeutic window of BZDs.

SEROTONERGIC SYSTEM

Serotonin (5-HT), is a neurotransmitter that plays a complex role in the modulation of several psychological, emotional, and cognitive processes. Moreover, 5-HT affects long-term and short-term memory and cognitive function through the regulating of many other neurotransmitters, such as ACh, DA, GABA, and glutamate (Rodríguez et al., 2012). The principal 5-HT-source in the human brain comes from neurons in the raphe nuclei, with various projections throughout the CNS (Vertes, 1991; Vertes et al., 1999). There are seven main 5-HTRs, which can be divided into two major classes: the G-protein coupled receptors (5-HTR$_{1,2,4-7}$) and the ligand-gated cation channels (5-HTR$_3$), many of which have also several subcategories (Hoyer et al., 2002). For the 'normal' physiological and pharmacological role of these receptors, readers are referred to several reviews on the topic (Barnes and Sharp, 1999; Hoyer et al., 2002; Niesler et al., 2008). An overall reduction of the serotonergic system in AD pathology, likely reflecting the loss of serotonergic projections from the raphe nuclei, has been demonstrated (Bowen et al., 1983; Chen et al., 1996, 2000). Interestingly, loss of function seems more extensive in early onset AD than in later-onset AD, which may be due to compensating systems (Arai et al., 1992; Halliday et al., 1992). More specifically, marked reduction of the 5-HTR$_{1A}$, which is expressed in brain areas known for their role in memory and learning, has been noted in the hippocampus and the frontal cortex during AD progression (Lai et al., 2003). This may, however, reflect a compensatory mechanism for reduction of cholinergic receptors in the AD brain, since inhibition of the 5-HTR$_{1A}$ has been implicated in the release of ACh (Millan et al., 2004; Kehr et al., 2010; Rodríguez et al., 2012). Another receptor that is affected during AD progression is 5-HTR$_{2A}$, with reductions being noted in the frontal, temporal, parietal and enthorinal cortex and the hippocampus (Crow et al., 1984; Procter et al., 1988; Dewar et al., 1990). In a review by Rodríguez et al. (2012) it was suggested that a decrease in 5-HTR$_{2A}$ may effect cognitive functions in AD patients. A positive correlation between cognitive decline and 5-HTR$_{2A}$ related decrease in the frontal cortex has indeed been noted (Lai et al., 2005). Moreover, it was implied that decrease in 5-HTR$_{2A}$ density may be due to pathological accumulation of Aβ (Christensen et al., 2008; Holm et al., 2010). Stimulation of the 5-HTR$_4$ may lead to an increase of the non-amyloidogenic pathway *in vitro* (Consolo et al., 1994;

Robert and Benoit, 2008), indication for an important role in APP metabolism. Other 5-HTRs with marked reduction in AD are 5-HTR$_{1B}$, 5-HTR$_{1D}$, and 5-HTR$_6$ (Garcia-Alloza et al., 2004; Lorke et al., 2006). Additionally, reduction of the former two correlates well with the cognitive decline in AD (Garcia-Alloza et al., 2004). Significant decrease (up to 25%) in binding sites of the 5-HTT during AD progression is also to be noted (Bowen et al., 1983; Ouchi et al., 2009). As part of the monoamine transporter family, the SERT is responsible for removal of serotonin from the synaptic cleft. There seems, however, no correlation between the reduced density of this transporter and BPSD symptoms, as seen in AD (Tsang et al., 2010).

Most drugs targeting the serotonergic system are used as adjuvant therapy, combatting BPSD symptoms by inhibition of SERT and/or the norepinephrine transporter. Recent meta-analyses have proven their efficacy in treating these behavioral symptoms in AD (Ballard and Corbett, 2010; Henry et al., 2011). Some serotonin reuptake inhibitors have, however, also been evaluated for their possible cognitive enhancement in AD patients (See **Table**). Likewise, increasing interest has been noted for 5-HTR drugs that are able to improve cognition and/or memory in AD. 5-HT$_1$-, 5-HT$_4$-, and 5-HT$_6$ receptors are hereby of particular interest, due to their important role in learning and memory processes (Geldenhuys and Van der Schyf, 2011), effects which are most likely due to their modulation on glutamatergic and cholinergic transmission, or, in the case of 5-HT-4, due to an enhanced release of ACh upon stimulation of this receptor (Rodríguez et al., 2012). An overview of trials that have looked into the clinical benefit of serotonergic drugs on cognitive impairment in AD patients is given in **Table** .

Although much progress has been made in the development of PET- and SPECT radioligands for visualization of the serotonergic system (Paterson et al., 2013), only a few radiolabeled compounds have been evaluated on AD patients

TABLE | Enhancement of cognitive functions in AD by drugs that modulate serotonergic neurotransmission (Geldenhuys and Van der Schyf, 2011; Ramirez et al., 2014).

Drug	Mechanism	Trial (Phase)	Outcome	Reference/ongoing trail
Lecozotan (SRR-333)	5-HTR$_{1A}$ antagonist	2	Unsuccessful due to adverse effects	Sabbagh, 2009
Xailiproden (SRR57746A)	5-HTR$_{1A}$ antagonist	3	Unsuccessful to demonstrate efficacy	Sabbagh, 2009
PRX-03140	5-HTR$_4$ agonist	2	Improvement on ADAS-cog scale	Sabbagh, 2009
SB-742457	5-HTR$_6$ antagonist	2	Improvement on CIBIC+ score and ADAS-cog scale	Maher-Edwards et al., 2010
Lu-AE-58054 (SGS-518)	5-HTR$_6$ antagonist	2	Improvement on ADAS-cog scale and ADL	Rodríguez et al., 2012
		3	Ongoing	NCT02079246
		3	Ongoing	NCT02006654
		3	Ongoing	NCT02006641
		3	Ongoing	NCT01955161
PF-05212377 (SAM-760)	5-HTR$_6$ antagonist	2	Ongoing	Rodríguez et al., 2012/NCT01712074
SUVN-502	5-HTR$_6$ antagonist	2	Ongoing	Geldenhuys and Van der Schyf, 2011/ NCT02580305
Citolapram	SSRI	4 weeks	Improvement on ADL	Nyth and Gottfries, 1990
Fluoxetine	SSRI	8 weeks	Improvement on MMSE	Mowla et al., 2007
Sertraline	SSRI	12 weeks	Improvement on ADL	Lyketsos et al., 2003

ADAS-cog, Alzheimer's Disease Assessment Scale-cognitive subscale; CIBIC+, Clinician's Interview-Based Impression of Change; ADL, Activity of Daily Living; MMSE, Mini-Mental State Examination; SSRI, Selective Serotonin Reuptake Inhibitor.

thus far. In the group of the 5-HT_{1A}R, only one PET radioligand, 4-[^{18}F]fluoro-N-{2-[4-(2-methoxyphenyl)-1-piperazinyl]ethyl}-N-(2-pyridinyl)benzamide ([^{18}F]MPPF, **Figure**), a reversible, competitive 5-HT_{1A}R antagonist, was investigated in patients with MCI and AD (Kepe et al., 2006; Truchot et al., 2008). Decrease of [^{18}F]MPPF binding was noticed in the hippocampus and raphe nuclei of AD patients (as compared to HCs). Furthermore, loss of receptor density in the hippocampus was strongly correlated to a decline in the MMSE score. In patients with MCI, only a small loss of 5-HT_{1A}R density was noticed, correlated to only small cognitive decline (Kepe et al., 2006). [^{18}F]MPPF is one of many fluoro-analogs of [^{11}C]WAY100635, the latter one being excessively studied in humans. Yet, no studies on AD patients were performed with [^{11}C]WAY100635, mainly due its rapid metabolism, making kinetic modeling difficult (Paterson et al., 2013). [^{18}F]MPPF does not suffer from these limitations, but is on the other hand a substrate of the P-gp, which could limit its further use in clinic (Kumar and Mann, 2014). Imaging of the 5-HT_2R in AD patients was done by one SPECT- and three PET radiolabeled 5-HT_2R antagonists, namely 4-amino-N-{1-[3-(4-fluorophenyl)propyl]-4-methylpiperidin-4-yl}-5-[^{123}I]iodo-2-methoxybenzamide ([^{123}I]-R91150), 6-(2-{4-[4-[^{18}F]fluorobenzoyl]piperidin-1-yl}ethyl)-7-methyl-2H,3H,5H-[1,3]thiazolo[3,2-a]pyrimidin-5-one ([^{18}F]setoperone), 3-(2-{4-[4-[^{18}F]fluorobenzoyl]piperidin-1-yl}ethyl)-2-sulfanylidene-1,2,3,4-tetrahydroquinazolin-4-one ([^{18}F]altanserin) and 3-(2-{4-[4-[^{18}F]fluorobenzoyl]piperidin-1-yl}(2,2-^{2}H2)ethyl)-2-sulfanylidene-1,2,3,4-tetrahydroquinazolin-4-one ([^{18}F]deuteroaltanserin) (**Figure**). In agreement with previous postmortem studies, an overall significant reduction in the cerebral cortex was noted in mild to severe AD patients, compared to their age-matched controls (Blin et al., 1993; Versijpt et al., 2003; Santhosh et al., 2009; Marner et al., 2012). In the 5-HT_4R class though, one PET ligand was evaluated on AD patients: [1-[^{11}C]methylpiperidin-4-yl]methyl 8-amino-7-chloro-2,3-dihydro-1,4-benzodioxine-5-carboxylate ([^{11}C]SB207145), a 5-HT_4R antagonist (**Figure**). This radioligand did not display significant

differences between mild AD cases and their HCs, although a positive correlation was found with the Aβ density (as measured by [^{11}C]PiB). Moreover, a negative correlation was noticed between [^{11}C]SB207145's binding potential and the MMSE score. Authors suggested that upregulation of 5-HT_4R may take place at a preclinical stage of AD (this in contrast to the other 5-HTRs) and that this may continue through the later AD stages (Madsen et al., 2011). Finally, (3-amino-4-(2-dimethylamino-methyl-phenylsulfanyl)-benzonitrile) ([^{11}C]DASB, **Figure**), a SERT tracer, displayed a more outspoken decrease (25%) of binding in the subcortical serotonergic projection region in depressed, as compared to non-depressed AD patients (mean MMSE score of 18) (Ouchi et al., 2009). Yet, in another clinical study on patients with mild AD (not corrected for depression) no such reduction was found (Marner et al., 2012). Authors of the latter study suggest that this discrepancy may, however, lay in both differences in dementia severity as well as methodological differences between these studies (Marner et al., 2012). For a more detailed discussion about the current state of other 5-HT PET- and SPECT radioligands, readers are referred to some excellent reviews (Saulin et al., 2012; Paterson et al., 2013; Billard et al., 2014; Kumar and Mann, 2014). These compounds can be used for evaluation of inclusion- and outcome criteria, but also in dose-occupancy studies.

DOPAMINERGIC SYSTEM

The activity of DA, a catecholamine, is mediated through five dopaminergic, metabotropic, G-protein coupled receptors. They are divided into two classes: D_1-like receptors (D_1R and D_5R) and D_2-like receptors (D_{2-4}R), depending on the downstream signaling cascade. Levels of DA are regulated through the activity of the presynaptic DAT, which removes DA from the synaptic cleft to terminate its activity (Mitchell et al., 2011). Dopaminergic neurons are largely located in the midbrain, with many projections throughout the brain (Martorana and Koch, 2014),

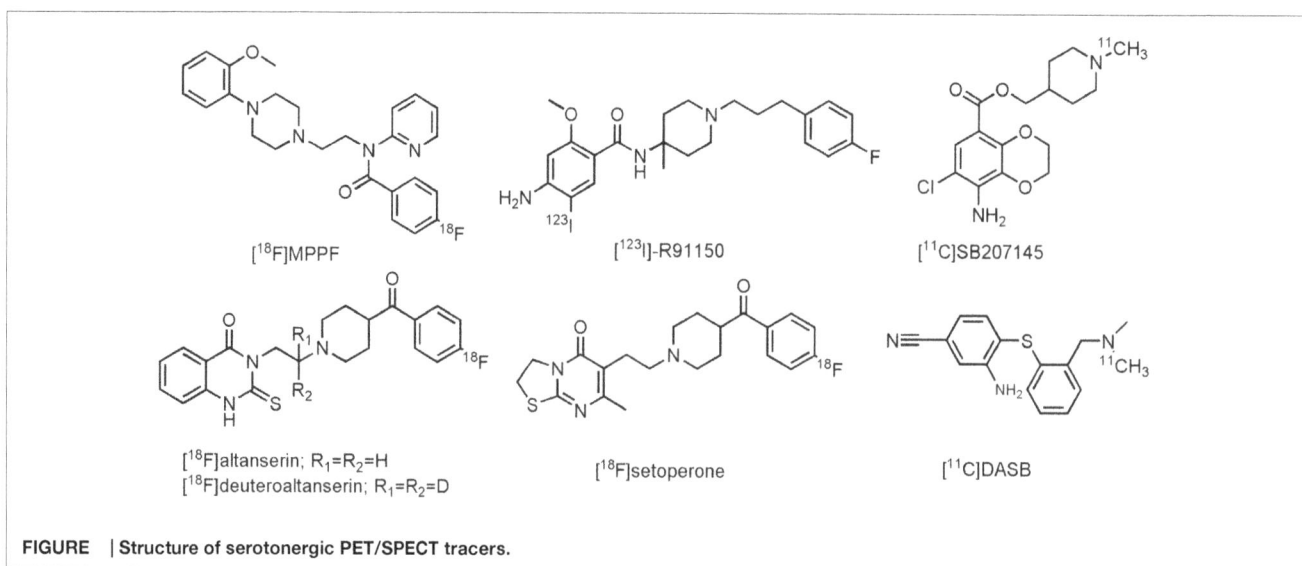

FIGURE | Structure of serotonergic PET/SPECT tracers.

where they are involved in various neurological processes. Of particular importance here is their role in motivation, cognition, and learning (Xu et al., 2012). Indeed, around 35–40% of AD patients exhibit extrapyramidal symptoms and more than 70% display extensive apathy (Lopez et al., 1997; Mitchell et al., 2011). These symptoms might be explained by the significantly reduced levels of DA and its precursor L-3,4-dihydroxyphenylalanine (L-DOPA) (Storga et al., 1996). Although large involvement of DA in AD is still under debate (Portet et al., 2009; Trillo et al., 2013), several noticeable changes have been documented in the DA receptor density. More specifically, a significant reduced expression of D_1- and D_2-like receptors has been documented in the prefrontal cortex and the hippocampus of AD patients (Kemppainen et al., 2003; Kumar and Patel, 2007). Furthermore, alterations of the D_2R in AD seems positively correlated to BPSD and verbal memory performance (Kemppainen et al., 2003; Tanaka et al., 2003). Conflicting results are, however, reported for the D_2R density in AD patients (see further) (Piggott et al., 1999; Piggott et al., 2007). Contradictory results are also reported for changes in the DAT levels in AD patients (Murray et al., 1995; Ceravolo et al., 2004). Despite some discrepancy, it is clear that there are important DA changes in the AD brains. Finally, it is to be noted that several *in vivo* experiments on mice, expressing AD like pathology, show that significant behavioral and cognitive deficits can be restored by administering DA reuptake inhibitors and L-DOPA (Ambree et al., 2009; Guzman-Ramos et al., 2012). Aβ oligomers may indeed have an early impact on catecholaminergic transmission (Mura et al., 2010).

There are several modes of interventions toward the failing dopaminergic system in AD patients, mostly used to address apathy (the most common BPSD symptom) and extrapyramidal symptoms. One of many approaches is the use of MAO-B inhibitors, which are discussed in Section "Monoamine Oxidase B" of this review. Another therapeutic method is modulation of the DAT transporter, and thus increasing synaptic DA levels. This was done by methylphenidate and dextroamphetamine in several clinical AD studies (Galynker et al., 1997; Herrmann et al., 2008; Lanctot et al., 2008). Although not selective for

the dopaminergic system, an overall improvement was noted in symptoms of apathy on the Apathy Evaluation Scale (AES). There are, however, some concerns about the tolerability of methylphenidate (Padala et al., 2010). Other drugs that are frequently used to treat BPSD symptoms in clinical trials (and routine practice) involving AD patients are the antipsychotic drugs quetiapine, aripiprazole, olanzapine, and risperidone. As FDA- and EMA-approved drugs, these drugs act as partial DA receptor agonist or partial DA receptor antagonist (among often interaction with many other targets). Overall improvement on BPSD symptoms was recorded in a large meta-analysis of the use of antipsychotics in AD patients (Ballard and Waite, 2006). Nevertheless, caution was advised by the FDA with these drugs, as they were associated with an increase in risk of death, and other severe side effects, among elder people with dementia (Ballard and Waite, 2006; De Deyn et al., 2013). Yet another drug, rotigotine, a D_2R- and D_3R agonist, was able to show cognitive enhancement on probable AD patients, compared to their age-matched HCs by measuring the cortical excitability and central cholinergic transmission (Martorana et al., 2013).

Imaging of the dopaminergic system can be done by a number of PET- and SPECT radioligands. Conflicting results are, however, reported between several clinical studies on AD patients, using different PET- and/or SPECT tracers. In a combined PET study, reduced striatal expression of D_1R, but not D_2R was seen with D_2R antagonist 3,5-dichloro-N-{[(2S)-1-ethyl pyrrolidin-2-yl]methyl}-2-hydroxy-6-[^{11}C]methoxybenzamide ([^{11}C]raclopride) and D_1R antagonist (5R)-8-chloro-5-(2,3-dihydro-1-benzofuran-7-yl)-3-[^{11}C]methyl-2,3,4,5-tetrahydro-1H-3-benzazepin-7-ol ([^{11}C]NNC 756) in AD patients (**Figure**), compared to age-matched HCs (Kemppainen et al., 2000). Striatal uptake of 2-amino-3-[2-[^{18}F]fluoro-4,5-dihydroxyphenyl]propanoic acid ([^{18}F]FDOPA), a fluorinated form of L-DOPA (**Figure**), was also unchanged in AD patients, compared to HCs (Tyrrell et al., 1990). Conversely, decreased striatal expression of D_2R with [^{11}C]raclopride was demonstrated in AD patients (with BPSD symptoms) as compared to their HCs (Tanaka et al.,

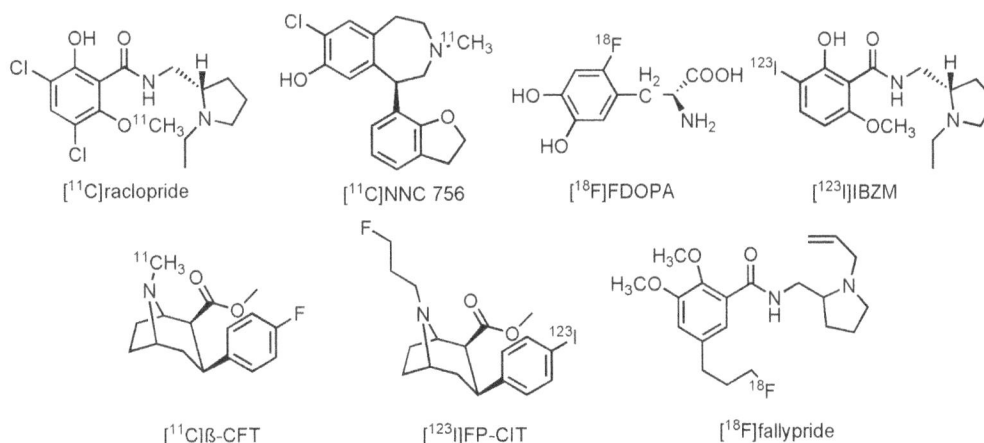

FIGURE | Structure of dopaminergic PET/SPECT tracers.

2003). Similar studies, using N-{[(2S)-1-ethylpyrrolidin-2-yl]methyl}-2-hydroxy-3-[^{123}I]iodo-6-methoxybenzamide ([^{123}I]IBZM) (**Figure**), a D_2R antagonist, or methyl (2S,3S)-3-(4-fluorophenyl)-8-[^{11}C]methyl-8-azabicyclo[3.2.1]octane-2-carboxylate ([^{11}C]β-CFT) (**Figure**), a cocaine derivative which binds to DAT, showed, respectively, a reduced expression of D_2R and a reduced DA reuptake (Pizzolato et al., 1996; Rinne et al., 1998). Reduction of DA reuptake sites, as measured by [^{11}C]β-CFT, was hereby positively correlated to the severity of the extrapyramidal symptoms of AD patients, whereas in the study with [^{123}I]IBZM, patients did not exhibit any extrapyramidal symptoms. Likewise, a decrease in [^{18}F]FDOPA striatal uptake was noticed in another study on AD patients, a decrease which was correlated to the cognitive scores of the AD patients (Itoh et al., 1994). On the other hand, even more confusing, is the fact that in yet another clinical study involving AD patients an increase in D_2R expression in the striatum was now measured with [^{11}C]raclopride (Reeves et al., 2009). Discrepancies between these different studies might, however, be explained by different study populations, and the degree of dementia, since time-dependent dopaminergic receptor changes were also seen in patients with PD (Brooks, 1993). Another role for dopaminergic neuroimaging was displayed by methyl (2S,3S)-8-(3-fluoropropyl)-3-[4-[^{123}I]iodophenyl]-8-azabicyclo[3.2.1]octane-2-carboxylate ([^{123}I]FP-CIT) (**Figure**), an analog of [^{11}C]β-CFT. [^{123}I]FP-CIT was able to differentiate, with high accuracy, patients with AD, and patients with DLB (Colloby et al., 2008; Spehl et al., 2015). Overall reduced striatal uptake was noticed in both diseases, but lower binding potentials of [^{123}I]FP-CIT were reported in DLB than in the case of the AD patients. These scans can greatly improve differential diagnosis between the different neurodegenerative diseases, which often display similar clinical presentations. [^{123}I]FP-CIT SPECT scans are already used in clinical routine to distinguish DLB- from AD patients (Spehl et al., 2015). Finally, 5-[3-[^{18}F]fluoropropyl]-2,3-dimethoxy-N-{[1-(prop-2-en-1-yl)pyrrolidin-2-yl]methyl}benzamide ([^{18}F]fallypride) (**Figure**), a D_2R/D_3R antagonist, could be used to assess the ideal therapeutic window for the use of antipsychotic drugs (Clark-Papasavas et al., 2014), since, as mentioned before, elder people are very sensitive to these drugs. [^{18}F]fallypride PET scans could consequently assist in antipsychotic dose-occupancy studies, and thus help to provide an ideal antipsychotic strategy in AD patients with extensive BPSD symptoms.

NEUROINFLAMMATION

Translocator Protein

Formerly known as PBR, the 18 kDa TSPO, is located on the outer membrane of the mitochondria, predominantly in glial cells. As part of a multimeric complex, which is comprised of a VDAC and an adenine nucleotide carrier (McEnery et al., 1992; Casellas et al., 2002; Cosenza-Nashat et al., 2009), several functions are associated with TSPO (Midzak et al., 2015). They play an essential role in neurosteriod synthesis, by facilitating the transport of cholesterol from the outer to the inner membrane of the mitochondria (Papadopoulos et al., 2006a,b), and hence potentiate the GABAergic neurotransmission through allosteric modulation of the $GABA_A$ receptor by neurosteroids (Belelli and Lambert, 2005; Hosie et al., 2006; Rudolph and Mohler, 2006). Furthermore, TSPO may have a crucial function in a variety of cellular processes, such as cell proliferation (Miettinen et al., 1995; Hardwick et al., 1999), mitochondrial respiration (Hirsch et al., 1989) and cell apoptosis (Kugler et al., 2008). In light of TSPO's association with the pathophysiology of neurodegenerative diseases, it has been well established that part of the neurotoxicity caused by tau and Aβ deposits in AD is induction of a neuroinflammatory response (McGeer and McGeer, 1995; Hoozemans et al., 2011), which triggers the upregulation of TSPO in activated microglia and astrocytes. Moreover, this upregulation clearly correlates with the degree of neuroinflammation, making TSPO a valuable target for drug monitoring (Venneti et al., 2006). Interestingly, in a review by Chua et al. (2014), it was suggested that TSPO ligands may provide effective tools for treatment of AD through activation of neuroprotective pathways of increased expression of astrocytes and microglial cells, since these mechanisms may have a protective phagocytic role in early AD (Morgan et al., 2005). Once a more progressed AD state has been reached, neuroinflammation turns chronic and becomes harmful (Hickman et al., 2008). This view is in contrast with numerous clinical trials, using anti-inflammatory drugs that failed to produce significant improvement in AD patients (Streit, 2010; Venigalla et al., 2015), although this failure may be attributed to a 'wrong' stage of the disease when therapy was initiated (Moreira et al., 2006). There are currently no drugs in clinical trials that interact with the TSPO receptor in AD. Drugs that are already described are mainly used for their use against BPSD symptoms (Rupprecht et al., 2009; Owen et al., 2011). TSPO is, however, an important marker for neuroinflammation, which makes it an interesting target for neuroimaging. PET tracers in this class will thus mainly be used to assess inclusion- and outcome criteria in clinical trials with anti-neuroinflammatory drugs in AD.

The most studied TSPO tracer in patients with CNS disorder is without a doubt N-[(2R)-butan-2-yl]-1-(2-chlorophenyl)-N-[^{11}C]methylisoquinoline-3-carboxamide ([^{11}C]PK11195) (**Figure**), despite its low specific binding and minimal brain uptake (Damont et al., 2013). Nonetheless, conflicting results are reported with [^{11}C]PK11195, but also with several other clinical TPSO tracers, such as N-{[2-[^{11}C]methoxyphenyl]methyl}-N-(4-phenoxypyridin-3-yl)acetamide ([^{11}C]PBR28), N-(5-fluoro-2-phenoxyphenyl)-N-{[2-[^{11}C]methoxy-5-methoxyphenyl]methyl}acetamide ([^{11}C]DAA1106), (2-[^{11}C])ethyl (15S,19S)-15-ethyl-1,11-diazapentacyclo[9.6.2.0^{2,7}0^{8,18}.0^{15,19}]nonadeca-2,4,6,8(18),16-pentaene-17-carboxylate ([^{11}C]vinpocetine), N-({2-[2-[^{18}F]fluor-ethoxy]-5-methoxyphenyl}methyl)-N-[2-(4-methoxyphenoxy)pyridin-3-yl]acetamide ([^{18}F]FEMPA), N-({2-[2-[^{18}F]fluoroethoxy]-5-methoxyphenyl}methyl)-N-(2-phenoxyphenyl)acetamide ([^{18}F]FEDAA1106) and N,N-diethyl-2-(2-{4-[2-[^{18}F]fluoroethoxy]phenyl}-5,7-dimethylpyrazolo[1,5-a]pyrimidin-3-yl)acetamide ([^{18}F]DPA-714) (**Figure**).

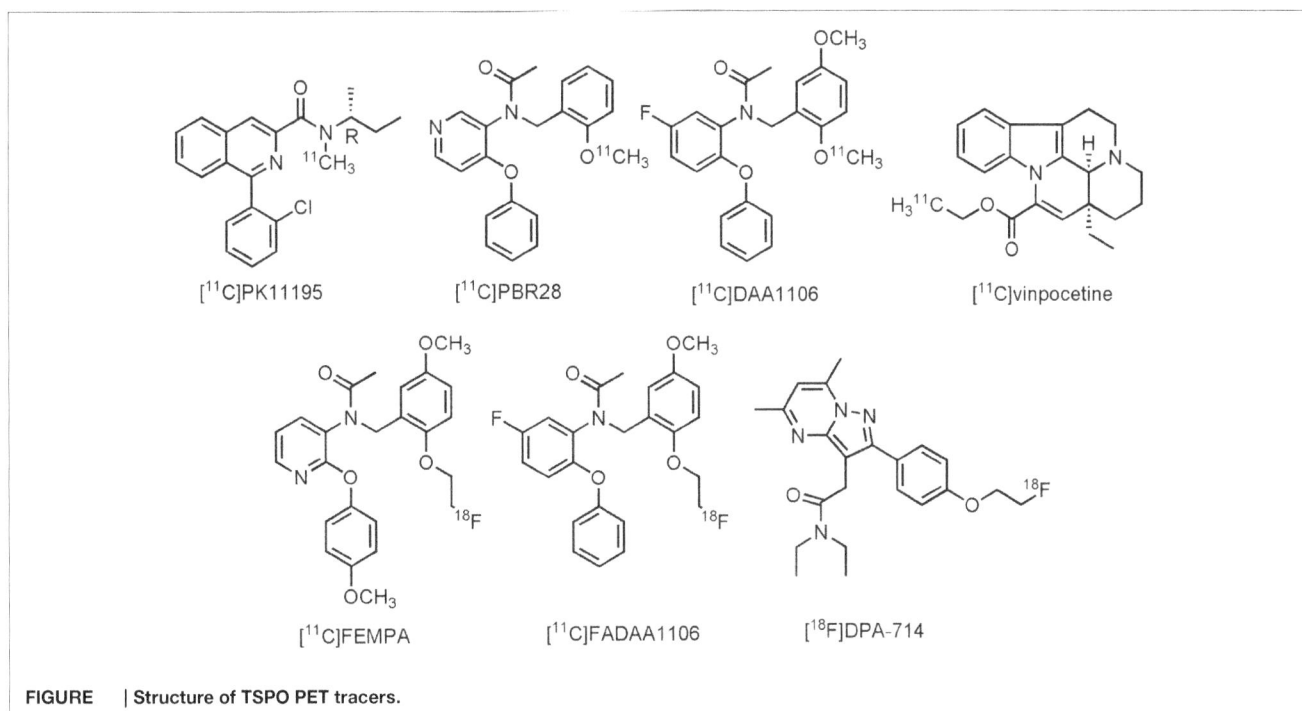

FIGURE | Structure of TSPO PET tracers.

While a majority of clinical trials was able to show significant tracer uptake in at least one brain area in AD patients, several other studies failed to differentiate MCI or even HCs from AD (Varley et al., 2015; Stefaniak and O'Brien, 2016). Apart from low signal-to-noise ratios and low brain uptake of some of these compounds, there are many possible explanations for the discrepancies in TSPO expression, as measured by PET in these clinical trials involving AD patients (Janssen et al., 2016). It is, however, important to realize, as suggested before (Janssen et al., 2016), that many patients exhibit different TSPO expression levels, depending on the specific polymorphism in the TSPO gene, resulting in intersubject variability in the binding affinities of TSPO PET tracers (Owen et al., 2012). Increasing efforts have therefore been focused toward compounds that are insensitive toward TSPO polymorphism, but also toward compounds for other neuroinflammatory targets (such as MAO-B, see Section Monoamine Oxidase B). Furthermore, overexpression of TSPO in both astrocytes and microglial cells make it difficult to differentiate MCI from AD patients (Ekonomou et al., 2015; Janssen et al., 2016). Nevertheless, [^{18}F]DPA-714 is currently being used to assess the degree of neuroinflammation in AD patients in two clinical trials (CTI: NCT02377206 and NCT02062099). For a more detailed discussion of the current status of PET development for TSPO, or neuroinflammation in general, readers are referred to several other reviews (Ory et al., 2014; Varley et al., 2015; Janssen et al., 2016).

Monoamine Oxidase B

Monoamine oxidases are mitochondrial bound enzymes, as a member of the flavin-containing amine oxidoreductases protein family, in the CNS primarily found in astrocytes. They are responsible for oxidative deamination of monamines of both

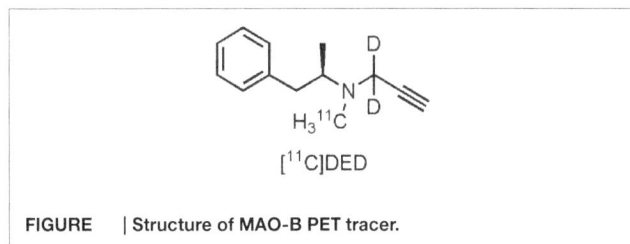

FIGURE | Structure of MAO-B PET tracer.

endogenous and exogenous sources, regulating the physiological activity of neurotransmitters as serotonin, DA, and noradrenaline (Strolin and Dostert, 1989). There are two types of isoforms, MAO-A and MAO-B, which differ in inhibitor sensitivity and substrate selectivity, although there is an overlap to some degree (Bortolato et al., 2008). Increased MAO-B activity has been noted in AD in both brain and blood platelets (Adolfsson et al., 1980; Alexopoulos et al., 1987; Sparks et al., 1991), the severe upregulation in the brain mainly being a consequence of a plaque associated neuroinflammatory response by reactive astrocytes (Jossan et al., 1991; Saura et al., 1994). Furthermore, during their catalytic deamination, MAOs produce neurotoxic byproducts such as hydrogen peroxide, which are one of the main culprits in oxidative stress, contributing to the formation of amyloid plaques (Huang et al., 2012; Zheng et al., 2012). Since MAOs play a key role in the regulation of several important neurotransmitters, cognitive impairment, due to pathological upregulation of MAOs has also been demonstrated (Delumeau et al., 1994). MAO inhibitors may therefore have a significant neuroprotective role in AD. Since MAO-B is the main isoform present in brain (Riederer et al., 1978; Sonsalla and Golbe, 1988) and inhibition of MAO-B proved to be useful as therapeutic approach in PD, focus has mainly been targeted toward MAO-B inhibition in AD (Thomas, 2000). So far, five different drugs have inhibited MAOs in clinical trials involving AD patients (Cai, 2014). Two of them, selegiline (L-deprenyl) and rasagiline (Azilect), irreversible MAO-B selective inhibitors, are established drugs in the treatment of PD, delaying the need for DA replacement therapy (Birkmayer et al., 1977; Lees et al., 1977; Weinreb et al., 2010). While selegiline initially showed promise in clinical trials involving AD patients, demonstrating modest improvements on cognitive and behavioral functions (Filip and Kolibas, 1999), a comprehensive meta-analysis showed no justification for the use of selegiline in the treatment of AD, since there was a lack of overall significant benefit (Birks and Flicker, 2003). The beneficial effect of rasagiline is yet to be evaluated in AD patients. A Phase II proof of concept trial in patients with mild to moderate AD is, however, underway (CTI: NCT02359552). Interestingly, rasagiline formed the basis of two other multi-target drugs, ladogistil (TV3326), and M-30. The former drug is a MAO-B inhibitor and AChE inhibitor, the latter a MAO-A and MAO-B inhibitor (Youdim, 2013). Both compounds are thought to modulate APP expression levels (by stimulating the non-amyloidogenic pathway) and both may have neuroprotective and neurorestorative functions (Riederer et al., 2004; Youdim, 2013). Phase II trials with ladogistil on mild to moderate AD patients have been completed, but results are yet to be published (CTI: NCT01354691). These drugs may hold promise as multi-target approach for treatment of AD, being able to tackle various pathophysiological changes at once (Youdim, 2013). Finally, EVT 301 (RO4477478), a reversible MAO-B inhibitor was evaluated on four AD patients (MMSE score: not specified) in a dose-finding study, using [^{11}C]deprenyl-D2 ([^{11}C]DED) PET (See further, **Figure**   ) to assess MAO-B occupancy levels. Seven days of treatment resulted hereby in an almost complete dose-occupancy of MAO-B (Hirvonen et al., 2009). No further clinical trials, to our knowledge, have since been performed with this drug.

Only one MAO binding PET tracer has been elevated on AD patients thus far: [^{11}C]methyl[(2R)-1-phenylpropan-2-yl][(1,1-^{2}H2)prop-2-yn-1-yl]amine ([^{11}C]DED), an irreversible MAO-B inhibitor (Hirvonen et al., 2009; Carter et al., 2012; Choo et al., 2014). Increased uptake of [^{11}C]DED was observed in patients with MCI (who responded positively to a [^{11}C]PIB scan), suggesting that astrocytocis may be an early event in the development of AD. Clinical AD studies with other emerging (fluorine-18 labeled) MAO radiotracers are yet to be published (Ory et al., 2014; Fowler et al., 2015).

AD. Important to notice is that each of these pathways is linked to the pathophysiological processes of (often many) other targets, hence a multi-target approach, addressing various pathophysiological changes at once, will be the way forward. Concordant neuroimaging techniques, such as PET and SPECT, could hereby greatly improve therapeutic monitoring, but also significantly aid with the proposal of current inclusion- and outcome criteria in large clinical studies. Moreover, once a disease altering drug has been found, PET/SPECT could eventually be used as standard test to assess and follow up disease progression (Barthel et al., 2015). Still, there are a few important factors to take in consideration. One of them is the need for quantitative PET assessment, especially during evaluation of novel therapies, to allow quantitative and accurate evaluations. Visual inspection or simplified models (such as SUV) are indeed less robust, as they are influenced by several physiological and technical factors (Boellaard, 2009; Tomasi et al., 2012). The other side of the coin is, however, that quantitative PET assessment is very time-consuming, which limits capacity and throughput which are essential in large multi-center trials. Another crucial issue is the loss of BBB function during AD progression, which could greatly affect drug dosage and bioavailability of novel AD therapeutics. One way of monitoring the viability of the BBB is by looking at the P-gp function. Several promising PET candidates are now under development for this purpose (Syvanen and Eriksson, 2013), and a pilot study to assess the P-gp function in AD patients is currently ongoing (ECT: 2013-001724-19). Finally, there is a great need for a thorough preclinical evaluation of the mechanism of action. This could not be better demonstrated than by the rise and fall of dimebon. Initially developed as an antihistaminic drug in the former USSR, dimebon demonstrated significant improvement on the ADAS-cog-, MMSE-, and CIBIC+ scales in a 6-month Phase II trial on AD patients in Russia (Bezprozvanny, 2010). Consequently, a multi-national Phase III trial was launched, but this trial failed to show any significant improvement on mild to moderate AD patients, as compared to placebo (Bezprozvanny, 2010). In a synopsis by Bezprozvanny (Bezprozvanny, 2010), failure was largely attributed to poor understanding of the proper mechanism of action in preclinical studies and the lack of objective biomarkers to assess the true therapeutic response in clinical trials. In the last decade, most clinical trials aiming to find AD combatting drugs ultimately failed to produce (convincing) positive results. Although there may be many explanations for this overall failure, thorough preclinical assessment remains an important factor.

CONCLUSION

This review demonstrates that there are multiple approaches to be considered when developing disease altering drugs for

AUTHOR CONTRIBUTIONS

LD wrote the manuscript. RV, KVL, AV, and GB reviewed it, corrected it and made suggestions.

REFERENCES

Adolfsson, R., Gottfries, C. G., Oreland, L., Wiberg, A., and Winblad, B. (1980). Increased activity of brain and platelet monoamine oxidase in dementia of Alzheimer type. *Life Sci.* 27, 1029–1034. doi: 10.1016/0024-3205(80)90025-9

Ahmed, R. M., Paterson, R. W., Warren, J. D., Zetterberg, H., O'Brien, J. T., Fox, N. C., et al. (2014). Biomarkers in dementia: clinical utility and new directions. *J. Neurol. Neurosurg. Psychiatry* 85, 1426–1434. doi: 10.1136/jnnp-2014-307662

Alexopoulos, G. S., Young, R. C., Lieberman, K. W., and Shamoian, C. A. (1987). Platelet MAO activity in geriatric patients with depression and dementia. *Am. J. Psychiatry* 144, 1480–1483. doi: 10.1176/ajp.144.11.1480

Ambree, O., Richter, H., Sachser, N., Lewejohann, L., Dere, E., de Souza Silva, M. A., et al. (2009). Levodopa ameliorates learning and memory deficits in a murine model of Alzheimer's disease. *Neurobiol. Aging* 30, 1192–1204. doi: 10.1016/j.neurobiolaging.2007.11.010

Anandatheerthavarada, H. K., Biswas, G., Robin, M. A., and Avadhani, N. G. (2003). Mitochondrial targeting and a novel transmembrane arrest of Alzheimer's amyloid precursor protein impairs mitochondrial function in neuronal cells. *J. Cell Biol.* 161, 41–54. doi: 10.1083/jcb.200207030

Andersson, J. D., and Halldin, C. (2013). PET radioligands targeting the brain GABAA /benzodiazepine receptor complex. *J. Labelled Comp. Radiopharm.* 56, 196–206. doi: 10.1002/jlcr.3008

Aprahamian, I., Stella, F., and Forlenza, O. V. (2013). New treatment strategies for Alzheimer's disease: is there a hope? *Indian J. Med. Res.* 138, 449–460.

Apter, J. T., Shastri, K., and Pizano, K. (2015). Update on disease-modifying/preventive therapies in Alzheimer's disease. *Curr. Geriatr. Rep.* 4, 312–317. doi: 10.1007/s13670-015-0141-x

Arai, H., Ichimiya, Y., Kosaka, K., Moroji, T., and Iizuka, R. (1992). Neurotransmitter changes in early- and late-onset Alzheimer-type dementia. *Prog. Neuropsychopharmacol. Biol. Psychiatry* 16, 883–890. doi: 10.1016/0278-5846(92)90106-O

Asuni, A. A., Boutajangout, A., Quartermain, D., and Sigurdsson, E. M. (2007). Immunotherapy targeting pathological tau conformers in a tangle mouse model reduces tangle pathology with associated functional improvements. *J. Neurosci.* 27, 9115–9129. doi: 10.1523/JNEUROSCI.2361-07.2007

Ballard, C., and Corbett, A. (2010). Management of neuropsychiatric symptoms in people with dementia. *CNS Drugs* 24, 729–739. doi: 10.2165/11319240-000000000-00000

Ballard, C., Gauthier, S., Corbett, A., Brayne, C., Aarsland, D., and Jones, E. (2011). Alzheimer's disease. *Lancet* 377, 1019–1031. doi: 10.1016/S0140-6736(10)61349-9

Ballard, C., and Waite, J. (2006). The effectiveness of atypical antipsychotics for the treatment of aggression and psychosis in Alzheimer's disease. *Cochrane Database Syst. Rev.* 25:CD003476. doi: 10.1002/14651858.CD003476.pub2

Ballatore, C., Lee, V. M., and Trojanowski, J. Q. (2007). Tau-mediated neurodegeneration in Alzheimer's disease and related disorders. *Nat. Rev. Neurosci.* 8, 663–672. doi: 10.1038/nrn2194

Bancher, C., Braak, H., Fischer, P., and Jellinger, K. A. (1993). Neuropathological staging of Alzheimer lesions and intellectual status in Alzheimer's and Parkinson's disease patients. *Neurosci. Lett.* 162, 179–182. doi: 10.1016/0304-3940(93)90590-H

Bancher, C., Jellinger, K., Lassmann, H., Fischer, P., and Leblhuber, F. (1996). Correlations between mental state and quantitative neuropathology in the Vienna Longitudinal Study on Dementia. *Eur. Arch. Psychiatry Clin. Neurosci.* 246, 137–146. doi: 10.1007/BF02189115

Banks, W. A., Terrell, B., Farr, S. A., Robinson, S. M., Nonaka, N., and Morley, J. E. (2002). Passage of amyloid beta protein antibody across the blood-brain barrier in a mouse model of Alzheimer's disease. *Peptides* 23, 2223–2226. doi: 10.1016/S0196-9781(02)00261-9

Barage, S. H., and Sonawane, K. D. (2015). Amyloid cascade hypothesis: pathogenesis and therapeutic strategies in Alzheimer's disease. *Neuropeptides* 52, 1–18. doi: 10.1016/j.npep.2015.06.008

Barnes, N. M., and Sharp, T. (1999). A review of central 5-HT receptors and their function. *Neuropharmacology* 38, 1083–1152. doi: 10.1016/S0028-3908(99)00010-6

Barnham, K. J., Haeffner, F., Ciccotosto, G. D., Curtain, C. C., Tew, D., Mavros, C., et al. (2004). Tyrosine gated electron transfer is key to the toxic mechanism of Alzheimer's disease beta-amyloid. *FASEB J.* 18, 1427–1429. doi: 10.1096/fj.04-1890fje

Barthel, H., Gertz, H. J., Dresel, S., Peters, O., Bartenstein, P., Buerger, K., et al. (2011). Cerebral amyloid-beta PET with florbetaben (18F) in patients with Alzheimer's disease and healthy controls: a multicentre phase 2 diagnostic study. *Lancet Neurol.* 10, 424–435. doi: 10.1016/S1474-4422(11)700771

Barthel, H., Seibyl, J., and Sabri, O. (2015). The role of positron emission tomography imaging in understanding Alzheimer's disease. *Expert Rev. Neurother.* 15, 395–406. doi: 10.1586/14737175.2015.1023296

Bartus, R. T. (2000). On neurodegenerative diseases, models, and treatment strategies: lessons learned and lessons forgotten a generation following the cholinergic hypothesis. *Exp. Neurol.* 163, 495–529. doi: 10.1006/exnr.2000.7397

Bartus, R. T., Dean, R. L. III, Beer, B., and Lippa, A. S. (1982). The cholinergic hypothesis of geriatric memory dysfunction. *Science* 217, 408–414. doi: 10.1126/science.7046051

Belelli, D., and Lambert, J. J. (2005). Neurosteroids: endogenous regulators of the GABA(A) receptor. *Nat. Rev. Neurosci.* 6, 565–575. doi: 10.1038/nrn1703

Benadiba, M., Luurtsema, G., Wichert-Ana, L., Buchpigel, C. A., and Busatto, F. G. (2012). New molecular targets for PET and SPECT imaging in neurodegenerative diseases. *Rev. Bras. Psiquiatr.* 34(Suppl. 2), S125–S136. doi: 10.1016/j.rbp.2012.07.002

Berg, S., Bergh, M., Hellberg, S., Hogdin, K., Lo-Alfredsson, Y., Soderman, P., et al. (2012). Discovery of novel potent and highly selective glycogen synthase kinase-3beta (GSK3beta) inhibitors for Alzheimer's disease: design, synthesis, and characterization of pyrazines. *J. Med. Chem.* 55, 9107–9119. doi: 10.1021/jm201724m

Bezprozvanny, I. (2010). The rise and fall of Dimebon. *Drug News Perspect* 23, 518–523. doi: 10.1358/dnp.2010.23.8.1500435

Billard, T., Le, B. D., and Zimmer, L. (2014). PET radiotracers for molecular imaging of serotonin 5-HT1A receptors. *Curr. Med. Chem.* 21, 70–81. doi: 10.2174/09298673113209990215

Billings, L. M., Oddo, S., Green, K. N., McGaugh, J. L., and Laferla, F. M. (2005). Intraneuronal Abeta causes the onset of early Alzheimer's disease-related cognitive deficits in transgenic mice. *Neuron* 45, 675–688. doi: 10.1016/j.neuron.2005.01.040

Binder, L. I., Frankfurter, A., and Rebhun, L. I. (1986). Differential localization of MAP-2 and tau in mammalian neurons in situ. *Ann. N. Y. Acad. Sci.* 466, 145–166. doi: 10.1111/j.1749-6632.1986.tb38392.x

Birkmayer, W., Riederer, P., Ambrozi, L., and Youdim, M. B. (1977). Implications of combined treatment with 'Madopar ' and L-deprenil in Parkinson's disease, A long-term study. *Lancet* 1, 439–443. doi: 10.1016/S0140-6736(77)91940-7

Birks, J., and Flicker, L. (2003). Selegiline for Alzheimer's disease. *Cochrane Database Syst. Rev.* CD000442. doi: 10.1002/14651858.CD000442

Blin, J., Baron, J. C., Dubois, B., Crouzel, C., Fiorelli, M., Attar-Levy, D., et al. (1993). Loss of brain 5-HT2 receptors in Alzheimer's disease. In vivo assessment with positron emission tomography and [18F]setoperone. *Brain* 116(Pt 3), 497–510. doi: 10.1093/brain/116.3.497

Bodick, N. C., Offen, W. W., Levey, A. I., Cutler, N. R., Gauthier, S. G., Satlin, A., et al. (1997). Effects of xanomeline, a selective muscarinic receptor agonist, on cognitive function and behavioral symptoms in Alzheimer disease. *Arch. Neurol.* 54, 465–473. doi: 10.1001/archneur.1997.00550160091022

Boellaard, R. (2009). Standards for PET image acquisition and quantitative data analysis. *J. Nucl. Med.* 50(Suppl. 1), 11S–20S. doi: 10.2967/jnumed.108.057182

Bonner, T. I. (1989). The molecular basis of muscarinic receptor diversity. *Trends Neurosci.* 12, 148–151. doi: 10.1016/0166-2236(89)90054-4

Bonner, T. I., Buckley, N. J., Young, A. C., and Brann, M. R. (1987). Identification of a family of muscarinic acetylcholine receptor genes. *Science* 237, 527–532. doi: 10.1126/science.3037705

Bonner, T. I., Young, A. C., Brann, M. R., and Buckley, N. J. (1988). Cloning and expression of the human and rat m5 muscarinic acetylcholine receptor genes. *Neuron* 1, 403–410. doi: 10.1016/0896-6273(88)90190-0

Bortolato, M., Chen, K., and Shih, J. C. (2008). Monoamine oxidase inactivation: from pathophysiology to therapeutics. *Adv. Drug Deliv. Rev.* 60, 1527–1533. doi: 10.1016/j.addr.2008.06.002

Bowen, D. M., Allen, S. J., Benton, J. S., Goodhardt, M. J., Haan, E. A., Palmer, A. M., et al. (1983). Biochemical assessment of serotonergic and cholinergic dysfunction and cerebral atrophy in Alzheimer's disease. *J. Neurochem.* 41, 266–272. doi: 10.1111/j.1471-4159.1983.tb11838.x

Braak, H., and Braak, E. (1991). Neuropathological stageing of Alzheimer-related changes. *Acta Neuropathol.* 82, 239–259. doi: 10.1007/BF00308809

Bremner, J. D., Baldwin, R., Horti, A., Staib, L. H., Ng, C. K., Tan, P. Z., et al. (1999). Quantitation of benzodiazepine receptor binding with PET [11C]iomazenil and SPECT [123I]iomazenil: preliminary results of a direct comparison in healthy human subjects. *Psychiatry Res.* 91, 79–91. doi: 10.1016/S0925-4927(99) 00015-3

Bresjanac, M., Smid, L. M., Vovko, T. D., Petric, A., Barrio, J. R., and Popovic, M. (2003). Molecular-imaging probe 2-(1-[6-[(2-fluoroethyl)(methyl) amino]-2-naphthyl]ethylidene) malononitrile labels prion plaques in vitro. *J. Neurosci.* 23, 8029–8033.

Broich, K., Grunwald, F., Kasper, S., Klemm, E., Biersack, H. J., and Moller, H. J. (1998). D2-dopamine receptor occupancy measured by IBZM-SPECT in relation to extrapyramidal side effects. *Pharmacopsychiatry* 31, 159–162. doi: 10.1055/s-2007-979321

Brookmeyer, R., Johnson, E., Ziegler-Graham, K., and Arrighi, H. M. (2007). Forecasting the global burden of Alzheimer's disease. *Alzheimers Dement.* 3, 186–191. doi: 10.1016/j.jalz.2007.04.381

Brooks, D. J. (1993). Functional imaging in relation to parkinsonian syndromes. *J. Neurol. Sci.* 115, 1–17. doi: 10.1016/0022-510X(93)90061-3

Brown, D., Chisholm, J. A., Owens, J., Pimlott, S., Patterson, J., and Wyper, D. (2003). Acetylcholine muscarinic receptors and response to anti-cholinesterase therapy in patients with Alzheimer's disease. *Eur. J. Nucl. Med. Mol. Imaging* 30, 296–300. doi: 10.1007/s00259-002-1028-6

Brun, A., and Englund, E. (1981). Regional pattern of degeneration in Alzheimer's disease: neuronal loss and histopathological grading. *Histopathology* 5, 549–564. doi: 10.1111/j.1365-2559.1981.tb01818.x

Bruno, G., Mohr, E., Gillespie, M., Fedio, P., and Chase, T. N. (1986). Muscarinic agonist therapy of Alzheimer's disease. A clinical trial of RS-86. *Arch. Neurol.* 43, 659–661. doi: 10.1001/archneur.1986.00520070017009

Buckingham, S. D., Jones, A. K., Brown, L. A., and Sattelle, D. B. (2009). Nicotinic acetylcholine receptor signalling: roles in Alzheimer's disease and amyloid neuroprotection. *Pharmacol. Rev.* 61, 39–61. doi: 10.1124/pr.108.000562

Bulic, B., Pickhardt, M., Mandelkow, E. M., and Mandelkow, E. (2010). Tau protein and tau aggregation inhibitors. *Neuropharmacology* 59, 276–289. doi: 10.1016/j.neuropharm.2010.01.016

Bulic, B., Pickhardt, M., and Schmidt, B. (2009). Development of tau aggregation inhibitors for Alzheimer's disease. *Angew. Chem. Int. Ed. Engl.* 48, 1740–1752. doi: 10.1002/anie.200802621

Burns, A., Rossor, M., Hecker, J., Gauthier, S., Petit, H., Moller, H. J., et al. (1999). The effects of donepezil in Alzheimer's disease - results from a multinational trial. *Dement. Geriatr. Cogn. Disord.* 10, 237–244. doi: 10.1159/000017126

Butner, K. A., and Kirschner, M. W. (1991). Tau protein binds to microtubules through a flexible array of distributed weak sites. *J. Cell Biol.* 115, 717–730. doi: 10.1083/jcb.115.3.717

Buxbaum, J. D., Oishi, M., Chen, H. I., Pinkas-Kramarski, R., Jaffe, E. A., Gandy, S. E., et al. (1992). Cholinergic agonists and interleukin 1 regulate processing and secretion of the Alzheimer beta/A4 amyloid protein precursor. *Proc. Natl. Acad. Sci. U.S.A.* 89, 10075–10078. doi: 10.1073/pnas.89.21.10075

Cai, Z. (2014). Monoamine oxidase inhibitors: promising therapeutic agents for Alzheimer's disease (Review). *Mol. Med. Rep.* 9, 1533–1541. doi: 10.3892/mmr.2014.2040

Carter, S. F., Scholl, M., Almkvist, O., Wall, A., Engler, H., Langstrom, B., et al. (2012). Evidence for astrocytosis in prodromal Alzheimer disease provided by 11C-deuterium-L-deprenyl: a multitracer PET paradigm combining 11C-Pittsburgh compound B and 18F-FDG. *J. Nucl. Med.* 53, 37–46. doi: 10.2967/jnumed.110.087031

Casellas, P., Galiegue, S., and Basile, A. S. (2002). Peripheral benzodiazepine receptors and mitochondrial function. *Neurochem. Int.* 40, 475–486. doi: 10.1016/S0197-0186(01)00118-8

Caspersen, C., Wang, N., Yao, J., Sosunov, A., Chen, X., Lustbader, J. W., et al. (2005). Mitochondrial Abeta: a potential focal point for neuronal metabolic dysfunction in Alzheimer's disease. *FASEB J.* 19, 2040–2041. doi: 10.1096/fj.05-3735fje

Castelan, F., Castillo, M., Mulet, J., Sala, S., Sala, F., Dominguez Del, T. E., et al. (2008). Molecular characterization and localization of the RIC-3 protein, an effector of nicotinic acetylcholine receptor expression. *J. Neurochem.* 105, 617–627. doi: 10.1111/j.1471-4159.2007.05169.x

Ceravolo, R., Volterrani, D., Gambaccini, G., Bernardini, S., Rossi, C., Logi, C., et al. (2004). Presynaptic nigro-striatal function in a group of Alzheimer's disease patients with parkinsonism: evidence from a dopamine transporter imaging study. *J. Neural Transm. (Vienna)* 111, 1065–1073.

Chalon, S., Vercouillie, J., Guilloteau, D., Suzenet, F., and Routier, S. (2015). PET tracers for imaging brain alpha7 nicotinic receptors: an update. *Chem. Commun. (Camb.)* 51, 14826–14831. doi: 10.1039/c5cc04536c

Chebib, M., and Johnston, G. A. (1999). The 'ABC' of GABA receptors: a brief review. *Clin. Exp. Pharmacol. Physiol.* 26, 937–940. doi: 10.1046/j.1440-1681.1999.03151.x

Chen, C. P., Alder, J. T., Bowen, D. M., Esiri, M. M., McDonald, B., Hope, T., et al. (1996). Presynaptic serotonergic markers in community-acquired cases of Alzheimer's disease: correlations with depression and neuroleptic medication. *J. Neurochem.* 66, 1592–1598. doi: 10.1046/j.1471-4159.1996.66041592.x

Chen, C. P., Eastwood, S. L., Hope, T., McDonald, B., Francis, P. T., and Esiri, M. M. (2000). Immunocytochemical study of the dorsal and median raphe nuclei in patients with Alzheimer's disease prospectively assessed for behavioural changes. *Neuropathol. Appl. Neurobiol.* 26, 347–355. doi: 10.1046/j.1365-2990.2000.00254.x

Chien, D. T., Bahri, S., Szardenings, A. K., Walsh, J. C., Mu, F., Su, M. Y., et al. (2012). Early clinical PET imaging results with the novel PHF-tau tadioligand [F-18]-T807. *J. Alzheimers Dis.* 34, 457–468. doi: 10.3233/JAD-122059

Chien, D. T., Szardenings, A. K., Bahri, S., Walsh, J. C., Mu, F., Xia, C., et al. (2013). Early clinical PET imaging results with the novel PHF-tau radioligand [F18]-T808. *J. Alzheimers Dis.* 38, 171–184. doi: 10.3233/JAD-130098

Choo, I. L., Carter, S. F., Scholl, M. L., and Nordberg, A. (2014). Astrocytosis measured by (1)(1)C-deprenyl PET correlates with decrease in gray matter density in the parahippocampus of prodromal Alzheimer's patients. *Eur. J. Nucl. Med. Mol. Imaging* 41, 2120–2126. doi: 10.1007/s00259-014-2859-7

Christensen, R., Marcussen, A. B., Wortwein, G., Knudsen, G. M., and Aznar, S. (2008). Abeta(1-42) injection causes memory impairment, lowered cortical and serum BDNF levels, and decreased hippocampal 5-HT(2A) levels. *Exp. Neurol.* 210, 164–171. doi: 10.1016/j.expneurol.2007.10.009

Chua, S. W., Kassiou, M., and Ittner, L. M. (2014). The translocator protein as a drug target in Alzheimer's disease. *Expert Rev. Neurother.* 14, 439–448. doi: 10.1586/14737175.2014.896201

Clark-Papasavas, C., Dunn, J. T., Greaves, S., Mogg, A., Gomes, R., Brownings, S., et al. (2014). Towards a therapeutic window of D2/3 occupancy for treatment of psychosis in Alzheimer's disease, with [18F]fallypride positron emission tomography. *Int. J. Geriatr. Psychiatry* 29, 1001–1009. doi: 10.1002/gps.4090

Colloby, S. J., Firbank, M. J., Pakrasi, S., Lloyd, J. J., Driver, I., McKeith, I. G., et al. (2008). A comparison of 99mTc-exametazime and 123I-FP-CIT SPECT imaging in the differential diagnosis of Alzheimer's disease and dementia with Lewy bodies. *Int. Psychogeriatr.* 20, 1124–1140. doi: 10.1017/S1041610208007709

Connolly, C. N., Krishek, B. J., McDonald, B. J., Smart, T. G., and Moss, S. J. (1996). Assembly and cell surface expression of heteromeric and homomeric gamma-aminobutyric acid type A receptors. *J. Biol. Chem.* 271, 89–96. doi: 10.1074/jbc.271.1.89

Consolo, S., Bertorelli, R., Russi, G., Zambelli, M., and Ladinsky, H. (1994). Serotonergic facilitation of acetylcholine release in vivo from rat dorsal hippocampus via serotonin 5-HT3 receptors. *J. Neurochem.* 62, 2254–2261. doi: 10.1046/j.1471-4159.1994.62062254.x

Contestabile, A. (2011). The history of the cholinergic hypothesis. *Behav. Brain Res.* 221, 334–340. doi: 10.1016/j.bbr.2009.12.044

Cooper, S. T., and Millar, N. S. (1997). Host cell-specific folding and assembly of the neuronal nicotinic acetylcholine receptor alpha7 subunit. *J. Neurochem.* 68, 2140–2151. doi: 10.1046/j.1471-4159.1997.68052140.x

Cosenza-Nashat, M., Zhao, M. L., Suh, H. S., Morgan, J., Natividad, R., Morgello, S., et al. (2009). Expression of the translocator protein of 18 kDa by microglia, macrophages and astrocytes based on immunohistochemical localization in abnormal human brain. *Neuropathol. Appl. Neurobiol.* 35, 306–328. doi: 10.1111/j.1365-2990.2008.01006.x

Covington, J. S. (1975). Alleviating agitation, apprehension, and related symptoms in geriatric patients: a double-blind comparison of a phenothiazine and a benzodiazepien. *South. Med. J.* 68, 719–724. doi: 10.1097/00007611-197506000-00015

Coyle, J. T., Price, D. L., and DeLong, M. R. (1983). Alzheimer's disease: a disorder of cortical cholinergic innervation. *Science* 219, 1184–1190. doi: 10.1126/science.6338589

Criado, M., Mulet, J., Gerber, S., Sala, S., and Sala, F. (2011). A small cytoplasmic region adjacent to the fourth transmembrane segment of the alpha7 nicotinic receptor is essential for its biogenesis. *FEBS Lett.* 585, 2477–2480. doi: 10.1016/j.febslet.2011.06.028

Crow, T. J., Cross, A. J., Cooper, S. J., Deakin, J. F., Ferrier, I. N., Johnson, J. A., et al. (1984). Neurotransmitter receptors and monoamine metabolites in the brains of patients with Alzheimer-type dementia and depression, and suicides. *Neuropharmacology* 23, 1561–1569. doi: 10.1016/0028-3908(84)90100-X

Cummings, J. L. (2008). Optimizing phase II of drug development for disease-modifying compounds. *Alzheimers Dement.* 4, S15–S20. doi: 10.1016/j.jalz.2007.10.002

Dahlgren, K. N., Manelli, A. M., Stine, W. B. Jr., Baker, L. K., Krafft, G. A., and LaDu, M. J. (2002). Oligomeric and fibrillar species of amyloid-beta peptides differentially affect neuronal viability. *J. Biol. Chem.* 277, 32046–32053. doi: 10.1074/jbc.M201750200

Damont, A., Roeda, D., and Dolle, F. (2013). The potential of carbon-11 and fluorine-18 chemistry: illustration through the development of positron emission tomography radioligands targeting the translocator protein 18 kDa. *J. Labelled Comp. Radiopharm.* 56, 96–104. doi: 10.1002/jlcr.2992

Dani, M., Brooks, D. J., and Edison, P. (2015). Tau imaging in neurodegenerative diseases. *Eur. J. Nucl. Med. Mol. Imaging* doi: 10.1007/s00259-015-3231-2 [Epub ahead of print].

Darreh-Shori, T., Hosseini, S. M., and Nordberg, A. (2014). Pharmacodynamics of cholinesterase inhibitors suggests add-on therapy with a low-dose carbamylating inhibitor in patients on long-term treatment with rapidly reversible inhibitors. *J. Alzheimers Dis.* 39, 423–440. doi: 10.3233/JAD-130845

Davies, P., and Maloney, A. J. (1976). Selective loss of central cholinergic neurons in Alzheimer's disease. *Lancet* 2:1403. doi: 10.1016/S0140-6736(76)91936-X

de Calignon, A., Polydoro, M., Suarez-Calvet, M., William, C., Adamowicz, D. H., Kopeikina, K. J., et al. (2012). Propagation of tau pathology in a model of early Alzheimer's disease. *Neuron* 73, 685–697. doi: 10.1016/j.neuron.2011.11.033

De Deyn, P. P., Drenth, A. F., Kremer, B. P., Oude Voshaar, R. C., and Van, D. D. (2013). Aripiprazole in the treatment of Alzheimer's disease. *Expert Opin. Pharmacother.* 14, 459–474. doi: 10.1517/14656566.2013.764989

de Souza, L. C., Sarazin, M., Teixeira-Junior, A. L., Caramelli, P., Santos, A. E., and Dubois, B. (2014). Biological markers of Alzheimer's disease. *Arq. Neuropsiquiatr.* 72, 227–231. doi: 10.1590/0004-282X20130233

Deardorff, W. J., Shobassy, A., and Grossberg, G. T. (2015). Safety and clinical effects of EVP-6124 in subjects with Alzheimer's disease currently or previously receiving an acetylcholinesterase inhibitor medication. *Expert Rev. Neurother.* 15, 7–17. doi: 10.1586/14737175.2015.995639

Decker, M. W., and McGaugh, J. L. (1991). The role of interactions between the cholinergic system and other neuromodulatory systems in learning and memory. *Synapse* 7, 151–168. doi: 10.1002/syn.890070209

Defrancesco, M., Marksteiner, J., Fleischhacker, W. W., and Blasko, I. (2015). Use of benzodiazepines in Alzheimer's disease: a systematic review of literature. *Int. J. Neuropsychopharmacol.* 18:pyv055. doi: 10.1093/ijnp/pyv055

Delumeau, J. C., Bentue-Ferrer, D., Gandon, J. M., Amrein, R., Belliard, S., and Allain, H. (1994). Monoamine oxidase inhibitors, cognitive functions and neurodegenerative diseases. *J. Neural Transm. Suppl.* 41, 259–266.

Devi, L., Prabhu, B. M., Galati, D. F., Avadhani, N. G., and Anandatheerthavarada, H. K. (2006). Accumulation of amyloid precursor protein in the mitochondrial import channels of human Alzheimer's disease brain is associated with mitochondrial dysfunction. *J. Neurosci.* 26, 9057–9068. doi: 10.1523/JNEUROSCI.1469-06.2006

Dewar, D., Graham, D. I., and McCulloch, J. (1990). 5 HT2 receptors in dementia of Alzheimer type: a quantitative autoradiographic study of frontal cortex and hippocampus. *J. Neural Transm. Park Dis. Dement. Sect.* 2, 129–137. doi: 10.1007/BF02260900

Dineley, K. T., Bell, K. A., Bui, D., and Sweatt, J. D. (2002). beta-Amyloid peptide activates alpha 7 nicotinic acetylcholine receptors expressed in *Xenopus oocytes*. *J. Biol. Chem.* 277, 25056–25061. doi: 10.1074/jbc.M200066200

Dubois, B., Feldman, H. H., Jacova, C., Hampel, H., Molinuevo, J. L., Blennow, K., et al. (2014). Advancing research diagnostic criteria for Alzheimer's disease: the IWG-2 criteria. *Lancet Neurol.* 13, 614–629. doi: 10.1016/S1474-4422(14)700900

Dunbar, G. C., Inglis, F., Kuchibhatla, R., Sharma, T., Tomlinson, M., and Wamsley, J. (2007). Effect of ispronicline, a neuronal nicotinic acetylcholine receptor partial agonist, in subjects with age associated memory impairment (AAMI). *J. Psychopharmacol.* 21, 171–178. doi: 10.1177/0269881107066855

Dunbar, G. C., Kuchibhatla, R. V., and Lee, G. (2011). A randomized double-blind study comparing 25 and 50 mg TC-1734 (AZD3480) with placebo, in older subjects with age-associated memory impairment. *J. Psychopharmacol.* 25, 1020–1029. doi: 10.1177/0269881110367727

Dunker, A. K., Silman, I., Uversky, V. N., and Sussman, J. L. (2008). Function and structure of inherently disordered proteins. *Curr. Opin. Struct. Biol.* 18, 756–764. doi: 10.1016/j.sbi.2008.10.002

Duyckaerts, C., Bennecib, M., Grignon, Y., Uchihara, T., He, Y., Piette, F., et al. (1997). Modeling the relation between neurofibrillary tangles and intellectual status. *Neurobiol. Aging* 18, 267–273. doi: 10.1016/S0197-4580(97)80306-5

Duyckaerts, C., Potier, M. C., and Delatour, B. (2008). Alzheimer disease models and human neuropathology: similarities and differences. *Acta Neuropathol.* 115, 5–38. doi: 10.1007/s00401-007-03128

Eckelman, W. C. (2001). Radiolabeled muscarinic radioligands for in vivo studies. *Nucl. Med. Biol.* 28, 485–491. doi: 10.1016/S0969-8051(01)00217-7

Eckelman, W. C. (2002). Accelerating drug discovery and development through in vivo imaging. *Nucl. Med. Biol.* 29, 777–782. doi: 10.1016/S0969-8051(02)00345-1

Ekonomou, A., Savva, G. M., Brayne, C., Forster, G., Francis, P. T., Johnson, M., et al. (2015). Stage-specific changes in neurogenic and glial markers in Alzheimer's disease. *Biol. Psychiatry* 77, 711–719. doi: 10.1016/j.biopsych.2014.05.021

Eldar-Finkelman, H., and Martinez, A. (2011). GSK-3 inhibitors: preclinical and clinical focus on CNS. *Front. Mol. Neurosci.* 4:32. doi: 10.3389/fnmol.2011.00032

Ellis, J. R., Villemagne, V. L., Nathan, P. J., Mulligan, R. S., Gong, S. J., Chan, J. G., et al. (2008). Relationship between nicotinic receptors and cognitive function in early Alzheimer's disease: a 2-[18F]fluoro-A-85380 PET study. *Neurobiol. Learn. Mem.* 90, 404–412. doi: 10.1016/j.nlm.2008.05.006

Engler, H., Santillo, A. F., Wang, S. X., Lindau, M., Savitcheva, I., Nordberg, A., et al. (2008). In vivo amyloid imaging with PET in frontotemporal dementia. *Eur. J. Nucl. Med. Mol. Imaging* 35, 100–106. doi: 10.1007/s00259-007-0523-1

Farde, L., Suhara, T., Halldin, C., Nyback, H., Nakashima, Y., Swahn, C. G., et al. (1996). PET study of the M1-agonists [11C]xanomeline and [11C]butylthio-TZTP in monkey and man. *Dementia* 7, 187–195.

Farlow, M., Anand, R., Messina, J. Jr., Hartman, R., and Veach, J. (2000). A 52-week study of the efficacy of rivastigmine in patients with mild to moderately severe Alzheimer's disease. *Eur. Neurol.* 44, 236–241. doi: 10.1159/000008243

Filip, V., and Kolibas, E. (1999). Selegiline in the treatment of Alzheimer's disease: a long-term randomized placebo-controlled trial. Czech and slovak senile dementia of alzheimer type study group. *J. Psychiatry Neurosci.* 24, 234–243.

Fisher, A., Heldman, E., Gurwitz, D., Haring, R., Karton, Y., Meshulam, H., et al. (1996). M1 agonists for the treatment of Alzheimer's disease. Novel properties and clinical update. *Ann. N. Y. Acad. Sci.* 777, 189–196. doi: 10.1111/j.1749-6632.1996.tb34418.x

Fodero-Tavoletti, M. T., Okamura, N., Furumoto, S., Mulligan, R. S., Connor, A. R., McLean, C. A., et al. (2011). 18F-THK523: a novel in vivo tau imaging ligand for Alzheimer's disease. *Brain* 134, 1089–1100. doi: 10.1093/brain/awr038

Fowler, J. S., Logan, J., Shumay, E., Alia-Klein, N., Wang, G. J., and Volkow, N. D. (2015). Monoamine oxidase: radiotracer chemistry and human studies. *J. Labelled Comp. Radiopharm.* 58, 51–64. doi: 10.1002/jlcr.3247

Francis, P. T., Palmer, A. M., Snape, M., and Wilcock, G. K. (1999). The cholinergic hypothesis of Alzheimer's disease: a review of progress. *J. Neurol. Neurosurg. Psychiatry* 66, 137–147. doi: 10.1136/jnnp.66.2.137

Frankle, W. G., Cho, R. Y., Mason, N. S., Chen, C. M., Himes, M., Walker, C., et al. (2012). [11C]flumazenil binding is increased in a dose-dependent manner with tiagabine-induced elevations in GABA levels. *PLoS ONE* 7:e32443. doi: 10.1371/journal.pone.0032443

Frankle, W. G., Cho, R. Y., Narendran, R., Mason, N. S., Vora, S., Litschge, M., et al. (2009). Tiagabine increases [11C]flumazenil binding in cortical brain regions in healthy control subjects. *Neuropsychopharmacology* 34, 624–633. doi: 10.1038/npp.2008.104

Frolich, L., Ashwood, T., Nilsson, J., and Eckerwall, G. (2011). Effects of AZD3480 on cognition in patients with mild-to-moderate Alzheimer's disease: a phase IIb dose-finding study. *J. Alzheimers Dis.* 24, 363–374. doi: 10.3233/JAD-2011-101554

Fukuchi, K., Hashikawa, K., Seike, Y., Moriwaki, H., Oku, N., Ishida, M., et al. (1997). Comparison of iodine-123-iomazenil SPECT and technetium-99m-HMPAO-SPECT in Alzheimer's disease. *J. Nucl. Med.* 38, 467–470.

Galynker, I., Ieronimo, C., Miner, C., Rosenblum, J., Vilkas, N., and Rosenthal, R. (1997). Methylphenidate treatment of negative symptoms in patients with dementia. *J. Neuropsychiatry Clin. Neurosci.* 9, 231–239. doi: 10.1176/jnp.9.2.231

Garcia-Alloza, M., Hirst, W. D., Chen, C. P., Lasheras, B., Francis, P. T., and Ramirez, M. J. (2004). Differential involvement of 5-HT(1B/1D) and 5-HT6 receptors in cognitive and non-cognitive symptoms in Alzheimer's disease. *Neuropsychopharmacology* 29, 410–416. doi: 10.1038/sj.npp.1300330

Gatto, G. J., Bohme, G. A., Caldwell, W. S., Letchworth, S. R., Traina, V. M., Obinu, M. C., et al. (2004). TC-1734: an orally active neuronal nicotinic acetylcholine receptor modulator with antidepressant, neuroprotective and long-lasting cognitive effects. *CNS Drug Rev.* 10, 147–166. doi: 10.1111/j.1527-3458.2004.tb00010.x

Geldenhuys, W. J., and Van der Schyf, C. J. (2011). Role of serotonin in Alzheimer's disease: a new therapeutic target? *CNS Drugs* 25, 765–781. doi: 10.2165/11590190-000000000-00000

Ghezzi, L., Scarpini, E., and Galimberti, D. (2013). disease-modifying drugs in Alzheimer's disease. *Drug Des. Devel. Ther.* 7, 1471–1478. doi: 10.2147/DDDT.S41431

Gilmor, M. L., Erickson, J. D., Varoqui, H., Hersh, L. B., Bennett, D. A., Cochran, E. J., et al. (1999). Preservation of nucleus basalis neurons containing choline acetyltransferase and the vesicular acetylcholine transporter in the elderly with mild cognitive impairment and early Alzheimer's disease. *J. Comp. Neurol.* 411, 693–704. doi: 10.1002/(SICI)1096-9861(19990906)411:4<693::AID-CNE13>3.0.CO;2-D

Goedert, M., and Jakes, R. (1990). Expression of separate isoforms of human tau protein: correlation with the tau pattern in brain and effects on tubulin polymerization. *EMBO J.* 9, 4225–4230.

Gomez-Isla, T., Hollister, R., West, H., Mui, S., Growdon, J. H., Petersen, R. C., et al. (1997). Neuronal loss correlates with but exceeds neurofibrillary tangles in Alzheimer's disease. *Ann. Neurol.* 41, 17–24. doi: 10.1002/ana.410410106

Gotti, C., and Clementi, F. (2004). Neuronal nicotinic receptors: from structure to pathology. *Prog. Neurobiol.* 74, 363–396. doi: 10.1016/j.pneurobio.2004.09.006

Gozes, I., Stewart, A., Morimoto, B., Fox, A., Sutherland, K., and Schmeche, D. (2009). Addressing Alzheimer's disease tangles: from NAP to AL-108. *Curr. Alzheimer Res.* 6, 455–460. doi: 10.2174/156720509789207895

Graeber, M. B., and Mehraein, P. (1999). Reanalysis of the first case of Alzheimer's disease. *Eur. Arch. Psychiatry Clin. Neurosci.* 249(Suppl. 3), 10–13. doi: 10.1007/PL00014167

Grant, M. K., and El-Fakahany, E. E. (2005). Persistent binding and functional antagonism by xanomeline at the muscarinic M5 receptor. *J. Pharmacol. Exp. Ther.* 315, 313–319. doi: 10.1124/jpet.105.090134

Greenberg, S. M., Tennis, M. K., Brown, L. B., Gomez-Isla, T., Hayden, D. L., Schoenfeld, D. A., et al. (2000). Donepezil therapy in clinical practice: a randomized crossover study. *Arch. Neurol.* 57, 94–99. doi: 10.1001/archneur.57.1.94

Grober, E., Dickson, D., Sliwinski, M. J., Buschke, H., Katz, M., Crystal, H., et al. (1999). Memory and mental status correlates of modified Braak staging. *Neurobiol. Aging* 20, 573–579. doi: 10.1016/S0197-4580(99)00063-9

Guzman-Ramos, K., Moreno-Castilla, P., Castro-Cruz, M., McGaugh, J. L., Martinez-Coria, H., Laferla, F. M., et al. (2012). Restoration of dopamine release deficits during object recognition memory acquisition attenuates cognitive impairment in a triple transgenic mice model of Alzheimer's disease. *Learn. Mem.* 19, 453–460. doi: 10.1101/lm.026070.112

Haass, C. (2004). Take five—BACE and the gamma-secretase quartet conduct Alzheimer's amyloid beta-peptide generation. *EMBO J.* 23, 483–488. doi: 10.1038/sj.emboj.7600061

Haass, C., and Selkoe, D. J. (2007). Soluble protein oligomers in neurodegeneration: lessons from the Alzheimer's amyloid beta-peptide. *Nat. Rev. Mol. Cell Biol.* 8, 101–112. doi: 10.1038/nrm2101

Halliday, G. M., McCann, H. L., Pamphlett, R., Brooks, W. S., Creasey, H., McCusker, E., et al. (1992). Brain stem serotonin-synthesizing neurons in Alzheimer's disease: a clinicopathological correlation. *Acta Neuropathol.* 84, 638–650. doi: 10.1007/BF00227741

Hampel, H., Blennow, K., Shaw, L. M., Hoessler, Y. C., Zetterberg, H., and Trojanowski, J. Q. (2010). Total and phosphorylated tau protein as biological markers of Alzheimer's disease. *Exp. Gerontol.* 45, 30–40. doi: 10.1016/j.exger.2009.10.010

Hampel, H., Ewers, M., Burger, K., Annas, P., Mortberg, A., Bogstedt, A., et al. (2009). Lithium trial in Alzheimer's disease: a randomized, single-blind, placebo-controlled, multicenter 10-week study. *J. Clin. Psychiatry* 70, 922–931. doi: 10.4088/JCP.08m04606

Hampel, H., and Teipel, S. J. (2004). Total and phosphorylated tau proteins: evaluation as core biomarker candidates in frontotemporal dementia. *Dement. Geriatr. Cogn. Disord.* 17, 350–354. doi: 10.1159/000077170

Han, S. H., and Mook-Jung, I. (2014). Diverse molecular targets for therapeutic strategies in Alzheimer's disease. *J. Korean Med. Sci.* 29, 893–902. doi: 10.3346/jkms.2014.29.7.893

Harada, R., Okamura, N., Furumoto, S., Furukawa, K., Ishiki, A., Tomita, N., et al. (2016). 18F-THK5351: a novel PET radiotracer for imaging neurofibrillary pathology in Alzheimer's disease. *J. Nucl. Med.* 57, 208–214. doi: 10.2967/jnumed.115.164848

Hardwick, M., Fertikh, D., Culty, M., Li, H., Vidic, B., and Papadopoulos, V. (1999). Peripheral-type benzodiazepine receptor (PBR) in human breast cancer: correlation of breast cancer cell aggressive phenotype with PBR expression, nuclear localization, and PBR-mediated cell proliferation and nuclear transport of cholesterol. *Cancer Res.* 59, 831–842.

Hardy, J. (2006). Has the amyloid cascade hypothesis for Alzheimer's disease been proved? *Curr. Alzheimer Res.* 3, 71–73. doi: 10.2174/156720506775697098

Hardy, J. (2009). The amyloid hypothesis for Alzheimer's disease: a critical reappraisal. *J. Neurochem.* 110, 1129–1134. doi: 10.1111/j.1471-4159.2009.06181.x

Hardy, J. A., and Higgins, G. A. (1992). Alzheimer's disease: the amyloid cascade hypothesis. *Science* 256, 184–185. doi: 10.1126/science.1566067

Heiss, W. D., Sobesky, J., Smekal, U., Kracht, L. W., Lehnhardt, F. G., Thiel, A., et al. (2004). Probability of cortical infarction predicted by flumazenil binding and diffusion-weighted imaging signal intensity: a comparative positron emission tomography/magnetic resonance imaging study in early ischemic stroke. *Stroke* 35, 1892–1898. doi: 10.1161/01.STR.0000134746.93535.9b

Henry, G., Williamson, D., and Tampi, R. R. (2011). Efficacy and tolerability of antidepressants in the treatment of behavioral and psychological symptoms of dementia, a literature review of evidence. *Am. J. Alzheimers Dis. Other Demen.* 26, 169–183. doi: 10.1177/1533317511402051

Hernandez, C. M., Kayed, R., Zheng, H., Sweatt, J. D., and Dineley, K. T. (2010). Loss of alpha7 nicotinic receptors enhances beta-amyloid oligomer accumulation, exacerbating early-stage cognitive decline and septohippocampal pathology in a mouse model of Alzheimer's disease. *J. Neurosci.* 30, 2442–2453. doi: 10.1523/JNEUROSCI.5038-09.2010

Herrmann, N., Rothenburg, L. S., Black, S. E., Ryan, M., Liu, B. A., Busto, U. E., et al. (2008). Methylphenidate for the treatment of apathy in Alzheimer disease: prediction of response using dextroamphetamine challenge. *J. Clin. Psychopharmacol.* 28, 296–301. doi: 10.1097/JCP.0b013e318172b479

Hevers, W., and Luddens, H. (1998). The diversity of GABAA receptors. Pharmacological and electrophysiological properties of GABAA channel subtypes. *Mol. Neurobiol.* 18, 35–86. doi: 10.1007/BF02741459

Hickman, S. E., Allison, E. K., and El, K. J. (2008). Microglial dysfunction and defective beta-amyloid clearance pathways in aging Alzheimer's disease mice. *J. Neurosci.* 28, 8354–8360. doi: 10.1523/JNEUROSCI.0616-08.2008

Hirsch, J. D., Beyer, C. F., Malkowitz, L., Beer, B., and Blume, A. J. (1989). Mitochondrial benzodiazepine receptors mediate inhibition of mitochondrial respiratory control. *Mol. Pharmacol.* 35, 157–163.

Hirvonen, J., Kailajarvi, M., Haltia, T., Koskimies, S., Nagren, K., Virsu, P., et al. (2009). Assessment of MAO-B occupancy in the brain with PET and [11C]-L-deprenyl-D2: a dose-finding study with a novel MAO-B inhibitor, EVT 301. *Clin. Pharmacol. Ther.* 85, 506–512. doi: 10.1038/clpt.2008.241

Hock, C., Maddalena, A., Heuser, I., Naber, D., Oertel, W., von der, K. H., et al. (2000). Treatment with the selective muscarinic agonist talsaclidine decreases cerebrospinal fluid levels of total amyloid beta-peptide in patients with

Alzheimer's disease. *Ann. N. Y. Acad. Sci.* 920, 285–291. doi: 10.1111/j.1749-6632.2000.tb06937.x

Holm, P., Ettrup, A., Klein, A. B., Santini, M. A., El-Sayed, M., Elvang, A. B., et al. (2010). Plaque deposition dependent decrease in 5-HT2A serotonin receptor in AbetaPPswe/PS1dE9 amyloid overexpressing mice. *J. Alzheimers Dis.* 20, 1201–1213. doi: 10.3233/JAD-2010-100117

Holman, B. L., Gibson, R. E., Hill, T. C., Eckelman, W. C., Albert, M., and Reba, R. C. (1985). Muscarinic acetylcholine receptors in Alzheimer's disease. In vivo imaging with iodine 123-labeled 3-quinuclidinyl-4-iodobenzilate and emission tomography. *JAMA* 254, 3063–3066. doi: 10.1001/jama.254.21.3063

Hong, M., Zhukareva, V., Vogelsberg-Ragaglia, V., Wszolek, Z., Reed, L., Miller, B. I., et al. (1998). Mutation-specific functional impairments in distinct tau isoforms of hereditary FTDP-17. *Science* 282, 1914–1917. doi: 10.1126/science.282.5395.1914

Hoozemans, J. J., Rozemuller, A. J., van Haastert, E. S., Eikelenboom, P., and van Gool, W. A. (2011). Neuroinflammation in Alzheimer's disease wanes with age. *J. Neuroinflammation* 8, 171.

Hoshi, M., Sato, M., Matsumoto, S., Noguchi, A., Yasutake, K., Yoshida, N., et al. (2003). Spherical aggregates of beta-amyloid (amylospheroid) show high neurotoxicity and activate tau protein kinase I/glycogen synthase kinase-3beta. *Proc. Natl. Acad. Sci. U.S.A.* 100, 6370–6375. doi: 10.1073/pnas.1237107100

Hosie, A. M., Wilkins, M. E., da Silva, H. M., and Smart, T. G. (2006). Endogenous neurosteroids regulate GABAA receptors through two discrete transmembrane sites. *Nature* 444, 486–489. doi: 10.1038/nature05324

Hoyer, D., Hannon, J. P., and Martin, G. R. (2002). Molecular, pharmacological and functional diversity of 5-HT receptors. *Pharmacol. Biochem. Behav.* 71, 533–554. doi: 10.1016/S0091-3057(01)00746-8

Huang, L., Lu, C., Sun, Y., Mao, F., Luo, Z., Su, T., et al. (2012). Multitarget-directed benzylideneindanone derivatives: anti-beta-amyloid (Abeta) aggregation, antioxidant, metal chelation, and monoamine oxidase B (MAO-B) inhibition properties against Alzheimer's disease. *J. Med. Chem.* 55, 8483–8492. doi: 10.1021/jm300978h

Hyman, B. T., Phelps, C. H., Beach, T. G., Bigio, E. H., Cairns, N. J., Carrillo, M. C., et al. (2012). National institute on aging-Alzheimer's association guidelines for the neuropathologic assessment of Alzheimer's disease. *Alzheimers Dement.* 8, 1–13. doi: 10.1016/j.jalz.2011.10.007

Imbimbo, B. P., and Giardina, G. A. (2011). gamma-secretase inhibitors and modulators for the treatment of Alzheimer's disease: disappointments and hopes. *Curr. Top. Med. Chem.* 11, 1555–1570. doi: 10.2174/156802611795860942

Iqbal, K., and Grundke-Iqbal, I. (2008). Alzheimer neurofibrillary degeneration: significance, etiopathogenesis, therapeutics and prevention. *J. Cell Mol. Med.* 12, 38–55. doi: 10.1111/j.1582-4934.2008.00225.x

Irie, T., Fukushi, K., Akimoto, Y., Tamagami, H., and Nozaki, T. (1994). Design and evaluation of radioactive acetylcholine analogs for mapping brain acetylcholinesterase (AchE) in vivo. *Nucl. Med. Biol.* 21, 801–808. doi: 10.1016/0969-8051(94)90159-7

Ishiki, A., Okamura, N., Furukawa, K., Furumoto, S., Harada, R., Tomita, N., et al. (2015). Longitudinal assessment of tau pathology in patients with Alzheimer's disease using [18F]THK-5117 positron emission tomography. *PLoS ONE* 10:e0140311. doi: 10.1371/journal.pone.0140311

Itoh, M., Meguro, K., Fujiwara, T., Hatazawa, J., Iwata, R., Ishiwata, K., et al. (1994). Assessment of dopamine metabolism in brain of patients with dementia by means of 18F-fluorodopa and PET. *Ann. Nucl. Med.* 8, 245–251. doi: 10.1007/BF03165027

Iyo, M., Namba, H., Fukushi, K., Shinotoh, H., Nagatsuka, S., Suhara, T., et al. (1997). Measurement of acetylcholinesterase by positron emission tomography in the brains of healthy controls and patients with Alzheimer's disease. *Lancet* 349, 1805–1809. doi: 10.1016/S0140-6736(96)09124-6

Jack, C. R. Jr., Barrio, J. R., and Kepe, V. (2013). Cerebral amyloid PET imaging in Alzheimer's disease. *Acta Neuropathol.* 126, 643–657. doi: 10.1007/s00401-013-1185-7

Jack, C. R. Jr., Knopman, D. S., Jagust, W. J., Shaw, L. M., Aisen, P. S., Weiner, M. W., et al. (2010). Hypothetical model of dynamic biomarkers of the Alzheimer's pathological cascade. *Lancet Neurol.* 9, 119–128. doi: 10.1016/S1474-4422(09)70299-6

Jack, C. R. Jr., Lowe, V. J., Senjem, M. L., Weigand, S. D., Kemp, B. J., Shiung, M. M., et al. (2008). 11C PiB and structural MRI provide complementary information

in imaging of Alzheimer's disease and amnestic mild cognitive impairment. *Brain* 131, 665–680. doi: 10.1093/brain/awm336

Jack, C. R. Jr., Lowe, V. J., Weigand, S. D., Wiste, H. J., Senjem, M. L., Knopman, D. S., et al. (2009). Serial PIB and MRI in normal, mild cognitive impairment and Alzheimer's disease: implications for sequence of pathological events in Alzheimer's disease. *Brain* 132, 1355–1365. doi: 10.1093/brain/awp062

James, O. G., Doraiswamy, P. M., and Borges-Neto, S. (2015). PET imaging of tau pathology in Alzheimer's disease and tauopathies. *Front. Neurol.* 6:38. doi: 10.3389/fneur.2015.00038

Janssen, B., Vugts, D. J., Funke, U., Molenaar, G. T., Kruijer, P. S., van Berckel, B. N., et al. (2016). Imaging of neuroinflammation in Alzheimer's disease, multiple sclerosis and stroke: recent developments in positron emission tomography. *Biochim. Biophys. Acta* 1862, 425–441. doi: 10.1016/j.bbadis.2015.11.011

Jaworski, T., Dewachter, I., Lechat, B., Gees, M., Kremer, A., Demedts, D., et al. (2011). GSK-3alpha/beta kinases and amyloid production in vivo. *Nature* 480, E4–E5. doi: 10.1038/nature10615

Jones, G. M., Sahakian, B. J., Levy, R., Warburton, D. M., and Gray, J. A. (1992). Effects of acute subcutaneous nicotine on attention, information processing and short-term memory in Alzheimer's disease. *Psychopharmacology (Berl.)* 108, 485–494. doi: 10.1007/BF02247426

Jossan, S. S., Gillberg, P. G., Gottfries, C. G., Karlsson, I., and Oreland, L. (1991). Monoamine oxidase B in brains from patients with Alzheimer's disease: a biochemical and autoradiographical study. *Neuroscience* 45, 1–12. doi: 10.1016/0306-4522(91)90098-9

Jurgensen, S., and Ferreira, S. T. (2010). Nicotinic receptors, amyloid-beta, and synaptic failure in Alzheimer's disease. *J. Mol. Neurosci.* 40, 221–229. doi: 10.1007/s12031-009-92370

Kaasinen, V., Nagren, K., Jarvenpaa, T., Roivainen, A., Yu, M., Oikonen, V., et al. (2002). Regional effects of donepezil and rivastigmine on cortical acetylcholinesterase activity in Alzheimer's disease. *J. Clin. Psychopharmacol.* 22, 615–620. doi: 10.1097/00004714-200212000-00012

Kadir, A., Almkvist, O., Wall, A., Langstrom, B., and Nordberg, A. (2006). PET imaging of cortical 11C-nicotine binding correlates with the cognitive function of attention in Alzheimer's disease. *Psychopharmacology (Berl.)* 188, 509–520. doi: 10.1007/s00213-006-04477

Kadir, A., Darreh-Shori, T., Almkvist, O., Wall, A., Langstrom, B., and Nordberg, A. (2007). Changes in brain 11C-nicotine binding sites in patients with mild Alzheimer's disease following rivastigmine treatment as assessed by PET. *Psychopharmacology (Berl.)* 191, 1005–1014. doi: 10.1007/s00213-007-0725-z

Karlin, A. (2002). Emerging structure of the nicotinic acetylcholine receptors. *Nat. Rev. Neurosci.* 3, 102–114. doi: 10.1038/nrn731

Katsifis, A., and Kassiou, M. (2004). Development of radioligands for in vivo imaging of GABA(A)-benzodiazepine receptors. *Mini. Rev. Med. Chem.* 4, 909–921. doi: 10.2174/1389557043403332

Kayed, R., Head, E., Thompson, J. L., McIntire, T. M., Milton, S. C., Cotman, C. W., et al. (2003). Common structure of soluble amyloid oligomers implies common mechanism of pathogenesis. *Science* 300, 486–489. doi: 10.1126/science.1079469

Kehr, J., Hu, X. J., Yoshitake, T., Wang, F. H., Osborne, P., Stenfors, C., et al. (2010). The selective 5-HT(1A) receptor antagonist NAD-299 increases acetylcholine release but not extracellular glutamate levels in the frontal cortex and hippocampus of awake rat. *Eur. Neuropsychopharmacol.* 20, 487–500. doi: 10.1016/j.euroneuro.2010.03.003

Kemp, P. M., Holmes, C., Hoffmann, S., Wilkinson, S., Zivanovic, M., Thom, J., et al. (2003). A randomised placebo controlled study to assess the effects of cholinergic treatment on muscarinic receptors in Alzheimer's disease. *J. Neurol. Neurosurg. Psychiatry* 74, 1567–1570. doi: 10.1136/jnnp.74.11.1567

Kempermann, N., Laine, M., Laakso, M. P., Kaasinen, V., Nagren, K., Vahlberg, T., et al. (2003). Hippocampal dopamine D2 receptors correlate with memory functions in Alzheimer's disease. *Eur. J. Neurosci.* 18, 149–154. doi: 10.1046/j.1460-9568.2003.02716.x

Kemppainen, N., Ruottinen, H., Nagren, K., and Rinne, J. O. (2000). PET shows that striatal dopamine D1 and D2 receptors are differentially affected in AD. *Neurology* 55, 205–209. doi: 10.1212/WNL.55.2.205

Kemppainen, N. M., Aalto, S., Wilson, I. A., Nagren, K., Helin, S., Bruck, A., et al. (2006). Voxel-based analysis of PET amyloid ligand

[11C]PIB uptake in Alzheimer disease. *Neurology* 67, 1575–1580. doi: 10.1212/01.wnl.0000240117.55680.0a

Kendziorra, K., Wolf, H., Meyer, P. M., Barthel, H., Hesse, S., Becker, G. A., et al. (2011). Decreased cerebral alpha4beta2* nicotinic acetylcholine receptor availability in patients with mild cognitive impairment and Alzheimer's disease assessed with positron emission tomography. *Eur. J. Nucl. Med. Mol. Imaging* 38, 515–525. doi: 10.1007/s00259-010-1644-5

Kepe, V., Barrio, J. R., Huang, S. C., Ercoli, L., Siddarth, P., Shoghi-Jadid, K., et al. (2006). Serotonin 1A receptors in the living brain of Alzheimer's disease patients. *Proc. Natl. Acad. Sci. U.S.A.* 103, 702–707. doi: 10.1073/pnas.0510237103

Kepe, V., Bordelon, Y., Boxer, A., Huang, S. C., Liu, J., Thiede, F. C., et al. (2013). PET imaging of neuropathology in tauopathies: progressive supranuclear palsy. *J. Alzheimers Dis.* 36, 145–153. doi: 10.3233/JAD-130032

Kepe, V., Ghetti, B., Farlow, M. R., Bresjanac, M., Miller, K., Huang, S. C., et al. (2010). PET of brain prion protein amyloid in Gerstmann-Straussler-Scheinker disease. *Brain Pathol.* 20, 419–430. doi: 10.1111/j.1750-3639.2009.00306.x

Keverne, E. B. (1999). GABA-ergic neurons and the neurobiology of schizophrenia and other psychoses. *Brain Res. Bull.* 48, 467–473. doi: 10.1016/S0361-9230(99)00025-8

Kilbourn, M. R., Snyder, S. E., Sherman, P. S., and Kuhl, D. E. (1996). In vivo studies of acetylcholinesterase activity using a labeled substrate, N-[11C]methylpiperdin-4-yl propionate ([11C]PMP). *Synapse* 22, 123–131. doi: 10.1002/(SICI)1098-2396(199602)22:2<123::AID-SYN5>3.0.CO;2-F

Kim, S. Y., Choi, S. H., Rollema, H., Schwam, E. M., McRae, T., Dubrava, S., et al. (2014). Phase II crossover trial of varenicline in mild-to-moderate Alzheimer's disease. *Dement. Geriatr. Cogn. Disord.* 37, 232–245. doi: 10.1159/0003 55373

King, M. K., Pardo, M., Cheng, Y., Downey, K., Jope, R. S., and Beurel, E. (2014). Glycogen synthase kinase-3 inhibitors: rescuers of cognitive impairments. *Pharmacol. Ther.* 141, 1–12. doi: 10.1016/j.pharmthera.2013.07.010

Kirven, L. E., and Montero, E. F. (1973). Comparison of thioridazine and diazepam in the control of nonpsychotic symptoms associated with senility: double-blind study. *J. Am. Geriatr. Soc.* 21, 546–551. doi: 10.1111/j.1532-5415.1973.tb01661.x

Kitazawa, M., Oddo, S., Yamasaki, T. R., Green, K. N., and Laferla, F. M. (2005). Lipopolysaccharide-induced inflammation exacerbates tau pathology by a cyclin-dependent kinase 5-mediated pathway in a transgenic model of Alzheimer's disease. *J. Neurosci.* 25, 8843–8853. doi: 10.1523/JNEUROSCI.2868-05.2005

Koo, J., and Byun, Y. (2013). Current status of PET-imaging probes of beta-amyloid plaques. *Arch. Pharm. Res.* 36, 1178–1184. doi: 10.1007/s12272-013-01934

Korczyn, A. D. (2008). The amyloid cascade hypothesis. *Alzheimers. Dement.* 4, 176–178. doi: 10.1016/j.jalz.2007.11.008

Kugler, W., Veenman, L., Shandalov, Y., Leschiner, S., Spanier, I., Lakomek, M., et al. (2008). Ligands of the mitochondrial 18 kDa translocator protein attenuate apoptosis of human glioblastoma cells exposed to erucylphosphohomocholine. *Cell Oncol.* 30, 435–450.

Kuhl, D. E., Minoshima, S., Frey, K. A., Foster, N. L., Kilbourn, M. R., and Koeppe, R. A. (2000). Limited donepezil inhibition of acetylcholinesterase measured with positron emission tomography in living Alzheimer cerebral cortex. *Ann. Neurol.* 48, 391–395. doi: 10.1002/1531-8249(200009)48:3<391::AID-ANA17>3.3.CO;2-8

Kumar, J. S., and Mann, J. J. (2014). PET tracers for serotonin receptors and their applications. *Cent. Nerv. Syst. Agents Med. Chem.* 14, 96–112. doi: 10.2174/1871524914666141030124316

Kumar, U., and Patel, S. C. (2007). Immunohistochemical localization of dopamine receptor subtypes (D1R-D5R) in Alzheimer's disease brain. *Brain Res.* 1131, 187–196. doi: 10.1016/j.brainres.2006.10.049

Lai, M. K., Tsang, S. W., Alder, J. T., Keene, J., Hope, T., Esiri, M. M., et al. (2005). Loss of serotonin 5-HT2A receptors in the postmortem temporal cortex correlates with rate of cognitive decline in Alzheimer's disease. *Psychopharmacology (Berl.)* 179, 673–677. doi: 10.1007/s00213-004-2077-2

Lai, M. K., Tsang, S. W., Francis, P. T., Esiri, M. M., Keene, J., Hope, T., et al. (2003). Reduced serotonin 5-HT1A receptor binding in the temporal cortex correlates with aggressive behavior in Alzheimer disease. *Brain Res.* 974, 82–87. doi: 10.1016/S0006-8993(03)02554-X

Lanctot, K. L., Herrmann, N., Black, S. E., Ryan, M., Rothenburg, L. S., Liu, B. A., et al. (2008). Apathy associated with Alzheimer disease: use of

dextroamphetamine challenge. *Am. J. Geriatr. Psychiatry* 16, 551–557. doi: 10.1097/JGP.0b013e318170a6d1

Lanctot, K. L., Herrmann, N., Mazzotta, P., Khan, L. R., and Ingber, N. (2004). GABAergic function in Alzheimer's disease: evidence for dysfunction and potential as a therapeutic target for the treatment of behavioural and psychological symptoms of dementia. *Can. J. Psychiatry* 49, 439–453.

Lee, V. M., Goedert, M., and Trojanowski, J. Q. (2001). Neurodegenerative tauopathies. *Annu. Rev. Neurosci.* 24, 1121–1159. doi: 10.1146/annurev.neuro.24.1.1121

Lees, A. J., Shaw, K. M., Kohout, L. J., Stern, G. M., Elsworth, J. D., Sandler, M., et al. (1977). Deprenyl in Parkinson's disease. *Lancet* 2, 791–795. doi: 10.1016/S0140-6736(77)90725-5

Lemere, C. A. (2013). Immunotherapy for Alzheimer's disease: hoops and hurdles. *Mol. Neurodegener.* 8:36. doi: 10.1186/1750-1326-8-36

Levin, E. D. (1992). Nicotinic systems and cognitive function. *Psychopharmacology (Berl.)* 108, 417–431. doi: 10.1007/BF02247415

Liao, C. F., Themmen, A. P., Joho, R., Barberis, C., Birnbaumer, M., and Birnbaumer, L. (1989). Molecular cloning and expression of a fifth muscarinic acetylcholine receptor. *J. Biol. Chem.* 264, 7328–7337.

Limon, A., Reyes-Ruiz, J. M., and Miledi, R. (2012). Loss of functional GABA(A) receptors in the Alzheimer diseased brain. *Proc. Natl. Acad. Sci. U.S.A.* 109, 10071–10076. doi: 10.1073/pnas.1204606109

Lleo, A., Greenberg, S. M., and Growdon, J. H. (2006). Current pharmacotherapy for Alzheimer's disease. *Annu. Rev. Med.* 57, 513–533. doi: 10.1146/annurev.med.57.121304.131442

Lopez, O. L., Wisnieski, S. R., Becker, J. T., Boller, F., and DeKosky, S. T. (1997). Extrapyramidal signs in patients with probable Alzheimer disease. *Arch. Neurol.* 54, 969–975. doi: 10.1001/archneur.1997.00550200033007

Lorke, D. E., Lu, G., Cho, E., and Yew, D. T. (2006). Serotonin 5-HT2A and 5-HT6 receptors in the prefrontal cortex of Alzheimer and normal aging patients. *BMC Neurosci.* 7:36. doi: 10.1186/1471-2202-7-36

Lovestone, S., Boada, M., Dubois, B., Hull, M., Rinne, J. O., Huppertz, H. J., et al. (2015). A phase II trial of tideglusib in Alzheimer's disease. *J. Alzheimers Dis.* 45, 75–88. doi: 10.3233/JAD-141959

Lowe, V. J., Kemp, B. J., Jack, C. R. Jr., Senjem, M., Weigand, S., Shiung, M., et al. (2009). Comparison of 18F-FDG and PiB PET in cognitive impairment. *J. Nucl. Med.* 50, 878–886. doi: 10.2967/jnumed.108.058529

Luo, Y., Bolon, B., Kahn, S., Bennett, B. D., Babu-Khan, S., Denis, P., et al. (2001). Mice deficient in BACE1, the Alzheimer's beta-secretase, have normal phenotype and abolished beta-amyloid generation. *Nat. Neurosci.* 4, 231–232. doi: 10.1038/85059

Lustbader, J. W., Cirilli, M., Lin, C., Xu, H. W., Takuma, K., Wang, N., et al. (2004). ABAD directly links Abeta to mitochondrial toxicity in Alzheimer's disease. *Science* 304, 448–452. doi: 10.1126/science.1091230

Lyketsos, C. G., DelCampo, L., Steinberg, M., Miles, Q., Steele, C. D., Munro, C., et al. (2003). Treating depression in Alzheimer disease: efficacy and safety of sertraline therapy, and the benefits of depression reduction: the DIADS. *Arch. Gen. Psychiatry* 60, 737–746. doi: 10.1001/archpsyc.60.7.737

Madsen, K., Neumann, W. J., Holst, K., Marner, L., Haahr, M. T., Lehel, S., et al. (2011). Cerebral serotonin 4 receptors and amyloid-beta in early Alzheimer's disease. *J. Alzheimers Dis.* 26, 457–466. doi: 10.3233/JAD-2011-110056

Maher-Edwards, G., Zvartau-Hind, M., Hunter, A. J., Gold, M., Hopton, G., Jacobs, G., et al. (2010). Double-blind, controlled phase II study of a 5-HT6 receptor antagonist, SB-742457, in Alzheimer's disease. *Curr. Alzheimer Res.* 7, 374–385. doi: 10.2174/156720510791383831

Maqbool, M., Mobashir, M., and Hoda, N. (2016). Pivotal role of glycogen synthase kinase-3: a therapeutic target for Alzheimer's disease. *Eur. J. Med. Chem.* 107, 63–81. doi: 10.1016/j.ejmech.2015.10.018

Marczynski, T. J. (1998). GABAergic deafferentation hypothesis of brain aging and Alzheimer's disease revisited. *Brain Res. Bull.* 45, 341–379. doi: 10.1016/S0361-9230(97)00347-X

Marner, L., Frokjaer, V. G., Kalbitzer, J., Lehel, S., Madsen, K., Baare, W. F., et al. (2012). Loss of serotonin 2A receptors exceeds loss of serotonergic projections in early Alzheimer's disease: a combined [11C]DASB and [18F]altanserin-PET study. *Neurobiol. Aging* 33, 479–487. doi: 10.1016/j.neurobiolaging.2010.03.023

Martin, L., Latypova, X., and Terro, F. (2011). Post-translational modifications of tau protein: implications for Alzheimer's disease. *Neurochem. Int.* 58, 458–471. doi: 10.1016/j.neuint.2010.12.023

Martorana, A., Di, L. F., Esposito, Z., Lo, G. T., Bernardi, G., Caltagirone, C., et al. (2013). Dopamine D(2)-agonist rotigotine effects on cortical excitability and central cholinergic transmission in Alzheimer's disease patients. *Neuropharmacology* 64, 108–113. doi: 10.1016/j.neuropharm.2012.07.015

Martorana, A., and Koch, G. (2014). Is dopamine involved in Alzheimer's disease? *Front. Aging Neurosci.* 6:252. doi: 10.3389/fnagi.2014.00252

Maruyama, M., Shimada, H., Suhara, T., Shinotoh, H., Ji, B., Maeda, J., et al. (2013). Imaging of tau pathology in a tauopathy mouse model and in Alzheimer patients compared to normal controls. *Neuron* 79, 1094–1108. doi: 10.1016/j.neuron.2013.07.037

Masters, C. L., Cappai, R., Barnham, K. J., and Villemagne, V. L. (2006). Molecular mechanisms for Alzheimer's disease: implications for neuroimaging and therapeutics. *J. Neurochem.* 97, 1700–1725. doi: 10.1111/j.1471-4159.2006.03989.x

Maziere, M. (1995). Cholinergic neurotransmission studied in vivo using positron emission tomography or single photon emission computerized tomography. *Pharmacol. Ther.* 66, 83–101. doi: 10.1016/0163-7258(95)00003-Y

McEnery, M. W., Snowman, A. M., Trifiletti, R. R., and Snyder, S. H. (1992). Isolation of the mitochondrial benzodiazepine receptor: association with the voltage-dependent anion channel and the adenine nucleotide carrier. *Proc. Natl. Acad. Sci. U.S.A.* 89, 3170–3174. doi: 10.1073/pnas.89.8.3170

McGeer, P. L., and McGeer, E. G. (1995). The inflammatory response system of brain: implications for therapy of Alzheimer and other neurodegenerative diseases. *Brain Res. Brain Res. Rev.* 21, 195–218. doi: 10.1016/0165-0173(95)00011-9

Mecocci, P., and Polidori, M. C. (2012). Antioxidant clinical trials in mild cognitive impairment and Alzheimer's disease. *Biochim. Biophys. Acta* 1822, 631–638. doi: 10.1016/j.bbadis.2011.10.006

Mehta, A. K., and Ticku, M. K. (1999). An update on GABAA receptors. *Brain Res. Brain Res. Rev.* 29, 196–217. doi: 10.1016/S0165-0173(98)00052-6

Meyer, P. M., Tiepolt, S., Barthel, H., Hesse, S., and Sabri, O. (2014). Radioligand imaging of alpha4beta2* nicotinic acetylcholine receptors in Alzheimer's disease and Parkinson's disease. *Q. J. Nucl. Med. Mol. Imaging* 58, 376–386.

Midzak, A., Zirkin, B., and Papadopoulos, V. (2015). Translocator protein: pharmacology and steroidogenesis. *Biochem. Soc. Trans.* 43, 572–578. doi: 10.1042/BST20150061

Miettinen, H., Kononen, J., Haapasalo, H., Helen, P., Sallinen, P., Harjuntausta, T., et al. (1995). Expression of peripheral-type benzodiazepine receptor and diazepam binding inhibitor in human astrocytomas: relationship to cell proliferation. *Cancer Res.* 55, 2691–2695.

Millan, M. J., Gobert, A., Roux, S., Porsolt, R., Meneses, A., Carli, M., et al. (2004). The serotonin1A receptor partial agonist S15535 [4-(benzodioxan-5-yl)1-(indan-2-yl)piperazine] enhances cholinergic transmission and cognitive function in rodents: a combined neurochemical and behavioral analysis. *J. Pharmacol. Exp. Ther.* 311, 190–203. doi: 10.1124/jpet.104.069625

Minati, L., Edginton, T., Bruzzone, M. G., and Giaccone, G. (2009). Current concepts in Alzheimer's disease: a multidisciplinary review. *Am. J. Alzheimers. Dis. Other Demen.* 24, 95–121. doi: 10.1177/1533317508328602

Mitchell, R. A., Herrmann, N., and Lanctot, K. L. (2011). The role of dopamine in symptoms and treatment of apathy in Alzheimer's disease. *CNS Neurosci. Ther.* 17, 411–427. doi: 10.1111/j.1755-5949.2010.00161.x

Moreira, P. I., Zhu, X., Nunomura, A., Smith, M. A., and Perry, G. (2006). Therapeutic options in Alzheimer's disease. *Expert Rev. Neurother.* 6, 897–910. doi: 10.1586/14737175.6.6.897

Morgan, D., Gordon, M. N., Tan, J., Wilcock, D., and Rojiani, A. M. (2005). Dynamic complexity of the microglial activation response in transgenic models of amyloid deposition: implications for Alzheimer therapeutics. *J. Neuropathol. Exp. Neurol.* 64, 743–753. doi: 10.1097/01.jnen.0000178444.33972.e0

Mowla, A., Mosavinasab, M., and Pani, A. (2007). Does fluoxetine have any effect on the cognition of patients with mild cognitive impairment? A double-blind, placebo-controlled, clinical trial. *J. Clin. Psychopharmacol.* 27, 67–70. doi: 10.1097/JCP.0b013e31802e0002

Mura, E., Lanni, C., Preda, S., Pistoia, F., Sara, M., Racchi, M., et al. (2010). Beta-amyloid: a disease target or a synaptic regulator affecting age-related neurotransmitter changes? *Curr. Pharm. Des.* 16, 672–683. doi: 10.2174/138161210790883723

Murray, A. M., Weihmueller, F. B., Marshall, J. F., Hurtig, H. I., Gottleib, G. L., and Joyce, J. N. (1995). Damage to dopamine systems differs between Parkinson's disease and Alzheimer's disease with parkinsonism. *Ann. Neurol.* 37, 300–312. doi: 10.1002/ana.410370306

Nelson, L. D., Siddarth, P., Kepe, V., Scheibel, K. E., Huang, S. C., Barrio, J. R., et al. (2011). Positron emission tomography of brain beta-amyloid and tau levels in adults with Down syndrome. *Arch. Neurol.* 68, 768–774. doi: 10.1001/archneurol.2011.104

Nelson, P. T., Alafuzoff, I., Bigio, E. H., Bouras, C., Braak, H., Cairns, N. J., et al. (2012). Correlation of Alzheimer disease neuropathologic changes with cognitive status: a review of the literature. *J. Neuropathol. Exp. Neurol.* 71, 362–381. doi: 10.1097/NEN.0b013e31825018f7

Neve, R. L., Harris, P., Kosik, K. S., Kurnit, D. M., and Donlon, T. A. (1986). Identification of cDNA clones for the human microtubule-associated protein tau and chromosomal localization of the genes for tau and microtubule-associated protein 2. *Brain Res.* 387, 271–280. doi: 10.1016/0169-328X(86)90033-1

Niesler, B., Kapeller, J., Hammer, C., and Rappold, G. (2008). Serotonin type 3 receptor genes: HTR3A, B, C, D, E. *Pharmacogenomics* 9, 501–504. doi: 10.2217/14622416.9.5.501

Nitsch, R. M., Slack, B. E., Wurtman, R. J., and Growdon, J. H. (1992). Release of Alzheimer amyloid precursor derivatives stimulated by activation of muscarinic acetylcholine receptors. *Science* 258, 304–307. doi: 10.1126/science.1411529

Noble, W., Planel, E., Zehr, C., Olm, V., Meyerson, J., Suleman, F., et al. (2005). Inhibition of glycogen synthase kinase-3 by lithium correlates with reduced tauopathy and degeneration in vivo. *Proc. Natl. Acad. Sci. U.S.A.* 102, 6990–6995. doi: 10.1073/pnas.0500466102

Noble, W., Pooler, A. M., and Hanger, D. P. (2011). Advances in tau-based drug discovery. *Expert Opin. Drug Discov.* 6, 797–810. doi: 10.1517/17460441.2011.586690

Nordberg, A., Amberla, K., Shigeta, M., Lundqvist, H., Viitanen, M., Hellstrom-Lindahl, E., et al. (1998). Long-term tacrine treatment in three mild Alzheimer patients: effects on nicotinic receptors, cerebral blood flow, glucose metabolism, EEG, and cognitive abilities. *Alzheimer Dis. Assoc. Disord.* 12, 228–237. doi: 10.1097/00002093-199809000-00017

Nordberg, A., Hartvig, P., Lilja, A., Viitanen, M., Amberla, K., Lundqvist, H., et al. (1990). Decreased uptake and binding of 11C-nicotine in brain of Alzheimer patients as visualized by positron emission tomography. *J. Neural Transm. Park. Dis. Dement. Sect.* 2, 215–224. doi: 10.1007/BF02257652

Nordberg, A., Lilja, A., Lundqvist, H., Hartvig, P., Amberla, K., Viitanen, M., et al. (1992). Tacrine restores cholinergic nicotinic receptors and glucose metabolism in Alzheimer patients as visualized by positron emission tomography. *Neurobiol. Aging* 13, 747–758. doi: 10.1016/0197-4580(92)90099-J

Nordberg, A., Lundqvist, H., Hartvig, P., Andersson, J., Johansson, M., Hellstrom-Lindahl, E., et al. (1997). Imaging of nicotinic and muscarinic receptors in Alzheimer's disease: effect of tacrine treatment. *Dement. Geriatr. Cogn. Disord.* 8, 78–84. doi: 10.1159/000106611

Nordberg, A., Lundqvist, H., Hartvig, P., Lilja, A., and Langstrom, B. (1995). Kinetic analysis of regional (S)(-)11C-nicotine binding in normal and Alzheimer brains-in vivo assessment using positron emission tomography. *Alzheimer Dis. Assoc. Disord.* 9, 21–27. doi: 10.1097/00002093-199505000-00006

Nykanen, N. P., Kysenius, K., Sakha, P., Tammela, P., and Huttunen, H. J. (2012). gamma-Aminobutyric acid type A (GABAA) receptor activation modulates tau phosphorylation. *J. Biol. Chem.* 287, 6743–6752. doi: 10.1074/jbc.M111.309385

Nyth, A. L., and Gottfries, C. G. (1990). The clinical efficacy of citalopram in treatment of emotional disturbances in dementia disorders. A Nordic multicentre study. *Br. J. Psychiatry* 157, 894–901. doi: 10.1192/bjp.157.6.894

O'Brien, J. T., Colloby, S. J., Pakrasi, S., Perry, E. K., Pimlott, S. L., Wyper, D. J., et al. (2007). Alpha4beta2 nicotinic receptor status in Alzheimer's disease using 123I-5IA-85380 single-photon-emission computed tomography. *J. Neurol. Neurosurg. Psychiatry* 78, 356–362. doi: 10.1136/jnnp.2006.108209

Oddo, S., Caccamo, A., Shepherd, J. D., Murphy, M. P., Golde, T. E., Kayed, R., et al. (2003). Triple-transgenic model of Alzheimer's disease with plaques and tangles: intracellular Abeta and synaptic dysfunction. *Neuron* 39, 409–421. doi: 10.1016/S0896-6273(03)00434-3

Oddo, S., and Laferla, F. M. (2006). The role of nicotinic acetylcholine receptors in Alzheimer's disease. *J. Physiol. Paris* 99, 172–179. doi: 10.1016/j.jphysparis.2005.12.080

Okada, H., Ouchi, Y., Ogawa, M., Futatsubashi, M., Saito, Y., Yoshikawa, E., et al. (2013). Alterations in alpha4beta2 nicotinic receptors in cognitive decline in Alzheimer's aetiopathology. *Brain* 136, 3004–3017. doi: 10.1093/brain/awt195

Okamura, N., Furumoto, S., Fodero-Tavoletti, M. T., Mulligan, R. S., Harada, R., Yates, P., et al. (2014a). Non-invasive assessment of Alzheimer's disease neurofibrillary pathology using 18F-THK5105 PET. *Brain* 137, 1762–1771. doi: 10.1093/brain/awu064

Okamura, N., Harada, R., Furumoto, S., Arai, H., Yanai, K., and Kudo, Y. (2014b). Tau PET imaging in Alzheimer's disease. *Curr. Neurol. Neurosci. Rep.* 14:500. doi: 10.1007/s11910-014-0500_6

Okello, A., Koivunen, J., Edison, P., Archer, H. A., Turkheimer, F. E., Nagren, K., et al. (2009). Conversion of amyloid positive and negative MCI to AD over 3 years: an 11C-PIB PET study. *Neurology* 73, 754–760. doi: 10.1212/WNL.0b013e3181b23564

Orgogozo, J. M., Gilman, S., Dartigues, J. F., Laurent, B., Puel, M., Kirby, L. C., et al. (2003). Subacute meningoencephalitis in a subset of patients with AD after Abeta42 immunization. *Neurology* 61, 46–54. doi: 10.1212/01.WNL.0000073623.84147.A8

Ory, D., Celen, S., Verbruggen, A., and Bormans, G. (2014). PET radioligands for in vivo visualization of neuroinflammation. *Curr. Pharm. Des.* 20, 5897–5913. doi: 10.2174/1381612820666140613120212

Ouchi, Y., Yoshikawa, E., Futatsubashi, M., Yagi, S., Ueki, T., and Nakamura, K. (2009). Altered brain serotonin transporter and associated glucose metabolism in Alzheimer disease. *J. Nucl. Med.* 50, 1260–1266. doi: 10.2967/jnumed.109.063008

Owen, D. R., Lewis, A. J., Reynolds, R., Rupprecht, R., Eser, D., Wilkins, M. R., et al. (2011). Variation in binding affinity of the novel anxiolytic XBD173 for the 18 kDa translocator protein in human brain. *Synapse* 65, 257–259. doi: 10.1002/syn.20884

Owen, D. R., Yeo, A. J., Gunn, R. N., Song, K., Wadsworth, G., Lewis, A., et al. (2012). An 18-kDa translocator protein (TSPO) polymorphism explains differences in binding affinity of the PET radioligand PBR28. *J. Cereb. Blood Flow Metab.* 32, 1–5. doi: 10.1038/jcbfm.2011.147

Padala, P. R., Burke, W. J., Shostrom, V. K., Bhatia, S. C., Wengel, S. P., Potter, J. F., et al. (2010). Methylphenidate for apathy and functional status in dementia of the Alzheimer type. *Am. J. Geriatr. Psychiatry* 18, 371–374. doi: 10.1097/JGP.0b013e3181cabcf6

Pagani, L., and Eckert, A. (2011). Amyloid-Beta interaction with mitochondria. *Int. J. Alzheimers Dis.* 2011, 925050. doi: 10.4061/2011/925050

Pakrasi, S., Colloby, S. J., Firbank, M. J., Perry, E. K., Wyper, D. J., Owens, J., et al. (2007). Muscarinic acetylcholine receptor status in Alzheimer's disease assessed using (R, R) 123I-QNB SPECT. *J. Neurol.* 254, 907–913. doi: 10.1007/s00415-006-04738

Palacios, J. M., Bolliger, G., Closse, A., Enz, A., Gmelin, G., and Malanowski, J. (1986). The pharmacological assessment of RS 86 (2-ethyl-8-methyl-2,8-diazaspiro-[4,5]-decan-1,3-dion hydrobromide). A potent, specific muscarinic acetylcholine receptor agonist. *Eur. J. Pharmacol.* 125, 45–62. doi: 10.1016/0014-2999(86)90082-8

Palacios, J. M., Mengod, G., Vilaro, M. T., Wiederhold, K. H., Boddeke, H., Alvarez, F. J., et al. (1990). Cholinergic receptors in the rat and human brain: microscopic visualization. *Prog. Brain Res.* 84, 243–253. doi: 10.1016/S0079-6123(08)60909-7

Panza, F., Frisardi, V., Solfrizzi, V., Imbimbo, B. P., Logroscino, G., Santamato, A., et al. (2012). Immunotherapy for Alzheimer's disease: from anti-beta-amyloid to tau-based immunization strategies. *Immunotherapy* 4, 213–238. doi: 10.2217/imt.11.170

Papadopoulos, V., Baraldi, M., Guilarte, T. R., Knudsen, T. B., Lacapere, J. J., Lindemann, P., et al. (2006a). Translocator protein (18kDa): new nomenclature for the peripheral-type benzodiazepine receptor based on its structure and molecular function. *Trends Pharmacol. Sci.* 27, 402–409. doi: 10.1016/j.tips.2006.06.005

Papadopoulos, V., Lecanu, L., Brown, R. C., Han, Z., and Yao, Z. X. (2006b). Peripheral-type benzodiazepine receptor in neurosteroid biosynthesis, neuropathology and neurological disorders. *Neuroscience* 138, 749–756. doi: 10.1016/j.neuroscience.2005.05.063

Pappata, S., Varrone, A., Vicidomini, C., Milan, G., De, F. C., Sansone, V., et al. (2010). SPECT imaging of GABA(A)/benzodiazepine receptors and cerebral perfusion in mild cognitive impairment. *Eur. J. Nucl. Med. Mol. Imaging* 37, 1156–1163. doi: 10.1007/s00259-010-1409-1

Passchier, J., Gee, A., Willemsen, A., Vaalburg, W., and van, W. A. (2002). Measuring drug-related receptor occupancy with positron emission tomography. *Methods* 27, 278–286. doi: 10.1016/S1046-2023(02)00084-1

Paterson, D., and Nordberg, A. (2000). Neuronal nicotinic receptors in the human brain. *Prog. Neurobiol.* 61, 75–111. doi: 10.1016/S0301-0082(99)00045-3

Paterson, L. M., Kornum, B. R., Nutt, D. J., Pike, V. W., and Knudsen, G. M. (2013). 5-HT radioligands for human brain imaging with PET and SPECT. *Med. Res. Rev.* 33, 54–111. doi: 10.1002/med.20245

Peralta, E. G., Ashkenazi, A., Winslow, J. W., Smith, D. H., Ramachandran, J., and Capon, D. J. (1987). Distinct primary structures, ligand-binding properties and tissue-specific expression of four human muscarinic acetylcholine receptors. *EMBO J.* 6, 3923–3929.

Piggott, M., Owens, J., O'Brien, J., Paling, S., Wyper, D., Fenwick, J., et al. (2002). Comparative distribution of binding of the muscarinic receptor ligands pirenzepine, AF-DX 384, (R,R)-I-QNB and (R,S)-I-QNB to human brain. *J. Chem. Neuroanat.* 24, 211–223. doi: 10.1016/S0891-0618(02)00066-2

Piggott, M. A., Ballard, C. G., Rowan, E., Holmes, C., McKeith, I. G., Jaros, E., et al. (2007). Selective loss of dopamine D2 receptors in temporal cortex in dementia with Lewy bodies, association with cognitive decline. *Synapse* 61, 903–911. doi: 10.1002/syn.20441

Piggott, M. A., Marshall, E. F., Thomas, N., Lloyd, S., Court, J. A., Jaros, E., et al. (1999). Striatal dopaminergic markers in dementia with Lewy bodies, Alzheimer's and Parkinson's diseases: rostrocaudal distribution. *Brain* 122(Pt 8), 1449–1468. doi: 10.1093/brain/122.8.1449

Pimlott, S. L., Piggott, M., Owens, J., Greally, E., Court, J. A., Jaros, E., et al. (2004). Nicotinic acetylcholine receptor distribution in Alzheimer's disease, dementia with Lewy bodies, Parkinson's disease, and vascular dementia: in vitro binding study using 5-[(125)i]-a-85380. *Neuropsychopharmacology* 29, 108–116. doi: 10.1038/sj.npp.1300302

Pizzolato, G., Chierichetti, F., Fabbri, M., Cagnin, A., Dam, M., Ferlin, G., et al. (1996). Reduced striatal dopamine receptors in Alzheimer's disease: single photon emission tomography study with the D2 tracer [123I]-IBZM. *Neurology* 47, 1065–1068. doi: 10.1212/WNL.47.4.1065

Polidori, M. C., and Nelles, G. (2014). Antioxidant clinical trials in mild cognitive impairment and Alzheimer's disease - challenges and perspectives. *Curr. Pharm. Des.* 20, 3083–3092. doi: 10.2174/13816128113196660706

Portet, F., Scarmeas, N., Cosentino, S., Helzner, E. P., and Stern, Y. (2009). Extrapyramidal signs before and after diagnosis of incident Alzheimer disease in a prospective population study. *Arch. Neurol.* 66, 1120–1126. doi: 10.1001/archneurol.2009.196

Potter, A., Corwin, J., Lang, J., Piasecki, M., Lenox, R., and Newhouse, P. A. (1999). Acute effects of the selective cholinergic channel activator (nicotinic agonist) ABT-418 in Alzheimer's disease. *Psychopharmacology (Berl.)* 142, 334–342. doi: 10.1007/s002130050897

Procter, A. W., Lowe, S. L., Palmer, A. M., Francis, P. T., Esiri, M. M., Stratmann, G. C., et al. (1988). Topographical distribution of neurochemical changes in Alzheimer's disease. *J. Neurol. Sci.* 84, 125–140. doi: 10.1016/0022-510X(88)90118-9

Puzzo, D., and Arancio, O. (2013). Amyloid-beta peptide: Dr. Jekyll or Mr. Hyde? *J. Alzheimers Dis.* 33(Suppl. 1), S111–S120.

Pym, L., Kemp, M., Raymond-Delpech, V., Buckingham, S., Boyd, C. A., and Sattelle, D. (2005). Subtype-specific actions of beta-amyloid peptides on recombinant human neuronal nicotinic acetylcholine receptors (alpha7, alpha4beta2, alpha3beta4) expressed in *Xenopus laevis* oocytes. *Br. J. Pharmacol.* 146, 964–971. doi: 10.1038/sj.bjp.0706403

Qosa, H., Batarseh, Y. S., Mohyeldin, M. M., El Sayed, K. A., Keller, J. N., and Kaddoumi, A. (2015). Oleocanthal enhances amyloid-beta clearance from the brains of TgSwDI mice and in vitro across a human blood-brain barrier model. *ACS Chem. Neurosci.* 6, 1849–1859. doi: 10.1021/acschemneuro.5b00190

Rabinovici, G. D., Furst, A. J., O'Neil, J. P., Racine, C. A., Mormino, E. C., Baker, S. L., et al. (2007). 11C-PIB PET imaging in Alzheimer disease and frontotemporal lobar degeneration. *Neurology* 68, 1205–1212. doi: 10.1212/01.wnl.0000259035.98480.ed

Rabinovici, G. D., Jagust, W. J., Furst, A. J., Ogar, J. M., Racine, C. A., Mormino, E. C., et al. (2008). Abeta amyloid and glucose metabolism in three variants of primary progressive aphasia. *Ann. Neurol.* 64, 388–401. doi: 10.1002/ana.21451

Rafii, M. S., Walsh, S., Little, J. T., Behan, K., Reynolds, B., Ward, C., et al. (2011). A phase II trial of huperzine A in mild to moderate Alzheimer disease. *Neurology* 76, 1389–1394. doi: 10.1212/WNL.0b013e318216eb7b

Rahmim, A., and Zaidi, H. (2008). PET versus SPECT: strengths, limitations and challenges. *Nucl. Med. Commun.* 29, 193–207. doi: 10.1097/MNM.0b013e3282f3a515

Ramirez, M. J., Lai, M. K., Tordera, R. M., and Francis, P. T. (2014). Serotonergic therapies for cognitive symptoms in Alzheimer's disease: rationale and current status. *Drugs* 74, 729–736. doi: 10.1007/s40265-014-02175

Raskind, M. A., Peskind, E. R., Wessel, T., and Yuan, W. (2000). Galantamine in AD: a 6-month randomized, placebo-controlled trial with a 6-month extension. The Galantamine USA-1 Study Group. *Neurology* 54, 2261–2268. doi: 10.1212/WNL.54.12.2261

Ravasi, L., Tokugawa, J., Nakayama, T., Seidel, J., Sokoloff, L., Eckelman, W. C., et al. (2012). Imaging of the muscarinic acetylcholine neuroreceptor in rats with the M2 selective agonist [18F]FP-TZTP. *Nucl. Med. Biol.* 39, 45–55. doi: 10.1016/j.nucmedbio.2011.06.003

Reddy, P. H., and Beal, M. F. (2008). Amyloid beta, mitochondrial dysfunction and synaptic damage: implications for cognitive decline in aging and Alzheimer's disease. *Trends Mol. Med.* 14, 45–53. doi: 10.1016/j.molmed.2007.12.002

Reeves, S., Brown, R., Howard, R., and Grasby, P. (2009). Increased striatal dopamine (D2/D3) receptor availability and delusions in Alzheimer disease. *Neurology* 72, 528–534. doi: 10.1212/01.wnl.0000341932.21961.f3

Riederer, P., Danielczyk, W., and Grunblatt, E. (2004). Monoamine oxidase-B inhibition in Alzheimer's disease. *Neurotoxicology* 25, 271–277. doi: 10.1016/S0161-813X(03)001062

Riederer, P., Youdim, M. B., Rausch, W. D., Birkmayer, W., Jellinger, K., and Seemann, D. (1978). On the mode of action of L-deprenyl in the human central nervous system. *J. Neural Transm.* 43, 217–226. doi: 10.1007/BF01246958

Rigacci, S. (2015). Olive oil phenols as promising multi-targeting agents against Alzheimer's disease. *Adv. Exp. Med. Biol.* 863, 1–20. doi: 10.1007/978-3-319-18365-7_1

Rinne, J. O., Sahlberg, N., Ruottinen, H., Nagren, K., and Lehikoinen, P. (1998). Striatal uptake of the dopamine reuptake ligand [11C]beta-CFT is reduced in Alzheimer's disease assessed by positron emission tomography. *Neurology* 50, 152–156. doi: 10.1212/WNL.50.1.152

Rishton, G. M. (2008). Aggregator compounds confound amyloid fibrillization assay. *Nat. Chem. Biol.* 4, 159–160. doi: 10.1038/nchembio0308-159

Rissman, R. A., De Blas, A. L., and Armstrong, D. M. (2007). GABA(A) receptors in aging and Alzheimer's disease. *J. Neurochem.* 103, 1285–1292. doi: 10.1111/j.1471-4159.2007.04832.x

Roberds, S. L., Anderson, J., Basi, G., Bienkowski, M. J., Branstetter, D. G., Chen, K. S., et al. (2001). BACE knockout mice are healthy despite lacking the primary beta-secretase activity in brain: implications for Alzheimer's disease therapeutics. *Hum. Mol. Genet.* 10, 1317–1324. doi: 10.1093/hmg/10.12.1317

Robert, P. H., and Benoit, M. (2008). Neurochemistry of cognition: serotonergic and adrenergic mechanisms. *Handb. Clin. Neurol.* 88, 31–40. doi: 10.1016/S0072-9752(07)88002-X

Rodriguez, J. J., Noristani, H. N., and Verkhratsky, A. (2012). The serotonergic system in ageing and Alzheimer's disease. *Prog. Neurobiol.* 99, 15–41. doi: 10.1016/j.pneurobio.2012.06.010

Rodríguez-Puertas, R., Pascual, J., Vilaro, T., and Pazos, A. (1997). Autoradiographic distribution of M1, M2, M3, and M4 muscarinic receptor subtypes in Alzheimer's disease. *Synapse* 26, 341–350. doi: 10.1002/(SICI)1098-2396(199708)26:4<341::AID-SYN2>3.0.CO;2-6

Romano, M., and Buratti, E. (2013). Florbetapir F 18 for brain imaging of beta-amyloid plaques. *Drugs Today (Barc.)* 49, 181–193. doi: 10.1358/dot.2013.49.3.1937428

Rosler, M., Anand, R., Cicin-Sain, A., Gauthier, S., Agid, Y., Dal-Bianco, P., et al. (1999). Efficacy and safety of rivastigmine in patients with Alzheimer's disease: international randomised controlled trial. *BMJ* 318, 633–638. doi: 10.1136/bmj.318.7184.633

Rowe, C. C., Ackerman, U., Browne, W., Mulligan, R., Pike, K. L., O'Keefe, G., et al. (2008). Imaging of amyloid beta in Alzheimer's disease with 18F-BAY94-9172, a novel PET tracer: proof of mechanism. *Lancet Neurol.* 7, 129–135. doi: 10.1016/S1474-4422(08)70001-2

Rowe, C. C., Ng, S., Ackermann, U., Gong, S. J., Pike, K., Savage, G., et al. (2007). Imaging beta-amyloid burden in aging and dementia. *Neurology* 68, 1718–1725. doi: 10.1212/01.wnl.0000261919.22630.ea

Rowe, C. C., Pejoska, S., Mulligan, R. S., Jones, G., Chan, J. G., Svensson, S., et al. (2013). Head-to-head comparison of 11C-PiB and 18F-AZD4694 (NAV4694) for beta-amyloid imaging in aging and dementia. *J. Nucl. Med.* 54, 880–886. doi: 10.2967/jnumed.112.114785

Rowe, C. C., and Villemagne, V. L. (2013). Brain amyloid imaging. *J. Nucl. Med. Technol.* 41, 11–18. doi: 10.2967/jnumed.110.076315

Rudolph, U., and Mohler, H. (2006). GABA-based therapeutic approaches: GABAA receptor subtype functions. *Curr. Opin. Pharmacol.* 6, 18–23. doi: 10.1016/j.coph.2005.10.003

Rupprecht, R., Rammes, G., Eser, D., Baghai, T. C., Schule, C., Nothdurfter, C., et al. (2009). Translocator protein (18 kD) as target for anxiolytics without benzodiazepine-like side effects. *Science* 325, 490–493. doi: 10.1126/science.1175055

Sabbagh, M. N. (2009). Drug development for Alzheimer's disease: where are we now and where are we headed? *Am. J. Geriatr. Pharmacother.* 7, 167–185. doi: 10.1016/j.amjopharm.2009.06.003

Sabri, O., Kendziorra, K., Wolf, H., Gertz, H. J., and Brust, P. (2008). Acetylcholine receptors in dementia and mild cognitive impairment. *Eur. J. Nucl. Med. Mol. Imaging* 35(Suppl. 1), S30–S45. doi: 10.1007/s00259-007-0701-1

Sadigh-Eteghad, S., Majdi, A., Farhoudi, M., Talebi, M., and Mahmoudi, J. (2014). Different patterns of brain activation in normal aging and Alzheimer's disease from cognitional sight: meta analysis using activation likelihood estimation. *J. Neurol. Sci.* 343, 159–166. doi: 10.1016/j.jns.2014.05.066

Santa-Maria, I., Hernandez, F., Del, R. J., Moreno, F. J., and Avila, J. (2007). Tramiprosate, a drug of potential interest for the treatment of Alzheimer's disease, promotes an abnormal aggregation of tau. *Mol. Neurodegener.* 2:17. doi: 10.1186/1750-1326-2-17

Santhosh, L., Estok, K. M., Vogel, R. S., Tamagnan, G. D., Baldwin, R. M., Mitsis, E. M., et al. (2009). Regional distribution and behavioral correlates of 5-HT(2A) receptors in Alzheimer's disease with [(18)F]deuteroaltanserin and PET. *Psychiatry Res.* 173, 212–217. doi: 10.1016/j.pscychresns.2009.03.007

Saulin, A., Savli, M., and Lanzenberger, R. (2012). Serotonin and molecular neuroimaging in humans using PET. *Amino Acids* 42, 2039–2057. doi: 10.1007/s00726-011-10789

Saura, J., Luque, J. M., Cesura, A. M., Da, P. M., Chan-Palay, V., Huber, G., et al. (1994). Increased monoamine oxidase B activity in plaque-associated astrocytes of Alzheimer brains revealed by quantitative enzyme radioautography. *Neuroscience* 62, 15–30. doi: 10.1016/0306-4522(94)90311-5

Savic, I., Persson, A., Roland, P., Pauli, S., Sedvall, G., and Widen, L. (1988). In-vivo demonstration of reduced benzodiazepine receptor binding in human epileptic foci. *Lancet* 2, 863–866. doi: 10.1016/S0140-6736(88)92468-3

Savonenko, A., Xu, G. M., Melnikova, T., Morton, J. L., Gonzales, V., Wong, M. P., et al. (2005). Episodic-like memory deficits in the APPswe/PS1dE9 mouse model of Alzheimer's disease: relationships to beta-amyloid deposition and neurotransmitter abnormalities. *Neurobiol. Dis.* 18, 602–617. doi: 10.1016/j.nbd.2004.10.022

Schenk, D., Barbour, R., Dunn, W., Gordon, G., Grajeda, H., Guido, T., et al. (1999). Immunization with amyloid-beta attenuates Alzheimer-disease-like pathology in the PDAPP mouse. *Nature* 400, 173–177. doi: 10.1038/22124

Selkoe, D. J. (2001). Alzheimer's disease: genes, proteins, and therapy. *Physiol. Rev.* 81, 741–766.

Shah, M., and Catafau, A. M. (2014). Molecular imaging insights into neurodegeneration: focus on tau PET radiotracers. *J. Nucl. Med.* 55, 871–874. doi: 10.2967/jnumed.113.136069

Shinotoh, H., Aotsuka, A., Fukushi, K., Nagatsuka, S., Tanaka, N., Ota, T., et al. (2001). Effect of donepezil on brain acetylcholinesterase activity in patients with AD measured by PET. *Neurology* 56, 408–410. doi: 10.1212/WNL.56.3.408

Shinotoh, H., Fukushi, K., Nagatsuka, S., and Irie, T. (2004). Acetylcholinesterase imaging: its use in therapy evaluation and drug design. *Curr. Pharm. Des.* 10, 1505–1517. doi: 10.2174/1381612043384763

Shugart, J. (2016). *Rare but Severe Side Effects Sideline Some Phase 3 Encenicline Trials. Alzforum.* Available at: http://www.alzforum.org/news/research-news/rare-severe-side-effects-sideline-some-phase-3-encenicline-trials5-2-2016

Small, G. W., Kepe, V., Ercoli, L. M., Siddarth, P., Bookheimer, S. Y., Miller, K. J., et al. (2006). PET of brain amyloid and tau in mild cognitive impairment. *N. Engl. J. Med.* 355, 2652–2663. doi: 10.1056/NEJMoa054625

Small, G. W., Kepe, V., Siddarth, P., Ercoli, L. M., Merrill, D. A., Donoghue, N., et al. (2013). PET scanning of brain tau in retired national football league players: preliminary findings. *Am. J. Geriatr. Psychiatry* 21, 138–144. doi: 10.1016/j.jagp.2012.11.019

Snaedal, J., Johannesson, T., Jonsson, J. E., and Gylfadottir, G. (1996). The effects of nicotine in dermal plaster on cognitive functions in patients with Alzheimer's disease. *Dementia* 7, 47–52.

Sonsalla, P. K., and Golbe, L. I. (1988). Deprenyl as prophylaxis against Parkinson's disease? *Clin. Neuropharmacol.* 11, 500Ǔ511.

Soricelli, A., Postiglione, A., Grivet-Fojaja, M. R., Mainenti, P. P., Discepolo, A., Varrone, A., et al. (1996). Reduced cortical distribution volume of iodine-123 iomazenil in Alzheimer's disease as a measure of loss of synapses. *Eur. J. Nucl. Med.* 23, 1323–1328. doi: 10.1007/BF01367587

Sparks, D. L., Woeltz, V. M., and Markesbery, W. R. (1991). Alterations in brain monoamine oxidase activity in aging, Alzheimer's disease, and Pick's disease. *Arch. Neurol.* 48, 718–721. doi: 10.1001/archneur.1991.00530190064017

Spehl, T. S., Frings, L., Hellwig, S., Weiller, C., Hull, M., Meyer, P. T., et al. (2015). Role of semiquantitative assessment of regional binding potential in 123I-FP-CIT SPECT for the differentiation of frontotemporal dementia, dementia with Lewy bodies, and Alzheimer's dementia. *Clin. Nucl. Med.* 40, e27–e33. doi: 10.1097/RLU.0000000000000554

Spencer, B., and Masliah, E. (2014). Immunotherapy for Alzheimer's disease: past, present and future. *Front. Aging Neurosci.* 6:114. doi: 10.3389/fnagi.2014.00114

Stefaniak, J., and O'Brien, J. (2016). Imaging of neuroinflammation in dementia: a review. *J. Neurol. Neurosurg. Psychiatry* 87, 21–28. doi: 10.1136/jnnp-2015-311336

Storga, D., Vrecko, K., Birkmayer, J. G., and Reibnegger, G. (1996). Monoaminergic neurotransmitters, their precursors and metabolites in brains of Alzheimer patients. *Neurosci. Lett.* 203, 29–32. doi: 10.1016/0304-3940(95)12256-7

Streit, W. J. (2010). Microglial activation and neuroinflammation in Alzheimer's disease: a critical examination of recent history. *Front. Aging Neurosci.* 2:22. doi: 10.3389/fnagi.2010.00022

Strolin, B. M., and Dostert, P. (1989). Monoamine oxidase, brain ageing and degenerative diseases. *Biochem. Pharmacol.* 38, 555–561. doi: 10.1016/0006-2952(89)90198-6

Sunderland, T., Weingartner, H., Cohen, R. M., Tariot, P. N., Newhouse, P. A., Thompson, K. E., et al. (1989). Low-dose oral lorazepam administration in Alzheimer subjects and age-matched controls. *Psychopharmacology (Berl.)* 99, 129–133. doi: 10.1007/BF00634466

Syvanen, S., and Eriksson, J. (2013). Advances in PET imaging of P-glycoprotein function at the blood-brain barrier. *ACS Chem. Neurosci.* 4, 225–237. doi: 10.1021/cn3001729

Tanaka, Y., Meguro, K., Yamaguchi, S., Ishii, H., Watanuki, S., Funaki, Y., et al. (2003). Decreased striatal D2 receptor density associated with severe behavioral abnormality in Alzheimer's disease. *Ann. Nucl. Med.* 17, 567–573. doi: 10.1007/BF03006670

Tandon, R., Shipley, J. E., Greden, J. F., Mann, N. A., Eisner, W. H., and Goodson, J. A. (1991). Muscarinic cholinergic hyperactivity in schizophrenia. Relationship to positive and negative symptoms. *Schizophr. Res.* 4, 23–30. doi: 10.1016/0920-9964(91)90006-D

Tariot, P. N., and Aisen, P. S. (2009). Can lithium or valproate untie tangles in Alzheimer's disease? *J. Clin. Psychiatry* 70, 919–921. doi: 10.4088/JCP.09com05331

Tariot, P. N., Schneider, L. S., Cummings, J., Thomas, R. G., Raman, R., Jakimovich, L. J., et al. (2011). Chronic divalproex sodium to attenuate agitation and clinical progression of Alzheimer disease. *Arch. Gen. Psychiatry* 68, 853–861. doi: 10.1001/archgenpsychiatry.2011.72

Tariot, P. N., Solomon, P. R., Morris, J. C., Kershaw, P., Lilienfeld, S., and Ding, C. (2000). A 5-month, randomized, placebo-controlled trial of galantamine in AD. The Galantamine USA-10 Study Group. *Neurology* 54, 2269–2276. doi: 10.1212/WNL.54.12.2269

Tavitian, B., Pappata, S., Bonnot-Lours, S., Prenant, C., Jobert, A., Crouzel, C., et al. (1993). Positron emission tomography study of [11C]methyl-tetrahydroaminoacridine (methyl-tacrine) in baboon brain. *Eur. J. Pharmacol.* 236, 229–238. doi: 10.1016/0014-2999(93)90593-7

Terry, A. V. Jr., and Buccafusco, J. J. (2003). The cholinergic hypothesis of age and Alzheimer's disease-related cognitive deficits: recent challenges and their implications for novel drug development. *J. Pharmacol. Exp. Ther.* 306, 821–827. doi: 10.1124/jpet.102.041616

Thies, W., and Bleiler, L. (2013). 2013 Alzheimer's disease facts and figures. *Alzheimers Dement.* 9, 208–245. doi: 10.1016/j.jalz.2013.02.003

Thomas, T. (2000). Monoamine oxidase-B inhibitors in the treatment of Alzheimer's disease. *Neurobiol. Aging* 21, 343–348. doi: 10.1016/S0197-4580(00)00100-7

Tolboom, N., van der Flier, W. M., Yaqub, M., Boellaard, R., Verwey, N. A., Blankenstein, M. A., et al. (2009). Relationship of cerebrospinal fluid markers to 11C-PiB and 18F-FDDNP binding. *J. Nucl. Med.* 50, 1464–1470. doi: 10.2967/jnumed.109.064360

Tomasi, G., Turkheimer, F., and Aboagye, E. (2012). Importance of quantification for the analysis of PET data in oncology: review of current methods and trends for the future. *Mol. Imaging Biol.* 14, 131–146. doi: 10.1007/s11307-011-05142

Toyohara, J., Wu, J., and Hashimoto, K. (2010). Recent development of radioligands for imaging alpha7 nicotinic acetylcholine receptors in the brain. *Curr. Top. Med. Chem.* 10, 1544–1557. doi: 10.2174/156802610793176828

Trillo, L., Das, D., Hsieh, W., Medina, B., Moghadam, S., Lin, B., et al. (2013). Ascending monoaminergic systems alterations in Alzheimer's disease. translating basic science into clinical care. *Neurosci. Biobehav. Rev.* 37, 1363–1379. doi: 10.1016/j.neubiorev.2013.05.008

Trollor, J. N., Sachdev, P. S., Haindl, W., Brodaty, H., Wen, W., and Walker, B. M. (2006). Combined cerebral blood flow effects of a cholinergic agonist (milameline) and a verbal recognition task in early Alzheimer's disease. *Psychiatry Clin. Neurosci.* 60, 616–625. doi: 10.1111/j.1440-1819.2006.01567.x

Truchot, L., Costes, N., Zimmer, L., Laurent, B., Le, B. D., Thomas-Anterion, C., et al. (2008). A distinct [18F]MPPF PET profile in amnestic mild cognitive impairment compared to mild Alzheimer's disease. *Neuroimage* 40, 1251–1256. doi: 10.1016/j.neuroimage.2008.01.030

Tsang, S. W., Keene, J., Hope, T., Spence, I., Francis, P. T., Wong, P. T., et al. (2010). A serotoninergic basis for hyperphagic eating changes in Alzheimer's disease. *J. Neurol. Sci.* 288, 151–155. doi: 10.1016/j.jns.2009.08.066

Tsang, S. W., Lai, M. K., Kirvell, S., Francis, P. T., Esiri, M. M., Hope, T., et al. (2006). Impaired coupling of muscarinic M1 receptors to G-proteins in the neocortex is associated with severity of dementia in Alzheimer's disease. *Neurobiol. Aging* 27, 1216–1223. doi: 10.1016/j.neurobiolaging.2005.07.010

Tyrrell, P. J., Sawle, G. V., Ibanez, V., Bloomfield, P. M., Leenders, K. L., Frackowiak, R. S., et al. (1990). Clinical and positron emission tomographic studies in the 'extrapyramidal syndrome' of dementia of the Alzheimer type. *Arch. Neurol.* 47, 1318–1323. doi: 10.1001/archneur.1990.00530120062011

Valles, A. S., and Barrantes, F. J. (2012). Chaperoning alpha7 neuronal nicotinic acetylcholine receptors. *Biochim. Biophys. Acta* 1818, 718–729. doi: 10.1016/j.bbamem.2011.10.012

Vandenberghe, R., Adamczuk, K., and Van, L. K. (2013). The interest of amyloid PET imaging in the diagnosis of Alzheimer's disease. *Curr. Opin. Neurol.* 26, 646–655. doi: 10.1097/WCO.0000000000000036

Vandenberghe, R., Van, L. K., Ivanoiu, A., Salmon, E., Bastin, C., Triau, E., et al. (2010). 18F-flutemetamol amyloid imaging in Alzheimer disease and mild cognitive impairment: a phase 2 trial. *Ann. Neurol.* 68, 319–329. doi: 10.1002/ana.22068

Varley, J., Brooks, D. J., and Edison, P. (2015). Imaging neuroinflammation in Alzheimer's disease and other dementias: recent advances and future directions. *Alzheimers Dement.* 11, 1110–1120. doi: 10.1016/j.jalz.2014.08.105

Venigalla, M., Gyengesi, E., Sharman, M. J., and Munch, G. (2015). Novel promising therapeutics against chronic neuroinflammation and neurodegeneration in Alzheimer's disease. *Neurochem. Int.* doi: 10.1016/j.neuint.2015.10.011 [Epub ahead of print].

Venneti, S., Lopresti, B. J., and Wiley, C. A. (2006). The peripheral benzodiazepine receptor (Translocator protein 18kDa) in microglia: from pathology to imaging. *Prog. Neurobiol.* 80, 308–322. doi: 10.1016/j.pneurobio.2006.10.002

Versijpt, J., Van Laere, K. J., Dumont, F., Decoo, D., Vandecapelle, M., Santens, P., et al. (2003). Imaging of the 5-HT2A system: age-, gender-, and Alzheimer's disease-related findings. *Neurobiol. Aging* 24, 553–561. doi: 10.1016/S0197-4580(02)00137-9

Vertes, R. P. (1991). A PHA-L analysis of ascending projections of the dorsal raphe nucleus in the rat. *J. Comp Neurol.* 313, 643–668. doi: 10.1002/cne.903130409

Vertes, R. P., Fortin, W. J., and Crane, A. M. (1999). Projections of the median raphe nucleus in the rat. *J. Comp Neurol.* 407, 555–582. doi: 10.1002/(SICI)1096-9861(19990517)407:4<555::AID-CNE7>3.0.CO;2-E

Villemagne, V. L., Fodero-Tavoletti, M. T., Masters, C. L., and Rowe, C. C. (2015). Tau imaging: early progress and future directions. *Lancet Neurol.* 14, 114–124. doi: 10.1016/S1474-4422(14)702522

Villemagne, V. L., Furumoto, S., Fodero-Tavoletti, M. T., Mulligan, R. S., Hodges, J., Harada, R., et al. (2014). In vivo evaluation of a novel tau imaging tracer for Alzheimer's disease. *Eur. J. Nucl. Med. Mol. Imaging* 41, 816–826. doi: 10.1007/s00259-013-2681-7

Villemagne, V. L., Ong, K., Mulligan, R. S., Holl, G., Pejoska, S., Jones, G., et al. (2011). Amyloid imaging with (18)F-florbetaben in Alzheimer disease and other dementias. *J. Nucl. Med.* 52, 1210–1217. doi: 10.2967/jnumed.111.089730

Villemagne, V. L., Pike, K. E., Darby, D., Maruff, P., Savage, G., Ng, S., et al. (2008). Abeta deposits in older non-demented individuals with cognitive decline are indicative of preclinical Alzheimer's disease. *Neuropsychologia* 46, 1688–1697. doi: 10.1016/j.neuropsychologia.2008.02.008

Vogels, O. J., Broere, C. A., ter Laak, H. J., ten Donkelaar, H. J., Nieuwenhuys, R., and Schulte, B. P. (1990). Cell loss and shrinkage in the nucleus basalis Meynert complex in Alzheimer's disease. *Neurobiol. Aging* 11, 3–13. doi: 10.1016/0197-4580(90)90056-6

Wallin, A. K., Blennow, K., Andreasen, N., and Minthon, L. (2006). CSF biomarkers for Alzheimer's disease: levels of beta-amyloid, tau, phosphorylated tau relate to clinical symptoms and survival. *Dement. Geriatr. Cogn Disord.* 21, 131–138. doi: 10.1159/000090631

Weigand, S. D., Vemuri, P., Wiste, H. J., Senjem, M. L., Pankratz, V. S., Aisen, P. S., et al. (2011). Transforming cerebrospinal fluid Abeta42 measures into calculated Pittsburgh Compound B units of brain Abeta amyloid. *Alzheimers. Dement.* 7, 133–141. doi: 10.1016/j.jalz.2010.08.230

Weinberger, D. R., Gibson, R., Coppola, R., Jones, D. W., Molchan, S., Sunderland, T., et al. (1991). The distribution of cerebral muscarinic acetylcholine receptors in vivo in patients with dementia. A controlled study with 123IQNB and single photon emission computed tomography. *Arch. Neurol.* 48, 169–176. doi: 10.1001/archneur.1991.00530140061018

Weiner, M. W., Veitch, D. P., Aisen, P. S., Beckett, L. A., Cairns, N. J., Cedarbaum, J., et al. (2015). Impact of the Alzheimer's disease Neuroimaging Initiative, 2004 to 2014. *Alzheimers. Dement.* 11, 865–884. doi: 10.1016/j.jalz.2015.04.005

Weingarten, M. D., Lockwood, A. H., Hwo, S. Y., and Kirschner, M. W. (1975). A protein factor essential for microtubule assembly. *Proc. Natl. Acad. Sci. U.S.A.* 72, 1858–1862. doi: 10.1073/pnas.72.5.1858

Weinreb, O., Amit, T., Bar-Am, O., and Youdim, M. B. (2010). Rasagiline: a novel anti-Parkinsonian monoamine oxidase-B inhibitor with neuroprotective activity. *Prog. Neurobiol.* 92, 330–344. doi: 10.1016/j.pneurobio.2010.06.008

Wevers, A., and Schroder, H. (1999). Nicotinic acetylcholine receptors in Alzheimer's disease. *J. Alzheimers Dis.* 1, 207–219.

White, H. K., and Levin, E. D. (1999). Four-week nicotine skin patch treatment effects on cognitive performance in Alzheimer's disease. *Psychopharmacology (Berl.)* 143, 158–165. doi: 10.1007/s002130050931

Wilcock, G. K., Lilienfeld, S., and Gaens, E. (2000). Efficacy and safety of galantamine in patients with mild to moderate Alzheimer's disease: multicentre randomised controlled trial. Galantamine International-1 Study Group. *BMJ* 321, 1445–1449.

Wilson, A. L., Langley, L. K., Monley, J., Bauer, T., Rottunda, S., McFalls, E., et al. (1995). Nicotine patches in Alzheimer's disease: pilot study on learning, memory, and safety. *Pharmacol. Biochem. Behav.* 51, 509–514. doi: 10.1016/0091-3057(95)00043-V

Winblad, B., Engedal, K., Soininen, H., Verhey, F., Waldemar, G., Wimo, A., et al. (2001). A 1-year, randomized, placebo-controlled study of donepezil in patients with mild to moderate AD. *Neurology* 57, 489–495. doi: 10.1212/WNL.57.3.489

Winblad, B., Giacobini, E., Frolich, L., Friedhoff, L. T., Bruinsma, G., Becker, R. E., et al. (2010). Phenserine efficacy in Alzheimer's disease. *J. Alzheimers Dis.* 22, 1201–1208. doi: 10.3233/JAD-2010-101311

Wischik, C. M., Harrington, C. R., and Storey, J. M. (2014). Tau-aggregation inhibitor therapy for Alzheimer's disease. *Biochem. Pharmacol.* 88, 529–539. doi: 10.1016/j.bcp.2013.12.008

Wischik, C. M., Staff, R. T., Wischik, D. J., Bentham, P., Murray, A. D., Storey, J. M., et al. (2015). Tau aggregation inhibitor therapy: an exploratory phase 2 study in mild or moderate Alzheimer's disease. *J. Alzheimers. Dis.* 44, 705–720. doi: 10.3233/JAD-142874

Wolf, B. A., Wertkin, A. M., Jolly, Y. C., Yasuda, R. P., Wolfe, B. B., Konrad, R. J., et al. (1995). Muscarinic regulation of Alzheimer's disease amyloid precursor protein secretion and amyloid beta-protein production in human neuronal NT2N cells. *J. Biol. Chem.* 270, 4916–4922. doi: 10.1074/jbc.270.9.4916

Wu, T. Y., Chen, C. P., and Jinn, T. R. (2010). Alzheimer's disease: aging, insomnia and epigenetics. *Taiwan. J. Obstet. Gynecol.* 49, 468–472. doi: 10.1016/S1028-4559(10)60099-X

Wurtman, R. (2015). Biomarkers in the diagnosis and management of Alzheimer's disease. *Metabolism* 64, S47–S50. doi: 10.1016/j.metabol.2014.10.034

Wyper, D. J., Brown, D., Patterson, J., Owens, J., Hunter, R., Teasdale, E., et al. (1993). Deficits in iodine-labelled 3-quinuclidinyl benzilate binding in relation to cerebral blood flow in patients with Alzheimer's disease. *Eur. J. Nucl. Med.* 20, 379–386. doi: 10.1007/BF00208995

Xia, C. F., Arteaga, J., Chen, G., Gangadharmath, U., Gomez, L. F., Kasi, D., et al. (2013). [(18)F]T807, a novel tau positron emission tomography imaging agent for Alzheimer's disease. *Alzheimers Dement.* 9, 666–676. doi: 10.1016/j.jalz.2012.11.008

Xie, G., Gunn, R. N., Dagher, A., Daloze, T., Plourde, G., Backman, S. B., et al. (2004). PET quantification of muscarinic cholinergic receptors with [N-11C-methyl]-benztropine and application to studies of propofol-induced unconsciousness in healthy human volunteers. *Synapse* 51, 91–101. doi: 10.1002/syn.10292

Xu, Y., Yan, J., Zhou, P., Li, J., Gao, H., Xia, Y., et al. (2012). Neurotransmitter receptors and cognitive dysfunction in Alzheimer's disease and Parkinson's disease. *Prog. Neurobiol.* 97, 1–13. doi: 10.1016/j.pneurobio.2012.02.002

Yamada, M., Lamping, K. G., Duttaroy, A., Zhang, W., Cui, Y., Bymaster, F. P., et al. (2001). Cholinergic dilation of cerebral blood vessels is abolished in M(5) muscarinic acetylcholine receptor knockout mice. *Proc. Natl. Acad. Sci. U.S.A.* 98, 14096–14101. doi: 10.1073/pnas.251542998

Yang, L., Rieves, D., and Ganley, C. (2012). Brain amyloid imaging–FDA approval of florbetapir F18 injection. *N. Engl. J. Med.* 367, 885–887. doi: 10.1056/NEJMp1208061

Yiannopoulou, K. G., and Papageorgiou, S. G. (2013). Current and future treatments for Alzheimer's disease. *Ther. Adv. Neurol. Disord.* 6, 19–33. doi: 10.1177/1756285612461679

Youdim, M. B. (2013). Multi target neuroprotective and neurorestorative anti-Parkinson and anti-Alzheimer drugs ladostigil and m30 derived from rasagiline. *Exp. Neurobiol.* 22, 1–10. doi: 10.5607/en.2013.22.1.1

Zec, R. F., and Burkett, N. R. (2008). Non-pharmacological and pharmacological treatment of the cognitive and behavioral symptoms of Alzheimer disease. *NeuroRehabilitation* 23, 425–438.

Zhang, W., Arteaga, J., Cashion, D. K., Chen, G., Gangadharmath, U., Gomez, L. F., et al. (2012). A highly selective and specific PET tracer for imaging of tau pathologies. *J. Alzheimers Dis.* 31, 601–612. doi: 10.3233/JAD-2012-120712

Zheng, H., Fridkin, M., and Youdim, M. B. (2012). From antioxidant chelators to site-activated multi-target chelators targeting hypoxia inducing factor, beta-amyloid, acetylcholinesterase and monoamine oxidase A/B. *Mini Rev. Med. Chem.* 12, 364–370. doi: 10.2174/138955712800493898

Zimmer, E. R., Leuzy, A., Gauthier, S., and Rosa-Neto, P. (2014). Developments in tau PET imaging. *Can. J. Neurol. Sci.* 41, 547–553. doi: 10.1017/cjn.2014.15

Zorumski, C. F., and Isenberg, K. E. (1991). Insights into the structure and function of GABA-benzodiazepine receptors: ion channels and psychiatry. *Am. J. Psychiatry* 148, 162–173. doi: 10.1176/ajp.148.2.162

Conflict of Interest Statement: The authors declare that the research was conducted in the absence of any commercial or financial relationships that could be construed as a potential conflict of interest.

3

Cellular Imaging: A Key Phenotypic Screening Strategy for Predictive Toxicology

Jinghai J. Xu *

Merck and Co., Kenilworth, NJ, USA

Incorporating phenotypic screening as a key strategy enhances predictivity and translatability of drug discovery efforts. Cellular imaging serves as a "phenotypic anchor" to identify important toxicologic pathology that encompasses an array of underlying mechanisms, thus provides an effective means to reduce drug development failures due to insufficient safety. This mini-review highlights the latest advances in hepatotoxicity, cardiotoxicity, and genetic toxicity tests that utilized cellular imaging as a screening strategy, and recommends path forward for further improvement.

Keywords: hepatotoxicity, cardiotoxicity, genetic toxicology, cellular imaging, predictive toxicology, discovery toxicology, phenotypic screening

Edited by:
Nicolau Beckmann,
Novartis Institutes for BioMedical
Research, Switzerland

Reviewed by:
Peter James King,
Queen Mary University of London, UK
Mikael Varakun Persson,
H. Lundbeck A/S, Denmark
Paul Hockings,
Antaros Medical, Sweden

*Correspondence:
Jinghai J. Xu,
Merck and Co., 2000 Galloping Hill
Road, Kenilworth, NJ 07033, USA
jinghai_xu@merck.com

Introduction

Modern medicines have saved countless lives. One needs only to trace the discovery of antiretroviral drugs to marvel at its contribution to human health (Broder, 2010). However, new therapies are necessary to address still unmet medical needs while adhering to the timeless adage of "first doing no harm" to patients. Predictive toxicology meets the latter challenge by offering accurate and timely predictions to minimize drug toxicity (Xu and Urban, 2010). It is recognized as a frontier for identifying better medicines in a more cost-effective manner by biopharmaceutical research and regulatory communities (FDA, 2010).

To successfully practice predictive toxicology, one must adopt an integrated approach utilizing innovations from multiple fields of science and engineering. In recent years there is a resurgence of phenotypic screens in drug efficacy discovery (Moffat et al., 2014). Likewise to improve confidence in the translatability of toxicity predictions, one should also incorporate phenotypic screens as a key strategy. This is because the "phenotype" of a specific safety signal can be caused by many underlying mechanisms and pathways, thus a reductionist "one gene/protein/mechanism to one toxicity" approach most likely will not be sufficient. This does not mean that one should revert to simple cell death measurements. Instead, more specific cellular functions that are vital to sustain physiological homeostasis can serve as translational links between non-clinical tests and clinical observations. Among many practical choices of phenotypic screens, cellular imaging technologies can be applied as "phenotypic anchors" to identify the same histopathology that occurs *in vivo*. Cellular imaging encompasses the techniques that allow quantitative detection and measurement of cellular structures and components including organelles and biomolecules ranging from macromolecules to small ions, often aided by automated microscopes, digitized cameras, and image analysis algorithms. Since "seeing is believing," this "phenotype first" approach assures an unbiased study for compounds that affect important cellular homeostasis without exhausting all possible mechanistic tests. Of course, "phenotype first" does not preclude mechanistic investigations to better understand the underlying reason(s) of drug safety findings. Often it is a holistic approach relying on mechanism-informed phenotypic test, coupled with pharmacokinetic and pharmacodynamics (PKPD) modeling that produces the best overall prediction toward clinical outcome.

Hepatic Toxicity Imaging

Hepatic toxicity ranked highest in research priorities among adverse drug reactions in the pharmaceutical industry, and current detection systems remain imperfect especially with regard to idiosyncratic hepatotoxicity (Opar, 2012). Key mechanisms of drug-induced liver injury (DILI) include oxidative stress and/or mitochondrial damage leading to apoptosis or steatosis, and hepatobiliary transporter inhibition leading to cholestasis (Kaplowitz, 2005; Tujios and Fontana, 2011).

Mechanism-informed phenotypic tests using cellular imaging have been developed to encompass these key DILI mechanisms. For example, a panel of fluorescent imaging probes has been applied to measure oxidative stress, mitochondrial function, glutathione content, and hepatocellular lipidosis simultaneously in primary human hepatocytes (Xu et al., 2008). It has demonstrated ~60% sensitivity and ~95% specificity for drugs that have caused idiosyncratic DILI. This hepatocyte imaging assay technology has been successfully applied to both differentiate compounds for the same pharmacologic target (e.g., p38 MAP kinase inhibitors), and study the mechanism of DILI signals observed in the clinic (e.g., Her2 receptor antagonist) (Xu et al., 2011). A similar imaging approach measuring oxidative stress in primary human hepatocytes resulted in 41% sensitivity and 86% specificity, and was shown to have better predictivity than HepG2 cell lines or HepG2 plus hepatic metabolism from the liver S9 fractions (Garside et al., 2013). These studies demonstrated the application of cellular imaging technology to predict DILI, and highlighted the need to enhance test sensitivity by recapitulating additional DILI mechanisms and pathways.

Since inhibition of a panel of hepatobiliary transporters is another known pathway of drug-induced cholestasis (Morgan et al., 2013), cellular imaging was applied to assess transporter functions. The assay utilized quantitative imaging of fluorescent bile acid and its disposition in the bile canaliculi compartment of the hepatocyte cultures (Xu et al., 2011). As protein trafficking and sorting disturbances also play an integral part of intrahepatic cholestasis (Hayashi and Sugiyama, 2013), whole cell systems as opposed to isolated membrane vesicles over-expressing one transporter at a time should continue to play a key role in phenotypic screening of cholestasis-inducing drugs.

Several improvements on these cellular imaging tests should be explored to further enhance accurate prediction of DILI:

1) Long-term: Adopt a longer-term test system that maintains differentiated metabolic functions of human liver. Recently with advancement in iPSC-derived hepatocyte cultures, multi-day testing appeared promising. However, these longer-term models still need to be assessed with more DILI negative drugs to fully assess specificity (Ware et al., 2015).

2) Diversity: Apply more than one human liver origin with defined genetic background to increase test sensitivity toward idiosyncratic DILI. Patient-derived hepatic stem cells that can be differentiated into adult hepatocyte cultures can be interesting models to explore idiosyncratic causes of DILI.

3) Probes: Expand fluorescent imaging probes to include additional bile acid analogs that are substrates of both NTCP and BSEP transporters, in addition to cholyl lysyl fluoresceine which is a more specific substrate for OATP/MRP transporters (de Waart et al., 2010).

4) Inflammatory and multi-cell systems: Explore the role of pro-inflammatory cytokines and/or Kupffer cells for possible synergistic effects in test sensitivity without sacrificing specificity (Cosgrove et al., 2009), and assess the potential benefit of 3D liver chip with controlled microfluidics.

5) Modeling: Mechanism-based PKPD modeling approaches should be applied to integrate any *in vitro* measurements into a holistic *in vivo* prediction (Woodhead et al., 2014). Predictions made by the more complex model should also be compared to simple *in vitro-in vivo* scaling or classification approaches based on exposure multiples or pre-defined safety margins.

Cardiac Toxicity Imaging

Adverse cardiovascular effects ranked highest among safety reasons for delayed approvals or non-approvals by the US Food and Drug Administration (FDA) between 2000 and 2012 (Sacks et al., 2014). Many drugs that prolong the QT interval in electrocardiograms block the delayed rectifier K^+ current (Ikr) by blocking one key ion channel, the hERG channel. However, not all hERG channel blockers cause QT interval prolongation nor translate to the more severe clinical concern, torsade de pointes [TdP, or twisting of the points in electrocardiograms (Vargas, 2010)]. So QT prolongation is a surrogate biomarker that is not very specific to TdP. In addition to TdP there are other mechanisms of cardiotoxicity. Cardiovascular functional abnormalities can also arise through impaired left ventricular function characterized by changes in cardiomyocyte contractility (Doherty et al., 2013). Therefore, a more holistic screening approach is needed. Since 2013, the FDA working with other international research communities have an on-going initiative to develop better preclinical tools to evaluate cardiovascular safety with the ultimate goal of preventing early stage compounds from being unnecessarily discontinued, while still screening out molecules that are either pro-arrhythmic or lead to changes in cardiomyocyte contractility (Sager et al., 2014).

Synchronously beating human cardiomyocytes should be explored as a key phenotypic screening model. Despite some limitations of iPSC-derived cardiomyocytes, they are the future for large-scale functional cardiotoxicity screening models in preclinical drug evaluation (Puppala et al., 2013). This is because there is a virtually unlimited supply of functionally competent cells, and there is the possibility to create cells from defined genetic background thus lending the model amenable to further mechanistic studies. Researchers have studied 131 drugs using iPSC-derived cardiomyocytes, using fast kinetic imaging-based Ca^{2+} flux as continuously cell-beating measurements (Sirenko et al., 2013). Each output (beat rate, peak characteristics, and cell viability) generated as a result of such cellular imaging assay has yielded a panel of imaging "signatures" for understanding the type of pathophysiological effect that a chemical may have on the heart. Not surprisingly, beat rate and several peak shape parameters were found to be better predictors than simple cell viability. In another study, video-based microscopic imaging recapitulated expected drug effects in stem-cell-derived cardiomyocytes without the use of exogenous labels and produced the same beat traces as patch clamp (Maddah et al., 2015). Recently, the throughput and accuracy of iPSC-based model to detect changes in cardiomyocyte contraction was found applicable in drug discovery screening, with a sensitivity and specificity of 87 and 70%, respectively (Pointon et al., 2015).

Tyrosine kinase inhibitors (TKIs) are efficacious against tumors harboring mutations and/or over-expressing such kinases. However, TKIs have been hampered by cardiotoxicity issues detected most frequently as changes in left-ventricular ejection fraction (LVEF), which were not predicted by hERG inhibition *per se*. Using multi-parameter cellular imaging it was demonstrated while crizotinib, sunitinib, and nilotinib disrupted the normal beat pattern of human iPSC-derived cardiomyocytes, erlotinib did not. These alterations in iPSC-cardiomyocyte beat pattern correlated well with known clinical cardiac outcomes of these drugs, demonstrating the potential to use this phenotypic screen as a routine test to identify safer compounds in a class of drug candidates (Doherty et al., 2013).

Several improvements on these cellular imaging screens should be explored to further enhance the overall prediction of cardiotoxicity:

1) beating disturbances by a variety of drugs with different cardiotoxic mechanisms
2) longer-term cellular models to study cardiac hypertrophy
3) drug metabolites by introducing hepatic metabolism (e.g., either hepatic S9 fraction or multi-cell systems)
4) more test qualification with large compound sets consisting of an equal number of positive and negatives that have been rigorously adjudicated. A balanced test set of compounds with more negative or clean compounds is critical to assess test specificity.

Genetic Toxicity Imaging

Carcinogenicity remained a major nonclinical safety finding among FDA non-approvals and delayed approvals between 2000 and 2012 (Sacks et al., 2014). In one of the largest retrospective analyses of pharmaceutical compounds to date, it was demonstrated that significant R&D time, resources, and animal usage can be reduced by relying on the near 100% negative predictive values (NPV) of combined tests evaluating genetic toxicity, hormonal perturbation, and evidence of neoplasia in chronic rat toxicology studies (Sistare et al., 2011). To minimize the impact of carcinogenicity findings in late-stage drug development, both mutational and chromosomal changes need to be evaluated as they can be caused by different underlying mechanisms (FDA, 2012).

Cellular imaging has greatly enhanced the efficiency and accuracy of measuring both mutational and chromosomal changes. The Ames test remains a cost-effective stethoscope to study genetic toxicology (Claxton et al., 2010). In order to enable rapid scoring of mutant bacterial colonies, the Salmonella strains used in the Ames test were engineered to express bioluminescent proteins (Aubrecht et al., 2007). The high-throughput imaging based on automated counting of the number of surviving bioluminescent colonies offered a far more accurate assessment of genotoxicity than bulk biomass measurements (Xu and Aubrecht, 2010).

With regard to chromosomal changes, the *in vitro* micronucleus test is an accepted test by regulatory authorities (EMA and FDA) (FDA, 2012). While traditional micronucleus test relied on manual counting of the number of micronuclei in thousands of cells per treatment sample and hundreds of samples per test compound, cellular imaging has made this task more efficient. The increased throughput and accuracy of computerized analysis of micronuclei frequency enabled rapid structure-activity profiling of drug candidates during lead optimization (Xu and Aubrecht, 2010).

Conclusion

From a systems perspective, since *in vitro* genotoxicity tests have near 100% negative predictive value toward *in vivo* genotoxicity outcome, are among the most cost-effective to operate (i.e., using bacterial strains and mammalian cell lines), and include both general cytotoxicity and cell growth inhibition as integral part of assay readouts, *in vitro* Ames and micronucleus should be employed as the foundational tests to select those "clean" compounds for further R&D investments. In the lead optimization stage of small-molecule drug discovery, these genotoxicity tests should be followed by cardiac and hepatic toxicity screening using primary cells or iPSCs next, then other organ-specific tests on an *ad hoc* basis last. The *ad hoc* tests are reserved for program-specific purposes, e.g., triggered by hypotheses about the mechanism-based toxicity or prior *in vivo* findings for previous compounds in the program. Examples of such *ad hoc* assays include: muscle, kidney, neural, teratonenic, developmental, myelotoxicity, and lymphotoxicity. The potential for multi-organ chip to improve toxicity prediction should also fall into this last category until its predictivity and throughput make it possible for front-loading (Bhatia and Ingber, 2014). The *ad hoc* assays can also include further investigation of previous positive findings, e.g., micronucleus positives can be imaged for other markers to differentiate chromosome breaks (clastogens) vs. chromosome loss (aneuploidy), where an acceptable safety margin can allow for further drug development

TABLE | A summary of imaging tests and their predictive values reviewed by this article.

Cell model (reference)	Imaging technique	Threshold for positives	Predictive value	Example image
Human hepatocyte (Xu et al., 2008)	Fluorescence imaging of oxidative stress, mitochondrial function, glutathione content and hepatocellular lipidosis	>2.5 fold above or <2.5 fold below the vehicle control mean values (depending on which fluorescence channel). Appropriate cut-off levels were selected using ROC curves	~60% sensitivity and ~95% specificity	
Human hepatocyte (Garside et al., 2013)	Fluorescence imaging of oxidative stress	>6 SD of the vehicle control mean values	41% sensitivity and 86% specificity	
Human hepatocyte (Xu et al., 2011)	Fluorescence imaging of bile acid and its disposition in bile canaliculi	<2.5 fold below the vehicle control mean values	TBD	
iPSC-derived human cardiomyocytes (Sirenko et al., 2013)	Fast kinetic imaging-based Ca^{2+} flux as continuously cell-beating measurements (beat rate, amplitude, and other beat parameters)	>1 SD of the vehicle control mean values	TBD	
iPSC-derived human cardiomyocytes (Pointon et al., 2015)	Fast kinetic imaging-based Ca^{2+} flux as continuously cell-beating measurements (peak count, average peak amplitude, average peak width, average peak rise time, average peak decay time, and average peak spacing)	The median of the positive and negative control wells were set at 0 and −100, respectively, and the signals from all wells scaled to this range. Appropriate cut-off levels were selected using ROC curves	87% sensitivity and 70% specificity, using peak count	
Ames (Xu and Aubrecht, 2010)	Automated counting of the number of surviving bioluminescent colonies	Same as manual counting	100% combined negative predictive value to carcinogenicity test	
In vitro micronucleus (Xu and Aubrecht, 2010)	Automated scoring of the micronucleus frequency	Same as manual scoring	100% combined negative predictive value to carcinogenicity test	

SD, standard deviation; ROC, receiver operator characteristic; TBD, to be determined.

(Cheung et al., 2014). In the complex business of defining drug safety, "clean" compound in all test systems are not always realistic. One should therefore use a balanced and holistic approach starting with defining an acceptable safety profile for a drug candidate, understanding the predictive value and limitation of each test system, and a "weight-of-evidence" approach integrating findings from human cells, *in vivo* animal testing, and human clinical trials. **Table** summarizes the imaging tests and their predictive values described in this mini-review.

Safety deficiencies account for more than half of delayed FDA approval or non-approval of new drug applications from 2000 to 2012 (Sacks et al., 2014). Predictive toxicology holds the key to reduce this attrition and make R&D investment more sustainable.

To realize its promise practitioners of predictive toxicology must continue to integrate diverse innovations from multiple fields of biomedical engineering, including:

1) Predictive and reliable cellular models: esp., evaluation, characterization, production, and standardization of predictive human cells
2) Mechanism-informed phenotypic screening strategy, including cellular imaging as a key component as it provides a phenotypic anchor and direct linkage to *in vivo* histopathology
3) Quantitative therapeutic window predictions: e.g., using mechanism-based scaling or predictive PKPD modeling

One may envision a future when the banking of pluripotent stem cells from individual human donor with defined genetic makeup and subsequent expansion into fully-functional organ parenchymal cells as a desirable model toward predicting personalized drug responses, for both drug efficacy and safety. But before we achieve that dream, the holistic applications of an integrated approach as highlighted above have already marched us a long way toward transforming toxicology to improve product safety.

Acknowledgments

The author acknowledges Drs. Timothy Johnson, Frank Sistare, Nicolau Beckmann, and three peer reviewers for critical review of the manuscript. The author sincerely apologizes that many scholars' publications cannot be cited in this mini-review due to space limitation.

References

Aubrecht, J., Osowski, J. J., Persaud, P., Cheung, J. R., Ackerman, J., Lopes, S. H., et al. (2007). Bioluminescent Salmonella reverse mutation assay: a screen for detecting mutagenicity with high throughput attributes. *Mutagenesis* 22, 335–342. doi: 10.1093/mutage/gem022

Bhatia, S. N., and Ingber, D. E. (2014). Microfluidic organs-on-chips. *Nat. Biotechnol.* 32, 760–772. doi: 10.1038/nbt.2989

Broder, S. (2010). The development of antiretroviral therapy and its impact on the HIV-1/AIDS pandemic. *Antiviral Res.* 85, 1–18. doi: 10.1016/j.antiviral.2009.10.002

Cheung, J. R., Dickinson, D. A., Moss, J., Schuler, M. J., Spellman, R. A., and Heard, P. L. (2014). Histone markers identify the mode of action for compounds positive in the TK6 micronucleus assay. *Mutat. Res. Genet. Toxicol. Environ. Mutagen.* 777, 7–16. doi: 10.1016/j.mrgentox.2014.11.002

Claxton, L. D., Umbuzeiro Gde, A., and DeMarini, D. M. (2010). The Salmonella mutagenicity assay: the stethoscope of genetic toxicology for the 21st century. *Environ. Health Perspect.* 118, 1515–1522. doi: 10.1289/ehp.1002336

Cosgrove, B. D., King, B. M., Hasan, M. A., Alexopoulos, L. G., Farazi, P. A., Hendriks, B. S., et al. (2009). Synergistic drug-cytokine induction of hepatocellular death as an *in vitro* approach for the study of inflammation-associated idiosyncratic drug hepatotoxicity. *Toxicol. Appl. Pharmacol.* 237, 317–330. doi: 10.1016/j.taap.2009.04.002

de Waart, D. R., Häusler, S., Vlaming, M. L., Kunne, C., Hanggi, E., Gruss, H. J., et al. (2010). Hepatic transport mechanisms of cholyl-L-lysyl-fluorescein. *J. Pharmacol. Exp. Ther.* 334, 78–86. doi: 10.1124/jpet.110.166991

Doherty, K. R., Wappel, R. L., Talbert, D. R., Trusk, P. B., Moran, D. M., Kramer, J. W., et al. (2013). Multi-parameter *in vitro* toxicity testing of crizotinib, sunitinib, erlotinib, and nilotinib in human cardiomyocytes. *Toxicol. Appl. Pharmacol.* 272, 245–255. doi: 10.1016/j.taap.2013.04.027

FDA. (2010). *Predictive Safety Testing Consortium*. Available online at: http://c-path.org/programs/pstc/

FDA. (2012). International Conference on Harmonisation; guidance on S2(R1) Genotoxicity Testing and Data Interpretation for Pharmaceuticals intended for Human Use; availability. Notice. *Fed. Regist.* 77, 33748–33749. Available online at: http://www.gpo.gov/fdsys/pkg/FR-2012-06-07/html/2012-13774.htm

Garside, H., Marcoe, K. F., Chesnut-Speelman, J., Foster, A. J., Muthas, D., Gerry Kenna, J. G., et al. (2013). Evaluation of the use of imaging parameters for the detection of compound-induced hepatotoxicity in 384-well cultures of HepG2 cells and cryopreserved primary human hepatocytes. *Toxicol. In Vitro* 28, 171–181. doi: 10.1016/j.tiv.2013.10.015

Hayashi, H., and Sugiyama, Y. (2013). Bile salt export pump (BSEP/ABCB11): trafficking and sorting disturbances. *Curr. Mol. Pharmacol.* 6, 95–103. doi: 10.2174/18744672113069990036

Kaplowitz, N. (2005). Idiosyncratic drug hepatotoxicity. *Nat. Rev. Drug Discov.* 4, 489–499. doi: 10.1038/nrd1750

Maddah, M., Heidmann, J. D., Mandegar, M. A., Walker, C. D., Bolouki, S., Conklin, B. R., et al. (2015). A non-invasive platform for functional characterization of stem-cell-derived cardiomyocytes with applications in cardiotoxicity testing. *Stem Cell Reports* 4, 621–631. doi: 10.1016/j.stemcr.2015.02.007

Moffat, J. G., Rudolph, J., and Bailey, D. (2014). Phenotypic screening in cancer drug discovery—past, present and future. *Nat. Rev. Drug Discov.* 13, 588–602. doi: 10.1038/nrd4366

Morgan, R. E., van Staden, C. J., Chen, Y., Kalyanaraman, N., Kalanzi, J., Dunn, R. T., et al. (2013). A multifactorial approach to hepatobiliary transporter assessment enables improved therapeutic compound development. *Toxicol. Sci.* 136, 216–241. doi: 10.1093/toxsci/kft176

Opar, A. (2012). Overtaking the DILI Model-T. *Nat. Rev. Drug Discov.* 11, 585–586. doi: 10.1038/nrd3818

Pointon, A., Harmer, A. R., Dale, I. L., Abi-Gerges, N., Bowes, J., Pollard, C., et al. (2015). Assessment of cardiomyocyte contraction in human-induced pluripotent stem cell-derived cardiomyocytes. *Toxicol. Sci.* 144, 227–237. doi: 10.1093/toxsci/kfu312

Puppala, D., Collis, L. P., Sun, S. Z., Bonato, V., Chen, X., Anson, B., et al. (2013). Comparative gene expression profiling in human-induced pluripotent stem cell-derived cardiocytes and human and cynomolgus heart tissue. *Toxicol. Sci.* 131, 292–301. doi: 10.1093/toxsci/kfs282

Sacks, L. V., Shamsuddin, H. H., Yasinskaya, Y. I., Bouri, K., Lanthier, M. L., and Sherman, R. E. (2014). Scientific and regulatory reasons for delay and denial of FDA approval of initial applications for new drugs, 2000-2012. *JAMA* 311, 378–384. doi: 10.1001/jama.2013.282542

Sager, P. T., Gintant, G., Turner, J. R., Pettit, S., and Stockbridge, N. (2014). Rechanneling the cardiac proarrhythmia safety paradigm: a meeting report from the cardiac safety research consortium. *Am. Heart J.* 167, 292–300. doi: 10.1016/j.ahj.2013.11.004

Sirenko, O., Cromwell, E. F., Crittenden, C., Wignall, J. A., Wright, F. A., and Rusyn, I. (2013). Assessment of beating parameters in human induced pluripotent stem cells enables quantitative *in vitro* screening for cardiotoxicity. *Toxicol. Appl. Pharmacol.* 273, 500–507. doi: 10.1016/j.taap.2013.09.017

Sistare, F. D., Morton, D., Alden, C., Christensen, J., Keller, D., Jonghe, S. D., et al. (2011). An analysis of pharmaceutical experience with decades of rat carcinogenicity testing: support for a proposal to modify current regulatory guidelines. *Toxicol. Pathol.* 39, 716–744. doi: 10.1177/0192623311406935

Tujios, S., and Fontana, R. J. (2011). Mechanisms of drug-induced liver injury: from bedside to bench. *Nat. Rev. Gastroenterol. Hepatol.* 8, 202–211. doi: 10.1038/nrgastro.2011.22

Vargas, H. M. (2010). A new preclinical biomarker for risk of Torsades de Pointes: drug-induced reduction of the cardiac electromechanical window. *Br. J. Pharmacol.* 161, 1441–1443. doi: 10.1111/j.1476-5381.2010.00980.x

Ware, B. R., Berger, D. R., and Khetani, S. R. (2015). Prediction of drug-induced liver injury in micropatterned co-cultures containing iPSC-derived human hepatocytes. *Toxicol. Sci.* 145, 252–262. doi: 10.1093/toxsci/kfv048

Woodhead, J. L., Yang, K., Siler, S. Q., Watkins, P. B., Brouwer, K. L., Barton, H. A., et al. (2014). Exploring BSEP inhibition-mediated toxicity with a mechanistic model of drug-induced liver injury. *Front. Pharmacol.* 5:240. doi: 10.3389/fphar.2014.00240

Xu, J. J., and Aubrecht, J. (2010). "Screening approaches for genetic toxicity," in *Predictive Toxicology in Drug Safety,* eds J. J. Xu and L. Urban (Cambridge, UK: Cambridge University Press), 18–33.

Xu, J. J., and Urban, L. (2010). *Predictive Toxicology in Drug Safety.* Cambridge, UK: Cambridge University Press.

Xu, J. J., Henstock, P. V., Dunn, M. C., Smith, A. R., Chabot, J. R., and de Graaf, D. (2008). Cellular imaging predictions of clinical drug-induced liver injury. *Toxicol. Sci.* 105, 97–105. doi: 10.1093/toxsci/kfn109

Xu, J., Dunn, M. C., Smith, A., and Tien, E. (2011). "Assessment of hepatotoxicity potential of drug candidate molecules including kinase inhibitors by hepatocyte imaging assay technology and bile flux imaging assay technology," in *Kinase Inhibitors: Methods in Molecular Biology,* Vol. 795, ed B. Kuster (Freising: Humana Press), 83–107.

Conflict of Interest Statement: The author is an employee of Merck and Co. However, views expressed in this mini-review are the author's own and do not reflect positions of any company or organization.

4

Immuno-Positron Emission Tomography with Zirconium-89-Labeled Monoclonal Antibodies in Oncology: What can we Learn from Initial Clinical Trials?

Yvonne W. S. Jauw [1]*, C. Willemien Menke-van der Houven van Oordt [2], Otto S. Hoekstra [3], N. Harry Hendrikse [3, 4], Danielle J. Vugts [3], Josée M. Zijlstra [1], Marc C. Huisman [3] and Guus A. M. S. van Dongen [3]

[1] Department of Hematology, VU University Medical Center, Amsterdam, Netherlands, [2] Department of Medical Oncology, VU University Medical Center, Amsterdam, Netherlands, [3] Department of Radiology and Nuclear Medicine, VU University Medical Center, Amsterdam, Netherlands, [4] Department of Clinical Pharmacology and Pharmacy, VU University Medical Center, Amsterdam, Netherlands

Edited by:
Nicolau Beckmann,
Novartis Institutes for BioMedical
Research, Switzerland

Reviewed by:
Sridhar Nimmagadda,
Johns Hopkins University, USA
Andrew Mark Scott,
Olivia Newton-John Cancer Research
Institute, Australia
Vania Kenanova,
121 Bio, LLC., USA

*Correspondence:
Yvonne W. S. Jauw
yws.jauw@vumc.nl

Selection of the right drug for the right patient is a promising approach to increase clinical benefit of targeted therapy with monoclonal antibodies (mAbs). Assessment of in vivo biodistribution and tumor targeting of mAbs to predict toxicity and efficacy is expected to guide individualized treatment and drug development. Molecular imaging with positron emission tomography (PET) using zirconium-89 (^{89}Zr)-labeled monoclonal antibodies also known as ^{89}Zr-immuno-PET, visualizes and quantifies uptake of radiolabeled mAbs. This technique provides a potential imaging biomarker to assess target expression, as well as tumor targeting of mAbs. In this review we summarize results from initial clinical trials with ^{89}Zr-immuno-PET in oncology and discuss technical aspects of trial design. In clinical trials with ^{89}Zr-immuno-PET two requirements should be met for each ^{89}Zr-labeled mAb to realize its full potential. One requirement is that the biodistribution of the ^{89}Zr-labeled mAb (imaging dose) reflects the biodistribution of the drug during treatment (therapeutic dose). Another requirement is that tumor uptake of ^{89}Zr-mAb on PET is primarily driven by specific, antigen-mediated, tumor targeting. Initial trials have contributed toward the development of ^{89}Zr-immuno-PET as an imaging biomarker by showing correlation between uptake of ^{89}Zr-labeled mAbs on PET and target expression levels in biopsies. These results indicate that ^{89}Zr-immuno-PET reflects specific, antigen-mediated binding. ^{89}Zr-immuno-PET was shown to predict toxicity of RIT, but thus far results indicating that toxicity of mAbs or mAb-drug conjugate treatment can be predicted are lacking. So far, one study has shown that molecular imaging combined with early response assessment is able to predict response to treatment with the antibody-drug conjugate trastuzumab-emtansine, in patients with human epithelial growth factor-2 (HER2)-positive breast cancer. Future studies would benefit from a standardized criterion to define positive tumor uptake, possibly supported by quantitative analysis, and validated by linking imaging data with corresponding clinical outcome. Taken together, these results encourage further studies to develop ^{89}Zr-immuno-PET as a predictive imaging biomarker to guide individualized treatment, as well as for potential application in drug development.

Keywords: molecular imaging, positron emission tomography, ^{89}zirconium, monoclonal antibodies, imaging biomarker, clinical oncology

INTRODUCTION

In recent years, monoclonal antibodies (mAbs) have become widely used for treatment of cancer. Immunotherapy with mAbs aims for specific targeting and therefore less toxicity compared to chemotherapy. Some mAbs have resulted in a significant improvement of survival, for example the anti-CD20 antibody rituximab for B cell lymphoma (Feugier et al., 2005). However, not all patients benefit from mAb treatment. Monotherapy with the anti-epidermal growth factor receptor (EGFR) antibody cetuximab results in clinical benefit for half of the patients with advanced colorectal cancer (without relevant gene mutations; RAS wild type; Peeters et al., 2015).

Improving response rates by quickly selecting the right drug for the right patient is paramount to reducing unnecessary toxicity and costs. In order to obtain clinical benefit from mAb treatment, the target antigen should be expressed in the tumor and the drug is required to reach and bind to the target (tumor targeting). Absence of target expression on normal tissue is important to limit toxicity of treatment.

Next generation mAbs are aiming for increased potency, for example antibody-drug conjugates (ADC's), mAbs capable of inhibiting immune checkpoints and multi-specific mAbs recognizing at least two different targets (Sliwkowski and Mellman, 2013; Evans and Syed, 2014; Reichert, 2016). The number of novel targeted treatment options increases, however drug development requires time, efforts and significant resources. In addition, investigational drugs are evaluated in large patient cohorts before successful introduction in routine clinical care.

Molecular imaging with ^{89}Zr-labeled mAbs, also known as ^{89}Zr-immuno-PET, provides a potential imaging biomarker to evaluate tumor targeting of mAbs. This technique is non-invasive and provides whole body information on both target expression and tumor targeting, as opposed to immunohistochemistry on a single biopsy, which only provides information on target expression. Prediction of efficacy and toxicity of mAb treatment by molecular imaging may be used to select individual patients or patient groups for a treatment, or to select promising candidate drugs and their dosing schedule (Ciprotti et al., 2015).

^{89}Zr-immuno-PET allows visualization and quantification of biodistribution and tumor uptake. ^{89}Zr is considered a suitable radioisotope for this purpose, due to its relatively long half-life ($t_{1/2} = 78.4$ h), which corresponds with the time a mAb needs to reach the target. The use of ^{89}Zr as a radiolabel and the coupling of ^{89}Zr to mAbs, under Good Manufacturing Practice conditions, have been described previously (Verel et al., 2003; Perk et al., 2010; Vosjan et al., 2010). Harmonization of quantitative ^{89}Zr-immuno-PET imaging has also been reported, allowing for broad scale application, e.g., in a multi-center setting (Makris et al., 2014).

Before starting clinical ^{89}Zr-immuno-PET trials, the following conditions are essential to allow appropriate interpretation of data. Prerequisites are that the radioimmunoconjugate of interest is stable and has the same binding and biodistribution characteristics as the unlabeled parental mAb. Imaging procedures should be standardized and validated in order to provide reliable quantification. Assuming these requirements are fulfilled, biodistribution and tumor uptake of a ^{89}Zr-mAb, defined on PET, can be used as an imaging biomarker for tumor targeting of the "cold" therapeutic antibody. These basic technical aspects of ^{89}Zr-immuno-PET have been extensively discussed in a recent review by van Dongen et al. (2015).

Until now, at least 15 clinical ^{89}Zr-immuno-PET trials have been reported, see **Table** , providing information on the clinical performance of ^{89}Zr-immuno-PET. Therefore, evaluation of the potential and current limitations of this imaging technique seems timely to enable optimal design of future trials. This review summarizes the results from initial clinical ^{89}Zr-immuno-PET in oncology, and technical aspects of trial design are discussed.

^{89}Zr-LABELED ANTI-CD44V6 MAB IN HEAD AND NECK CANCER

^{89}Zr-immuno-PET is considered to be an attractive imaging technique for whole body tumor detection, due to the combined sensitivity of PET and the specificity of the mAb. Assessment of the mAb biodistribution to confirm specificity is particularly of interest to qualify the suitability of the mAb for therapy.

Börjesson et al. reported on the first clinical ^{89}Zr-immuno-PET study ever (Börjesson et al., 2006). In this study, twenty pre-operative patients with head and neck squamous cell carcinoma (HNSCC) were included. Immuno-PET with ^{89}Zr-labeled chimeric mAb U36 (cmAb U36) was investigated in order to improve tumor detection of HNSCC, especially in lymph nodes, and to assess the targeting potential of the

Abbreviations: ADC, antibody-drug conjugate; cmAb U36, chimeric monoclonal antibody U36; EGFR, epidermal growth factor receptor; FDG, 18F-fluoro-deoxy-glucose; HNSCC, head and neck squamous cell carcinoma; HER2, human epidermal growth factor receptor 2; HSP90, Heat shock protein 90; mAb, monoclonal antibody; MSLN, membrane-bound surface glycoprotein mesothelin; NET, neuroendocrine tumors; NHL, non-Hodgkin lymphoma; PET, positron emission tomography; p.i., post injection; PSMA, prostate specific membrane antigen; RIT, radioimmunotherapy; T-DM1, trastuzumab-emtansine; TGF-β, Transforming growth factor-β; VEGF-A, vascular endothelial growth factor-A; ^{90}Y, yttrium-90; ^{89}Zr, zirconium-89.

TABLE | Summary of clinical studies on [89]Zr-immuno-PET in oncology.

Author	Year	Target	mAb	Tumor type	N
Börjesson	2006	CD44v6	cmAb U36	Head and neck cancer	20
	2009				
Dijkers	2010	HER2	trastuzumab	Breast cancer	14
Rizvi	2012	CD20	ibritumomab-tiuxetan	B-cell lymphoma	7
Gaykema	2013	VEGF-A	bevacizumab	Breast cancer	23
van Zanten	2013	VEGF-A	bevacizumab	Glioma	3
van Asselt	2014	VEGF-A	bevacizumab	Neuroendocrine tumors	14
Bahce	2014	VEGF-A	bevacizumab	Non-small cell lung cancer	7
Pandit-Taskar	2014	PSMA	Hu-J591	Prostate cancer	50
	2015				
Den Hollander	2015	TGF-β	fresolimumab	Glioma	12
Gaykema	2015	HER2	trastuzumab	Breast cancer	10
		VEGF-A	bevacizumab		6
Gebhart	2015	HER2	trastuzumab	Breast cancer	56
Lamberts	2015	MSLN	MMOT0530A	Pancreatic cancer	11
				Ovarian cancer	4
Menke-van der Houven van Oordt	2015	EGFR	cetuximab	Colorectal cancer	10
Muylle	2015	CD20	rituximab	B-cell lymphoma	5
Oosting	2015	VEGF-A	bevacizumab	Renal cell carcinoma	22

mAb for therapy. cmAb U36 targets the v6 region of CD44 (cluster of differentiation; CD44v6). Homogeneous expression of CD44v6 has been observed in several malignancies, including HNSCC, lung, skin, esophagus, and cervix carcinoma. Expression of CD44v6 has also been reported in normal epithelial tissues, such as skin, breast, and prostate myoepithelium, and bronchial epithelium.

Administration of 74 megabecquerel (MBq) [89]Zr-mAb U36 (10 mg) appeared to be safe, as no adverse reactions were observed. A human anti-chimeric antibody response was reported in 2 patients, which was not directed to the chelate, but to the protein part of the conjugate. [89]Zr-immuno-PET scans were visually scored. All primary tumors were detected and [89]Zr-immuno-PET performed equally to computed tomography (CT) and magnetic resonance imaging (MRI) for detection of lymph node metastasis. Although, biopsies were obtained in this study to confirm tumor localization, immunohistochemistry for CD44v6 was not performed, as in literature >96% of HNSCC show CD44v6 expression by at least 50% of the cells. This study shows that immuno-PET with [89]Zr-cmAb U36 can be used as an imaging modality for tumor detection. However, traditional imaging techniques as ^{18}F-fluoro-deoxy-glucose(FDG)-PET (Mak et al., 2011) and sentinel node procedures for assessment of lymph node status remain standard of care for tumor detection in HNSCC patients, as the added value of immuno-PET with [89]Zr-cmAb U36 has not been demonstrated.

In a separate publication, biodistribution, radiation dose and quantification of [89]Zr-labeled cmAb U36 were reported for the same patient cohort (Börjesson et al., 2009). [89]Zr-cmAb U36 in blood pool, lungs, liver, kidneys and spleen decreased over time. Increasing uptake of [89]Zr-cmAb U36 over time was seen only at tumor sites and in the thyroid of some patients (suggesting expression of CD44v6 in thyroid of these patients). Although expression of CD44v6 in normal epithelial tissue has been described, no obvious targeting of [89]Zr-mAb U36 was observed in the skin. However, Tijink et al. reported a fatal adverse event due to skin toxicity after treatment with the ADC bivatuzumab mertansine, a humanized anti-CD44v6 mAb conjugated to a potent maytansine derivate (Tijink et al., 2006). This toxicity profile, most probably due to expression of CD44v6 in the skin, was not predicted based on assessment of biodistribution of [89]Zr-cmAbU36 as reported by Börjesson et al. (2009). Among others, this may be due to detection limitations of PET, inter-individual differences in target expression, or differences in biodistribution between the mAb and the ADC.

A technical aspect of this first [89]Zr-immuno-PET study to be considered is the rationale for the total protein dose of cmAb U36 administered, since tumor uptake, tumor to non-tumor ratio's, as well as tumor visualization might be protein dose dependent. This protein dose of 10 mg was chosen as previous studies observed that biodistribution was not mAb-dose dependent within the range of 2–52 mg (de Bree et al., 1995; Colnot et al., 2000; Stroomer et al., 2000).

Finally, good agreement was reported for image-derived quantification of blood pool radioactivity as well as tumor uptake of [89]Zr-cmAb U36 compared to *ex vivo* radioactivity measurements in, respectively, venous blood samples and biopsies from surgical tumor resection. This is an important achievement in performance, showing accurate quantification of [89]Zr-mAb with PET.

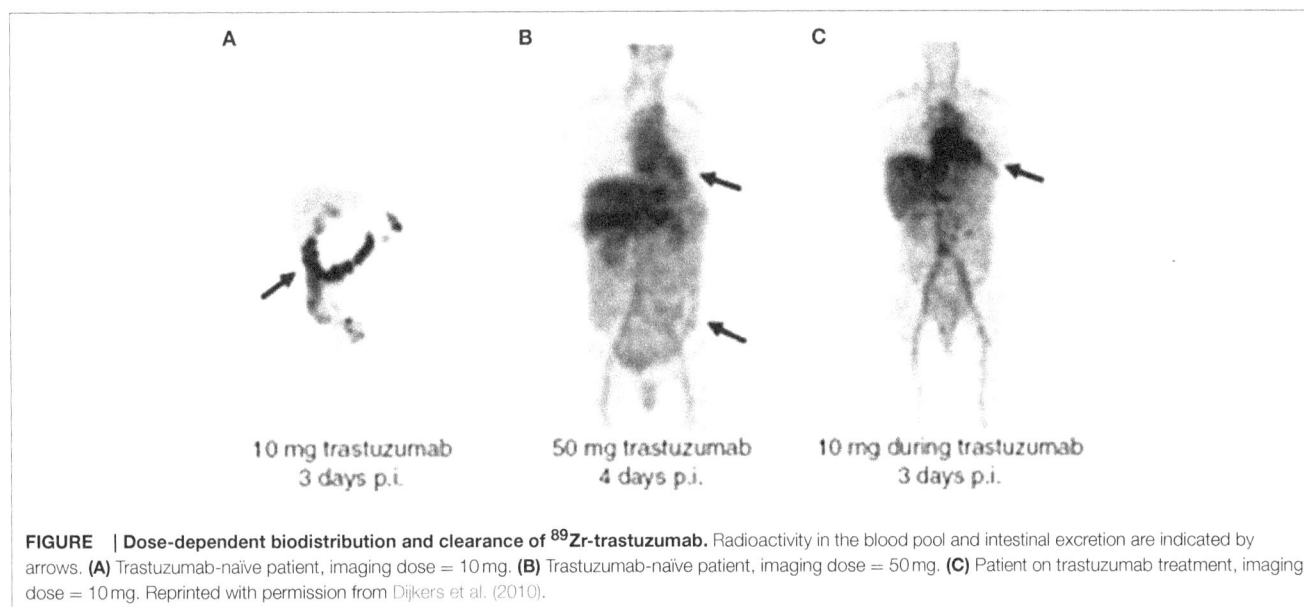

FIGURE | Dose-dependent biodistribution and clearance of ^{89}Zr-trastuzumab. Radioactivity in the blood pool and intestinal excretion are indicated by arrows. **(A)** Trastuzumab-naïve patient, imaging dose = 10 mg. **(B)** Trastuzumab-naïve patient, imaging dose = 50 mg. **(C)** Patient on trastuzumab treatment, imaging dose = 10 mg. Reprinted with permission from Dijkers et al. (2010).

^{89}Zr-LABELED TRASTUZUMAB IN BREAST CANCER

Treatment with trastuzumab, which targets the human epidermal growth factor receptor 2 (HER2), has improved the prognosis for patients with HER2-positive breast cancer (Moja et al., 2012) and gastric cancer (Gong et al., 2016). HER2 is involved in cell survival, proliferation, cell maturation, metastasis, angiogenesis and has anti-apoptotic effects. It is also expressed in other malignancies, including ovarian and endometrial carcinoma, and in normal epithelial cells and hematopoietic cells (Leone et al., 2003). It is known that the extracellular domain of HER2 can enter the circulation after shedding from the surface of tumor cells (Tse et al., 2012).

Currently assessment of HER2 status is performed with immunohistochemistry (IHC) or fluorescent in situ hybridization on tumor biopsies. Some studies have shown up to 15% intra-individual heterogeneity in HER2 status between primary tumors and metastases (Lindstrom et al., 2012) leading to the recommendation to repeat biopsies to assess HER2 status during the course of the disease. As some tumor lesions are inaccessible for biopsies and it is impossible to biopsy every tumor lesion to assess heterogeneity, there is a need for a non-invasive technique to assess whole body HER2 status for diagnosis, staging and to guide individualized treatment.

^{89}Zr-Trastuzumab-PET for Whole Body Assessment of HER2 Target Status

Dijkers et al. reported a feasibility study to determine optimal dosage and time of administration of ^{89}Zr-trastuzumab (37 MBq) to enable PET visualization and quantification of tumor lesions in 14 patients with HER2-positive metastatic breast cancer (Dijkers et al., 2010).

Trastuzumab naïve patients who received -^{89}Zr-trastuzumab (10 mg; $n = 2$), showed relatively high liver uptake and pronounced intestinal excretion, with low blood pool activity, indicating rapid clearance. This rapid clearance was most probably due to complex formation of trastuzumab with extracellular HER2 domains shed in the plasma. For optimal imaging, trastuzumab naïve patients required a total dose of 50 mg trastuzumab ($n = 5$). This resulted in less liver uptake, lower intestinal excretion and increased blood pool activity, as illustrated by **Figures** . This dose was considered the optimal dose, as good tumor-to-non-tumor ratio and favorable biodistribution were observed, although higher doses were not evaluated due to expected target saturation. Patients already on trastuzumab treatment received a dose of 10 mg trastuzumab. As these patients ($n = 7$) showed minimal intestinal excretion and slow blood clearance, this was considered an adequate dose, see **Figure** . This study illustrates a dose-dependent relationship between imaging dose and biodistribution of ^{89}Zr-trastuzumab.

Best timing for evaluation of tumor uptake of ^{89}Zr-trastuzumab was 4–5 days post injection (p.i.) while scans performed at day 6 or 7 p.i. yielded decreased image quality because of insufficient counting statistics.

^{89}Zr-trastuzumab-PET allowed detection of most of the known lesions and some that had remained unnoticed with CT, MRI or bone scans. In 6 of the 12 patients not all known lesions were detected. Liver lesions were missed in 3 out of 7 patients, possibly due to the high background activity in normal liver tissue, which is involved in mAb catabolism. Interestingly, while poor penetration of trastuzumab in the brain was expected, in 3 patients brain lesions could be visualized. This might be due to disruption of blood-brain barrier in brain metastasis. A limitation of this study was the lack of biopsies for confirmation of the HER2 status of immuno-PET negative lesions.

Tumor lesions showing no uptake of ^{89}Zr-trastuzumab may be due to suboptimal imaging conditions, as illustrated by a

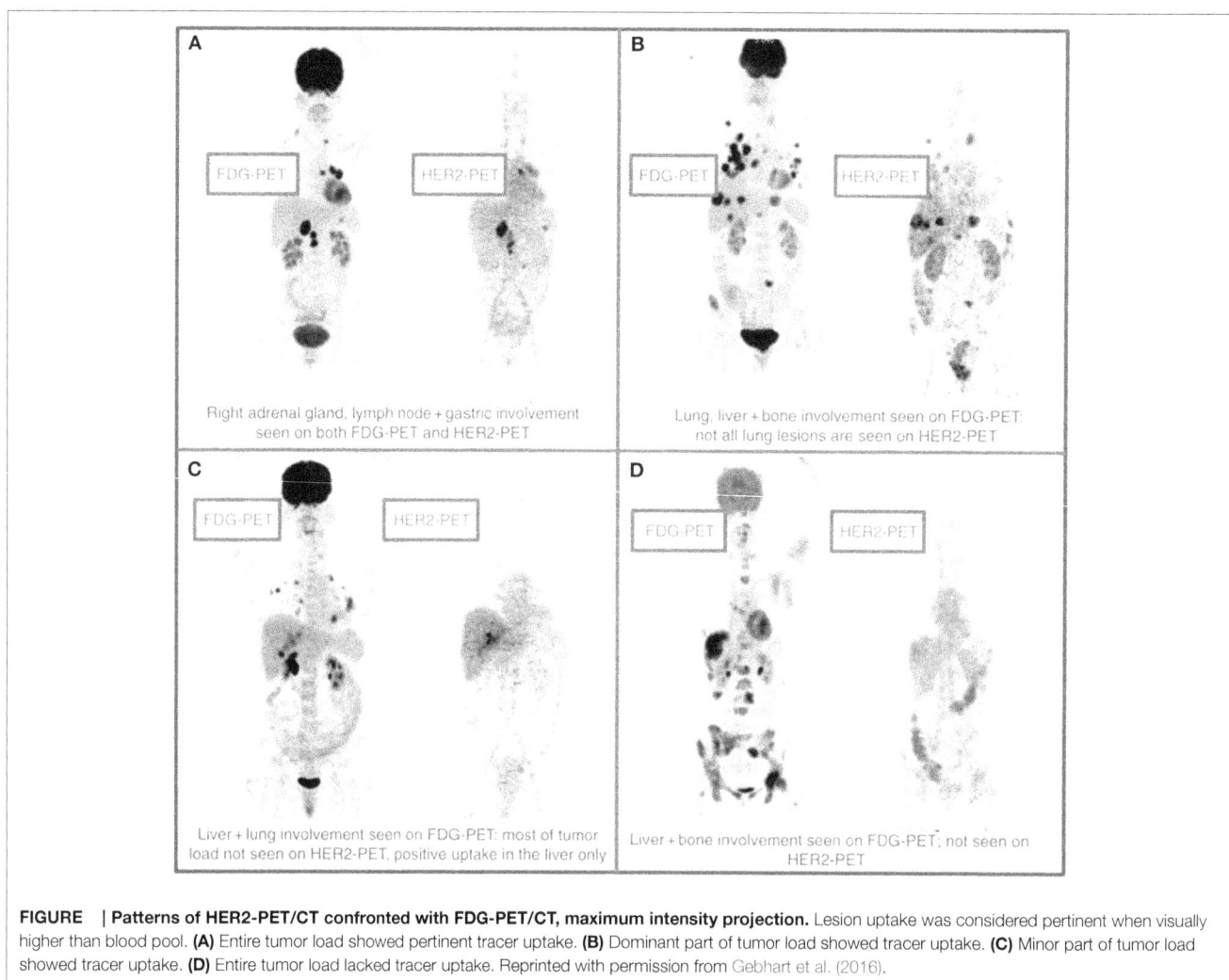

FIGURE | Patterns of HER2-PET/CT confronted with FDG-PET/CT, maximum intensity projection. Lesion uptake was considered pertinent when visually higher than blood pool. **(A)** Entire tumor load showed pertinent tracer uptake. **(B)** Dominant part of tumor load showed tracer uptake. **(C)** Minor part of tumor load showed tracer uptake. **(D)** Entire tumor load lacked tracer uptake. Reprinted with permission from Gebhart et al. (2016).

case report of a trastuzumab naïve breast cancer patient (Oude Munnink et al., 2010). Thirty seven MBq trastuzumab (50 mg) was administered and a PET scan was obtained 2 days p.i.. ^{89}Zr activity concentration in bloodpool was low, whereas massive uptake was observed in liver metastases (48% of the injected dose) as well as intestinal uptake, suggesting intestinal excretion. Known bone metastases were hardly visible. This might be the result of an extensive tumor load and/or soluble HER2, which reduces uptake in other tumor lesions, due to an insufficient amount of trastuzumab. After administration of 220 mg unlabeled trastuzumab, immediately followed by 10 mg ^{89}Zr-trastuzumab, liver uptake was lowered (33% of the injected dose) and an increase in uptake in the other tumor lesions, such as bone metastases, was observed. Based on a theoretical calculation the authors conclude that a dose of 280 mg trastuzumab could only saturate 47% of all HER2 present in the liver metastases of this patient, indicating a higher dose of trastuzumab is required to saturate lesions in case of extensive HER2-positive tumor load. Based on this important observation that pharmacokinetics and organ distribution can be influenced by the extent of tumor load, dosing of trastuzumab for metastastic

breast cancer should be reconsidered. An individualized dosing schedule of trastuzumab based on tumor load, guided by ^{89}Zr-trastuzumab-PET, instead of patient weight, might improve efficacy of treatment.

^{89}Zr-Trastuzumab to Assess Response by Alteration of Antigen Expression

Gaykema et al. evaluated ^{89}Zr-trastuzumab-PET to determine alteration of HER2 expression after anti-angiogenic treatment with the novel heat shock protein 90 (HSP90) inhibitor NVP-AUY922 in 10 patients with HER2-positive breast cancer (Gaykema et al., 2014). HSP90 inhibition can deplete client proteins like HER2. This study was performed with 37 MBq ^{89}Zr-trastuzumab (50 mg), while NVP-AUY922 was administered i.v. in a weekly schedule of 70 mg/m^2. Change in tumor uptake of ^{89}Zr-trastuzumab at baseline vs. 3 weeks on treatment was correlated to change in size on CT after 8 weeks treatment. This feasibility study suggests that ^{89}Zr-immuno-PET can be used to monitor alteration of antigen expression and supports further evaluation of ^{89}Zr-trastuzumab-PET in providing insight in treatment response of novel anti-cancer agents like the HSP90 inhibitor NVP-AUY922 in larger studies.

^{89}Zr-Trastuzumab-PET as Predictive Imaging Biomarker for ADC Treatment

Recently, the ADC trastuzumab-emtansine (T-DM1) was approved for treatment of patients with progression of HER2-positive breast cancer, previously treated with trastuzumab-based therapy. The ZEPHIR study investigated the use of ^{89}Zr-trastuzumab-PET, combined with early response assessment with FDG-PET, as a predictive imaging biomarker for treatment with T-DM1 (Gebhart et al., 2016). In this study intra- and interpatient heterogeneity in HER2 mapping of metastatic disease was also explored, see **Figure** . The study was performed by administration of 37 MBq ^{89}Zr-trastuzumab (50 mg). ^{89}Zr-trastuzumab-PET scans were acquired 4 days p.i. and visually scored. After 1 cycle of T-DM1 an early metabolic response was evaluated by FDG-PET. Clinical outcome after treatment with 3 cycles of T-DM1 was evaluated by CT.

For 55 evaluable patients with HER2-positive metastatic breast cancer, assessment of ^{89}Zr-trastuzumab uptake resulted in a positive predictive value of 72% and a negative predictive value of 88% for prediction of clinical outcome. For early metabolic response assessment with FDG-PET the positive predictive value was 96% and the negative predictive value was 83%. Intrapatient heterogeneity in tumor uptake was observed in 46% of patients, as illustrated by **Figure** . When combining ^{89}Zr-trastuzumab-PET with early FDG-PET response after 1 cycle of T-DM1, a negative predictive value of 100% was obtained for all concordant patients (with both a negative ^{89}Zr-trastuzumab-PET, as well as absence of response on early FDG-PET). This strategy of combining HER2-PET with early FDG-PET response monitoring was able to separate patients with a median time to treatment failure of 2.8 month from patients with a median time to treatment failure of 15 months.

It is not known why 2/16 patients with a negative ^{89}Zr-trastuzumab-PET did show response on treatment with T-DM1. Some possibilities are lack of receptor overexpression, receptor masking, or an induced response despite low HER2 expression due to the extreme potency of T-DM1. Another possibility is that DM1 becomes released in the circulation and exerts some antitumor activity. Absence of tumor uptake can also be explained by an insufficient tracer dose due to the extent of tumor load or the amount of soluble HER2 in these patients.

These results support that pre-treatment imaging of HER2-targeting is a promising tool to improve the understanding of tumor heterogeneity in metastatic breast cancer and to select patients who are deemed not to benefit from T-DM1. This might avoid toxicity and costs of T-DM1 and improve patient outcome by switching sooner to a more effective therapy (personalized medicine). A plausible explanation for the added value of early FDG-PET is that although target expression of HER2 is a prerequisite for clinical benefit, even with adequate targeting intracellular resistance mechanisms may be responsible for treatment failure. The authors recommend a future randomized trial with cost-effectiveness as secondary endpoint, to test the concept of interrupting T-DM1 treatment after 1 cycle in case of FDG-PET non-responsiveness, which can be expected in 20% of the patients. As such, this trial paved the road toward improved individualization of anti-HER2 therapy.

^{89}Zr-LABELED BEVACIZUMAB IN BREAST CANCER, LUNG CANCER, RENAL CELL CARCINOMA, NEUROENDOCRINE TUMORS, AND PONTINE GLIOMA

Another target for treatment of breast cancer and many other tumor types is vascular endothelial growth factor A (VEGF-A), which is involved in tumor angiogenesis. Overexpression of VEGF-A has been reported in malignant breast tumors and ductal carcinoma in situ and has been related to aggressiveness of the disease. Bevacizumab is a mAb that targets all splice variants of VEGF-A, both small isoforms which can diffuse freely in the circulation, as well as larger isoforms which are primarily matrix-bound. Despite the fact that VEGF-A is not a membrane target like HER2, it is partly associated with the tumor blood vessels and to some extent with the extracellular matrix of tumor cells, which could enable imaging of tumor lesions.

It can be hypothesized that local VEGF-A concentration reflects whether tumor progression is driven by angiogenesis and if anti-angiogenic treatment is likely to be effective. Therefore, ^{89}Zr-bevacizumab-PET is of interest for several applications: biological characterization of tumors, prediction of therapeutic outcome, and treatment evaluation of VEGF-A targeting drugs.

^{89}Zr-Labeled Bevacizumab in Breast Cancer

Gaykema et al. performed a study to assess whether VEGF-A can be visualized by ^{89}Zr-bevacizumab-PET in patients with primary breast cancer who were scheduled for surgery (Gaykema et al., 2013). In this study 37 MBq ^{89}Zr-labeled bevacizumab (5 mg) was administered and PET scans were acquired at 4 days p.i.. The same dose was used in a previous study with ^{111}Indium-labeled bevacizumab, which visualized all known melanoma lesions (Nagengast et al., 2011). Tumor uptake of ^{89}Zr-bevacizumab was observed in 25 of 26 tumors in 23 patients with primary breast cancer. The false-negative tumor was a 10 mm VEGF-A-positive invasive ductal carcinoma. Besides assessment of tumor uptake in the primary tumors, uptake of ^{89}Zr-bevacizumab in lymph node metastasis regions was evaluated. 4 of 10 metastasis-involved lymph node regions were detected in 9 patients. Zero of 4 axillary regions with lymph node metastases were detected by ^{89}Zr-bevacizumab-PET.

For all available tumors ($n = 25$) VEGF-A expression was quantified by enzyme-linked immunosorbent assay. ^{89}Zr-bevacizumab uptake in tumors correlated with the VEGF-A tumor levels measured. Microvessel density on immunohistochemistry was not correlated with ^{89}Zr-bevacizumab uptake. This was the first clinical study showing a significant correlation between antigen expression and tumor uptake of the mAb. The fact that VEGF-A is not/hardly expressed in normal tissue, while the antigen might be well accessible for mAbs in tumor tissue, might be favorable factors for finding such a correlation. This observation opens avenues for the use of [89]Zr-bevacizumab-PET for response monitoring in therapeutic strategies aiming to downregulate VEGF-A.

The effect of the HSP90 inhibitor NVP-AUY922 on alteration of VEGF-A status was evaluated in the same study discussed earlier for [89]Zr-trastuzumab in breast cancer (Gaykema et al., 2014). However, [89]Zr-bevacizumab-PET was not able to predict treatment outcome measured by CT in patients with estrogen-receptor-positive breast cancer ($n = 6$). Possible explanations are that most lesions found on [89]Zr-bevacizumab PET were bone lesions and not measurable on CT, and that HIF1a is likely a less prominent client protein of HSP90 than HER2. Target expression may be dependent on tumor type, as [89]Zr-bevacizumab uptake in breast tumors was consistently lower than in renal cell cancer.

[89]Zr-Labeled Bevacizumab in Lung Cancer

Bevacizumab is also used for treatment of non-small cell lung carcinoma and [89]Zr-bevacizumab is a potential predictive imaging biomarker for this patient group. In a pilot study it was evaluated whether tumor uptake of [89]Zr-bevacizumab could be visualized and quantified in 7 patients with lung cancer (Bahce et al., 2014). Moreover, in this study the correlation between tumor uptake of [89]Zr-bevacizumab and response to a bevacizumab-based treatment regimen was explored. [89]Zr-bevacizumab PET was performed at day 4 and 7 after injection of 37 MBq [89]Zr-labeled bevacizumab (5 mg), one week prior to start of induction therapy with carboplatin, paclitaxel and bevacizumab (15 mg/kg), followed by bevacizumab maintenance upon non-progression after 4 cycles.

All tumor lesions showed visible [89]Zr-bevacizumab uptake. Tumor-to-blood ratios increased from 1.2 ± 0.4 to 2.2 ± 1.2 between day 4 and 7 p.i.. Tumor lesions had an approximately four times higher [89]Zr-bevacizumab uptake compared to non-tumor background tissues (muscle, healthy lung and fatty tissue). A positive trend, but no significant correlation, was observed for tumor uptake and progression-free survival and overall survival after combined chemo-immunotherapy.

A limitation of this study design is that no distinction is possible between therapeutic contribution of chemotherapy and immunotherapy, as this is a combined treatment regimen. Therefore, further [89]Zr-bevacizumab-PET studies are required to assess VEGF-target status after combination treatment, as a response predictor for effectiveness of subsequent bevacizumab maintenance therapy.

As all lesions were visualized with a total protein dose of 5 mg [89]Zr-bevacizumab, and no targeting of normal tissues became apparent, there is no indication of an antigen sink for this mAb. A limitation of the current study was that no extra biopsies were obtained to confirm VEGF-A tumor expression as driver for [89]Zr-bevacizumab uptake and therapeutic response.

[89]Zr-Labeled Bevacizumab in Renal Cell Carcinoma

Oosting et al. investigated [89]Zr-bevacizumab-PET in patients with metastatic renal cell carcinoma as an imaging modality for treatment evaluation of anti-angiogenic drugs (Oosting et al., 2015).

Patients were randomized between treatment with bevacizumab (10 mg/kg intravenously every 14 days) combined with interferon-α (3 million IU, 3 times per week) ($n = 11$) or sunitinib (50 mg orally, daily for 4 weeks followed by 2 weeks off treatment) ($n = 11$), which is a multi-targeted receptor tyrosine kinase inhibitor. At baseline, and 2 and 6 weeks after treatment, PET scans were acquired after administration of 37 MBq [89]Zr-labeled bevacizumab (5 mg).

Tumor lesions were visualized in all patients (in total 125 lesions), including 35 that had not been detected by CT. 19 lesions were outside the field of view of the CT, including 5 brain lesions in 3 patients (two had known brain metastasis). Remarkable interpatient and intrapatient heterogeneity in tumor uptake of [89]Zr-bevacizumab was observed. A strong decrease in tumor uptake of -47.0% at week 2 was observed for patients on bevacizumab/interferon-α treatment, with an additional change of -9.7% at week 6. For patients on sunitinib treatment, a mean change in tumor uptake of -14.3% at week 2 and a rebound of $+72.6\%$ at week 6 was reported (after 2 drug-free weeks).

Change in tumor uptake of [89]Zr-bevacizumab did not correlate with time to progression. Baseline tumor uptake of [89]Zr-bevacizumab corresponded with longer time to progression. Although, reduced [89]Zr-bevacizumab tumor uptake after treatment might be caused by saturation due to treatment with unlabeled bevacizumab, other clinical studies have suggested that bevacizumab-induced vascular changes do occur after treatment.

Further studies are required to assess whether baseline tumor uptake of [89]Zr-bevacizumab can be used to predict benefit from anti-angiogenic treatment. Heterogeneity in tumor uptake of [89]Zr-bevacizumab may offer a possibility to differentiate patients groups based on tumor biology and to guide the choice between anti-angiogenic and other treatment strategies.

[89]Zr-Labeled Bevacizumab in Neuroendocrine Tumors

In another feasibility study with [89]Zr-bevacizumab, the effect of everolimus, a mammalian target of rapamycin inhibitor, on tumor uptake was investigated in patients with advanced progressive neuroendocrine tumors (NET) (van Asselt et al., 2014). As everolimus can reduce VEGF-A production, it was evaluated whether NET lesions can be visualized by [89]Zr-bevacizumab PET and whether tumor uptake of [89]Zr-bevacizumab decreases from baseline to week 2 and 12 during everolimus therapy (10 mg orally once daily). This study was also performed with 37 MBq [89]Zr-labeled bevacizumab (5 mg), with imaging 4 days p.i.. In 4 of 14 patients no tumor lesions could be visualized with [89]Zr-bevacizumab-PET, in the remaining patients only 19% of tumor lesions ≥ 1 cm (63 lesions in total) known by CT were positive at PET, demonstrating variable [89]Zr-bevacizumab tumor uptake in NET patients. [89]Zr-bevacizumab uptake diminished during everolimus treatment with a mean of -7% at 2 weeks and -35% at 12 weeks. Change in tumor uptake correlated with treatment outcome, assessed by CT after

3 months. There was no correlation between baseline tumor uptake and change of tumor size as assessed by CT, indicating that ^{89}Zr-bevacizumab-PET was not qualified for response prediction before therapy.

Interestingly, in 4 of 14 patients no visual uptake was observed, while no patient had progressive disease after 3 and 6 months of treatment with everolimus. This might indicate that everolimus exerts also other mechanisms of action than just reduction of VEGF-A, or reflect that NETs are slow growing tumors.

^{89}Zr-labeled Bevacizumab in Pontine Glioma

For brain tumors like diffuse intrinsic pontine glioma in children, it is not known whether targeted drugs actually can reach the tumor. Nevertheless, several studies are ongoing to investigate treatment with bevacizumab for this indication. The first report ever on molecular imaging in children, was a feasibility study on the therapeutic potential of bevacizumab and toxic risks, due to VEGF-A expression in normal organs in children with pontine glioma (van Zanten et al., 2013). 3 patients, aged 6, 7, and 17 years received 0.9 MBq/kg (range 18–37 MBq) ^{89}Zr–bevacizumab (0.1 mg/kg). Whole body PET scans were obtained at 1, 72, and 144 h p.i.. Tumor uptake of ^{89}Zr-bevacizumab was observed in 2 of 3 patients, limited to the T1-MRI contrast-enhanced part of the tumor. These findings suggest that disruption of the blood-brain barrier, as indicated by MRI contrast, is necessary for effective tumor targeting by ^{89}Zr-bevacizumab. Uptake in normal organs was highest in the liver, followed by the kidneys, lungs, and bone marrow. This study illustrates that also in children ^{89}Zr-immuno-PET is a feasible procedure, and has potential as a response and toxicity predictor for treatment with bevacizumab and other targeted drugs.

^{89}Zr-LABELED FRESOLIMUMAB IN HIGH-GRADE GLIOMA

As indicated before, mAbs might be prevented from reaching tumor lesions in the brain by impermeability of the blood-brain barrier, while tumor targeting is a prerequisite for effective treatment. An appealing target molecule for treatment of high-grade glioma is transforming growth factor β (TGF-β), which functions as a tumor promotor and induces proliferation and metastasis, while suppressing the immune response. TGF-β and its receptors are overexpressed in high-grade glioma and can be targeted with several types of TGF-β inhibitors. Fresolimumab is a mAb capable of neutralizing all mammalian isoforms of TGF-β (i.e., 1, 2, and 3) and has been investigated in phase I trials with patients with melanoma, renal cell carcinoma and in a phase II trial in patients with mesothelioma.

Den Hollander et al. investigated uptake of ^{89}Zr-fresolimumab in 12 patients with recurrent high-grade glioma and assessed clinical outcome after fresolimumab treatment (den Hollander et al., 2015). In this study an imaging dose of 37 MBq ^{89}Zr-fresolimumab (5 mg) was used before start of treatment (5 mg/kg

i.v. every 3 weeks) and PET scans were obtained for all patients on day 4 p.i., while 4 patients also received a scan at day 2 p.i..

In all patients uptake of ^{89}Zr-fresolimumab was observed in brain tumor lesions ($n = 16$), while in 8 patients not all known brain tumor lesions were visualized with ^{89}Zr-fresolimumab-PET (mostly small lesions, <10 mm on MRI). The three lesions larger than 10 mm that were missed by ^{89}Zr-fresolimumab-PET were suspected to represent radionecrosis instead of viable tumor tissue (therefore probably lacking TGF-β expression), based on previous irradiation or disappearance on follow-up MRI. Tumor-to-blood ratios increased from day 2 to 4 p.i. in patients who underwent whole body PET scans ($n = 4$), which was considered to be suggestive for tumor-specific TGF-β-driven mAb uptake. All patients showed progressive disease on fresolimumab treatment, therefore no correlation between tumor uptake of ^{89}Zr-fresolimumab and clinical response was observed. Because of absence of clinical benefit the study was closed after the first 12 patients.

In conclusion, this study showed that ^{89}Zr-fresolimumab reaches brain tumor lesions. mAb treatment with TGF-β targeting drugs remains an interesting approach for treatment of high-grade glioma, especially since targeting of brain tumor lesions has been observed by ^{89}Zr-fresolimumab-PET. Increase in tumor to blood ratios suggests specific tumor uptake, although non-specific antibody uptake due to disruption of the blood-brain barrier cannot be excluded.

^{89}Zr-LABELED CETUXIMAB IN COLORECTAL CARCINOMA

Another target antigen of interest is EGFR, which can be targeted with cetuximab. Binding of cetuximab to EGFR prevents growth factor binding to the receptor, induces receptor internalization, and causes inhibition of the receptor tyrosine kinase activity. In this way cetuximab interferes with cell growth, differentiation and proliferation, apoptosis and cellular invasiveness. Colorectal cancer with RAS wild type can be effectively treated with cetuximab, while it is known that patients with a K-RAS or N-RAS mutation do not respond to anti-EGFR treatment (van Cutsem et al., 2011). Only patients with RAS wild type colorectal cancer are eligible for anti-EGFR treatment. However, even in this selected patient group efficacy of single agent cetuximab remains limited, as clinical benefit is observed in only half of the patients (Peeters et al., 2015). Additional growth activating mutations or insufficient tumor targeting may affect clinical efficacy. As EGFR is highly expressed on hepatocytes in normal liver tissue, this might lead to sequestration of anti-EGFR-mAbs shortly after administration and interfere with effective tumor targeting.

Assuming that response to treatment is dependent on uptake of cetuximab in tumor lesions, only patients in whom tumor targeting can be confirmed will be susceptible to treatment. Menke-van der Houven van Oordt et al. performed a feasibility study in 10 patients with advanced colorectal cancer to investigate biodistribution and tumor uptake of ^{89}Zr-cetuximab and evaluated ^{89}Zr-cetuximab as a predictive imaging biomarker

(Menke-van der Houven van Oordt et al., 2015). While blood pool, spleen, kidney and lung activity decreased, uptake in the liver increased during the first 2 days, after which a plateau was reached. Total radioactivity derived from the whole body PET images decreased due to gastro-intestinal excretion, while no excretion via the bladder was observed.

Tumor uptake was visible in 6 of 10 patients, of which 4 had clinical benefit. In a patient with 2 lung lesions, one lesion could be visualized, while the other could not, possibly indicating intra-individual heterogeneity of receptor expression or an effect of tumor size (the lesion not visualized was smaller). Of the remaining 4 out of 10 patients without tumor uptake, 3 had progressive disease and 1 had clinical benefit without visible ^{89}Zr-cetuximab uptake. Possibly, the amount of cetuximab that reached the latter tumor was insufficient for visual detection, but did induce anti-tumor activity. This example indicates that for appropriate interpretation of tumor uptake-response relationships it is of paramount importance that ^{89}Zr-cetuximab and unlabeled cetuximab show exactly the same biodistribution.

Altogether these results support further investigations in a larger cohort to assess whether ^{89}Zr-cetuximab can discriminate between cetuximab responding and non-responding patients. Currently a follow-up study, including dose escalation for patients without visible tumor uptake of ^{89}Zr-cetuximab and assessment of cetuximab concentrations in tumor biopsies, is ongoing (ClinicalTrials.gov Identifier: NCT02117466). A limitation of ^{89}Zr-cetuximab-PET reported by the authors is its inability to detect tumor lesions in the liver. In contrast to ^{89}Zr-trastuzumab, ^{89}Zr-cetuximab specifically accumulates in normal liver tissue resulting in spillover when quantifying hepatic lesions. Important technical aspects to consider are whether the imaging dose (^{89}Zr-labeled cetuximab) and the therapeutic dose (unlabeled cetuximab) show similar biodistribution, and if the degree of similarity can be influenced by the sequence of administration.

In this study patients were treated with a cold therapeutic dose of cetuximab (500 mg/m^2), within 2 h followed by the infusion of 37 MBq ^{89}Zr-cetuximab (10 mg). It was assumed that within this time frame the therapeutic dose and the imaging dose behave as if injected simultaneously due to slow pharmacokinetics. Sequential administration was chosen to make radiation safety precautions during administration of ^{89}Zr-cetuximab easier.

Previous studies with ^{111}In-cetuximab (C225) in patients with squamous cell lung carcinoma have indicated a dose-dependent biodistribution, showing liver sequestration of ^{111}In-cetuximab, which decreased with increasing doses of unlabeled cetuximab (up to 300 mg), while tumor uptake increased (Divgi et al., 1991). To get better insight in the dose-dependent biodistribution of ^{89}Zr-cetuximab, Menke-van der Houven van Oordt et al. administered a scouting dose of 0.1 mg ^{89}Zr-cetuximab before the dose of unlabeled cetuximab in 3 patients (Menke-van der Houven van Oordt et al., 2015). Blood samples 2 and 3 h post injection of the scouting dose revealed that only <10% of the injected dose of ^{89}Zr-cetuximab was left in the blood circulation. When subsequently cold cetuximab (500 mg/m^2) was administered, ^{89}Zr-cetuximab reappeared in the blood, indicating that it can be reversibly

extracted, most probably by the liver. On the other hand, the biological half-life of ^{89}Zr-cetuximab, if administered directly after the unlabeled dose, was comparable with the half-life as reported for unlabeled cetuximab. This indicates that upon such sequential administration ^{89}Zr-cetuximab indeed reflects the biodistribution of unlabeled cetuximab. Future studies are required to assess to which extent sequential administration of imaging and therapeutic doses influences tumor biodistribution and tumor uptake of ^{89}Zr-cetuximab.

^{89}Zr-LABELED ANTI-PSMA IN PROSTATE CANCER

Current clinical challenges in imaging of metastatic prostate cancer include limited sensitivity and specificity to detect early metastases (especially in bone) and active disease and to monitor treatment of metastatic prostate cancer. The humanized mAb huJ591 targets the extracellular domain of prostate-specific membrane antigen (PSMA), a transmembrane glycoprotein expressed by both benign and malignant prostate epithelial cells. Nearly all prostate cancers express PSMA. Upon binding, the huJ591-PSMA complex becomes rapidly internalized. Binding of anti-PSMA mAbs to non-prostate tissue, as the liver, duodenal epithelial (brush border) cells and proximal tubule cells in the kidney, has been observed, as well as binding to tumor-associated neovasculature in other solid malignancies, including clear cell renal carcinoma, colon and breast carcinoma (Chang, 2004).

Recently, Pandit-Taskar et al. performed a clinical study with ^{89}Zr-labeled huJ591 in 50 patients with castrate-resistant metastatic prostate cancer (Pandit-Taskar et al., 2015). Results of the first 10 patients were reported separately, including assessment of optimal imaging time post-injection for lesion detection of ^{89}Zr-huJ591 PET imaging (Pandit-Taskar et al., 2014). These 10 patients received 4 scans within 8 days after injection. Based on optimal tumor-to-background ratios, the other 40 patients were imaged once at 6–8 days p.i.. In this ^{89}Zr-immuno-PET study a total mAb dose of 25 mg huJ591 was used, of which 1.7 mg was ^{89}Zr-labeled (203 MBq). This dose was based on prior studies with ^{111}In-J591 and ^{177}Lu-J591 that showed saturation of PSMA expressed by the normal liver at 25 mg of huJ591 (Morris et al., 2005). A dose-dependent uptake in the liver with increasing mAb dose was observed, and optimal trade off was reached at a mAb dose of 25 mg. The unlabeled dose of huJ591 was administered intravenously within 5 min, immediately followed by injection of ^{89}Zr-huJ591 within 1 min.

Pandit-Taskar et al. evaluated performance characteristics of ^{89}Zr-DFO-huJ591 PET/CT for detecting metastases compared to conventional imaging modalities (baseline FDG-PET, ^{99m}Tc-methylenediphosphonate (MDP) bone scans and CT scans) and pathology, to provide evidence for the use of ^{89}Zr-huJ591 as an imaging biomarker. In a lesion-based analysis ^{89}Zr-J591 imaging demonstrated superior visualization of bone lesions relative to conventional imaging, see **Figure** . However, detection of soft tissue lesions was suboptimal. A generalized lower tumor uptake was observed for soft tissue lesions compared to bone lesions. Low uptake was observed in normal bone and considered to be

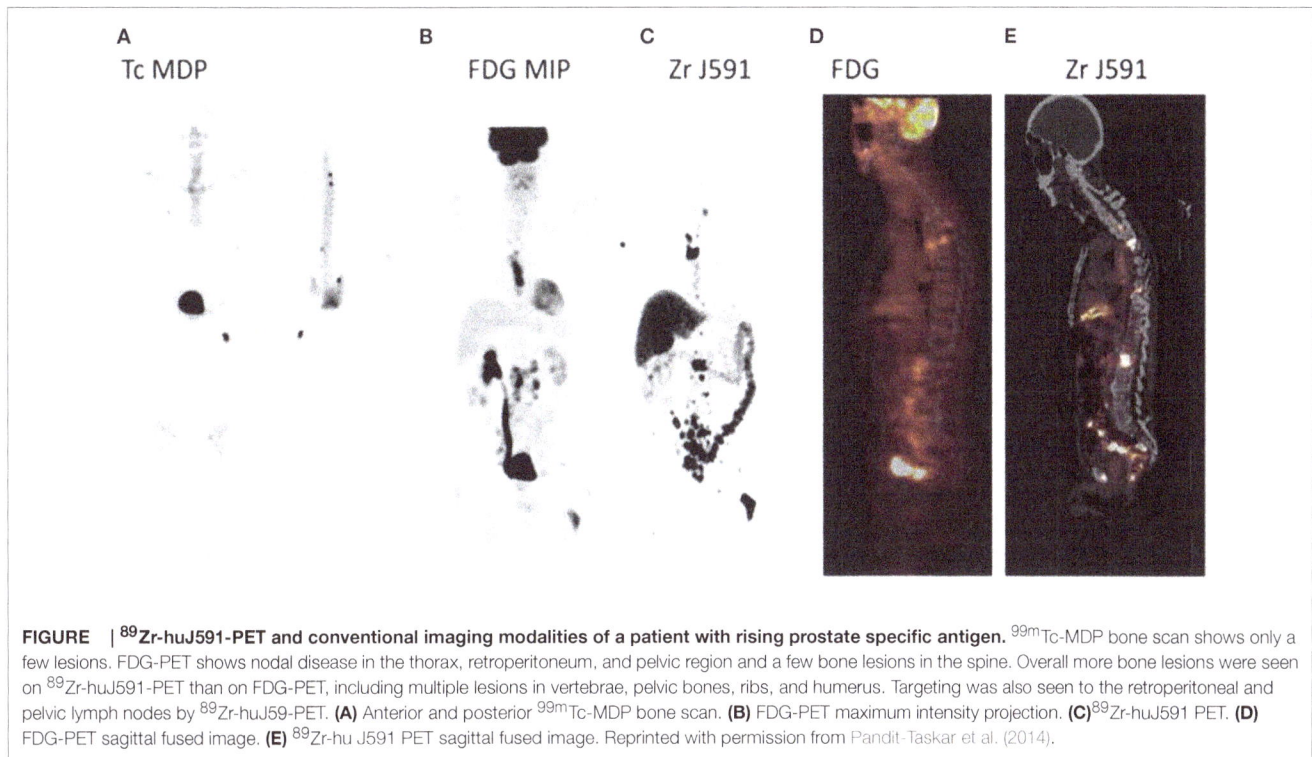

FIGURE | **^{89}Zr-huJ591-PET and conventional imaging modalities of a patient with rising prostate specific antigen.** ^{99m}Tc-MDP bone scan shows only a few lesions. FDG-PET shows nodal disease in the thorax, retroperitoneum, and pelvic region and a few bone lesions in the spine. Overall more bone lesions were seen on ^{89}Zr-huJ591-PET than on FDG-PET, including multiple lesions in vertebrae, pelvic bones, ribs, and humerus. Targeting was also seen to the retroperitoneal and pelvic lymph nodes by ^{89}Zr-huJ59-PET. **(A)** Anterior and posterior ^{99m}Tc-MDP bone scan. **(B)** FDG-PET maximum intensity projection. **(C)** ^{89}Zr-huJ591 PET. **(D)** FDG-PET sagittal fused image. **(E)** ^{89}Zr-hu J591 PET sagittal fused image. Reprinted with permission from Pandit-Taskar et al. (2014).

non-specific. Among the possibilities explaining a lower tumor uptake in soft tissue are: lower PSMA expression, absence of tumor in lesions presumed to be disease by CT and FDG-PET scan, or impaired accessibility of PSMA for intact mAbs. For the biopsy-confirmed lesions overall accuracy of ^{89}Zr-J591 was 95.2% (20/21) for osseous lesions and 60% (15/25) for soft-tissue lesions. No data is provided on ^{89}Zr-J591 uptake related to PSMA expression in tumor biopsies.

The authors conclude that ^{89}Zr-huJ591 imaging is able to detect active disease earlier than conventional imaging, making PSMA an attractive target for diagnosis of prostate cancer. Despite the fact that just a small proportion of lesions were biopsied, statistical arguments indicated that ^{89}Zr-huJ591 imaging detects 50% more bone lesions (occult disease) than bone scan. However, no single imaging modality can serve as gold standard, therefore a known site of disease was defined as any lesions identified by conventional imaging at baseline. Small lesions were most probably missed, while the treatment of patients after imaging was variable, which limits the detection of lesions through follow-up imaging.

The relatively long period post injection required for optimal imaging, may be a practical limitation of ^{89}Zr-immuno-PET for routine application in diagnosis. Promising alternative ligands for molecular imaging of prostate cancer are smaller molecules as radiolabeled minibodies or urea-based small peptides, although none have been validated in controlled clinical trials for routine clinical use (Viola-Villegas et al., 2014). The perspectives of ^{89}Zr-immuno-PET might be different when considering ^{89}Zr-huJ591 for therapeutic approaches.

^{89}Zr-LABELED ANTI-MSLN IN PANCREATIC AND OVARIAN CARCINOMA

For several tumor types, such as pancreatic and ovarian carcinoma, no important drug targets are available. Exploitation of tumor-specific membrane proteins, even those without a known role in oncogenesis, as targets for delivery of potent drugs by ADCs is a promising approach. In this respect, a potential target molecule, with largely unknown biological function, is membrane-bound surface glycoprotein mesothelin (MSLN). It is minimally expressed by normal mesothelial cells, lining pleural, pericardial and peritoneal surfaces. Besides in mesothelioma, it is also highly overexpressed in 80-100% of pancreatic and ovarian cancers (and some other cancers). In preclinical studies with MSLN-expressing tumor bearing mice, ^{89}Zr-anti-MSLN antibody MMOT0530A showed progressive and antigen-specific tumor uptake with micro-PET (Ter Weele et al., 2015).

Therefore, Lamberts et al. evaluated ^{89}Zr-labeled MMOT0530A as a predictive imaging biomarker for treatment (in a phase I setting) with the ADC DMOT4039A, containing the MSLN-antibody MMOT0530A combined with the cytotoxic agent monomethyl auristatin E (Lamberts et al., 2016). For such an approach either the ADC itself can be labeled with ^{89}Zr or the corresponding "naked" mAb, if available for human use. Labeling of the mAb part of the ADCs with ^{89}Zr is well possible, but requires advanced analytical tools to prove that labeling is performed inertly. Assuming that both types of conjugates demonstrate similar biodistribution, which is a research question as such, PET imaging of the target will provide insight into drug distribution (tissue exposure, but also expression of the target and internalization of the antibody). Ideally, clinical [89]Zr-immuno-PET studies with the "naked" mAb are performed before resources are put in the development of an ADC.

The aim of this imaging study was to assess biodistribution and tumor uptake, and the relationship between tumor uptake and MSLN expression, as well as response to treatment. Uptake in normal tissues was as expected, and did not indicate specific uptake, except for high hepatic uptake of [89]Zr-MMOT0530A. This might be due to normal hepatic catabolism of the antibody, maybe slightly elevated by complex formation of the mAb with MSLN antigen shed into the circulation, as MSLN is not expressed on normal liver. Nevertheless, the uptake level in liver was similar to that of other antibodies such as trastuzumab and huJ591. Significant clinical toxicity, reported as dose limiting toxicity, were hypophosphatemia and hyperglycaemia and liver function abnormalities occurred in less than 10% of these patients. Tumor uptake of [89]Zr-MMOT0530A was observed in 37 tumor lesions in 11 patients with pancreatic cancer and 4 patients with ovarian cancer, while 6 measurable tumor lesions visible on diagnostic CT in 4 patients were not detected by [89]Zr-immuno-PET. Within patients a mean 2.4 ± 1.1-fold difference in uptake between tumor lesions was observed, indicating interlesional heterogeneity of tumor uptake.

Tumor uptake of [89]Zr-MMOT0530A was correlated with MSLN expression levels determined with IHC scores (6 patients with pancreatic cancer and 4 patients with ovarian cancer). No correlation was found when the two tumor types were analyzed separately. Tumor uptake of [89]Zr-MMOT0530A was not correlated with progression free survival, on both patient and lesion-based analysis.

The imaging dose for this study was considered to be sufficient, since the amount of tracer still present at 7 days p.i. was enough to clearly visualize the circulation. A first cohort of two patients received 37 MBq [89]Zr-anti-MSLN (1 mg) and were imaged at days 2, 4 and 7 p.i.. Patients in the second cohort ($n = 10$) received a total protein dose of 10 mg mAb, administered as a co-infusion. The biological half-life of [89]Zr-anti-MSLN in cohort 1 was shorter than in cohort 2, most likely due to faster antibody clearance related to small amounts of shed MSLN antigen present in the circulation. Bioavailability of the imaging dose in the second cohort was considered sufficient to evaluate tumor uptake.

This was the first study aiming the use of [89]Zr-immuno-PET as an imaging biomarker for whole body target expression and organs at risk for toxicity, to ultimately guide dosing, confirm delivery, and predict efficacy of the ADC. At this stage of development, however, [89]Zr-immuno-PET was not able yet to add valuable information for individualized treatment decisions.

[89]Zr-LABELED ANTI-CD20 MABS IN B CELL LYMPHOMA

Especially when using mAbs for radioimmunotherapy (RIT), [89]Zr-immuno-PET may be applied to predict toxicity by assessment of biodistribution. This information may enable individualized treatment by optimizing dose schedules to limit unnecessary toxicity for patients.

RIT is used in the treatment of lymphoma, as this type of cancer is highly radiosensitive. More than 90% of B-cell non-Hodgkin lymphoma (NHL) express CD20, making it an attractive target for treatment. The transmembrane phosphoprotein CD20 is also expressed on mature B cells. The biological function of CD20 is still unclear. CD20 is highly expressed on the cell surface and is not rapidly internalized after antibody binding. The anti-CD20 antibody rituximab is widely used in both first-line, as well as subsequent treatment lines for patients with B-cell NHL. Anti-CD20 based RIT with yttrium-90 (^{90}Y)-labeled-ibritumomab tiuxetan is currently approved for treatment of relapsed and refractory NHL (Mondello et al., 2016). Bone marrow toxicity of RIT is dose-limiting, and especially patients with bone marrow infiltration may suffer excessive hematotoxicity.

Rizvi et al. published a clinical study on [89]Zr-immuno-PET to predict toxicity of RIT in NHL patients in order to guide individualized dose optimization (Rizvi et al., 2012). The aim of this study was to assess whether pre-therapy scout scans with [89]Zr-ibritumomab tiuxetan can be used to predict biodistribution of ^{90}Y-ibritumomab tiuxetan and the dose limiting organ during therapy. Patients received standard treatment of 250 mg/m^2 rituximab 1 week before and on the same day prior to both ^{90}Y-and/or [89]Zr-ibritumomab tiuxetan (70 MBq) administrations. The correlation between predicted pre-therapy and therapy organ absorbed doses as based on [89]Zr-ibritumomab tiuxetan images was high. Biodistribution of [89]Zr-ibritumomab tiuxetan was not influenced by simultaneous therapy with ^{90}Y-ibritumomab tiuxetan. Pre-therapy scout scans with [89]Zr-ibritumomab tiuxetan can therefore be used to predict biodistribution and dose-limiting organ during therapy. These results indicate that [89]Zr-immuno-PET may guide safe individualized therapy by optimizing the radioimmunotherapy dose of ^{90}Y-ibritumomab tiuxetan.

The standard treatment with a high amount of cold rituximab before anti-CD20 based RIT, also administered to the patients in the study of Rizvi et al., is common practice to enhance the therapeutic index for RIT. It is thought that the usage of excess unlabeled mAb before RIT may reduce toxicity, in particular bone marrow toxicity. Preloading with unlabeled mAb might prevent normal tissue toxicity by providing a more predictable biodistribution of ^{90}Y-labeled mAb, decreasing clearance rates, and prolonging its circulation half-life. This preload is assumed to clear the peripheral blood of circulating CD20-positive B cells and enhance tumor targeting of the ^{90}Y-labeled antibody to tumor cells. However, supportive data for this approach is limited. It is unclear whether the preload may block subsequently administered ^{90}Y-labeled anti-CD20 antibody, which might impair therapeutic effects.

Muylle et al. performed a study with [89]Zr-rituximab-PET to explore the influence of a preload with unlabeled rituximab in five patients with CD20-positive B-cell lymphoma, scheduled for subsequent RIT with ^{90}Y-labeled rituximab (Muylle et al., 2015). The aim of the study was to compare the distribution of [89]Zr-rituximab without and with a preload of unlabeled rituximab

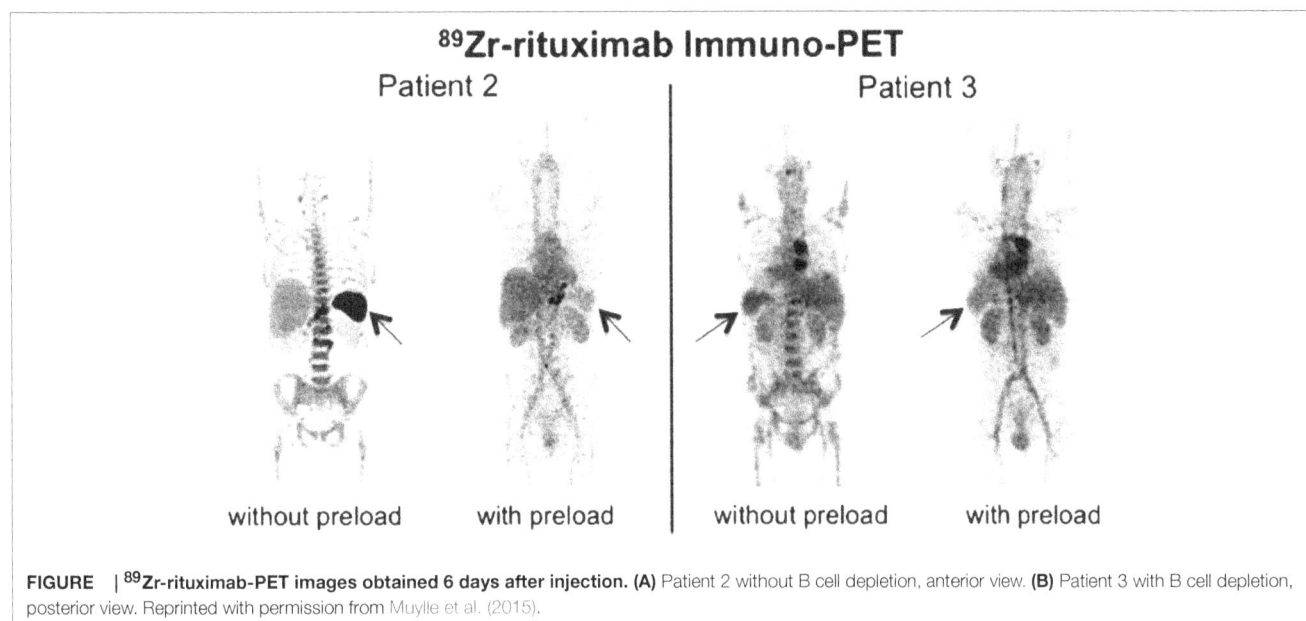

FIGURE | ^{89}Zr-rituximab-PET images obtained 6 days after injection. **(A)** Patient 2 without B cell depletion, anterior view. **(B)** Patient 3 with B cell depletion, posterior view. Reprinted with permission from Muylle et al. (2015).

(within the same patient) to assess the impact on tumor targeting and radiation dose of subsequent radioimmunotherapy with ^{90}Y-labeled rituximab. PET scans were obtained at baseline after administration of 111 MBq ^{89}Zr-labeled rituximab (10 mg). After 3 weeks, a standard preload of unlabeled rituximab (250 mg/m^2) was administered, immediately followed by administration of 10 mg ^{89}Zr-rituximab, and PET scans were acquired.

For the patients with B cell depletion ($n = 3$) tumor uptake without a preload was consistently higher. In patients with preserved circulating B cells ($n = 2$), 3 lesions showed less or no uptake without a preload, while other lesions showed higher uptake. The authors explain higher tumor uptake upon preload by improved biodistribution and prevention of sequestration of ^{89}Zr-rituximab in the "antigen-sink," consisting of CD20-positive B cells in the circulation and in the spleen. Impaired targeting of other tumor sites, however, is explained by partial saturation with unlabeled rituximab.

For patients with preserved circulating CD20-positive B-cells ($n = 2$) without a preload of unlabeled rituximab, an increase in whole-body radiation dose of 59 and 87% was observed mainly due to increased uptake in the spleen, see **Figure** . The effective dose of ^{89}Zr-rituximab was 0.50 milliSievert (mSv)/MBq without a preload and 0.41 mSv/MBq with a preload.

These results suggest that administration of the standard preload of unlabeled rituximab impairs tumor targeting of ^{89}Zr-rituximab in patients with B-cell depletion, due to previous treatment with rituximab. These data suggest that common practice of preloading with unlabeled rituximab before RIT should be re-evaluated and reconsidered.

CONCLUSIONS AND FUTURE DIRECTIONS

In clinical trials with ^{89}Zr-immuno-PET, two requirements should be met in order to realize its full potential. One requirement is that the biodistribution of the ^{89}Zr-mAb (imaging dose) should reflect the biodistribution of the drug during treatment (therapeutic dose). An important pitfall to eliminate is a "false negative" ^{89}Zr-immuno-PET due to absence of tumor uptake of the imaging dose, while there is tumor targeting of the therapeutic dose of unlabeled mAb. This situation may occur in case of expression of target antigen on normal tissue, or in case of a large tumor load with antigen expression. This causes an "antigen sink" that absorbs the tracer dose, leaving insufficient ^{89}Zr-mAb to target all tumor lesions. Therefore, for each mAb, information should be obtained to assess whether a dose-dependent correlation between imaging dose and tumor uptake exists. Preferably a pilot study with different dose levels, within the same patient, is used to define the optimal ^{89}Zr-mAb dose for imaging, i.e., the dose that reflects the therapeutic dose best. With respect to this, in case of co-administration of ^{89}Zr-labeled and cold mAb, it should also be confirmed whether simultaneous administration is needed, or whether sequential administration immediate after each other is allowed.

Another requirement is that tumor uptake of the ^{89}Zr-mAb reflects specific, antigen-mediated, tumor targeting. Next to specific uptake, also non-antigen mediated tumor uptake can occur, possibly caused by enhanced permeability and retention in tumor tissue. Even when tracer uptake is visualized in the tumor, no biological effect can be expected if tumor uptake is not primarily antigen-mediated (a "false positive" ^{89}Zr-immuno-PET). Two clinical studies have reported a correlation between tumor uptake on PET and target expression in biopsies (Gaykema et al., 2013; Lamberts et al., 2016) indicating that tumor uptake on ^{89}Zr-immuno-PET reflects specific, antigen-mediated binding. This would allow the use of ^{89}Zr-immuno-PET as an imaging biomarker to assess target expression, as well as tumor targeting. However, for every mAb-antigen combination this has to be confirmed. In order to evaluate to which extent tumor uptake is driven by nonspecific and/or specific binding, studies correlating tumor uptake to target expression in biopsies, as well as exploration of kinetic modeling, may provide further insight.

Assuming these two crucial requirements are met, ^{89}Zr-immuno-PET can be expected to predict toxicity and response to treatment.

For RIT, it was shown that biodistribution of ^{89}Zr-rituximab can be used to predict biodistribution and the dose-limiting organ for subsequent treatment with ^{90}Y-ibritumomab tiuxetan (Rizvi et al., 2012). This allows for future application of ^{89}Zr-immuno-PET for individualized doze optimization of RIT with the aim to reduce the risk for toxicity. However, so far no clinical studies reported that ^{89}Zr-immuno-PET predicted toxicity of mAb or mAb conjugate treatment.

Prediction of response to treatment for mAbs, is based on the assumption that the drug can only be effective if the target antigen is reached. Although, this is no guarantee for efficacy, as therapy failure may occur due to inadequate dosing of the mAb or intrinsic resistance mechanisms. On the other hand efficacy might occur at low antigen expression levels which is not visualized by ^{89}Zr-immuno-PET. To improve prediction of efficacy of treatment, confirmation of tumor targeting of the drug can be combined with early response assessment. This combined approach may be able to predict whether adequate tumor targeting is followed by sufficient cytotoxicity. Clinical application of molecular imaging to guide individualized treatment may ideally consist of the following 3-step approach:

1. Tumor detection and staging of the disease with conventional imaging (e.g., FDG-PET/diagnostic CT)
2. Assessment of tumor targeting of the drug with molecular imaging (e.g., ^{89}Zr-immuno-PET)
3. Early response assessment on treatment with conventional imaging (e.g., FDG-PET/diagnostic CT)

So far, the ZEPHIR study is the only study utilizing this 3-step approach, using an optimized ^{89}Zr-mAb dose for imaging, and a visual classification for tumor uptake (Gebhart et al., 2016). This study reported that molecular imaging combined with early response assessment is able to predict response to treatment with T-DM1 in patients with HER2-positive breast cancer, opening avenues to cost-effectiveness studies and individualized treatment protocols. Still, this promising result can possibly benefit from improving criteria of positive uptake by quantitative analysis.

Currently, no standardized scale for visual scoring of ^{89}Zr-immuno-PET is available, as opposed to scoring FDG-PET/CT scans by the Deauville criteria (Meignan et al., 2010). Imaging procedures, including data analysis and measurements of tumor uptake should be standardized and validated in order to use ^{89}Zr-immuno-PET in clinical practice. As an example, problems with partial volume effects should be solved. Ideally, by linking imaging data with corresponding clinical outcome of a large set of patients, a criterion for positive tumor uptake can be defined.

Overall, these initial clinical trials have provided indications of the potential of ^{89}Zr-immuno-PET as an imaging biomarker to assess target expression, as well as tumor targeting. The first results supporting application of molecular imaging for prediction of toxicity for RIT and response prediction for treatment with an ADC, form an important first step toward individualized treatment.

AUTHOR CONTRIBUTIONS

YJ, GV performed the literature search and drafted the manuscript. CW, OH, NH, DV, JZ, and MH contributed significantly to the writing. All authors revised the work critically.

ACKNOWLEDGMENTS

Financial support was provided by the Dutch Cancer Society, grant number VU 2013-5839 to YJ.

REFERENCES

Bahce, I., Huisman, M. C., Verwer, E. E., Ooijevaar, R., Boutkourt, F., Vugts, D. J., et al. (2014). Pilot study of ^{89}Zr-bevacizumab positron emission tomography in patients with advanced non-small cell lung cancer. *EJNMMI Res.* 4:35. doi: 10.1186/s13550-014-0035-5

Börjesson, P. K., Jauw, Y. W., Boellaard, R., de Bree, R., Comans, E. F., Roos, J. C., et al. (2006). Performance of immuno-positron emission tomography with zirconium-89-labeled chimeric monoclonal antibody U36 in the detection of lymph node metastases in head and neck cancer patients. *Clin. Cancer Res.* 12, 2133–2140. doi: 10.1158/1078-0432.CCR-05-2137

Börjesson, P. K., Jauw, Y. W., de Bree, R., Roos, J. C., Castelijns, J. A., Leemans, C. R., et al. (2009). Radiation dosimetry of ^{89}Zr-labeled chimeric monoclonal antibody U36 as used for immuno-PET in head and neck cancer patients. *J. Nucl. Med.* 50, 1828–1836. doi: 10.2967/jnumed.109.065862

Chang, S. S. (2004). Overview of prostate-specific membrane antigen. *Rev. Urol.* 6 (Suppl. 10), S13–S18.

Ciprotti, M., Tebbutt, N. C., Lee, F. T., Lee, S. T., Gan, H. K., McKee, D. C., et al. (2015). Phase I imaging and pharmacodynamic trial of CS-1008 in patients with metastatic colorectal cancer. *J. Clin. Oncol.* 33, 2609–2616. doi: 10.1200/JCO.2014.60.4256

Colnot, D. R., Quak, J. J., Roos, J. C., van Lingen, A., Wilhelm, A. J., van Kamp, G. J., et al. (2000). Phase I therapy study of ^{186}Re-labeled chimeric monoclonal antibody U36 in patients with squamous cell carcinoma of the head and neck. *J. Nucl. Med.* 41, 1999–2010.

de Bree, R., Roos, J. C., Quak, J. J., den Hollander, W., Snow, G. B., and van Dongen, G. A. (1995). Radioimmunoscintigraphy and biodistribution of technetium-99m-labeled monoclonal antibody U36 in patients with head and neck cancer. *Clin. Cancer Res.* 1, 591–598.

den Hollander, M. W., Bensch, F., Glaudemans, A. W., Oude Munnink, T. H., Enting, R. H., den Dunnen, W. F., et al. (2015). TGF-β antibody uptake in recurrent high-grade glioma imaged with ^{89}Zr-fresolimumab PET. *J. Nucl. Med.* 56, 1310–1314. doi: 10.2967/jnumed.115.154401

Dijkers, E. C., Oude Munnink, T. H., Kosterink, J. G., Brouwers, A. H., Jager, P. L., de Jong, J. R., et al. (2010). Biodistribution of ^{89}Zr-trastuzumab and PET imaging of HER2-positive lesions in patients with metastatic breast cancer. *Clin. Pharmacol. Ther.* 87, 586–592. doi: 10.1038/clpt.2010.12

Divgi, C. R., Welt, S., Kris, M., Real, F. X., Yeh, S. D., Gralla, R., et al. (1991). Phase I and imaging trial of indium 111-labeled anti-epidermal growth factor receptor monoclonal antibody 225 in patients with squamous cell lung carcinoma. *J. Natl. Cancer Inst.* 83, 97–104. doi: 10.1093/jnci/83.2.97

Evans, J. B., and Syed, B. A. (2014). From the analyst's couch: next-generation antibodies. *Nat. Rev. Drug. Discov.* 13, 413–414. doi: 10.1038/nrd4255

Feugier, P., van Hoof, A., Sebban, C., Solal-Celigny, P., Bouabdallah, R., Ferme, C., et al. (2005). Long-term results of the R-CHOP study in the treatment of elderly patients with diffuse large B-cell lymphoma: a study by the Groupe d'Etude des Lymphomes de l'Adulte. *J. Clin. Oncol.* 23, 4117–4126. doi: 10.1200/JCO.2005.09.131

Gaykema, S. B., Brouwers, A. H., Lub-de Hooge, M. N., Pleijhuis, R. G., Timmer-Bosscha, H., Pot, L., et al. (2013). [89]Zr-bevacizumab PET imaging in primary breast cancer. *J. Nucl. Med.* 54, 1014–1018. doi: 10.2967/jnumed.112.117218

Gaykema, S. B., Schroder, C. P., Vitfell-Rasmussen, J., Chua, S., Oude Munnink, T. H., Brouwers, A. H., et al. (2014). [89]Zr-trastuzumab and [89]Zr-bevacizumab PET to evaluate the effect of the HSP90 inhibitor NVP-AUY922 in metastatic breast cancer patients. *Clin. Cancer Res.* 20, 3945–3954. doi: 10.1158/1078-0432.CCR-14-049

Gebhart, G., Lamberts, L. E., Wimana, Z., Garcia, C., Emonts, P., Ameye, L., et al. (2016). Molecular imaging as a tool to investigate heterogeneity of advanced HER2-positive breast cancer and to predict patient outcome under trastuzumab emtansine (T-DM1): the ZEPHIR trial. *Ann. Oncol.* 37, 619–624. doi: 10.1093/annonc/mdv577

Gong, J., Liu, T., Fan, Q., Bai, L., Bi, F., Qin, S., et al. (2016). Optimal regimen of trastuzumab in combination with oxaliplatin/capecitabine in first-line treatment of HER2-positive advanced gastric cancer (CGOG1001): a multicenter, phase II trial. *BMC Cancer.* 16:68. doi: 10.1186/s12885-016-2092-9

Lamberts, T. E., Menke-van der Houven van Oordt, C. W., Ter Weele, E. J., Bensch, F., Smeenk, M. M., Voortman, J., et al. (2016). ImmunoPET with anti-mesothelin antibody in patients with pancreatic and ovarian cancer before anti-mesothelin antibody-drug conjugate treatment. *Clin. Cancer Res.* 22, 1642–1652. doi: 10.1158/1078-0432

Leone, F., Perissinotto, E., Cavalloni, G., Fonsato, V., Bruno, S., Surrenti, N., et al. (2003). Expression of the c-ErbB-2/HER2 proto-oncogene in normal hematopoietic cells. *J. Leukoc. Biol.* 74, 593–601. doi: 10.1189/jlb.0203068

Lindstrom, L. S., Karlsson, E., Wilking, U. M., Johansson, U., Hartman, J., Lidbrink, E. K., et al. (2012). Clinically used breast cancer markers such as estrogen receptor, progesterone receptor, and human epidermal growth factor receptor 2 are unstable throughout tumor progression. *J. Clin. Oncol.* 30, 2601–2608. doi: 10.1200/JCO.2011.37.2482

Mak, D., Corry, J., Lau, E., Rischin, D., and Hicks, R. J. (2011). Role of FDG-PET/CT in staging and follow-up of head and neck squamous cell carcinoma. *Q. J. Nucl. Med. Mol. Imaging* 55, 487–499.

Makris, N. E., Boellaard, R., Visser, E. P., de Jong, J. R., Vanderlinden, B., Wierts, R., et al. (2014). Multicenter harmonization of [89]Zr PET/CT performance. *J. Nucl. Med.* 55, 264–267. doi: 10.2967/jnumed.113.130112

Meignan, M., Gallamini, A., Haioun, C., and Polliack, A. (2010). Report on the Second International Workshop on interim positron emission tomography in lymphoma held in Menton, France, 8-9 April 2010. *Leuk. Lymphoma.* 51, 2171–2180. doi: 10.3109/10428194.2010.529208

Menke-van der Houven van Oordt, C. W., Gootjes, E. C., Huisman, M. C., Vugts, D. J., Roth, C., Luik, A. M., et al. (2015). [89]Zr-cetuximab PET imaging in patients with advanced colorectal cancer. *Oncotarget* 6, 30384–30393. doi: 10.18632/oncotarget.4672

Moja, L., Tagliabue, L., Balduzzi, S., Parmelli, E., Pistotti, V., Guarneri, V., et al. (2012). Trastuzumab containing regimens for early breast cancer. *Cochrane Database Syst. Rev.* 4:CD006243. doi: 10.1002/14651858.CD006243.pub2

Mondello, P., Cuzzocrea, S., Navarra, M., and Mian, M. (2016). ^{90}Y-ibritumomab tiuxetan: a nearly forgotten opportunity. *Oncotarget* 7, 7597–7609. doi: 10.18632/oncotarget.6531

Morris, M. J., Divgi, C. R., Pandit-Taskar, N., Batraki, M., Warren, N., Nacca, A., et al. (2005). Pilot trial of unlabeled and indium-111-labeled anti-prostate-specific membrane antigen antibody J591 for castrate metastatic prostate cancer. *Clin. Cancer Res.* 11, 7454–7461. doi: 10.1158/1078-0432.CCR-05-0826

Muylle, K., Flamen, P., Vugts, D. J., Guiot, T., Ghanem, G., Meuleman, N., et al. (2015). Tumour targeting and radiation dose of radioimmunotherapy with ^{90}Y-rituximab in CD20+ B-cell lymphoma as predicted by [89]Zr-rituximab immuno-PET: impact of preloading with unlabelled rituximab. *Eur. J. Nucl. Med. Mol. Imaging* 42, 1304–1314. doi: 10.1007/s00259-015-3025-6

Nagengast, W. B., Hooge, M. N., van Straten, E. M., Kruijff, S., Brouwers, A. H., den Dunnen, W. F., et al. (2011). VEGF-SPECT with 111In-bevacizumab in stage III/IV melanoma patients. *Eur. J. Cancer.* 47, 1595–1602. doi: 10.1016/j.ejca.2011.02.009

Oosting, S. F., Brouwers, A. H., van Es, S. C., Nagengast, W. B., Oude Munnink, T. H., Lub-de Hooge, M. N., et al. (2015). [89]Zr-bevacizumab PET visualizes heterogeneous tracer accumulation in tumor lesions of renal cell carcinoma patients and differential effects of antiangiogenic treatment. *J. Nucl. Med.* 56, 63–69. doi: 10.2967/jnumed.114.144840

Oude Munnink, T. H., Dijkers, E. C., Netters, S. J., Lub-de Hooge, M. N., Brouwers, A. H., Haasjes, J. G., et al. (2010). Trastuzumab pharmacokinetics influenced by extent human epidermal growth factor receptor 2-positive tumor load. *J. Clin. Oncol.* 28, e355–e356. doi: 10.1200/JCO.2010.28.4604

Pandit-Taskar, N., O'Donoghue, J. A., Beylergil, V., Lyashchenko, S., Ruan, S., Solomon, S. B., et al. (2014). [89]Zr-huJ591 immuno-PET imaging in patients with advanced metastatic prostate cancer. *Eur. J. Nucl. Med. Mol. Imaging* 41, 2093–2105. doi: 10.1007/s00259-014-2830-7

Pandit-Taskar, N., O'Donoghue, J. A., Durack, J. C., Lyashchenko, S. K., Cheal, S. M., Beylergil, V., et al. (2015). A phase I/II study for analytic validation of [89]Zr-J591 immunoPET as a molecular imaging agent for metastatic prostate cancer. *Clin. Cancer Res.* 21, 5277–5285. doi: 10.1158/1078-0432.CCR-15-0552

Peeters, M., Karthaus, M., Rivera, F., Terwey, J. H., and Douillard, J. Y. (2015). Panitumumab in metastatic colorectal cancer: the importance of tumour RAS status. *Drugs* 75, 731–748. doi: 10.1007/s40265-015-0386-x

Perk, L. R., Vosjan, M. J., Visser, G. W., Budde, M., Jurek, P., Kiefer, G. E., et al. (2010). p-Isothiocyanatobenzyl-desferrioxamine: a new bifunctional chelate for facile radiolabeling of monoclonal antibodies with zirconium-89 for immuno-PET imaging. *Eur. J. Nucl. Med. Mol. Imaging.* 37, 250–259. doi: 10.1007/s00259-009-1263-1

Reichert, J. M. (2016). Antibodies to watch in 2016. *MAbs* 8, 197–204. doi: 10.1080/19420862.2015.1125583

Rizvi, S. N., Visser, O. J., Vosjan, M. J., van Lingen, A., Hoekstra, O. S., Zijlstra, J. M., et al. (2012). Biodistribution, radiation dosimetry and scouting of ^{90}Y-ibritumomab tiuxetan therapy in patients with relapsed B-cell non-Hodgkin's lymphoma using [89]Zr-ibritumomab tiuxetan and PET. *Eur. J. Nucl. Med. Mol. Imaging* 39, 512–520. doi: 10.1007/s00259-011-2008-5

Sliwkowski, M. X., and Mellman, I. (2013). Antibody therapeutics in cancer. *Science* 341, 1192–1198. doi: 10.1126/science.1241145

Stroomer, J. W., Roos, J. C., Sproll, M., Quak, J. J., Heider, K. H., Wilhelm, B. J., et al. (2000). Safety and biodistribution of 99mTechnetium-labeled anti-CD44v6 monoclonal antibody BIWA 1 in head and neck cancer patients. *Clin. Cancer Res.* 6, 3046–3055.

Ter Weele, E. J., van Scheltinga, A. G. T. T., Kosterink, J. G. W., Pot, L., Vedelaar, S. R., Lamberts, L. E., et al. (2015). Imaging the distribution of an antibody-drug conjugate constituent targeting mesothelin with [89]Zr and IRDye800CW in mice bearing human pancreatic tumor xenografts. *Oncotarget.* 6, 42081–42090. doi: 10.18632/oncotarget.5877

Tijink, B. M., Buter, J., de Bree, R., Giaccone, G., Lang, M. S., Staab, A., et al. (2006). A phase I dose escalation study with anti-CD44v6 bivatuzumab mertansine in patients with incurable squamous cell carcinoma of the head and neck or esophagus. *Clin. Cancer Res.* 12, 6064–6072. doi: 10.1158/1078-0432.CCR-06-0910

Tse, C., Gauchez, A. S., Jacot, W., and Lamy, P. J. (2012). HER2 shedding and serum HER2 extracellular domain: biology and clinical utility in breast cancer. *Cancer Treat. Rev.* 38, 133–142. doi: 10.1016/j.ctrv.2011.03.008

van Asselt, S. J., Oosting, S. F., Brouwers, A. H., Bongaerts, A. H., de Jong, J. R., Lub-de Hooge, M. N., et al. (2014). Everolimus reduces [89]Zr-bevacizumab tumor uptake in patients with neuroendocrine tumors. *J. Nucl. Med.* 55, 1087–1092. doi: 10.2967/jnumed.113.129056

van Cutsem, E., Kohne, C. H., Lang, I., Folprecht, G., Nowacki, M. P., Cascinu, S., et al. (2011). Cetuximab plus irinotecan, fluorouracil, and leucovorin as first-line treatment for metastatic colorectal cancer: updated analysis of overall survival according to tumor KRAS and BRAF mutation status. *J. Clin. Oncol.* 29, 2011–2019. doi: 10.1200/JCO.2010.33.5091

van Dongen, G. A., Huisman, M. C., Boellaard, R., Hendrikse, H. N., Windhorst, A. D., Visser, G. W., et al. (2015). [89]Zr-immuno-PET for imaging of long circulating drugs and disease targets: why, how and when to be applied? *Q. J. Nucl. Med. Mol. Imaging* 59, 18–38.

van Zanten, S., Jansen, M., van Vuurden, D., Huisman, M., Hoekstra, O., van Dongen, G. et al. (2013). Innovative molecular imaging in children with diffuse intrinsic pontine glioma. *Neuro Oncol.* 15:132.

Verel, I., Visser, G. W., Boellaard, R., Stigter-van Walsum, M., Snow, G. B., and van Dongen, G. A. (2003). [89]Zr immuno-PET: comprehensive procedures for the production of [89]Zr-labeled monoclonal antibodies. *J. Nucl. Med.* 44, 1271–1281.

Viola-Villegas, N. T., Sevak, K. K., Carlin, S. D., Doran, M. G., Evans, H. W., Bartlett, D. W., et al. (2014). Noninvasive Imaging of PSMA in prostate tumors with [89]Zr-labeled huJ591 engineered antibody fragments: the faster alternatives. *Mol. Pharm.* 11, 3965–3973. doi: 10.1021/mp500164r

Vosjan, M. J., Perk, L. R., Visser, G. W., Budde, M., Jurek, P., Kiefer, G. E., et al. (2010). Conjugation and radiolabeling of monoclonal antibodies with zirconium-89 for PET imaging using the bifunctional chelate p-isothiocyanatobenzyl-desferrioxamine. *Nat. Protoc.* 5, 739–743. doi: 10.1038/nprot.2010.13

Conflict of Interest Statement: The authors declare that the research was conducted in the absence of any commercial or financial relationships that could be construed as a potential conflict of interest.

5

S-thanatin Functionalized Liposome Potentially Targeting on *Klebsiella Pneumoniae* and its Application in Sepsis Mouse Model

Xiaobo Fan[1,2†], Juxiang Fan[2†], Xiyong Wang[2], Pengpeng Wu[1] and Guoqiu Wu[1]*

[1] *Center of Clinical Laboratory Medicine of Zhongda Hospital, Southeast University, Nanjing, China,* [2] *Medical School, Southeast University, Nanjing, China*

S-thanatin (Ts) was a short antimicrobial peptide with selective antibacterial activity. In this study, we aimed to design a drug carrier with specific bacterial targeting potential. The positively charged Ts was modified onto the liposome surface by linking Ts to the constituent lipids via a PEG linker. The benefits of this design were evaluated by preparing a series of liposomes and comparing their biological effects *in vitro* and *in vivo*. The particle size and Zeta potential of the constructed liposomes were measured with a Zetasizer Nano ZS system and a confocal laser scanning microscope. The *in vitro* drug delivery potential was evaluated by measuring the cellular uptake of encapsulated levofloxacin using HPLC. Ts-linked liposome or its conjugates with quantum dots favored bacterial cells, and increased the bacterial uptake of levofloxacin. In antimicrobial assays, the Ts and levofloxacin combination showed a synergistic effect, and Ts-LPs-LEV exhibited excellent activity against the quality control stain *Klebsiella pneumoniae* ATCC 700603 and restored the susceptibility of multidrug-resistant *K. pneumoniae* clinical isolates to levofloxacin *in vitro*. Furthermore, Ts-LPs-LEV markedly reduced the lethality rate of the septic shock and resulted in rapid bacterial clearance in mouse models receiving clinical multidrug resistant (MDR) isolates. These results suggest that the Ts-functionalized liposome may be a promising antibiotic delivery system for clinical infectious disorders caused by MDR bacteria, in particular the sepsis related diseases.

Keywords: targeting delivery, sepsis, antimicrobial peptide, liposome, multidrug resistance

Edited by:
Albert D. Windhorst,
VU University Medical Center,
Netherlands

Reviewed by:
Rink-Jan Lohman,
The University of Queensland,
Australia
Ghanshyam Upadhyay,
The City University of New York, USA

*Correspondence:
Guoqiu Wu
nationball@163.com

† These authors have contributed equally to this work.

INTRODUCTION

Increasing data from clinics has revealed the wide spreading of multidrug resistant (MDR) *Klebsiella pneumoniae* resistant to almost all conventional antibiotics with different structures, such as cephalosporins, carbapenems, fluoroquinolones, lincosamides, and aminoglycosides (Datta et al., 2012; Leone et al., 2012; Kronman et al., 2014). Developing antibiotics with new antimicrobial mechanisms has again become a matter of emergency (Bassetti and Righi, 2015).

Antimicrobial peptides (AMPs) exhibit a broad antimicrobial activity independent of current drug resistance (da Costa et al., 2015). AMPs are considered as a promising solution for the drug resistance and are expected to reach a good synergistic effect when in combination with the traditional antibiotics due to their unique antimicrobial mechanism. In our previous study, we reported a novel antimicrobial peptide of S-thanatin that exhibited selective antimicrobial activity (Wu et al., 2010a,b; Bassetti and Righi, 2015). Notably, Ts showed lipopolysaccharide (LPS) binding affinity, indicating its great potential as a treatment for blood infections (Wu et al., 2010a,b). Ts was proved active against numerous Gram-negative bacteria including MDR but barely active over the Gram-positive species (Wu et al., 2011). The antimicrobial activity of Ts is structure dependent. Ts is a random coil with limited or none antimicrobial activity but adopts a beta-sheet form after activation (Wu et al., 2010a,b). Ts kills bacteria in a membrane-dependent manner. Negatively charged components such as LPS on the cell wall of Gram-negative bacteria and negatively charged lipids on bacterial cytoplastic membranes, can attract Ts electrostatically and thus promote the intercalation of Ts into the cytoplastic membrane. The cytoplastic membrane becomes leaky, which subsequently disintegrates the bacterial respiration and energization (Wu et al., 2010b).

Liposomes have been widely used as pharmaceutical carriers in the past decade due to their merits, such as reducing potential toxicity, prolonging circulation half-life *in vivo*, and enabling controlled release and active or passive targeting of specific cells, tissues, or organs (Kibria et al., 2013). Liposomes have been reported to serve as carriers for antibiotics (Furneri et al., 2000; Muppidi et al., 2011), improving the pharmacokinetics of the encapsulated antibiotics. However, to the best of our knowledge, the coupling of AMPs, such as Ts, to an antibiotic-loaded liposome and the application on bacterial cells have not been reported.

The Ts functioned liposomes were prepared by linking the Ts to the constituent lipids with a PEG linker. Ts played dual-role in this design as a targeting carrier and a bactericidin as well. The preparations were tested *in vitro* and *in vivo* for antimicrobial activities against clinical MDR isolates.

MATERIALS AND METHODS

Chemical Reagents

Hydrogenated soybean phosphatidylcholine (HSPC), cholesterol (CHO), and 3-(N-succinimidyloxyglutaryl) aminopropyl-polyethyleneglycol (2000)-carbamyldistearoyl phosphatidyl ethanolamine (NHS-PEG2000-DSPE) were purchased from Avanti Polar Lipids (Alabaster, AL, USA). The antimicrobial peptide Ts (GSKKPVPIIYCNRRSGKCQRM) was synthesized, refolded and purified, as previously reported (Wu et al., 2010a,b). Ts was conjugated with NHS-PEG2000-DSPE using a method similar to the synthesis of RGD (arginine-glycine-aspartic acid) peptide conjugation (Kibria et al., 2013). Briefly, the Ts peptide was coupled with NHS-PEG-DSPE (1.2:1molar ratio) in deionized water at room temperature for 24 h. The conjugation was purified by HPLC using an appropriate 0–60% acetonitrile gradient in 0.1% trifluoroacetic acid, supplemented with 10 mg/ml of dihydroxy benzoic acid. The purity of the resulting product was 95% or higher. Carbonyl cyanide m-chlorophenyl hydrazone (CCCP, C9H5ClN4, CAS: 555-60-2), bis-(1,3-dibutylbarbituric acid) trimethineoxonol [DiBAC4(3)],

propidium iodide (PI) and 1-(3-dimethylaminopropyl)-3-ethyl-carbodiimide (EDC) were obtained from Sigma (St. Louis, MO, USA). Carboxyl near-infrared quantum dots (QDs605) were purchased from Jiayuan QD Tech Ins (Wuhan, China).

Microorganisms

In this study, a total of 17 clinical isolates of *K. pneumoniae* were used for the antimicrobial assay. These isolates were collected between February and May 2013 in the Center of Medical Laboratory of Zhongda Hospital (Southeast University, China). The VITEK2 system with AST-GN13 cards and GN/CE strips (bio Mérieux, Marcy l'Etoile, France) was used to confirm the identities and susceptibilities of bacteria. *K. pneumonia* ATCC 700603 from the Health Administrate of the People's Republic of China was used as a reference.

Animals

Adult male ICR mice (30–33 g) were obtained from the Experimental Animal Center of Yangzhou, China and reared in the Animal Environmental Control Unit under $23 \pm 3°C$, $50 \pm 10\%$ relative humidity, and a 12-h light-dark cycle. The animal experiments were carried out according to the guideline from the Medical Ethics Committee of Southeast University, China (Permit Number: 2013ZDSYLL109.0).

Preparation of the Liposomes and Encapsulation Efficiency Measurement

The lipids formula, levofloxacin dosage, ammonium sulfate concentration, drug-loading temperature and time for liposome preparation were optimized. HSPC, CHO, and Ts-PEG2000-DSPE were mixed at different ratio for the Ts-LPs liposome preparation with the lipid film hydration method. Levofloxacin was loaded into liposome with the ammonium sulfate gradient method (see Supplementary Methods).

The liposome loaded levofloxacin was measured by HPLC to assess the optimization methods (Furneri et al., 2000) (see Supplementary Methods). A standard curve was made by measuring levofloxacin standard concentration series (Supplementary Figure). A solution containing 0-60% gradient acetonitrile supplemented with 0.1% trifluoroacetic acid was used as the mobile phase for HPLC. The injection volume was fixed to 20 μL. The results were assessed by the encapsulation efficiency (EE), which was calculated as follows: $EE\% = C1/C0^*100\%$, where $C0$ is the amount of total drug, and $C1$ is the amount of drug entrapped in the liposomes. Levofloxacin-loaded liposome without TS (LEV-LPs) was prepared in a similar way.

Liposome Properties

The liposome size, zeta potential, and polydispersity index (PDI) of the liposome emulsion were measured using a Zetasizer Nano ZS system (Malvern Instruments Ltd, Worcestershire, UK).

The shape and size were also examined by transmission electron microscopy (TEM). The liposome suspension was placed on copper grids with films, stained with 2% (w/v) phosphotungstic acid, air-dried for 10 min, and finally examined using a JEM-1010 transmission electron microscope (JEOL, Tokyo, Japan) to determine the morphology of the liposome.

Antimicrobial Activity Assay

MICs were used to evaluate the antimicrobial activity of Ts, levofloxacin, LPs-LEV, Ts-LPs, and Ts-LPs-LEV, according to the broth microdilution guidelines from the Clinical and Laboratory Standards Institute (CLSI) (Anonymous, 2001). LPs-LEV and Ts-LPs-LEV liposome concentrations were calculated as the levofloxacin-containing concentrations which were measured by a similar method as the EE assay. Ts-LPs concentration was calculated as the Ts-containing concentration. The final concentration for Ts, free levofloxacin, LPs-LEV or Ts-LPs-LEV in the tested wells ranged from 2 to 256 µg/mL. After incubation at 37°C for 16–24 h, the bacterial culture optical density (OD) value was measured using a microplate reader with a wavelength of 630 nm (MRX, Dynex). MICs are defined as the lowest concentration where 100% bacterial growth inhibition was reached. Each of the experiments was performed in triplicate. The combination of Ts with conventional antibiotics such as silver nitrate, ampicillin and kanamycin was tested for a synergistic effect (see Supplementary Methods).

Bacterial Targeting of Ts and Ts-LPs

The carboxyl near-infrared quantum dot QDs605 was used to determine the bacterial targeting of Ts. QDs605 and Ts (molar ratio: 1:10) were co-incubated in a solution containing 1 mg/ml EDC for linkage for 2 h at room temperature. The prepared conjugate, Ts-QDs605 was rinsed twice with PBS (0.1M, pH7.4) and stored at 4°C before usage. The Ts-functionalized liposome containing coumarin (Ts-LPs-CM) was prepared using a similar method as described above. The cells pretreated with Ts-QDs605 or Ts-LPs-CM were imaged using a confocal microscope (Olympus, Japan) with excitation/emission wavelengths of 470/505 nm for coumarin and 388/605 nm for QDs605. The photographic parameters were chosen from default and no changes for relative measurements.

Effects of Ts and Ts-LPs on Membrane Permeability and Potential

A single colony of *K. pneumonia* ATCC 700603 was inoculated in Luria-Bertani (LB) broth and cultured at 37°C to reach log-phase. A sample containing approximate 10^7 cells/ml medium was prepared and added with 100 µg/ml Ts or Ts-LPs plus 10 mM CCCP (carbonyl cyanide m-chlorophenyl hydrazone, $C_9H_5ClN_4$, a type of respiratory inhibitor) followed by an incubation at 37°C for 60 min. PBS was used as a negative control. The bacterial cells were retrieved and washed twice with PBS (0.1M, pH7.4). The lipophilic anionic membrane potential-sensitive dye DiBAC4(3) or nucleic acid dye PI was added at a final concentration of 10 µg/ml and incubated for 10 min at room temperature before flow cytometric analysis by BD FACS Canto (Becton Drive, NJ, USA). The excitation/emission wavelengths were 470/510 nm and 488/630 nm for DiBAC4(3) and PI, respectively. The photographic exposure time was set to 500 ms for all measurements.

TABLE | Zeta potential versus Ts-PEG2000-DSPE dosage (w/w).

C_{lip}	C_T	Zeta potential
100%	0%	−29.43 ± 1.32 mV
99%	1%	+8.56 ± 2.43 mV
95%	5%	+20.68 ± 1.72 mV

The liposome formula was optimized as shown in Supplementary Tables S1 and S2. Ts-PEG2000-DSPE was incorporated into the formula at different concentrations to produce positively charged liposomes. The Zeta potential increased along with the concentration of Ts-PEG2000-DSPE in the liposome. At 5% (w/w) concentration, the zeta potential reached +20.68 ± 1.72 mV. C_{lip} represented the total weight ratio of HSPC:cholesterol (CHO) (7:3) used in the liposome preparation, and C_T was the ratio of Ts-PEG2000-DSPE.

Electron Microscopy Studies of *K. pneumoniae* Treated with Ts-LPs-LEV

Transmission electron microscopy (TEM) was employed to confirm the cellular morphological changes after Ts-LPs-LEV treatment (Chapple et al., 1998). Cells were retrieved after receiving saline or Ts-LPs-LEV, and slices were made from cell pellets (see Supplementary Methods). The slices were pre-stained with aqueous uranyl acetate and lead citrate before being sent for examination with a JEM-1010 transmission electron microscope (JEOL, Tokyo, Japan).

Drug Uptake

The accumulation of free levofloxacin and levofloxacin liposomes (LPs-LEV) was determined as previously reported (Furneri et al., 2000). The cellular levofloxacin was retrieved by destruction of the bacterial cells and measured by HPLC, as described for the liposome EE assay. The extracellular levofloxacin concentration in the supernatant was measure by HPLC as well.

Septic Shock Model

Sixty male ICR mice were randomly grouped (15 animals in each group), and intraperitoneally inoculated with 2.5×10^7 cells of clinical MDR isolate CI 130702215 of *K. pneumonia* (MIC > 256 µg/mL for levofloxacin, refer to **Table**). Immediately after the bacterial challenge, the animals were intravenously administrated with levofloxacin, LPs-LEV or Ts-LPs-LEV. Levofloxacin in all forms were equal at the dosage of levofloxacin of 10 mg/kg. The survival rate was monitored and

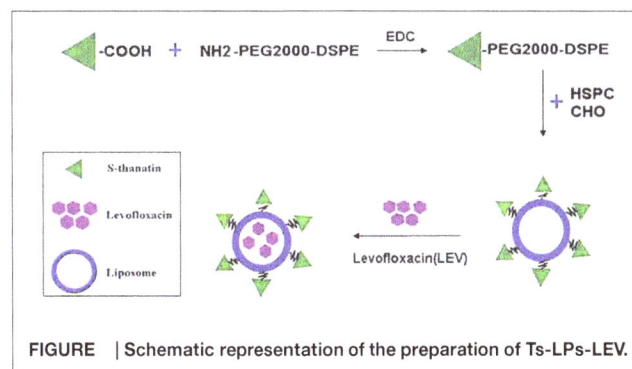

FIGURE | Schematic representation of the preparation of Ts-LPs-LEV.

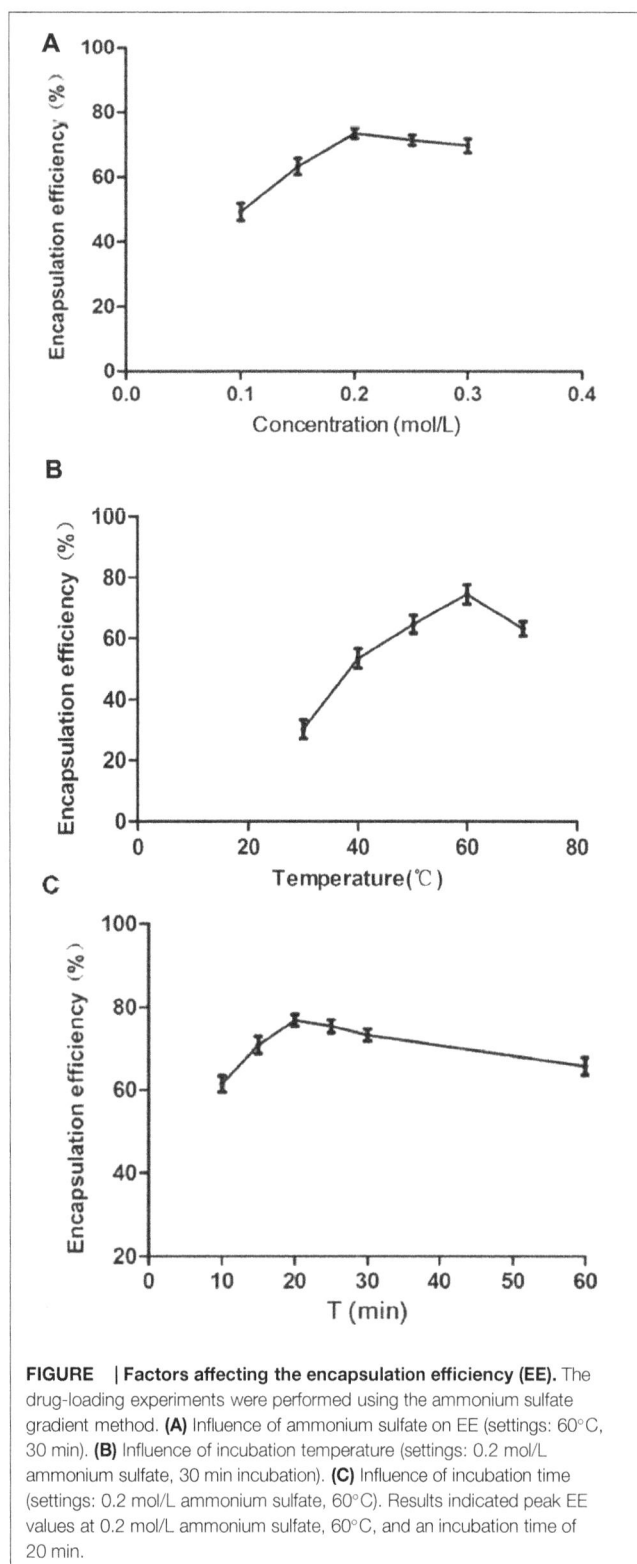

FIGURE | Factors affecting the encapsulation efficiency (EE). The drug-loading experiments were performed using the ammonium sulfate gradient method. **(A)** Influence of ammonium sulfate on EE (settings: 60°C, 30 min). **(B)** Influence of incubation temperature (settings: 0.2 mol/L ammonium sulfate, 30 min incubation). **(C)** Influence of incubation time (settings: 0.2 mol/L ammonium sulfate, 60°C). Results indicated peak EE values at 0.2 mol/L ammonium sulfate, 60°C, and an incubation time of 20 min.

TABLE | Liposome properties by ZetasizerNano ZS system.

Liposome	Diameter size (nm)	PDI	Zeta potential (mV)
LPs	161.3 ± 4.5	0.293	−29.43
Ts-LPs	151.1 ± 2.4	0.216	+20.68
Ts-LPs-LEV	152.5 ± 3.2	0.254	+5.3

A volume of 10 μL liposome sample mixed with 990 μL saline was placed in the cuvette and equilibrated for 10 min before measurement at 25°C. The result was the mean value taken from three repeats for each measurement.

intraperitoneal puncture at 10 min after an intraperitoneal injection of 2 mL sterile saline. Bacterial counting was performed by spreading the samples onto blood agar plates after series dilution of the samples in sterile saline. The plates were incubated overnight at 37°C for bacterial colony counting.

Statistical Analysis

MICs are presented as the mean value from three independent measurements. The quantitative evaluations of levofloxacin accumulation in bacteria and bacterial counting in the intra-abdominal fluid and blood cultures are expressed as the means ± standard deviations (SDs). The analysis of variance (ANOVA) was used for comparison between groups. The mortality rate differences between groups were compared using Fisher's exact test. In all the analyses, $P < 0.05$ was considered statistical significant.

RESULTS

Preparation and Characterization of the Liposomes

The prepared liposome consisted of HSPC, CHO, and Ts-PEG2000-DSPE, with Ts anchored on the surface. The scheme for the preparation of Ts-LP-LEV is showed in **Figure** . As shown in **Table** , Supplementary Tables and **Figure** , the liposome preparation of Ts-LPs-LEV was optimized as follows: (1) Formula: 30 mg/ml HSPC:CHO (4:1, w/w) plus 5% Ts-PEG2000-DSPE; (2) levofloxacin:lipids = 1:4 (mol/mol); (3) drug loading parameters: using 0.2 mol/L ammonium sulfate, incubation at 60°C for 20 min. The drug loading efficiency EE% reached 76.8 ± 2.7% after optimization. As shown in **Table** and **Figure** , the prepared Ts-LEV-LPs with a PDI of 0.254 were 152.5 ± 3.2 nm in diameter showing a good homogeneity, and were positively charged as expected. The blank liposome without levofloxacin was +20.68 mV in zeta potential. The Ts-LPs-LEV possessed a zeta potential of +4.6–5.9 mV. The positive charge indicated the presence of the positively charged Ts on the surface. The liposomes were confirmed of a spherical shape with a diameter of ∼86.9 nm by TEM (**Figure**). The TEM showed decreased size because the TEM imaging was performed in a high-vacuum environment causing liposome shrinkage. The prepared liposomes showed a very good stability in aqueous buffer. No apparent changes or degradation were

blood samples were taken by tail-vein puncture every 6 h for the next 3 days.

Approximately 24 h after bacterial challenge, 0.5 mL abdominal lavage fluid was collected using a long needle through

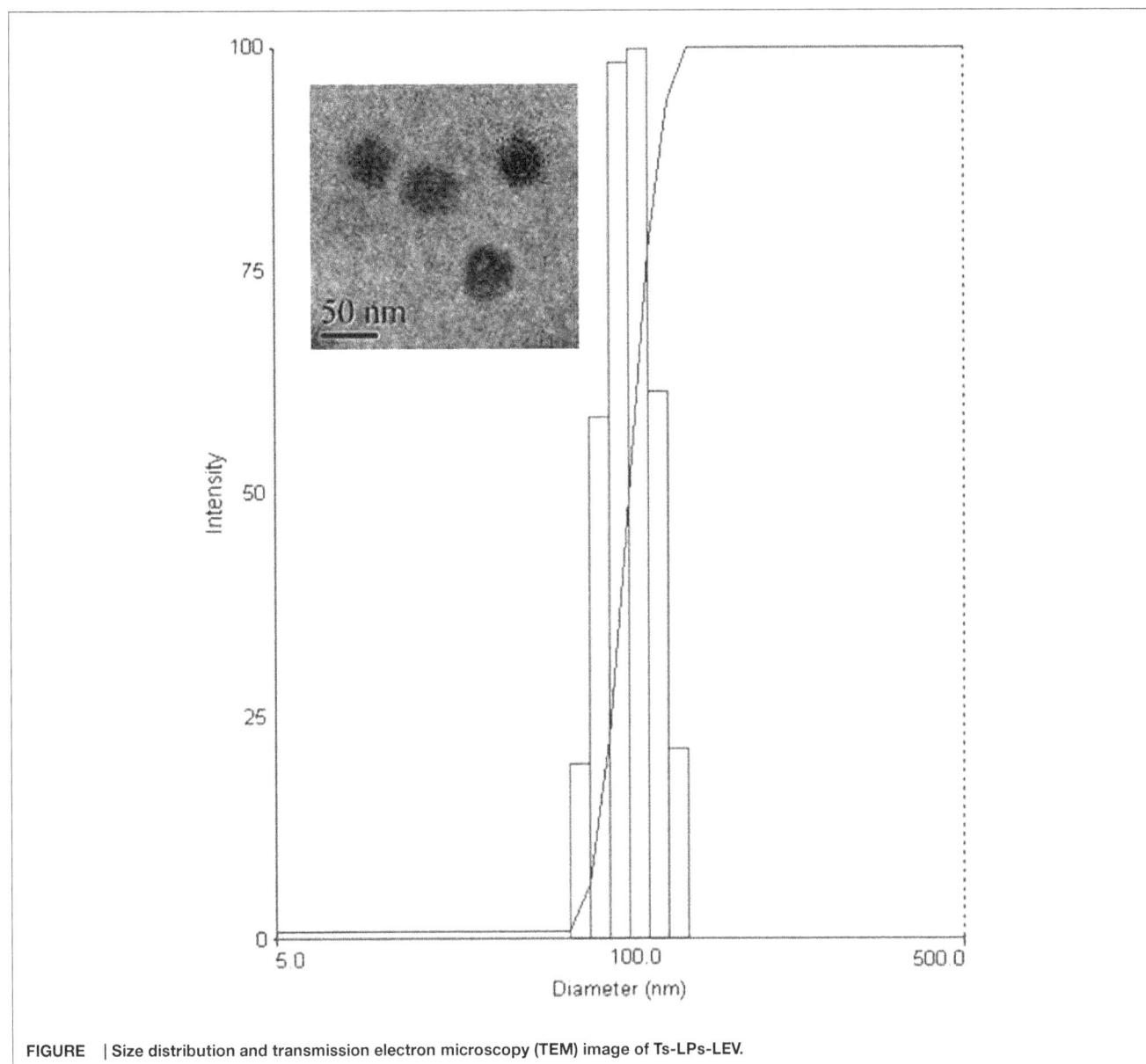

FIGURE | Size distribution and transmission electron microscopy (TEM) image of Ts-LPs-LEV.

observed after the liposomes were stored for 2 months (data not shown).

Confocal Laser Scanning Microscopy (CLSM)

Ts was labeled with the near-infrared quantum dots to confirm the bacterial uptake of Ts. Bacteria were co-incubated with Ts-QDs605 for 60 min before being sent for microscope. The CLSM results indicated that bacteria received Ts-QDs605 gave out stronger fluorescence than that of bacteria receiving QDs605 (**Figures** ,). The uptake of Ts-LPs in the bacteria was also assessed by CLSM using coumarin (CM)-loaded liposome. As shown in **Figures** , , Ts-LPs-CM treated bacterial cells exhibited higher fluorescence intensity than in the LP-CM treated cells.

Effects of Ts and Ts-LPs on Membrane Permeability and Potential by Flow Cytometric Determination

Flow cytometry was employed to investigate the effects of Ts and Ts-LPs on the membrane permeability and potential. The results of the bacteria exposed to PI or DiBAC4(3) were shown in **Figure** . After adding Ts or Ts-LPs, the cell percentages of the dye-associated fluorescence significantly increased ($P < 0.01$). Bactericidal kinetics experiment indicated Ts and Ts-LPs had a rapid bactericidal effect and killed 99% bacteria within the first 10 min (Supplementary Figure). The CCCP with a capacity of reducing energization and respiration in cells dramatically decreased Ts- or Ts-LPs-induced uptake of PI ($P < 0.05$) and DiBAC4(3) ($P < 0.01$; **Figures** ,).

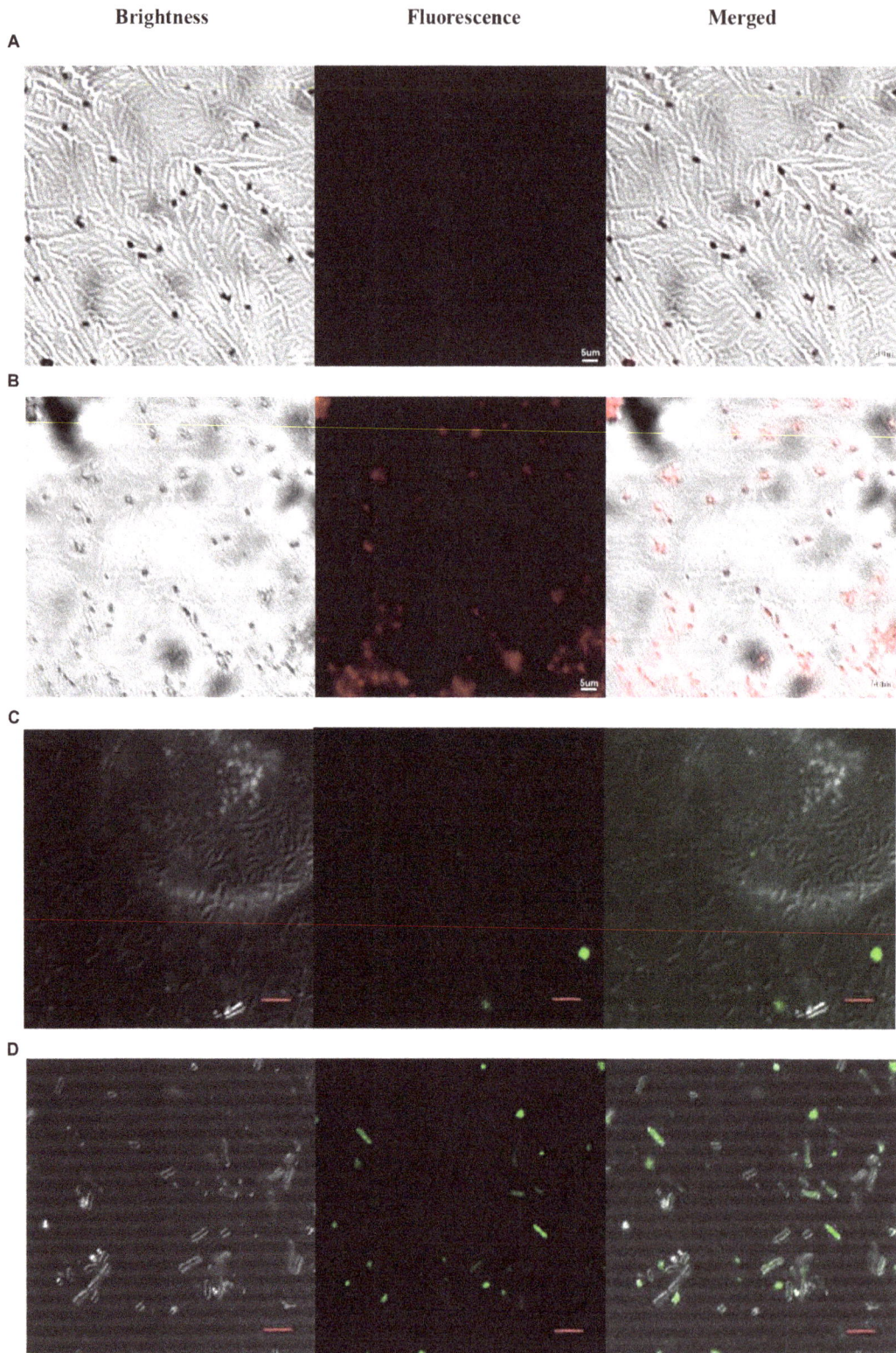

FIGURE | **Ts-QDs605 and Ts-LPs-CM selectively targeting *Klebsiella pneumoniae* cells.** The cell-targeting of Ts to *K. pneumoniae* ATCC 700603 observed by confocal laser scanning microscopy (CLSM) using quantum dots (QD) or coumarin (CM)-loaded liposomes (LPs): **(A)** QDs605. **(B)** Ts-QDs605. **(C)** LPs-CM. **(D)** Ts-LPs-CM. *K. pneumonia* ATCC 700603 cells (approximately 1×10^5 bacteria/ml) were first incubated with Ts-QDs605 (10 nM) for 2 h at 37°C followed by trice rinse with PBS, and then placed on slides. A solution containing 4% (wt/vol) paraformaldehyde was added for sample fixation for 30 min. Ts-LPs-CM were used at 20 nM but different from Ts-QDs605 assay, the cells receiving Ts-LPs-CM were sent to CLSM without washing with PBS. The bar indicated scale of 5 μm.

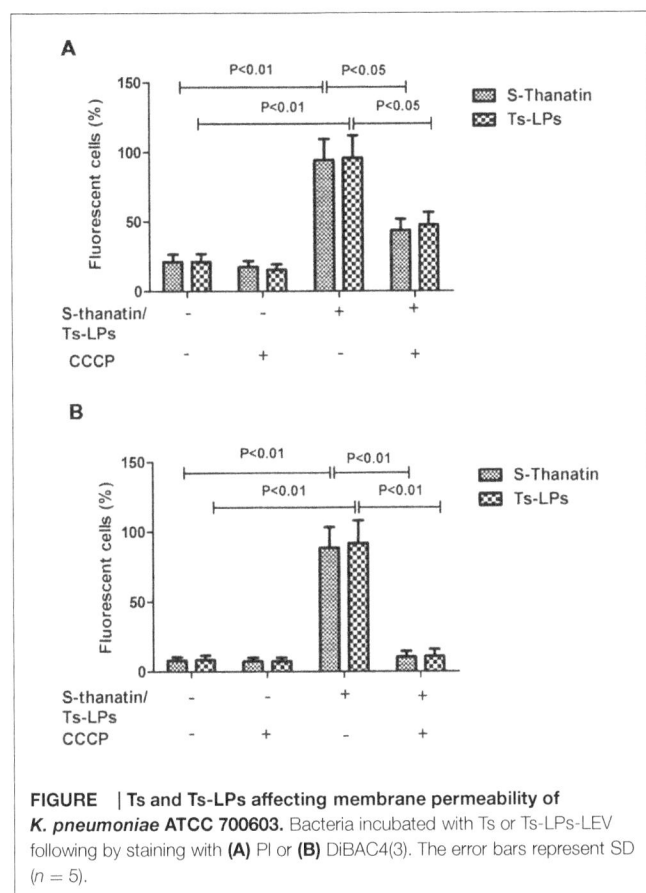

FIGURE | Ts and Ts-LPs affecting membrane permeability of *K. pneumoniae* ATCC 700603. Bacteria incubated with Ts or Ts-LPs-LEV following by staining with (A) PI or (B) DiBAC4(3). The error bars represent SD ($n = 5$).

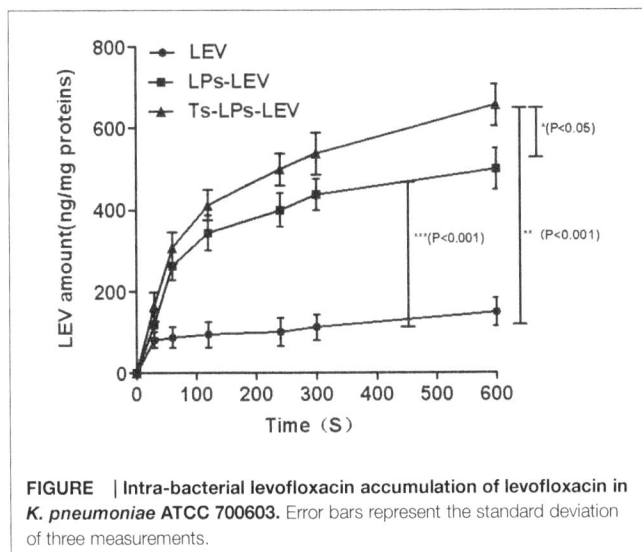

FIGURE | Intra-bacterial levofloxacin accumulation of levofloxacin in *K. pneumoniae* ATCC 700603. Error bars represent the standard deviation of three measurements.

Bacteria Uptake of Levofloxacin

HPLC was used to measure the intracellular levofloxacin level. The levofloxacin accumulation in different groups was presented in **Figure** . A gradual uptake of levofloxacin following a rapid accumulation was observed in the LPs-LEV and Ts-LPs-LEV treated groups. No apparent uptake

was observed after 10 min (data not shown), and Ts and its conjugates killed 99% bacteria within 10 min by CFU counting assay (Supplementary Figure). A significant difference was observed between the Ts-LPs-LEV and LPs-LEV groups with intracellular concentrations of 657 ± 47 and 500 ± 52 ng/mg protein, respectively ($P < 0.05$). Compared with the free drug group (150 ± 35 ng/mg protein), levofloxacin in liposome formulations reached significantly higher intracellular accumulations ($P < 0.001$).

In Vitro Antimicrobial Activities Against Clinical MDR-isolates

All 17 *K. pneumoniae* clinical isolates were multi-drug-resistant, and their MICs to levofloxacin ranged from 8 to >256 μg/mL. Their *in vitro* susceptibilities to Ts, free levofloxacin, LPs-LEV and Ts-LPs-LEV were listed in **Table** . The application of liposome as a drug carrier greatly improved the efficacy of levofloxacin, and incorporation of Ts again improved the efficacy of the LPs-LEV liposome. The MICs of the LPs-LEV and Ts-LPs-LEV were 1-2- and 2-16-dilution lower than that of the free drug, respectively. Drug-free Ts-LPs showed a decreased efficacy compared to Ts. No antimicrobial activity was observed in the blank liposome (data not shown). Ts showed at least additive effects when in combination with the conventional antimicrobial agents. Levofloxacin in combination with 0.2X MIC of Ts reached a synergistic effect (Supplementary Table).

The Bactericidal Effect by Transmission Electron Microscope

Log-phase bacterial cells were exposed to the liposome for 1 h to characterize the antimicrobial effect of Ts-LPs-LEV. Remarkable changes were observed with electron microscope (**Figure**) such as chaotic membrane morphology, vacuolization, chromatin concentration, and cell debris that was similar to the effects of Ts as we reported before.

In Vivo Antimicrobial Activities

A septic shock model was established by intraperitoneal injection of MDR clinical isolate and treatment with the free drug, LPs-LEV or Ts-LPs-LEV, respectively. The lethality rate at 24 h was 100% in both the saline-treated group and free levofloxacin-treated group, whereas it was 73.3 or 6.7% for the LPs-LEV-treated group or for the Ts-LPs-LEV-treated group, respectively. All the animals from the LPs-LEV-treated group were dead within 36 h, whereas 93.3% of the animals from the Ts-LPs-LEV-treated group survived at 72 h (**Figure**).

The bacterial culture results were showed in **Table** . At 24 h, all animals were positive for bacterial culture of the blood and peritoneal fluid samples, but colony count in the groups treated with LPs-LEV and Ts-LPs-LEV was significantly less than that of the saline and levofloxacin treated groups ($P < 0.05$). The Ts-LPs-LEV showed an improved efficacy on bacteria clearance compared to LPs-LEV ($P < 0.05$). To our surprise, levofloxacin used alone showed none priority over saline to bacterial clearance ($P > 0.2$).

TABLE | The susceptibilities of to *Klebsiella pneumoniae* standard strain and clinical isolates to LEV, LPs-LEV, and Ts-LPs-LEV.

Strains and clinical isolate no[a]	Source	AMP	SAM	TZP	CFZ	CTT	CRO	CAZ	FEP	ATM	ETP	AMI	IPM	GEN	TOB	CIP	NIT	SMZ[b]	MICs (μg/ml)[c,#]				
																			LEV	LPs-LEV	Ts-LPs-LEV[d]	Ts	Ts-LPs[e]
ATCC 700603		R	I	S	S	S	S	R	S	S	S	I	S	I	–	S	S	–	8	<2	<2	8	32
CI 130218317	Drainage fluid	R	R	R	R	S	R	S	S	R	S	S	S	R	–	R	R	R	>256	128	16	32	256
CI 130322206	Sputum	R	R	S	R	R	R	R	–	R	S	S	S	R	–	S	R	R	16	8	4	16	–
CI 130130102	Secretion	R	R	R	S	S	R	R	R	R	S	S	S	R	R	R	R	S	32	16	8	16	–
CI 130205205	Blood	R	S	R	S	R	S	R	S	S	R	S	S	S	R	R	S	R	16	8	4	16	–
CI 130305114	Secretion	R	R	S	R	S	R	R	R	R	S	R	S	R	–	R	S	R	64	16	8	32	–
CI 130400215	Sputum	R	S	S	R	R	R	S	R	R	R	R	R	R	R	R	R	R	8	4	2	8	–
CI 130401230	Sputum	R	R	R	S	R	R	S	S	S	R	R	R	S	S	R	S	R	128	32	8	16	–
CI 130411303	Throat swab	R	S	S	S	S	S	R	S	S	S	S	S	S	R	S	R	S	128	64	8	16	–
CI 130411422	Sputum	R	R	S	R	S	S	R	R	S	R	S	S	S	S	R	S	S	16	8	2	8	–
CI 130501235	Secretion	R	R	S	–	R	S	S	R	R	S	S	S	S	S	S	S	S	16	16	4	16	–
CI 130612312	Sputum	R	R	R	S	S	R	S	R	R	S	S	S	S	S	R	S	R	64	16	4	16	–
CI 130615203	Sputum	R	S	S	S	R	S	S	S	S	S	S	S	R	S	S	–	S	16	8	4	8	–
CI 130702215	Sputum	R	S	R	R	R	S	R	R	R	R	R	R	R	–	S	–	R	>256	64	16	32	–
CI 130814222	Sputum	R	S	S	R	R	S	S	R	R	S	S	S	R	S	S	R	R	64	32	4	16	–
CI 130830204	Sputum	R	R	S	R	S	S	R	S	S	S	R	R	R	R	R	S	S	64	16	4	16	–
CI 130931234	Secretion	R	S	S	S	S	R	R	R	S	S	R	S	R	R	S	R	S	128	64	8	16	–
CI 130901155	Secretion	R	R	R	R	R	S	R	R	R	S	S	R	R	R	R	–	R	16	8	4	8	–

[a] ATCC, American type culture collection; CI, clinical isolate. [b] R, resistant; S, sensitive; I, intermediate; —, not determined; AMP, ampicillin; SAM, ampicillin–sulbactam; TZP, piperacillin–tazobactam; CFZ, cefazolin; CTT, cefotetan; CRO, ceftriaxome; CAZ, ceftazidime; FEP, cefepime; ATM, aztreonam; ETP, ertapenem; AMI, amikacin; IPM, imipenem; GEN, gentamicin; TOB, tobramycin; CIP, ciprofloxacin; NIT, furadantin; SMZ, cotrimoxazole; LEV, levofloxacin. [c] Free drug or LEV concentration entrapped in liposomes. [d] Ts:LEV = 1:1(w/w). [e] Ts-LPs was calculated as the Ts-containing concentration. LPs-LEV and Ts-LPs-LEV liposome concentrations were calculated as the levofloxacin-containing concentrations. [#] We used two times dilution method to determine the MIC values, and the MICs were from triple replicates. In most of the cases, the MICs from three replicates were the same, so there were no SD values.

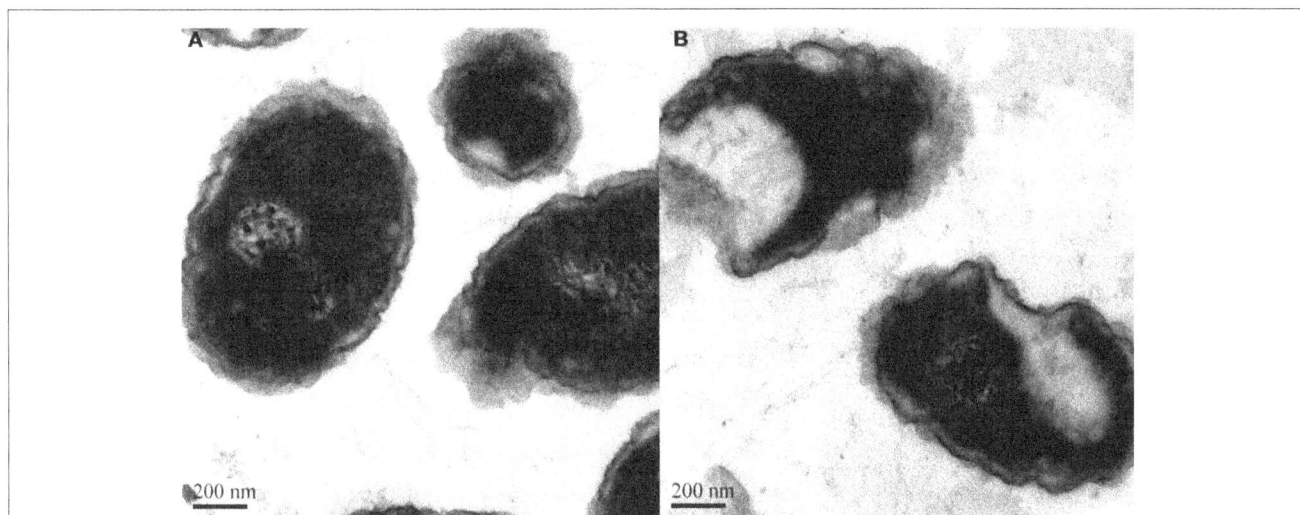

FIGURE | **Bactericidal effect of Ts-LPs-LEV.** Electron micrographs of *K. pneumoniae* ATCC 700603 incubated for 1 h after receiving **(A)** saline or **(B)** Ts-LPs-LEV. The length of the scale bar in the TEM image is 200 nm.

DISCUSSION

The designed liposome Ts-LPs was stable and met multiple requirements for a drug carrier. The liposome properties were closely affected by lipid species and their composition. CHO is the most comprehensive example. CHO comprises up to 50% of the total lipids of mammal cell membrane but rarely present in bacterial cells. CHO renders the lipid bilayer flexibility as well as stability. Incorporation of CHO into liposome formula can reduce unfavorable liposomal leakage and prohibit membrane fusion in artificial systems (Shimanouchi et al., 2009). Charge on the liposome surface prevents self-contact and self-fusion improving the stability of the liposome. A proper charge on the liposome surface introduced by Ts was another guarantee that the produced liposome remained stable for at least 2 months, and allowed the electrostatic attraction between the liposomes with negatively charged components from the bacterial membrane. The incorporation of DSPE and HSPC was meant to stabilize the liposome and to mediate the fusion of the liposome with bacterial membranes (Ma et al., 2010). PEGylation is a mature technique and has been widely applied in pharmaceutical industry. PEGylation reduced non-specific interactions between drugs with proteins and cells, and thus decreases the drug degradation and prolongs the drug circulation in the bloodstream (Anonymous, 2007). The drug metabolism and pharmacokinetics of the liposomes would be an interesting topic for the next step.

Levofloxacin was loaded to the liposomes using the ammonium sulfate gradient method (Haran et al., 1993) and reached a high EE. The carrier capacity is an important parameter to evaluate a drug delivery system for effective antibacterial chemotherapy. The ammonium sulfate gradient method has several advantages, including a shorter preparation period, milder conditions and higher drug EE than those of other methods (Fritze et al., 2006). Our results demonstrated that the levofloxacin EE (%) of Ts-LPs-LEV was ~76% using the ammonium sulfate gradient method, which was higher than that of the reverse phase evaporation method, ethanol injection method, or citric acid gradient method (data not shown).

Ts and levofloxacin combination against *K. pneumoniae* showed at least additive effects and it reached synergism when levofloxacin was used in combination with 0.2X MIC of Ts (Supplementary Table). Similarly, the antimicrobial activity assay demonstrated that the MICs of Ts-LPs-LEV against 17 *K. pneumoniae* clinical isolates were 2–16-fold lower than that of the free drug (**Table**). This was consistent with the drug uptake results, and was attributed to the distinguishing mechanism of action between Ts and Levofloxacin that we would discussed later. It was reasonable that Ts showed decreased activity when it was immobilized onto the liposome because such immobilization reduced the flexibility and geometrically prohibited the interaction between Ts monomers which was called self-promoting interaction during the unique membrane intercalation process of AMPs (Prado Montes de Oca, 2013). Different *K. pneumoniae* strains varied in susceptibility to Ts. It may be due to the modification at the cell envelope of wild type bacteria after receiving antibiotic treatment, particularly the LPS and/or negatively charged content. The selectivity of AMPs is largely dependent on the electrostatic interaction. Such a modification on the charge content at the cell envelope altered the susceptibility of the bacteria to Ts. However, the measurement of cellular charge of bacterial cells seemed infeasible. We tried several times but got totally different results for different cultures from the same colony. A pure study in artificial systems such as the liposome suggested the correlationship between charge and AMP efficiency (Prado Montes de Oca, 2013).

The bacterial uptake of coumarin (CM)-loaded Ts-LPs-CM was imaged by CLSM (Dong and Feng, 2007; Ma et al., 2010). The result was similar to that observed in the drug uptake assay by HPLC. The drug uptake assay revealed that the liposome delivery system was very effective. The liposome

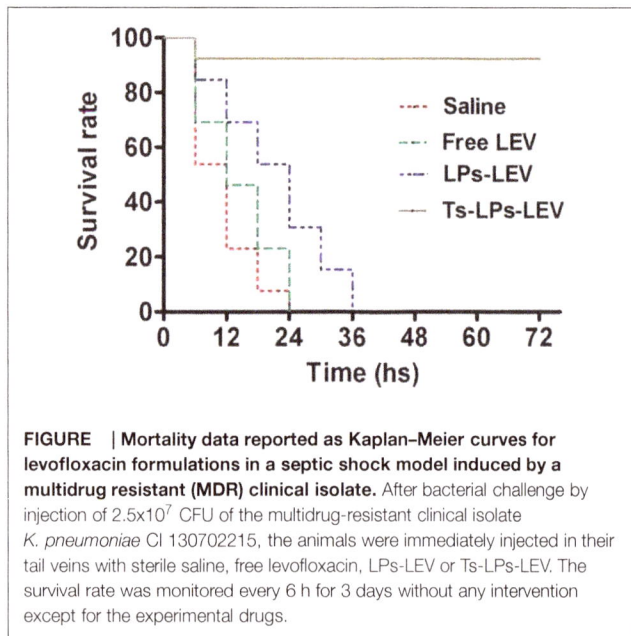

FIGURE | Mortality data reported as Kaplan–Meier curves for levofloxacin formulations in a septic shock model induced by a multidrug resistant (MDR) clinical isolate. After bacterial challenge by injection of 2.5×10^7 CFU of the multidrug-resistant clinical isolate *K. pneumoniae* CI 130702215, the animals were immediately injected in their tail veins with sterile saline, free levofloxacin, LPs-LEV or Ts-LPs-LEV. The survival rate was monitored every 6 h for 3 days without any intervention except for the experimental drugs.

TABLE | Bacterial clearance and mouse survival in septic shock models.

Treatment	Lethality [dead/total (%)]	Bacterial count in blood (CFU/mL)	Bacterial count in peritoneal fluid (CFU/mL)
Saline	15/15 (100)	$5.1 \pm 2.0 \times 10^6$	$7.8 \pm 3.1 \times 10^7$
Free LEV	15/15 (100)	$4.7 \pm 1.5 \times 10^6$	$6.3 \pm 2.5 \times 10^7$
LPs-LEV	11/15 (73.3)	$2.7 \pm 1.1 \times 10^{3*}$	$2.2 \pm 1.0 \times 10^{4*}$
Ts-LPs-LEV	1/15 (6.7)*#	$1.4 \pm 0.4 \times 10^{1*\#}$	$5.6 \pm 1.3 \times 10^{1*\#}$

*The samples were collected at 24 h or immediately after the dead mouse was observed. Mice were observed every 6 h. Error is represented as the standard deviation (n = 15). *P < 0.05 vs. the saline or the free LEV groups. #P < 0.05 vs. the LPs-LEV group.*

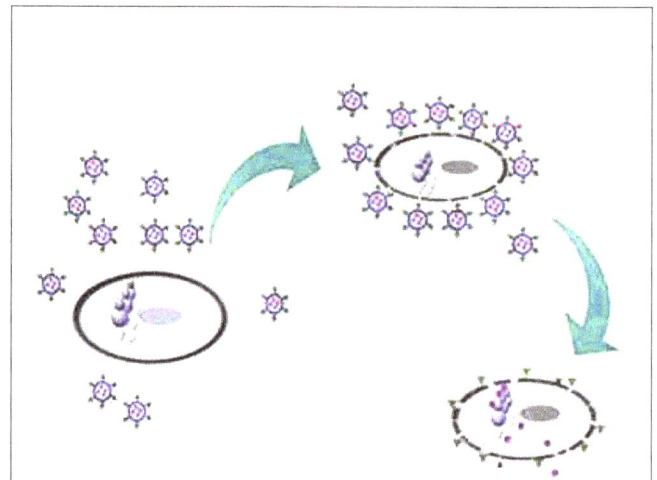

FIGURE | Schematic representation of Ts-LPs-LEV killing bacteria process. Briefly, when Ts-LPs-LEV co-incubated with the bacteria, Ts carried a large amount of levofloxacin-loaded liposomes to the bacterial surface and anchored in the outer membrane by combination with LPS and/or negatively charged components. Then, the liposomes fused with the bacterial cell outer membrane, which could enhance levofloxacin entry through hydrophobic and/or self-promoted pathway or contact release. Meanwhile, Ts perturbed the membrane lipid bilayers of the bacteria and removed the electrical potential of the membrane, affecting the activity of the drug efflux pumps and thus resulting in an intra-bacterial levofloxacin accumulation. The cells finally became dead and broken.

benefited the drug uptake by bacteria, and Ts could improve such effect resulting into relative higher uptake by bacteria for Ts-LPs-LEV/Ts-LPs-CM. Theoretically, Ts-LPs would result into a more promising effect if it was used *in vivo* where Ts-LPs could distinguish mammal cells from bacteria while the liposome without Ts might be distracted by mammal cells. In view of our previous study, highly positively charged Ts could selectively target bacterial cells through electrostatic interaction with negatively charged components present on the outer bacterial membranes, i.e., saccharide moieties of various natures, phospholipids, glycosphingolipids, peptidoglycan, and in particular the LPS that was proved to show affinity with Ts by ELISA assay (Wu et al., 2010b). By contrast, Ts showed a very limited cytotoxicity on mammal cells (Wu et al., 2010b).

The HPLC might not be a proper method to determine the cellular drug uptake. The Ts intercalated into the cellular membrane linking/fusing the liposomes with the cells. So it is impossible to separate the Ts-LPs from the cells by centrifugation or dialysis. Therefore, the HPLC measured the drug both inside the cells and in the surface adherent liposomes. We could not determine whether the drug remained in the liposomes or

entered into the cells. However, fusion or linkage between the liposomes and the cellular membrane would greatly facilitate the drug uptake by the bacterial cells, and the drug would later enter into the cells by membrane fusion. The size of the liposome is about 100 nm while the cell is about 500–2000 nm. The CLSM image did not provide information about cellular location of the liposomes due to the limited resolution. It was hard to tell whether the liposomes entered inside or still remained at the surface. The subcellular structures of the cells are visible under electronic microscope but the electronic microscopy lacks discernment between the liposomes and cells. An image indicating the cellular location of the liposomes would be helpful to understand more details.

The *in vivo* test using mouse model after bacterial challenge indicated the multiple functions of Ts in the liposome complex. Bacterial challenge would first evoke a systematic inflammation and finally developed a multiple organ failure that killed the mice. Antibiotics treatment is not prioritized for septic patients. The serious inflammation induced by endotoxin/exotoxin is highly concerned. From the results, the merits of using Ts were very convincible. Ts resulted into a better bacterial clearance in peritoneal fluid and blood compared with free levofloxacin and LPs-LEV (P < 0.05; **Table**), and greatly improved the survival rate probably through prohibiting the LPS-mediated inflammation.

It has been suggested that transport across the gram negative bacterial cell wall might be achieved by three different ways, namely, hydrophilic transport through porin channels

(Nikaido and Vaara, 1985), hydrophobic adsorption through the lipid membrane (Kotera et al., 1991) and self-promoted uptake (Chapman and Georgopapadakou, 1988). Drug properties such as the hydrophobicity, size and molecular structure can affect the hydrophilic and hydrophobic pathway. The self-promoted uptake route is based on the displacement of divalent cations from the LPSs on the bacterial outer membrane.

It is well known that the non-specific drug efflux and low outer membrane permeability are the major mechanisms for bacterial resistance to fluoroquinolone antibiotics (Nikaido and Vaara, 1985; Srikumar et al., 1998; Srinivasan et al., 2014). The flow cytometry results suggested that the membrane permeability of bacteria was increased by the addition of Ts or Ts-LPs. These findings indicated that Ts killed bacteria at least partially by exhausting the transmembrane potential that is closely related to the bacterial respiration and energization.

Our results are consistent with the following proposed mechanism of TS-LPs-LEV action : (1) Ts led levofloxacin-loaded liposomes to the bacterial surface by interacting with negatively charged content on the bacterial envelop such as LPS; (2) liposomes fused with the bacterial cell outer membrane, which could enhance drug entry through the hydrophobic and/or self-promoted pathway; (3) the integrity of the bacterial cytoplasmic membrane and the respiration chain located on the cytoplasmic membrane was compromised due to Ts insertion resulting into more drug uptake and active efflux failure; and (4) liposomes gave a contact release of levofloxacin (Furneri et al., 2000) close to the bacterial cell surface, resulting in a higher drug uptake than the free drug (**Figure**).

In summary, we successfully developed an antimicrobial-peptide-functionalized levofloxacin-loaded liposome (Ts-LPs-LEV). The liposome showed bacterial selectivity *in vitro* and

exhibited an excellent therapeutic effect in the septic mouse model induced by MDR *K. pneumoniae* clinic isolate. We presented a very promising approach to design a novel antibiotics deliver of targeting potential. The clinical application of this promising antibiotic delivery approach deserves further exploration.

AUTHOR CONTRIBUTIONS

XF discussed the results, did the *in vitro* antimicrobial assays and revised the paper; JF and PW did most of the *in vivo* and *in vitro* experiments and drafted the paper; XW helped to revise the manuscript; GW was the group leader offering supervision and financial support.

ACKNOWLEDGMENTS

We thank the National Natural Science Foundation of China (No. 30970809, 81271636), the Natural Science Foundation of Jiangsu Province (No. BK2009274) and the Special Fund of Clinical Medicine, Jiangsu Province, China (No. BL2012063) for the financial support of this work.

SUPPLEMENTARY MATERIAL

The Supplementary Material for this article can be found online at: http://journal.frontiersin.org/article/10.3389/fphar. 2015.00249

REFERENCES

Anonymous (ed). (2001). *National Committee for Clinical Laboratory Standards(2001) Methods for Dilution Antimicrobial Susceptibility Tests for Bacteria That Grow Aerobically*, 5th Edn. Wayne, PA: National Committee for Clinical Laboratory Standards.

Anonymous (2007). Drug discovery today: technologies (2007) volume 4 issues 3/4. *Drug Discov. Today Technol.* 4:e89–e108. doi: 10.1016/j.ddtec.2009. 07.001

Bassetti, M., and Righi, E. (2015). Development of novel antibacterial drugs to combat multiple resistant organisms. *Langenbecks Arch. Surg.* 400, 153–165. doi: 10.1007/s00423-015-1280-4

Chapman, J. S., and Georgopapadakou, N. H. (1988). Routes of quinolone permeation in *Escherichia coli. Antimicrob. Agents Chemother.* 32, 438–442. doi: 10.1128/AAC.32.4.438

Chapple, D. S., Mason, D. J., Joannou, C. L., Odell, E. W., Gant, V., and Evans, R. W. (1998). Structure-function relationship of antibacterial synthetic peptides homologous to a helical surface region on human lactoferrin against *Escherichia coli* serotype O111. *Infect. Immun.* 66, 2434–2440.

da Costa, J. P., Cova, M., Ferreira, R., and Vitorino, R. (2015). Antimicrobial peptides: an alternative for innovative medicines? *Appl. Microbiol. Biotechnol.* 99, 2023–2040. doi: 10.1007/s00253-015-6375-x

Datta, S., Wattal, C., Goel, N., Oberoi, J. K., Raveendran, R., and Prasad, K. J. (2012). A ten year analysis of multi-drug resistant blood stream infections caused by *Escherichia coli* & *Klebsiella pneumoniae* in a tertiary care hospital. *Indian J. Med. Res.* 135, 907–912.

Dong, Y., and Feng, S. S. (2007). In vitro and in vivo evaluation of methoxy polyethylene glycol-polylactide (MPEG-PLA) nanoparticles for small-molecule drug chemotherapy. *Biomaterials* 28, 4154–4160. doi: 10.1016/j.biomaterials.2007.05.026

Fritze, A., Hens, F., Kimpfler, A., Schubert, R., and Peschka-Suss, R. (2006). Remote loading of doxorubicin into liposomes driven by a transmembrane phosphate gradient. *Biochim. Biophys. Acta* 1758, 1633–1640. doi: 10.1016/j.bbamem.2006.05.028

Furneri, P. M., Fresta, M., Puglisi, G., and Tempera, G. (2000). Ofloxacin-loaded liposomes: in vitro activity and drug accumulation in bacteria. *Antimicrob. Agents Chemother.* 44, 2458–2464. doi: 10.1128/AAC.44.9.2458-246 4.2000

Haran, G., Cohen, R., Bar, L. K., and Barenholz, Y. (1993). Transmembrane ammonium sulfate gradients in liposomes produce efficient and stable entrapment of amphipathic weak bases. *Biochim. Biophys. Acta* 1151, 201–215. doi: 10.1016/0005-2736(93)90105-9

Kibria, G., Hatakeyama, H., Ohga, N., Hida, K., and Harashima, H. (2013). The effect of liposomal size on the targeted delivery of doxorubicin to Integrin alphavbeta3-expressing tumor endothelial cells. *Biomaterials* 34, 5617–5627. doi: 10.1016/j.biomaterials.2013.03.094

Kotera, Y., Watanabe, M., Yoshida, S., Inoue, M., and Mitsuhashi, S. (1991). Factors influencing the uptake of norfloxacin by *Escherichia coli. J. Antimicrob. Chemother.* 27, 733–739. doi: 10.1093/jac/27.6.733

Kronman, M. P., Zerr, D. M., Qin, X., Englund, J., Cornell, C., Sanders, J. E., et al. (2014). Intestinal decontamination of multidrug-resistant *Klebsiella pneumoniae* after recurrent infections in an immunocompromised host. *Diagn. Microbiol. Infect. Dis.* 80, 87–89. doi: 10.1016/j.diagmicrobio.2014.06.006

Leone, I., Mungo, E., Bisignano, G., Chirillo, M. G., and Savoia, D. (2012). *Klebsiella pneumoniae*: emergence of multi-drug-resistant strains in Northwest Italy. *J. Infect.* 64, 535–537. doi: 10.1016/j.jinf.2012. 01.009

Ma, Y., Zheng, Y., Liu, K., Tian, G., Tian, Y., Xu, L., et al. (2010). Nanoparticles of Poly(Lactide-Co-Glycolide)-d-a-Tocopheryl Polyethylene Glycol 1000 Succinate Random Copolymer for Cancer Treatment. *Nanoscale Res. Lett.* 5, 1161–1169. doi: 10.1007/s11671-010-9620-3

Muppidi, K., Wang, J., Betageri, G., and Pumerantz, A. S. (2011). PEGylated liposome encapsulation increases the lung tissue concentration of vancomycin. *Antimicrob. Agents Chemother.* 55, 4537–4542. doi: 10.1128/AAC.00713-11

Nikaido, H., and Vaara, M. (1985). Molecular basis of bacterial outer membrane permeability. *Microbiol. Rev.* 49, 1–32.

Prado Montes de Oca, E. (2013). Antimicrobial peptide elicitors: new hope for the post-antibiotic era. *Innate Immun.* 19, 227–241. doi: 10.1177/1753425912460708

Shimanouchi, T., Ishii, H., Yoshimoto, N., Umakoshi, H., and Kuboi, R. (2009). Calcein permeation across phosphatidylcholine bilayer membrane: effects of membrane fluidity, liposome size, and immobilization. *Colloids Surf. B Biointerfaces* 73, 156–160. doi: 10.1016/j.colsurfb.2009. 05.014

Srikumar, R., Kon, T., Gotoh, N., and Poole, K. (1998). Expression of *Pseudomonas aeruginosa* multidrug efflux pumps MexA-MexB-OprM and MexC-MexD-OprJ in a multidrug-sensitive *Escherichia coli* strain. *Antimicrob. Agents Chemother.* 42, 65–71.

Srinivasan, V. B., Singh, B. B., Priyadarshi, N., Chauhan, N. K., and Rajamohan, G. (2014). Role of novel multidrug efflux pump involved in drug resistance in *Klebsiella pneumoniae. PLoS ONE* 9:e96288. doi: 10.1371/journal.pone.0096288

Wu, G., Fan, X., Li, L., Wang, H., Ding, J., Hongbin, W., et al. (2010a). Interaction of antimicrobial peptide s-thanatin with lipopolysaccharide in vitro and in an experimental mouse model of septic shock caused by a multidrug-resistant clinical isolate of *Escherichia coli. Int. J. Antimicrob. Agents* 35, 250–254. doi: 10.1016/j.ijantimicag.2009.11.009

Wu, G., Wu, H., Fan, X., Zhao, R., Li, X., Wang, S., et al. (2010b). Selective toxicity of antimicrobial peptide S-thanatin on bacteria. *Peptides* 31, 1669–1673. doi: 10.1016/j.peptides.2010.06.009

Wu, G. Q., Li, X. F., Fan, X. B., Wu, H. B., Wang, S. L., Shen, Z. L., et al. (2011). The activity of antimicrobial peptide S-thanatin is independent on multidrug-resistant spectrum of bacteria. *Peptides* 32, 1139–1145. doi: 10.1016/j.peptides.2011.03.019

Conflict of Interest Statement: The authors declare that the research was conducted in the absence of any commercial or financial relationships that could be construed as a potential conflict of interest.

6

Preclinical *In vivo* Imaging for Fat Tissue Identification, Quantification, and Functional Characterization

Pasquina Marzola[1]*, Federico Boschi[1], Francesco Moneta[2], Andrea Sbarbati[3] and Carlo Zancanaro[3]

[1] Department of Computer Science, University of Verona, Verona, Italy, [2] Preclinical Imaging Division – Bruker BioSpin, Bruker Italia s.r.l, Milano, Italy, [3] Department of Neurosciences, Biomedicine and Movement Sciences, University of Verona, Verona, Italy

Edited by:
Nicolau Beckmann,
Novartis Institutes for BioMedical Research, Switzerland

Reviewed by:
Denis Richard,
Laval University, Canada
Rex Anthony Moats,
University of Southern California, USA

*Correspondence:
Pasquina Marzola
pasquina.marzola@univr.it

Localization, differentiation, and quantitative assessment of fat tissues have always collected the interest of researchers. Nowadays, these topics are even more relevant as obesity (the excess of fat tissue) is considered a real pathology requiring in some cases pharmacological and surgical approaches. Several weight loss medications, acting either on the metabolism or on the central nervous system, are currently under preclinical or clinical investigation. Animal models of obesity have been developed and are widely used in pharmaceutical research. The assessment of candidate drugs in animal models requires non-invasive methods for longitudinal assessment of efficacy, the main outcome being the amount of body fat. Fat tissues can be either quantified in the entire animal or localized and measured in selected organs/regions of the body. Fat tissues are characterized by peculiar contrast in several imaging modalities as for example Magnetic Resonance Imaging (MRI) that can distinguish between fat and water protons thank to their different magnetic resonance properties. Since fat tissues have higher carbon/hydrogen content than other soft tissues and bones, they can be easily assessed by Computed Tomography (CT) as well. Interestingly, MRI also discriminates between white and brown adipose tissue (BAT); the latter has long been regarded as a potential target for anti-obesity drugs because of its ability to enhance energy consumption through increased thermogenesis. Positron Emission Tomography (PET) performed with ^{18}F-FDG as glucose analog radiotracer reflects well the metabolic rate in body tissues and consequently is the technique of choice for studies of BAT metabolism. This review will focus on the main, non-invasive imaging techniques (MRI, CT, and PET) that are fundamental for the assessment, quantification and functional characterization of fat deposits in small laboratory animals. The contribution of optical techniques, which are currently regarded with increasing interest, will be also briefly described. For each technique the physical principles of signal detection will be overviewed and some relevant studies will be summarized. Far from being exhaustive, this review has the purpose to highlight some strategies that can be adopted for the *in vivo* identification, quantification, and functional characterization of adipose tissues mainly from the point of view of biophysics and physiology.

Keywords: fat, BAT, MRI imaging, CT imaging, PET imaging

INTRODUCTION

Fat Tissue: General Characteristics

Fat tissue, or adipose tissue, is a type of connective tissue whose predominant cell type is the fat cell, or the adipocyte. In mammals there are two types of fat tissues: the white adipose tissue (WAT) and the brown adipose tissue (BAT) (Cinti, 2000). BAT is characterized by special fat cells showing a multilocular lipid deposit, wherein thermogenesis takes place by "burning" fatty acids in uncoupled mitochondria (Cannon and Nedergaard, 2004). Instead, WAT cells typically present one lipid vacuole and are the major site for body lipids storage, especially triglycerides, serving as an energy deposit from which fatty acids may be delivered through the bloodstream to meet the body's energy requirements during fast or intense, enduring physical activity. Moreover, fat cells are plastic enough so that fat tissue may serve as an aid to prevent trauma injuries; fat cells may act as a heat insulator layer as well. Other cell types are found in fat tissue, e.g., preadipocytes, endothelial cells, pericytes (Rosen and Spiegelman, 2000), immune cells (lymphocytes, T-cells, macrophages, neutrophils), and multipotent stem cells (Tchoukalova et al., 2004; Carmon et al., 2008; Kintscher et al., 2008; Cawthorn et al., 2012). Overall, these cell types over number fat cells in adipose tissue; nevertheless, fat cells represent about 90% of tissue volume due to their large size ranging 20–200 microns. Fat tissue also represents an endocrine tissue by producing a variety of adipokines (e.g., leptin, visfatin, adipolin, and many others). Adipokines act at the autocrine/paracrine and endocrine level (Ronti et al., 2006). Adipokines participate in the regulation of glucose and lipid metabolism, energy homeostasis, feeding behavior, insulin sensitivity, and adipogenesis; they are also involved in the regulation of vascular function and coagulation (Romacho et al., 2014). Fat tissue also has a role in the immune function. In non-obese subjects, immune cells resident in fat tissue have housekeeping functions such as apoptotic cell clearance, extracellular matrix remodeling, and angiogenesis (Mathis, 2013). In obese subjects, excess of adipocytes produces danger signals mimicking bacterial infection, and drives a prototypic T helper 1 inflammatory response (Grant and Dixit, 2015).

Fat Tissue: Body Distribution

Fat tissue is distributed in several discrete anatomical deposits in the body (Shen et al., 2003). It is well known that women generally show higher adiposity than men. Moreover, there is a sexual dimorphism in fat tissue distribution, men accumulate more fat in the trunk region and women accumulate more in the gluteofemoral region (Geer and Shen, 2009). Ethnicity is also a factor that influences body fat distribution (Carroll et al., 2008). Over the last decades it became clear that adipose tissue is not a single homogeneous compartment; instead, it is a tissue with specific regional depots whose biological functions may vary (Vanderburgh, 1992; Schoen et al., 1996) and individual adipose tissue deposits are more closely correlated with physiological and pathological processes than total adipose tissue mass (Kelley et al., 2000). In humans, the largest fat tissue deposit is the subcutaneous adipose tissue, representing about 80% of body fat (Frayn and Karpe, 2014). Within subcutaneous adipose tissue different sub-deposits have been identified: the abdominal, gluteal, and femoral sub-deposits. The subcutaneous adipose tissue is divided into superficial and deep layers by the *fascia superficialis*. These layers have different functions and different correlations with metabolic complications of obesity (Smith et al., 2001). Visceral adipose tissue is found around organs in the thoracic and, to a greater extent, in the abdominal cavity. It has morphological and functional differences from subcutaneous adipose tissue. For example, visceral adipose tissue contains larger, insulin-resistant adipocytes, presents a well-developed vasculature and abundant innervation, and it is more sensitive to lipolysis. On the other hand, subcutaneous fat shows smaller, insulin-sensitive fat cells with less developed vasculature and nerve supply (Mårin et al., 1992; Bjorntorp, 2000). Subcutaneous and visceral adipose tissues have peculiar adipokine expression and secretion profiles (Kershaw and Flier, 2004). Visceral adipose tissue releases larger amounts of pro-inflammatory cytokines in the vena porta, which directly impacts liver metabolism; in its turn, subcutaneous adipose tissue releases more leptin and larger amounts of adiponectin, an anti-inflammatory and insulin-sensitizing adipokine (Ibrahim, 2010). Therefore, the ability to identify and quantify different adipose deposits non-invasively, which is a peculiar feature of *in vivo* imaging techniques, appears relevant to obesity research.

Triglycerides may also be deposited within cells of non-adipose tissue that normally contain only small amounts of fat; this is called ectopic fat deposition (Shulman, 2014) and it is usually associated with obesity and positive energy balance. Excess lipids can accumulate in the heart, liver, skeletal muscle, and pancreas probably because the adipose tissue is no longer capable of sequestering nutritional lipids. Ectopic fat deposits have been claimed as risk factors for disease development (Mathieu et al., 2014).

Fat Tissue: Body Composition Analysis

In the context of body composition analysis, fat (adipose) tissue and body fat are not synonymous. When the five levels (I, atomic; II, molecular; III, cellular; IV, tissue/system; V, whole body) approach to body composition is adopted (Wang et al., 1992), fat tissue is considered at level IV as a specialized loose connective tissue containing lipid-laden adipocytes as well as intra- and extracellular water, interstitial cells, blood vessels, etc. Instead, body fat at level II is considered as the total mass of body lipids (especially triglycerides). These lipids are mainly contained in the lipidic droplets of fat tissue adipocytes, but also in intermuscular adipocytes, in sparse adipocytes of interstitial tissue as well as in muscle cells, hepatocytes, cell membranes, etc. As a result, the total amount of fat tissue and body lipids may be similar, but not identical (Tothill et al., 1996). Traditionally, body fat has been evaluated with a two-compartment model, i.e., subdividing body mass in fat mass and fat-free mass (lean mass). For decades, the standard method for determining fat mass has been underwater weighing; later on, body water dilution, bioelectrical impedance, and air-displacement plethysmography have been used (Pietrobelli et al., 1998) until three-dimensional anthropometry (Wells et al., 2008; Giachetti et al., 2015). In parallel, several imaging techniques emerged as useful tools for body composition analysis on a multi-compartmental basis, e.g., magnetic resonance imaging (MRI), computed tomography (CT), ultrasounds (US), and positron emission tomography (PET).

Adipose Tissue as a Target for Anti-obesity Drugs

Obesity is nowadays recognized as a real pathological state requiring pharmacological and in some cases even surgical treatment. Several drugs for obesity treatment have been marketed over the past few years, but their efficacy was limited and severe adverse effects have often been reported. Anti-obesity drugs on the market or in clinical trials have been recently reviewed (Giordano et al., 2016). Their mechanism of action broadly falls in two categories: drugs that reduce nutrients absorption and anorexic drugs that act on the central nervous system to induce sense of satiety. An innovative mechanism of action for anti-obesity drugs has been more recently proposed and it consists in promoting conversion of WAT into BAT (Giordano et al., 2016). Indeed, it is well known that adult WAT can convert into BAT (browning), this conversion being triggered by several conditions including low ambient temperature, physical exercise or β3-adrenoceptor stimulation. White adipocytes converted to brown adipocytes are considered a new type of brown fat cells named beige adipocytes. A number of molecular targets that can potentially promote conversion of WAT into BAT have been identified recently and reviewed (Giordano et al., 2016). Interestingly, the target of such adipose conversion is the visceral WAT, which is inflamed in obese subjects and possibly involved in most of the adverse clinical correlates of obesity, e.g., metabolic syndrome. In the context of pharmacological research in anti-obesity drugs, suitable animal models and related imaging techniques are needed. In this review, we will examine the contribution of different imaging techniques to the issue of *in vivo* fat tissue identification, quantification, and functional characterization. While most of such imaging studies have been carried out in humans, longitudinal, mechanistic investigations of the metabolic and health correlates of excess/paucity of body fat are better performed in experimental animals. Small rodents, especially mice and rats, are extensively used in preclinical studies aimed at clarifying the causes and mechanisms of metabolic syndrome, diabetes, and obesity (Rees and Alcolado, 2005; Varga et al., 2010; Kanasaki and Koya, 2011) as well as in studies aimed at defining the effect of candidate drugs. Since BAT appears a potential new target tissue for anti-obesity drugs, special attention will be devoted to imaging techniques allowing for identification, quantification, and functional state assessment of BAT.

IMAGING TECHNIQUES FOR DETECTION OF FAT TISSUES IN PRECLINICAL STUDIES

Preclinical imaging has been widely employed in the study of obesity and metabolism. Preclinical protocols for assessing whole body and regional adipose tissue content have been reported using MRI, CT, and Dual-energy X-ray Absorptiometry (DXA) (Sjögren et al., 2001; Sasser et al., 2012; Metzinger et al., 2014). While DXA has been used to accurately estimate lean and fat mass in rodents, as a bi-dimensional radiological technique, it does not provide tridimensional information on fat volume and distribution (Luu et al., 2009); accordingly results obtained with DXA are not reported in this review. The interested reader is referred to the excellent reviews from Albanese et al. (2003) and Toombs et al. (2012). US has been used as an effective and economic technique to assess body composition in humans although its accuracy is strongly dependent on the operator proficiency (Wang et al., 2014). Moreover, applications of US to animal models of obesity and metabolic disorders are still limited; consequently US will not be discussed in this review. [18]FDG-PET has been employed in studies of BAT and metabolic disease (van der Veen et al., 2012). Preclinical imaging provides longitudinal imaging of obesity models, studies of molecular mechanisms of obesity and evaluation of candidate obesity therapeutics. Far from being exhaustive, this review has the purpose to highlight some strategies that can be adopted for the *in vivo* identification, quantification, and functional characterization of adipose tissues mainly from the point of view of biophysics and physiology.

MR-Techniques

Magnetic Resonance Imaging and Magnetic Resonance Spectroscopy (MRS) are currently considered to be the most comprehensive tools for quantification of fat in living organisms (Hu and Kan, 2013). Of note, MRI and MRS can be performed by a single instrument and within the same experimental setup. MRI and MRS have the same underlying concepts and exploit the difference in the resonance frequency between water and fat protons, a phenomenon known as chemical shift. Representative *ex vivo* and *in vivo* spectra obtained from WAT in mice are reported in **Figures**   where several proton resonances attributable to different chemical environments can be distinguished. The water proton resonance occurring at 4.7 ppm is barely visible in the WAT tissue. The signal at 1.3 ppm corresponds to the CH_2 methylene protons of the lipid chain, shown in **Figure**   , and represents the bigger component in the triglyceride spectrum (Bley et al., 2010). The spectrum reported in **Figure**   has been obtained after carefully shimming over a small Volume-of-Interest (VOI) and its spectral resolution is comparable to the resolution of the *ex vivo* spectrum reported in **Figure**   . However in most experimental setups only a few of the triglyceride spectral lines can be detected (see e.g., the typical liver spectrum in Figure   of Reeder et al., 2011). Consequently, in most of applications of MRS for determination of water/fat content, two peaks are considered: the water peak (4.7 ppm) and the CH_2 protons of the lipid chain peak (1.3 ppm), the latter

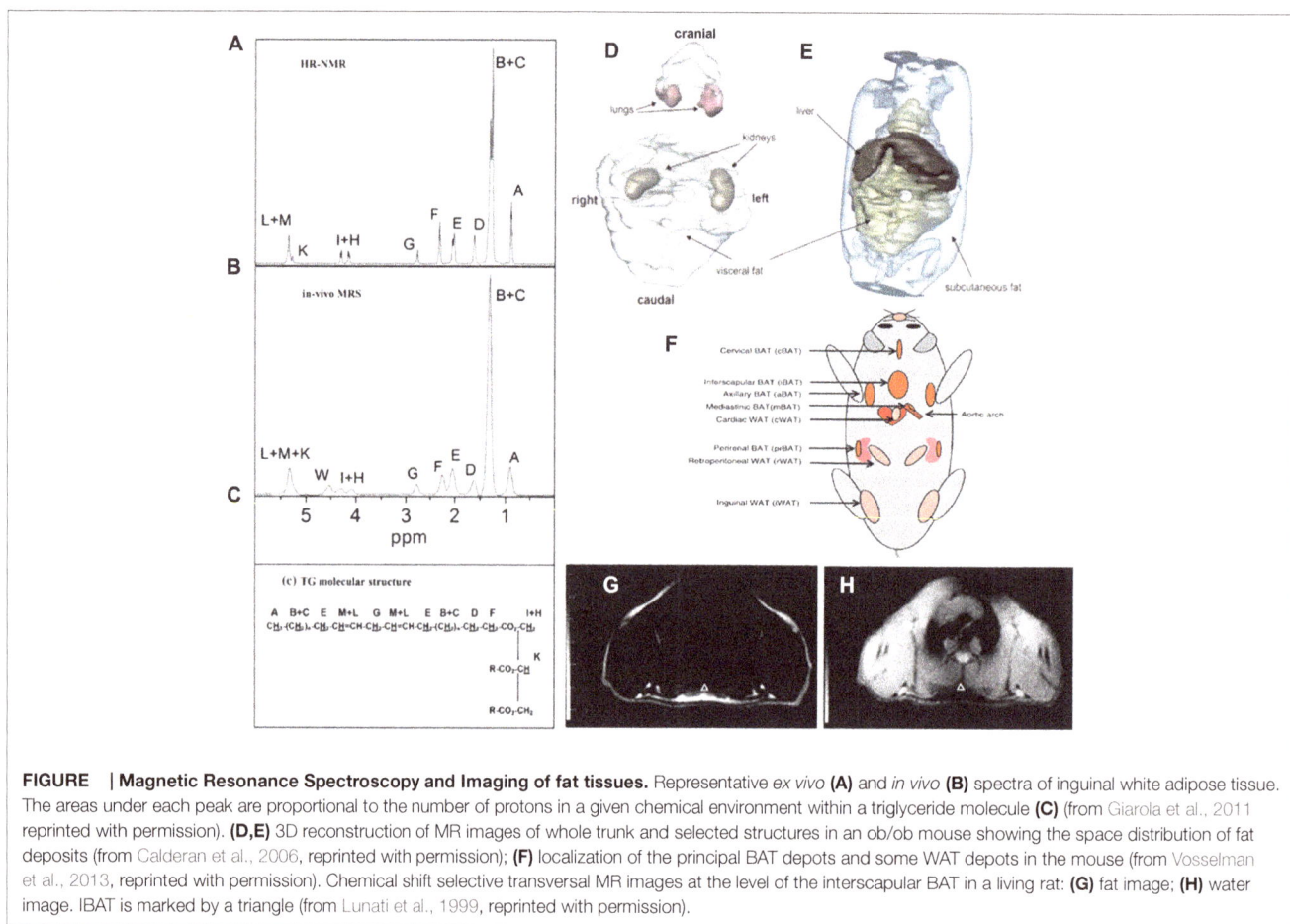

FIGURE | Magnetic Resonance Spectroscopy and Imaging of fat tissues. Representative *ex vivo* **(A)** and *in vivo* **(B)** spectra of inguinal white adipose tissue. The areas under each peak are proportional to the number of protons in a given chemical environment within a triglyceride molecule **(C)** (from Giarola et al., 2011 reprinted with permission). **(D,E)** 3D reconstruction of MR images of whole trunk and selected structures in an ob/ob mouse showing the space distribution of fat deposits (from Calderan et al., 2006, reprinted with permission); **(F)** localization of the principal BAT depots and some WAT depots in the mouse (from Vosselman et al., 2013, reprinted with permission). Chemical shift selective transversal MR images at the level of the interscapular BAT in a living rat: **(G)** fat image; **(H)** water image. IBAT is marked by a triangle (from Lunati et al., 1999, reprinted with permission).

containing more than 10 times the signal of any other fat peak (Bley et al., 2010). The fat and water content of a given tissue can be estimated from proton spectra as the ratio between the area of the water and CH_2 protons peaks.

Proton spectra acquired with high spectral resolution are used to chemically characterize lipid molecules *in vivo* (Giarola et al., 2011; Mosconi et al., 2011; Ye et al., 2012) in terms of unsaturation, poly-unsaturation index, and mean chain length. Quantification of protons corresponding to a certain chemical species requires suitable spectra analysis generally performed using commercial software (Giarola et al., 2011; Mosconi et al., 2011, 2014). To the best of our knowledge, ours was one of the first groups to suggest that *in vivo* MRS can provide information about fat composition in living animals (Lunati et al., 2001). Afterward, Mosconi et al. (2011) demonstrated that WAT in obese Zucker rats, a widely used experimental model for diabetes and obesity, is characterized by lower unsaturation and polyunsaturation index compared with controls (lean Zucker rats) thereby confirming the hypothesis that obese and lean Zucker rats have different adipose tissue composition. Ye et al. (2012) applied MRS to study lipids in the liver of ob/ob mice at 9.4 T and demonstrated that the mean chain length was significantly longer and the fraction of monounsaturated lipids higher in ob/ob mice than in control.

The fact that water and methylene lipid spectral lines are separated by about 3.5 ppm (corresponding to 420, 700, 1043 Hz at 3, 4.7, and 7 T, respectively) is the base for fat/water selective imaging. Several reviews have been recently published describing details of MRI techniques used to obtain water and fat separation (Bley et al., 2010; Reeder et al., 2011; Hu and Kan, 2013). Briefly, these techniques can be divided into frequency-selective or phase-selective. In frequency-selective imaging, the excitation pulse is shaped to selectively excite water or fat proton signal prior to acquisition. In this case the signal will be detected only from water or fat. In a different approach, frequency-selective pulses are first applied to suppress water or fat signal and then the signal of the unsuppressed chemical species is acquired. Fat selective excitation has been used to characterize the water/fat content of interscapular BAT and visceral WAT in the laboratory animal (Lunati et al., 1999) and it is routinely applied to suppress fat signal in clinical examinations where the high intensity signal coming from fat can mask the signal coming from other organs or pathologies.

The same physical property, i.e., chemical shift of water and methylene protons, is exploited in the phase-selective imaging methods originally proposed by Dixon (1984). A review of methods and applications of phase selective imaging has been recently published (Hu and Kan, 2013).

Compared to tissue water protons, fat protons are characterized by short longitudinal relaxation time (T1) and long transversal relaxation time (T2). Indeed, the T1 relaxation time of fat tissues is one of the shortest measurable *in vivo* (Hu and Kan, 2013). Accordingly, fat tissue appears brightest in T1 weighed images thereby allowing for easy quantification of fat volume trough threshold-based segmentation of images (Hu and Kan, 2013). This is defined the relaxometry-based approach while the above mentioned methods, based on the chemical shift difference between water and fat proton, are defined chemical shift-based approaches. Relaxometry-based approaches are widely applied in small animal imaging. Calderan et al. (2006) used this approach to study the fat distribution in ob/ob mice trough segmentation of T1 weighted images and 3D reconstruction of fat depots and internal organs (**Figures**). The same approach was applied in longitudinal studies of body fat accumulation in cathepsin K null mice and its wild type during treatment with high fat diet for 12 weeks (Funicello et al., 2007). The above mentioned differences in T1 and T2 values between water and fat protons permit analysis of body composition in awake small laboratory animals with simple acquisitions of the nuclear magnetic resonance (NMR) signal in the time domain from the whole body. Small bench top NMR instruments are now available that allow precise measurement of lean, fat, and free fluid content in laboratory animals which are widely used in pharmaceutical as well as in diabetes and obesity research. Such approach was used to measure body mass composition (fat, lean, and free fluids) in Ghrelin-receptor null transgenic mice in comparison to wild type, in order to comprehend the action mechanism of a new drug acting as a selective and potent antagonist of the Ghrelin receptor (Costantini et al., 2011).

The anatomical localization of the principal BAT and some WAT deposits are shown in **Figure** . It is noteworthy that MRI can distinguish between BAT and WAT. It has long been known that MRI findings correlate with ultrastructural patterns of BAT in laboratory animals (Osculati et al., 1991); this study was performed at different ages indicating that MRI is a reliable tool to investigate BAT tissue along its age-associated changes. Moreover, MRI allows for accurate determination of BAT deposits volume in living animals and reveals tissue changes associated with temperature manipulation, findings confirmed by histological and ultrastructural analysis (Sbarbati et al., 1991). Modification induced in BAT by interferon were studied with MRI and confirmed by histology and TEM. In particular, in treated mice, the interscapular BAT (iBAT) was found to be slightly enlarged and showed inhomogeneous areas of lipid accumulation (Sbarbati et al., 1995). As shown in **Figures** unequivocal definition of BAT deposits can be obtained using chemical shift selective imaging for fat and water protons; the experimental paradigm was validated in rats at 4.7 T (Sbarbati et al., 1997). MRI with fat selective excitation and correction for the T2 relaxation time was applied to quantify fat and water content in the iBAT of rats at 4.7 T in order to obtain lipidic maps of this tissue (Lunati et al., 1999). Chen et al. (2012) demonstrated the feasibility of estimating BAT volume and metabolic function *in vivo* in rats at a 9.4 T using sequences available from clinical MR scanners. Specifically, they measured

the volume distribution of BAT with MRI sequences showing strong fat-water contrast, and investigated BAT volume by utilizing spin-echo MRI sequences. MRI-estimated BAT volumes were compared with the mass of the excised samples. Moreover they were able to map the hemodynamic responses to changes in BAT metabolism induced pharmacologically by the β3-adrenergic receptor agonist, CL-316,243 in comparison with PET ^{18}F-FDG imaging, demonstrating the feasibility of BAT volume and functionality assessment with routinely used MRI sequences. It should be mentioned that over the past several years, BAT activity *in vivo* has been primarily assessed by PET (or PET-CT) scan following ^{18}F-FDG administration to measure glucose metabolism (see "PET imaging"). Another approach, the two-point magnitude MRI, based on a slightly modified standard MRI protocol, has been proposed to visualize mouse BAT differentiating it from surrounding WAT at 11.7 T (Lindenberg et al., 2014).

In order to discriminate between BAT and WAT in lean and ob/ob mice, T2* relaxation times and proton density fat-fraction values were measured in the two tissues (Hu et al., 2012). To determine differences in fat-signal fraction (FF) from chemical-shift-encoded water-fat MRI of iBAT, Smith et al. studied mice housed at different ambient temperatures. They found that lowering temperature leads to a significantly reduction in BAT-FF, in accordance with the expected BAT involvement in thermogenesis (Smith et al., 2013). Comparison between BAT and WAT fat fractions in ob, seipin, and Fsp27 gene knockout mice by chemical shift-selective imaging and (1)H-MR spectroscopy was reported by Peng et al. (2013). Finally, the effect of different diets on composition of intra-hepatocellular lipids as well intra-abdominal, subcutaneous and total adipose tissue, and BAT was measured *in vivo* with whole body 3D imaging (Bidar et al., 2012).

Several novel approaches have recently been explored to validate the *in vivo* quantification of BAT with MRI. In particular a dual-echo sequence, both with and without spectral presaturation inversion recovery (SPIR) fat suppression, was used at 1.5 T and validated through comparison with histology and ^{18}FDG-PET (Holstila et al., 2013). A new MRI method combined intermolecular double-quantum coherence and the chemical shift-encoded Dixon method in order to enable detection of BAT cells mixed to other cells. The contrast in this technique depends on the water-to-fat ratio at the cellular size scale, which is smaller than the imaging voxel size (Bao et al., 2013). Another method, based on the normally invisible intermolecular multiple-quantum coherence (1)H MR signal has been proposed (Branca et al., 2013). This method does not require special hardware modifications and can overcome the partial volume effect. Moreover, it exploits the characteristic structure of BAT adipocytes to selectively image them, even when they are intimately mixed with other cell types. The method was validated in mice using PET scans and histology. The patterns of oxygen consumption/perfusion were imaged by using blood-oxygen-level-dependent MRI upon BAT activation (Khanna and Branca, 2012) and a well-localized signal drop in BAT found, related to a substantial increase in oxygen consumption and the consequent increase in blood deoxyhemoglobin levels. Sbarbati et al. (2006)

used contrast enhanced MRI to study the effect of adrenergic stimulation on iBAT: adrenergic stimulation performed 40 s before MRI lead to a significantly higher enhancement of signal intensity in iBAT compared to unstimulated tissue, indicating that BAT stimulation is accompanied by increased blood flow.

The use of hyperpolarized nuclei for the identification and assessment of BAT function was proposed by two different groups. The first one (Lau et al., 2014) investigated the feasibility of using hyperpolarized (13)C imaging to quickly (<1 min) identify activated BAT in an *in vivo* rodent model following an infusion of pre-polarized [1-(13)C] pyruvate. Using hyperpolarized xenon gas, the second one (Branca et al., 2014) demonstrated a greater than 15-fold increase in xenon uptake by BAT during stimulation of thermogenesis, thereby, obtaining background-free maps of the tissue in both lean and obese mouse phenotypes.

Computed Tomography

X-ray computed tomography (also called X-ray CT or simply CT) is based on the combination of many X-ray images taken from different angles to produce tomographic images of a scanned object. For *in vivo* acquisitions, the most used construction principle involves scanners with X-ray detector and the radiation source mounted on a gantry that is rotated around the examined object. The majority of the marketed scanners use nano-microfocus X-ray tubes in which an electron beam is focused by several magnetic lenses onto a focal spot of 1–10 μm which interacts with a transmission target to produce the X-ray radiation. Passing through the samples, X-rays are differently absorbed by different materials; the transmitted radiation reaches scintillator crystals and is converted in light signals. The light is then lead by tapered glass fibers (Schambach et al., 2010) to a detector which is often a charge coupled device camera (CCD) and transformed in a digital image. A large series of two-dimensional radiographic images are taken around a single axis of rotation and trough suitable algorithms a three-dimensional image of the inside of the object can be generated. MicroCT systems are capable of volumetric CT analysis with isotropic voxels spacing 50–100 μm (Holdsworth and Thornton, 2002).

The different ability of the anatomical structures to attenuate the X-ray beam is responsible of the contrast in CT images. The adipose tissue has different X-ray attenuation compared to other soft tissues, and thus it has a distinct density in microCT images (**Figure**   ). Using microCT scanners with X-ray photon energies in the range 15–75 keV the principal modes of X-ray attenuation are photoelectric absorption and Compton scattering. Which mode predominates depends on the photon energy and the atomic number (Z) of the absorbing element (Evans, 1955, chapter 25, Figure   ). Photoelectric absorption predominates at low photon energies and in heavier elements, while higher photon energies and lower Z nuclei favor Compton scattering. Photoelectric absorption in materials is proportional to Z^4, this means an acute sensitivity of photoelectric absorption to elemental composition. Instead Compton scattering has unitary proportionality to Z. This

difference is important: it implies that photoelectric absorption gives much stronger absorption image contrast, based on material element composition, than Compton scattering. The elemental composition of soft tissue is predominantly hydrogen (H), carbon (C), nitrogen (N), and oxygen (O).

Elemental ratios in some representative biological tissues are shown in **Table**   . The content of C and O in fat is 57 and 30%, respectively, while in muscle (typical of soft tissues other than fat) the content of C and O is 12 and 73%, respectively.

The large difference in the carbon to oxygen ratio between fat and lean tissues accounts for the difference in X-ray absorption at X-ray energies where photoelectric absorption is the predominant interaction mechanism, i.e., at photon energies less than about 30 keV. C, N, and O are close to the boundary between predominance of photoelectric absorption and Compton scattering, at photon energies less than 50 keV so they can attenuate X-rays by both modalities. Decreasing X-ray photon energy, photoelectric absorption is favored and the Z-based contrast will increase. This means that fat can be imaged by microCT by using an appropriate X-ray energy without causing excessive radiation dose to the animal.

Computed tomography images can be treated with a set of software procedures (thresholds detection, segmentation) in order to enhance contrast, i.e., increase difference among anatomical structures enabling subsequent computational analysis. After segmentation of 2D images, volumetric reconstructions of different organs, including fat, can be obtained as reported in **Figures**

Computed tomography imaging has natural applications to bone imaging, with a special focus on bone architectures, bone density and vascular imaging, thanks to the implementation of novel vascular contrast agents (Holdsworth and Thornton, 2002). Moreover, it is also able to provide three-dimensional density maps with sufficient contrast to distinguish adipose tissue from other tissues, fluids and cavities without contrast agents (Luu et al., 2009). Noteworthy, it can not only measure the total volume of adipose tissue within an animal, but can also identify and quantify very small volumes of fat residing in discrete deposits (Luu et al., 2009). Indeed, acquiring high-resolution images based on the physical densities of the object allows discrimination of subcutaneous adipose tissue and visceral adipose tissue (Judex et al., 2010). As a non-invasive, *in vivo* technique CT provides measurement of the total, visceral, and subcutaneous adiposity in longitudinal studies (Luu et al., 2009). Adipose volumes determined by microCT and the weight of the explanted fat pads are highly correlated, demonstrating that CT can accurately monitor site-specific changes in adiposity (Judex et al., 2010). From the experimenter's point of view, it is important to note that voxel densities of fat are relatively uniform throughout the adipose tissue and partial volume effect in adipose tissue is less important than in bony structures. Instead, a greater effort is needed to set accurately voltage and current of the X-ray source to optimize the contrast.

Although fat tissue is spanned over the entire body, it was demonstrated that differences in total fat volume across various animal species are congruent with differences in their abdominal fat mass (Rubin et al., 2007). So scanning the entire mouse may

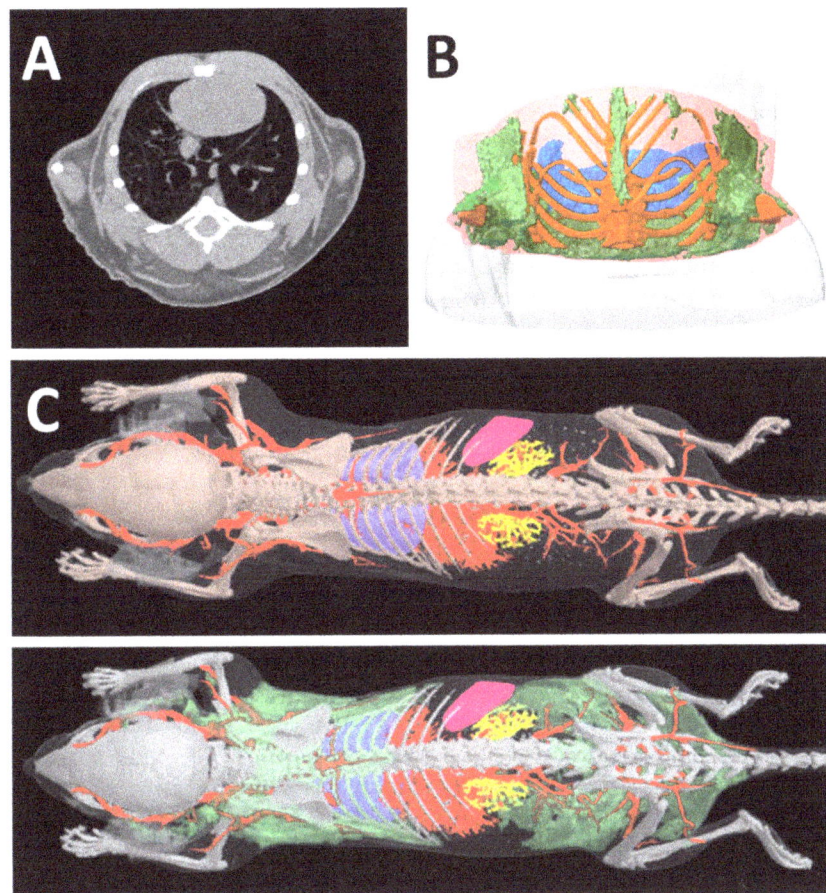

FIGURE | **Computed Tomography of fat tissues. (A)** In a reconstructed cross section of a microCT scan of a mouse thorax, the four tissues which are most readily distinguished in microCT images on the basis of differing x-ray attenuation are bone, lung, fat and "lean" or non-fat soft tissue. All four tissues are clearly visible in this image; the adipose tissue appears as the darker gray regions near the periphery of the thorax. Note that in this image lighter color means higher x-ray attenuation and "density," while darker color means low x-ray attenuation. Bone is saturated to white by narrowing of the reconstruction contrast limits to enhance soft tissue visual contrast. **(B)** A segment VOI of the mouse thorax selected for fat analysis relative to a lung landmark (branching of trachea) shows adipose tissue in green, lungs blue, bone gold. **(C)** Adipose tissue (green) in the lower surface rendered model image can be segmented and visualized on the basis of its lower X-ray density vs. "lean" soft tissues. (Courtesy of Bruker microCT NV, Kontich Belgium).

TABLE | **Biological tissue elemental ratios by mass percentage (modified from** Johns and Cunningham, 1983**).**

	H	C	N	O	Na	Mg	P	S	K	Ca
Atomic number Z	1	6	7	8	11	12	15	16	19	20
Fat	11.2	57.3	1.1	30.3				0.006		
Water	11.2			88.8						
Muscle	10.2	12.3	3.5	72.9	0.08	0.02	0.2	0.5	0.3	0.007
Bone	6.4	27.8	2.7	41.0		0.2	7.0	0.2		14.7

not be necessary and only the abdominal region can be acquired saving acquisition time and dose administered to the patient (Judex et al., 2010). For a quantitative analysis of discrete fat deposits, manual drawing of contour lines is very time consuming and does not yield adequate precision and accuracy; algorithms have been written and are now available based on automatic edge detection in the images, in order to obtain reproducible results (Judex et al., 2010). MicroCT can also allow determining the

degree of fat infiltration in liver by measuring the liver-to-spleen density ratio in a specific region around the intervertebral disk between the 13th thoracic and first lumbar vertebrae (Judex et al., 2010).

MicroCT was used to investigate the effect of high frequency and low intensity mechanical signals on adipogenesis in mice (Rubin et al., 2007). This study demonstrated that 15 weeks of brief, daily exposure to high-frequency mechanical signals of a magnitude well below that which would arise during walking, inhibits adipogenesis by 27% in C57BL/6J mice.

Using microCT scanning, a reduced percentage of adipose mass associated with decreased adipocyte cell size was found in mice null for Fyn (a member of the Src family of non-receptor tyrosine kinases). Such reduction was accompanied by a substantial reduction in fasting plasma glucose, insulin, triglycerides and free fatty acids, concomitant with decreased intrahepatocellular and intramyocellular lipid accumulation. For the quantification of total fat volume inside a volume of interest, freshly harvested fat pad from similar mouse, with identical scan settings, were imaged in order to identify the upper and lower thresholds useful to separate adipose tissues from other tissues and fluids (Bastie et al., 2007).

A study on BAT was conducted on rats exposed to room temperature (23–24°C) as the control condition and after 4 h of cold exposure (4°C), which is known to activate BAT. The CT Hounsfield units (which are related to the tissutal radiodensity) of BAT resulted higher (whiter density in the images) under the activated condition than under the control condition (Baba et al., 2010).

PET Imaging

Positron emission tomography is a nuclear medicine imaging technique used to reveal functional processes in living organisms. The main applications are in oncology, neuroimaging, cardiology, infectious disease, musculoskeletal imaging, and pharmacokinetics studies. PET is routinely used on humans and, in preclinical applications, on experimental animals. As far as fat imaging is concerned, applications of PET are limited to BAT.

Positron emission tomography instruments are able to detect pairs of gamma rays emitted in living bodies by i.v. injected radiotracers. The radiotracers used in PET contain positron-emitting isotopes, i.e., isotopes decaying by emitting positive charged electrons, called positrons. The positron can travel for about 1 mm in biological tissues before it loses most of its energy and encounters an electron. The interaction annihilates both particles producing two gamma rays emitted in opposite directions. The gamma rays are detected by scintillator crystals (of which the internal ring of the tomograph is made) generating bursts of light revealed by photomultiplier tubes (or avalanche photodiode) coupled with the crystals. Each light burst is then converted in electric signal. The detection of two different, almost simultaneous, events in crystals located approximately at 180 degrees with respect to the center of the tomograph is referred to as a coincidence and the signal is considered due to a real nuclear decay event. Noise or spurious events are attributable to the interaction of cosmic rays or natural radioactivity within the instrument.

The decay time of radioisotopes for PET applications is preferably chosen short enough to reduce the radiation exposure of patients, but at the same time, long enough to allow chemical synthesis and transport from the production site to the imaging facility. The most commonly used radiotracer in PET imaging is 2-deoxy-2-^{18}F-fluoro-D-glucose (^{18}F-FDG), an analog of glucose, which is labeled with 18 Fluorine. The half-life time of ^{18}F is 110 min. ^{18}F-FDG is internalized by cells in proportion to their metabolic activity so it accumulates preferentially in cancer cells, brain, heart, and kidney. Inside cells, ^{18}F-FDG cannot be further metabolized and it cannot move out of the cell before radioactive decay. Consequently, the distribution of ^{18}F-FDG reflects well metabolic rate in body tissues and consequently it is the most relevant radiotracer for studies of BAT metabolism.

Fueger et al. (2006) investigated the uptake of ^{18}F-FDG in BAT of mice under different experimental conditions. It is well known that BAT metabolism is activated in mice by low temperature to generate heat. Consequently, the uptake of ^{18}F-FDG in BAT was found to be higher at room temperature (21°C) than at thermoneutrality (30°C). ^{18}F-FDG uptake by BAT was reduced by fasting the animals overnight, in accordance with the well-known role of BAT in postprandial thermogenesis.

^{18}F-FDG uptake in BAT also increases in mice exposed to full-thickness thermal injury (30% of total body surface area), cold stress (4°C for 24 h) or cutaneous wounds (5-fold, 15-fold, and 15-fold, respectively), whereas the uptake in adjacent WAT is unchanged (Carter et al., 2011). Using a thermal imaging camera, a linear relationship between ^{18}F-FDG uptake and BAT temperature was demonstrated for the first time in *in vivo* studies (Carter et al., 2011).

^{18}F-FDG-PET imaging was used to investigate the diurnal rhythm of glucose uptake in C57Bl/6 mice: glucose uptake in iBAT peaks at approximately 9 h into the light phase of the 12 h light period. This result makes iBAT a candidate site of interaction between metabolic and circadian systems (van der Veen et al., 2012).

Pharmacological approaches were used to demonstrate that adrenergic pathway activation enhances BAT metabolism in rodents (Mirbolooki et al., 2011, 2013, 2014). BAT is innervated by sympathetic noradrenergic nerve fibers whose stimulation activates β3-adrenoreceptors in the target tissue resulting in enhancement of glycolysis. This probably increases the synthesis of cyclic AMP and the overexpression of uncoupling protein-1 (UCP1). In the first study, BAT activation was induced by administration of CL316243, a β3 adrenoceptor agonist in rats, and evaluated by ^{18}F-FDG-PET imaging (Mirbolooki et al., 2011). CL316243-induced activation of BAT was clearly visible in PET images, in particular in the interscapular, cervical, periaortic, and intercostal BAT deposits. The uptake of ^{18}F-FDG was enhanced by 12-fold in comparison to control animals, while low temperature (8°C for 120 min) increased the ^{18}F-FDG uptake only 1.1-fold (**Figure**). The uptake of ^{18}F-FDG in activated iBAT was greatly reduced (96.0%) by administration of the β-blocker propranolol. These results were confirmed by *ex vivo* ^{18}F-FDG autoradiography and histology. In a second study, the effect of presynaptic activation with atomoxetine on BAT metabolism was evaluated in rats (Mirbolooki et al., 2013). The existence of norepinephrine transporters in BAT was previously suggested by *in vivo* and *ex vivo* evaluations using ^{11}C-MRB, a highly selective norepinephrine transporter ligand for BAT imaging at room temperature in rats (Lin et al., 2012). It is noticeable that for this study the positron emitter ^{11}C with 20.3 min half-life was used. The results obtained in the studies previously mentioned were confirmed and extended to mice using three pharmacological approaches (atomoxetine,

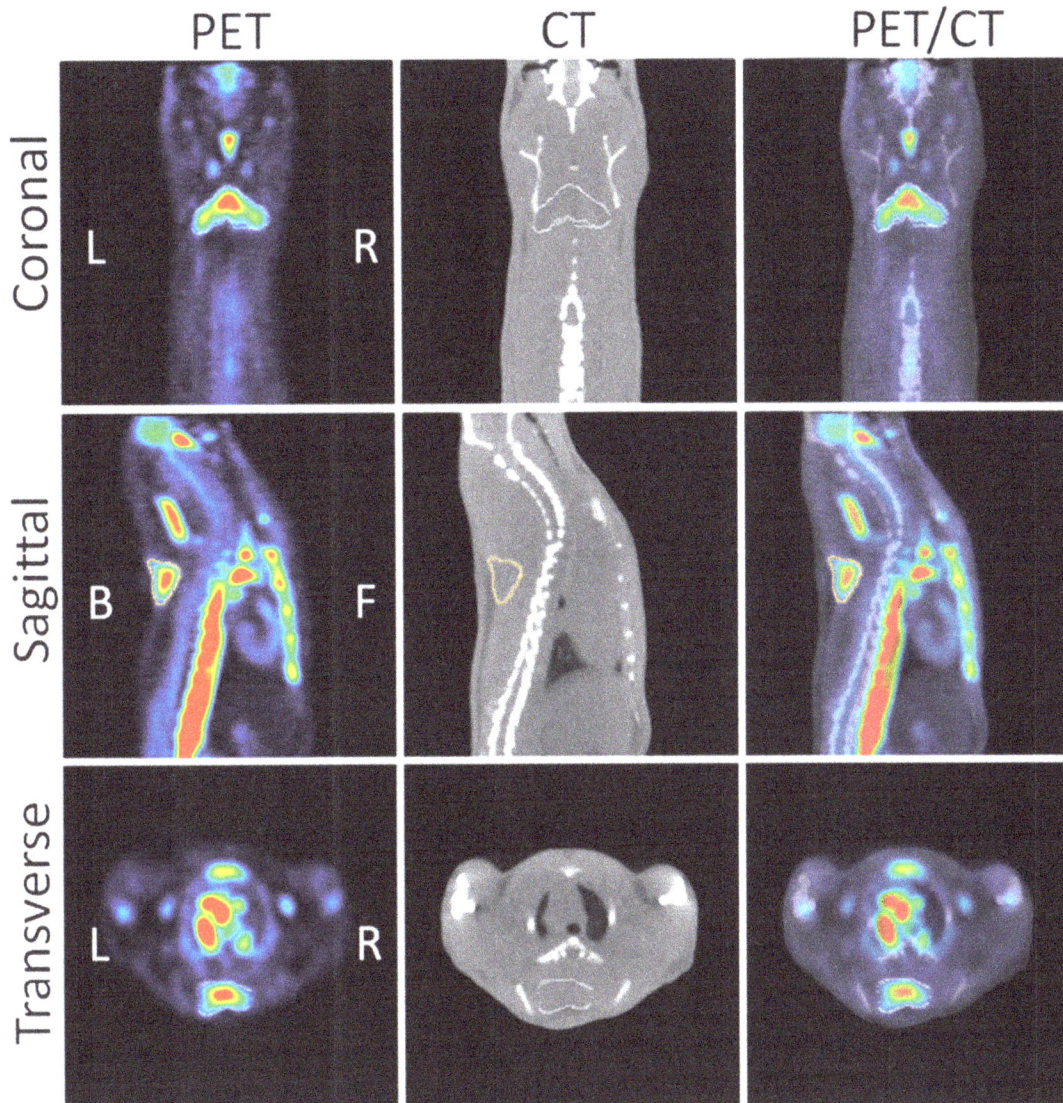

FIGURE | **Coronal, sagittal and transverse views of PET/CT images.** The images show CL316243 activated BATs in Sprague-Dawley rats: PET **(Left)**, CT **(Middle)**, and fused PET/CT **(Right)** (from Mirbolooki et al., 2011, reprinted with permission).

CL316243, and forskolin, an adenylyl cyclase enzyme activator) in a third study (Mirbolooki et al., 2014). Atomoxetine increased ^{18}F-FDG uptake of iBAT 1.7-fold vs. control mice. CL316243 increased ^{18}F-FDG uptake fivefold in IBAT, 2.4-fold in WAT and 2.7-fold in muscle vs. control mice. Finally, forskolin increased the uptake 1.9 in IBAT, 2.2-fold in WAT and 5.4-fold in heart compared to controls.

Beyond its role in thermal homeostasis (during both acute stress and cold acclimation), BAT is probably involved in energy homeostasis as a site of postprandial thermogenesis. The ablation of the essential protein for heat production in BAT namely, the uncoupling protein-1 (UCP-1), leads to an obese phenotype in mice housed at thermoneutral temperature (Feldmann et al., 2009). BAT was found to be involved in plasma triglyceride clearance (Bartelt et al., 2011) and glucose homeostasis (Guerra

et al., 2001; Gunawardana and Piston, 2012). Accordingly to Vosselman et al. (2013) these results highlight the antiobesity role of BAT in rodents, as well as its potential in obesity-related metabolic diseases (diabetes and cardiovascular disease).

Activation of BAT can be a new strategy to combat obesity and diabetes mellitus (DM). Wu et al. (2014) obtained models of obesity by feeding mice with a high fat diet for 8 weeks and models of DM by administration of streptozotocin to obese mice. Both obese and DM mice showed lower ^{18}F-FDG uptake in iBAT compared to controls. After 2 weeks of treatment with BRL37344 (a β3-adrenergic receptor agonist) the uptake was significantly increased in both animal models with a decrease of blood glucose levels and substantial weight loss in obese mice. Levothyroxine (the synthetic thyroid hormone) increased ^{18}F-FDG uptake in both obese and control mice, but not in DM mice. These results demonstrate that inhibition of BAT function found in obese and DM mice can be reversed by β3-adrenergic receptor agonist or thyroid hormone administration (Wu et al., 2014) and BAT activation may effectively lead to weight loss and blood glucose lowering.

To evaluate the significance of β3-adrenoreceptor agonist-induced BAT activation in obesity, a useful rat model is represented by the Zucker lean and obese rats. The effect of CL316243 administration on the BAT ¹⁸F-FDG uptake was investigated in both genotypes, resulting in fourfold increase of glucose uptake in Zucker lean with respect to saline-administered control rats and only a twofold increase in Zucker obese rats. The reduced CL316243 activation is consistent with the lower β3-adrenoreceptor levels in Zucker obese with respect Zucker lean rats (Schade et al., 2015).

A norepinephrine analog labeled with the 11C isotope ((11)C-meta-hydroxyephedrine, 11)C-MHED) was used to investigate the sympathetic nervous system (SNS) activity in BAT of lean and dietary obese mice, demonstrating that 11C-MHED is a specific marker of the SNS-mediated thermogenesis in BAT deposits, and that this radiotracer can detect *in vivo* the WAT-to-BAT conversion (Quarta et al., 2013).

Recently, concomitant application of ¹¹C-acetate, ¹⁸FDG, and ¹⁸F-fluoro-thiaheptadecanoic acid (¹⁸FTHA) has been reported in order to characterize BAT alterations in both clinical (Ouellet et al., 2012) and preclinical studies (Labbé et al., 2015, 2016). In preclinical studies, the effects of cold on BAT were investigated using ¹⁸F-FDG (for glucose uptake), ¹⁸FTHA (for non-esterified fatty acid–NEFA- uptake), and 11C-acetate (for oxidative activity). The experiment was performed in rats, adapted to 27°C, which were acutely subjected to cold (10°C) for 2 or 6 h and in rats chronically adapted to 10°C for 21 days, which were returned to 27°C for 2 or 6 h. Cold exposure (acute and chronic) led to increases in BAT oxidative activity, which was accompanied by concomitant increases in glucose and NEFA uptake (Labbé et al., 2015). The same radiotracers were used to investigate the metabolic activity of iBAT and "beige adipose tissue" in mice exposed to cold or to an adrenergic agonist

(CL) (Labbé et al., 2016) extending the results found in humans (Ouellet et al., 2012).

Finally, an experimental protocol for BAT functional imaging with ¹⁸F-FDG in mice was proposed by Wang et al. (2012) in order to standardize the imaging procedures, to uniform the post-images analysis and to quantify the FDG uptake in BAT as percentage of the injected dose per gram of tissue. The described method, which is based on a small animal- micro-PET/CT system, can be applied to screening drugs/compounds that modulate BAT activity, or to identify genes/pathways that are involved in BAT development and regulation in preclinical studies.

Other Imaging Techniques: Cerenkov Luminescence Imaging and Fluorescence Imaging

It has been recently reported that beta+ or beta− emitting radionuclides can be detected in living animals by Cerenkov Luminescence imaging (CLI) using standard optical imaging instrumentation (Boschi and Spinelli, 2014; Spinelli and Boschi, 2015). This methodology relies on the well-known Cerenkov effect. Briefly, while traveling in the biological tissues, the emitted particles polarize molecules of the medium which emit electromagnetic waves relaxing back to the equilibrium. If the particle travels with a speed greater than the speed of light in the medium, the electromagnetic waves interfere constructively producing a shock front, which can be detected in the UV-visible-near infrared range as Cerenkov radiation.

Brown adipose tissue and its activation can be studied by optical techniques via CLI, as shown by Zhang et al. (2013) after administration of ¹⁸F-FDG in mice. They demonstrated that CLI is able to detect iBAT *in vivo*. Data were confirmed by *ex vivo* radioactivity measurements; representative images are shown in **Figure** . Using norepinephrine as a stimulator, they found that norepinephrine-treated mice show significantly higher CLI signals compared to untreated mice. Moreover, in treated animals they observed an increase of the signal under short (5 min)

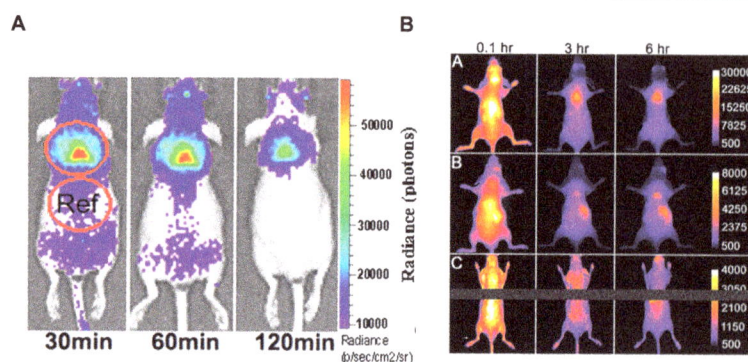

FIGURE | (A) Cerenkov luminescence images of a mouse at 30, 60, 120 min after 10.3 MBq ¹⁸F-FDG intravenous injection (from Zhang et al., 2013, reprinted with permission); (B) Fluorescence images of living SKH1 hairless mice after intravenous 10 nmol dose of SRFluor680 [A], IR780 [B], or Nile Red [C] and imaged periodically over a period of 6 h. The fluorescence pixel intensity scale bar applies to all images in the same row (arbitrary units) (from Rice et al., 2015, reprinted with permission).

isoflurane anesthesia (1.23-fold) and a greater increase after long (60 min) isoflurane anesthesia (2.47-fold). Finally, they reported a 39% increase in ^{18}F-FDG uptake in BAT of animals stimulated by cold exposure.

Fluorescence imaging is based on the detection of light coming from exogenous fluorochromes (dyes or genetically engineered fluorescent proteins) excited with light sources (laser or lamps). The photons escaping from the sample surface are generally detected by a charge CCD with high quantum efficiency. Excitation and emission wavelengths suitable for *in vivo* investigations are in the red-near infrared region (650–800 nm) where the biological tissues are optically thin. Outside this "transparency window" the substantial absorption of oxy- and deoxy-hemoglobin, melanin, water and fat reduces the light signal. Fluorescence imaging is a very simple, safe, and cost-effective technique, which has been implemented to obtain tomographic 3D reconstructions of the light sources inside the body (Beckmann et al., 2007).

A pure optical approach to the detection of BAT was recently reported by Rice et al. (2015) who administered mice with a micellar formulation of commercially available deep-red fluorescent probe (SRFluor680). They showed an extensive uptake of the fluorescent probe in iBAT, as clearly visible in **Figure** . The results were confirmed by ^{18}F-FDG PET imaging and *ex vivo* examinations. They explained the results by an irreversible translocation of the lipophilic fluorescent probe from the micelle nanocarrier to the adipocytes within the BAT. The authors suggest that combining optical methods with FDG/PET could constitute a path toward a new molecular imaging paradigm allowing non-invasive visualization of BAT mass and BAT metabolism in living subjects.

CONCLUSION

Magnetic Resonance Imaging, CT, and PET represent a panel of imaging techniques which are instrumental for the *in vivo* detection and quantification of fat tissues in cross sectional and longitudinal studies. Several qualitative and quantitative morphological and functional data can be extracted from images,

allowing for the investigation of fat tissue metabolism and drug response. Techniques based on MRI and MRS are considered the most comprehensive tools for quantification of fat in living organisms. MRI based techniques allow to investigate the anatomical distribution of adipose tissues, the presence of ectopic fat, and also chemical and functional state of fat deposits with high space resolution. MicroCT can discriminate fat tissue from remaining soft tissue in small laboratory animals with similar space resolution. PET suffers from limited space resolution (around 1 mm), from the need for expensive radiotracers and controlled environment, but it has been proven to be extremely sensitive in studies of BAT activation. Indeed MRI, CT and PET should be regarded as a set of complementary techniques. Much effort is currently in progress toward multimodal imaging approaches: hybrid instruments combining PET and MRI, or PET and CT, have been developed also for small animal imaging to overcome the limitations of individual techniques. MRI, CT, and PET are used in both clinical and preclinical fields, thereby enhancing the translational value of findings in experimental animals. A limitation of these techniques is the high cost of instrumentation and maintenance, and the need for specialized personnel. Accordingly, large studies employing tens or hundreds of animals are cumbersome. However, microCT, PET and, especially, MRI are non-invasive and allow for longitudinal studies where a reduced number of animals is sufficient in order to obtain statistically significant results. Recently other imaging techniques (CLI and fluorescence imaging) have been applied to these topics, but still await full validation.

AUTHOR CONTRIBUTIONS

All authors listed, have made substantial, direct and intellectual contribution to the work, and approved it for publication.

ACKNOWLEDGMENT

The authors acknowledge Miss Sara Domenici for language revision.

REFERENCES

Albanese, C. V., Diessel, E., and Genant, H. K. (2003). Clinical applications of body composition measurements using DXA. *J. Clin. Densitom.* 6, 75–85. doi: 10.1385/JCD:6:2:75

Baba, S., Jacene, H. A., Engles, J. M., Honda, H., and Wahl, R. L. (2010). CT Hounsfield units of brown adipose tissue increase with activation: preclinical and clinical studies. *J. Nucl. Med.* 51, 246–250. doi: 10.2967/jnumed.109.068775

Bao, J., Cui, X., Cai, S., Zhong, J., Cai, C., and Chen, Z. (2013). Brown adipose tissue mapping in rats with combined intermolecular double-quantum coherence and Dixon water-fat MRI. *NMR Biomed.* 26, 1663–1671. doi: 10.1002/nbm.3000

Bartelt, A., Bruns, O. T., Reimer, R., Hohenberg, H., Ittrich, H., Peldschus, K., et al. (2011). Brown adipose tissue activity controls triglyceride clearance. *Nat. Med.* 17, 200–205. doi: 10.1038/nm.2297

Bastie, C. C., Zong, H., Xu, J., Busa, B., Judex, S., Kurland, I. J., et al. (2007). Integrative metabolic regulation of peripheral tissue fatty acid oxidation by the SRC kinase family member Fyn *Cell Metab.* 5, 371–381. doi: 10.1016/j.cmet.2007.04.005

Beckmann, N., Kneuer, R., Gremlich, H. U., Karmouty-Quintana, H., Blé, F. X., and Muller, M. (2007). In vivo mouse imaging and spectroscopy in drug discovery. *NMR Biomed.* 20, 154–185. doi: 10.1002/nbm.1153

Bidar, A. W., Ploj, K., Lelliott, C., Nelander, K., Winzell, M. S., Böttcher, G., et al. (2012). In vivo imaging of lipid storage and regression in diet-induced obesity during nutrition manipulation. *Am. J. Physiol. Endocrinol. Metab.* 303, E1287–E1295. doi: 10.1152/ajpendo.00274.2012

Bjorntorp, P. (2000). Metabolic difference between visceral fat and subcutaneous abdominal fat. *Diabetes Metab.* 26, 10–12.

Bley, T. A., Wieben, O., François, C. J., Brittain, J. H., and Reeder, S. B. (2010). Fat and water magnetic resonance imaging. *J. Magn. Reson. Imaging* 31, 4–18. doi: 10.1002/jmri.21895

Boschi, F., and Spinelli, A. E. (2014). Cerenkov luminescence imaging at a glance. *Curr. Mol. Imaging* 3, 106–117. doi: 10.2174/2211555203666141128002406

Branca, R. T., He, T., Zhang, L., Floyd, C. S., Freeman, M., White, C., et al. (2014). Detection of brown adipose tissue and thermogenic activity in mice by hyperpolarized xenon MRI. *Proc. Natl. Acad. Sci. U.S.A.* 16, 18001–18006. doi: 10.1073/pnas.1403697111

Branca, R. T., Zhang, L., Warren, W. S., Auerbach, E., Khanna, A., Degan, S., et al. (2013). In vivo noninvasive detection of brown adipose tissue through intermolecular zero-quantum MRI. *PLoS ONE* 8:e74206. doi: 10.1371/journal.pone.0074206

Calderan, L., Marzola, P., Nicolato, E., Fabene, P. F., Milanese, C., Bernardi, P., et al. (2006). In vivo phenotyping of the ob/ob mouse by magnetic resonance imaging and 1H-magnetic resonance spectroscopy. *Obesity* 14, 405–414. doi: 10.1038/oby.2006.54

Cannon, B., and Nedergaard, J. (2004). Brown adipose tissue: function and physiological significance. *Physiol. Rev.* 84, 277–359. doi: 10.1152/physrev.00015.2003

Carmon, V. E., Rudich, A., Hadad, N., and Levy, R. (2008). Neutrophils transiently infiltrate intra-abdominal fat early in the course of high-fat feeding. *J. Lipid Res.* 49, 1894–1903. doi: 10.1194/jlr.M800132-JLR200

Carroll, J. F., Chiapa, A. L., Rodriquez, M., Phelps, D. R., Cardarelli, K. M., Vishwanatha, J. K., et al. (2008). Visceral fat, waist circumference, and BMI: impact of race/ethnicity. *Obesity* 16, 600–607. doi: 10.1038/oby.2007.92

Carter, E. A., Bonab, A. A., Paul, K., Yerxa, J., Tompkins, R. G., and Fischman, A. J. (2011). Association of heat production with 18F-FDG accumulation in murine brown adipose tissue after stress. *J. Nucl. Med.* 52, 1616–1620. doi: 10.2967/jnumed.111.090175

Cawthorn, W. P., Scheller, E. L., and MacDougald, O. A. (2012). Adipose tissue stem cells: the great WAT hope. *Trends Endocrinol. Metab.* 23, 270–277. doi: 10.1016/j.tem.2012.01.003

Chen, Y. I., Cypess, A. M., Sass, C. A., Brownell, A. L., Jokivarsi, K. T., Kahn, C. R., et al. (2012). Anatomical and functional assessment of brown adipose tissue by magnetic resonance imaging. *Obesity* 20, 1519–1526. doi: 10.1038/oby.2012.22

Cinti, S. (2000). Anatomy of the adipose organ. *Eat. Weight Disord.* 5, 132–142. doi: 10.1007/BF03354443

Costantini, V. J., Vicentini, E., Sabbatini, F. M., Valerio, E., Lepore, S., Tessari, M., et al. (2011). GSK1614343, a novel ghrelin receptor antagonist, produces an unexpected increase of food intake and body weight in rodents and dogs. *Neuroendocrinology* 94, 158–168. doi: 10.1159/000328968

Dixon, W. T. (1984). Simple proton spectroscopic imaging. *Radiology* 153, 189–194. doi: 10.1148/radiology.153.1.6089263

Evans, R. D. (1955). *The Atomic Nucleus.* New York, NY: McGraw-Hill.

Feldmann, H. M., Golozoubova, V., Cannon, B., and Nedergaard, J. (2009). UCP1 ablation induces obesity and abolishes diet-induced thermogenesis in mice exempt from thermal stress by living at thermoneutrality. *Cell Metab.* 9, 203–209. doi: 10.1016/j.cmet.2008.12.014

Frayn, K. N., and Karpe, F. (2014). Regulation of human subcutaneous adipose tissue blood flow. *Int. J. Obes.* 38, 1019–1026. doi: 10.1038/ijo.2013.200

Fueger, B. J., Czernin, J., Hildebrandt, I., Tran, C., Halpern, B. S., Stout, D., et al. (2006). Impact of animal handling on the results of 18F-FDG PET studies in mice. *J. Nucl. Med.* 47, 999–1006.

Funicello, M., Novelli, M., Ragni, M., Vottari, T., Cocuzza, C., Soriano-Lopez, J., et al. (2007). Cathepsin K null mice show reduced adiposity during the rapid accumulation of fat stores. *PLoS ONE* 2:e683. doi: 10.1371/journal.pone.0000683

Geer, E. B., and Shen, W. (2009). Gender differences in insulin resistance, body composition, and energy balance. *Gend. Med.* 6, 60–75. doi: 10.1016/j.genm.2009.02.002

Giachetti, A., Lovato, C., Piscitelli, F., Milanese, C., and Zancanaro, C. (2015). Robust automatic measurement of 3D scanned models for the human body fat estimation. *IEEE J. Biomed. Health Inform.* 19, 660–667. doi: 10.1109/JBHI.2014.2314360

Giarola, M., Rossi, B., Mosconi, E., Fontanella, M., Marzola, P., Scambi, I., et al. (2011). Fast and minimally invasive determination of the unsaturation index of white fat depots by micro-Raman spectroscopy. *Lipids* 46, 659–667. doi: 10.1007/s11745-011-3567-8

Giordano, A., Frontini, A., and Cinti, S. (2016). Convertible visceral fat as a therapeutic target to curb obesity. *Nat. Rev. Drug Discov.* 15, 405–424. doi: 10.1038/nrd.2016.31

Grant, R. W., and Dixit, V. D. (2015). Adipose tissue as an immunological organ. *Obesity* 23, 512–518. doi: 10.1002/oby.21003

Guerra, C., Navarro, P., Valverde, A., Arribas, M., Brüning, J., Kozak, L., et al. (2001). Brown adipose tissue-specific insulin receptor knockout shows diabetic phenotype without insulin resistance. *J. Clin. Invest.* 108, 1205–1213. doi: 10.1172/JCI13103

Gunawardana, S. C., and Piston, D. W. (2012). Reversal of type 1 diabetes in mice by brown adipose tissue transplant. *Diabetes Metab. Res. Rev.* 61, 674–682.

Holdsworth, D. W., and Thornton, M. M. (2002). Micro-CT in small animal and specimen imaging. *Trends Biotechnol.* 20, S34–S39. doi: 10.1016/S0167-7799(02)02004-8

Holstila, M., Virtanen, K. A., Grönroos, T. J., Laine, J., Lepomäki, V., Saunavaara, J., et al. (2013). Measurement of brown adipose tissue mass using a novel dual-echo magnetic resonance imaging approach: a validation study. *Metabolism* 62, 1189–1198. doi: 10.1016/j.metabol.2013.03.002

Hu, H. H., Hines, C. D., Smith, D. L. Jr., and Reeder, S. B. (2012). Variations in $T(2)^*$ and fat content of murine brown and white adipose tissues by chemical-shift MRI. *Magn. Reson. Imaging* 30, 323–329. doi: 10.1016/j.mri.2011.12.004

Hu, H. H., and Kan, H. E. (2013). Quantitative proton MR techniques for measuring fat. *NMR Biomed.* 26, 1609–1629. doi: 10.1002/nbm.3025

Ibrahim, M. M. (2010). Subcutaneous and visceral adipose tissue: structural and functional differences. *Obes. Rev.* 11, 11–18. doi: 10.1111/j.1467-789X.2009.00623.x

Johns, H. E., and Cunningham, J. R. (1983). *The Physics of Radiology*, 4th Edn. Springfield, IL: Charles C Thomas.

Judex, S., Luu, Y. K., Ozcivici, E., Adler, B., Lublinsky, S., and Rubin, C. T. (2010). Quantification of adiposity in small rodents using micro-CT. *Methods* 50, 14–19. doi: 10.1016/j.ymeth.2009.05.017

Kanasaki, K., and Koya, D. (2011). Biology of obesity: lessons from animal models of obesity. *J. Biomed. Biotechnol.* 2011:197636. doi: 10.1155/2011/197636

Kelley, D. E., Thaete, F. L., Troost, F., Huwe, T., and Goodpaster, B. H. (2000). Subdivisions of subcutaneous abdominal adipose tissue and insulin resistance. *Am. J. Physiol. Endocrinol. Metab.* 278, E941–E948.

Kershaw, E. E., and Flier, J. S. (2004). Adipose tissue as an endocrine organ. *J. Clin. Endocrinol. Metab.* 89, 2548–2556. doi: 10.1210/jc.2004-0395

Khanna, A., and Branca, R. T. (2012). Detecting brown adipose tissue activity with BOLD MRI in mice. *Magn. Reson. Med.* 68, 1285–1290. doi: 10.1002/mrm.24118

Kintscher, U., Hartge, M., Hess, K., Foryst-Ludwig, A., Clemenz, M., and Wabitsch, M. (2008). T-lymphocyte infiltration in visceral adipose tissue: a primary event in adipose tissue inflammation and the development of obesity-mediated insulin resistance. *Arterioscler. Thromb. Vasc. Biol.* 28, 1304–1310. doi: 10.1161/ATVBAHA.108.165100

Labbé, S. M., Caron, A., Bakan, I., Laplante, M., Carpentier, A. C., Lecomte, R., et al. (2015). In vivo measurement of energy substrate contribution to cold-induced brown adipose tissue thermogenesis. *FASEB J.* 29, 2046–2058. doi: 10.1096/fj.14-266247

Labbé, S. M., Caron, A., Chechi, K., Laplante, M., Lecomte, R., and Richard, D. (2016). Metabolic activity of brown, "beige" and white adipose tissues in response to chronic adrenergic stimulation in male mice. *Am. J. Physiol. Endocrinol. Metab.* 311, E260–E268. doi: 10.1152/ajpendo.00545.2015

Lau, A. Z., Chen, A. P., Gu, Y., Ladouceur-Wodzak, M., Nayak, K. S., and Cunningham, C. H. (2014). Noninvasive identification and assessment of functional brown adipose tissue in rodents using hyperpolarized ^{13}C imaging. *Int. J. Obes.* 38, 126–131. doi: 10.1038/ijo.2013.58

Lin, S. F., Fan, X., Yeckel, C. W., Weinzimmer, D., Mulnix, T., Gallezot, J. D., et al. (2012). Ex vivo and in vivo evaluation of the norepinephrine transporter ligand [(11)C]MRB for brown adipose tissue imaging. *Nucl. Med. Biol.* 39, 1081–1086. doi: 10.1016/j.nucmedbio.2012.04.005

Lindenberg, K. S., Weydt, P., Müller, H. P., Bornstedt, A., Ludolph, A. C., Landwehrmeyer, G. B., et al. (2014). Two-point magnitude MRI for rapid mapping of brown adipose tissue and its application to the R6/2 mouse model of Huntington disease. *PLoS ONE* 9:e105556. doi: 10.1371/journal.pone.0105556

Lunati, E., Farace, P., Nicolato, E., Righetti, C., Marzola, P., Sbarbati, A., et al. (2001). Polyunsaturated fatty acids mapping by (1)H MR-chemical shift imaging. *Magn. Reson. Med.* 46, 879–883. doi: 10.1002/mrm.1272

Lunati, E., Marzola, P., Nicolato, E., Fedrigo, M., Villa, M., and Sbarbati, A. (1999). In vivo quantitative lipidic map of brown adipose tissue by chemical shift imaging at 4.7 Tesla. *J. Lipid Res.* 40, 1395–1400.

Luu, Y. K., Lublinsky, S., Ozcivici, E., Capilla, E., Pessin, J. E., Rubin, C. T., et al. (2009). In vivo quantification of subcutaneous and visceral adiposity by micro-computed tomography in a small animal model. *Med. Eng. Phys.* 31, 34–41. doi: 10.1016/j.medengphy.2008.03.006

Mårin, P., Andersson, B., Ottosson, M., Olbe, L., Chowdhury, B., Kvist, H., et al. (1992). The morphology and metabolism of intra-abdominal adipose tissue in men. *Metabolism* 41, 1241–1248.

Mathieu, P., Boulanger, M. C., and Després, J. P. (2014). Ectopic visceral fat: a clinical and molecular perspective on the cardiometabolic risk. *Rev. Endocr. Metab. Disord.* 15, 289–298. doi: 10.1007/s11154-014-9299-3

Mathis, D. (2013). Immunological goings-on in visceral adipose tissue. *Cell Metab.* 4, 851–859. doi: 10.1016/j.cmet.2013.05.008

Metzinger, M. N., Miramontes, B., Zhou, P., Liu, Y., Chapman, S., Sun, L., et al. (2014). Correlation of X-ray computed tomography with quantitative nuclear magnetic resonance methods for pre-clinical measurement of adipose and lean tissues in living mice. *Sensors* 8, 18526–18542. doi: 10.3390/s141018526

Mirbolooki, M. R., Constantinescu, C. C., Pan, M. L., and Mukherjee, J. (2011). Quantitative assessment of brown adipose tissue metabolic activity and volume using [18 F]FDG PET/CT and β3-adrenergic receptor activation. *EJNMMI Res.* 1:30. doi: 10.1186/2191-219X-1-30

Mirbolooki, M. R., Constantinescu, C. C., Pan, M. L., and Mukherjee, J. (2013). Targeting presynaptic norepinephrine transporter in brown adipose tissue: a novel imaging approach and potential treatment for diabetes and obesity. *Synapse* 67, 79–93. doi: 10.1002/syn.21617

Mirbolooki, M. R., Upadhyay, S. K., Constantinescu, C. C., Pan, M. L., and Mukherjee, J. (2014). Adrenergic pathway activation enhances brown adipose tissue metabolism: a [18F]FDG PET/CT study in mice. *Nucl. Med. Biol.* 41, 10–16. doi: 10.1016/j.nucmedbio.2013.08.009

Mosconi, E., Fontanella, M., Sima, D. M., Van Huffel, S., Fiorini, S., Sbarbati, A., et al. (2011). Investigation of adipose tissues in Zucker rats using in vivo and ex vivo magnetic resonance spectroscopy. *J. Lipid Res.* 52, 330–336. doi: 10.1194/jlr.M011825

Mosconi, E., Sima, D. M., Osorio Garcia, M. I., Fontanella, M., Fiorini, S., Van Huffel, S., et al. (2014). Different quantification algorithms may lead to different results: a comparison using proton MRS lipid signals. *NMR Biomed.* 27, 431–443. doi: 10.1002/nbm.3079

Osculati, F., Sbarbati, A., Leclercq, F., Zancanaro, C., Accordini, C., Antonakis, K., et al. (1991). The correlation between magnetic resonance imaging and ultrastructural patterns of brown adipose tissue. *J. Submicrosc. Cytol. Pathol.* 23, 167–174.

Ouellet, V., Labbé, S. M., Blondin, D. P., Phoenix, S., Guérin, B., Haman, F., et al. (2012). Brown adipose tissue oxidative metabolism contributes to energy expenditure during acute cold exposure in humans. *J. Clin. Invest.* 122, 545–552. doi: 10.1172/JCI60433

Peng, X. G., Ju, S., Fang, F., Wang, Y., Fang, K., Cui, X., et al. (2013). Comparison of brown and white adipose tissue fat fractions in ob, seipin, and Fsp27 gene knockout mice by chemical shift-selective imaging and (1)H-MR spectroscopy. *Am. J. Physiol. Endocrinol. Metab.* 304, E160–E167. doi: 10.1152/ajpendo.00401.2012

Pietrobelli, A., Wang, Z., and Heymsfield, S. B. (1998). Techniques used in measuring human body composition. *Curr. Opin. Clin. Nutr. Metab. Care* 1, 439–448. doi: 10.1097/00075197-199809000-00013

Quarta, C., Lodi, F., Mazza, R., Giannone, F., Boschi, L., Nanni, C., et al. (2013). 11C-meta-hydroxyephedrine PET/CT imaging allows in vivo study of adaptive thermogenesis and white-to-brown fat conversion. *Mol. Metab.* 2, 153–160. doi: 10.1016/j.molmet.2013.04.002

Reeder, S. B., Cruite, I., Hamilton, G., and Sirlin, C. B. (2011). Quantitative assessment of liver fat with magnetic resonance imaging and spectroscopy. *J. Magn. Reson. Imaging* 34, 729–749. doi: 10.1002/jmri.22580

Rees, D. A., and Alcolado, J. C. (2005). Animal models of diabetes mellitus. *Diabet. Med.* 22, 359–370. doi: 10.1111/j.1464-5491.2005.01499.x

Rice, D. R., White, A. G., Leevy, W. M., and Smith, B. D. (2015). Fluorescence imaging of interscapular brown adipose tissue in living mice. *J. Mater. Chem. B* 3, 1979–1989. doi: 10.1039/C4TB01914H

Romacho, T., Elsen, M., Röhrborn, D., and Eckel, J. (2014). Adipose tissue and its role in organ crosstalk. *Acta Physiol.* 210, 733–753. doi: 10.1111/apha.12246

Ronti, T., Lupattelli, G., and Mannarino, E. (2006). The endocrine function of adipose tissue: an update. *Clin. Endocrinol.* 64, 355–365.

Rosen, E. D., and Spiegelman, B. M. (2000). Molecular regulation of adipogenesis. *Annu. Rev. Cell Dev. Biol.* 16, 145–171. doi: 10.1146/annurev.cellbio.16.1.145

Rubin, C. T., Capilla, E., Luu, Y. K., Busa, B., Crawford, H., Nolan, D. J., et al. (2007). Adipogenesis is inhibited by brief, daily exposure to high-frequency, extremely low-magnitude mechanical signals. *Proc. Natl. Acad. Sci. U.S.A.* 104, 17879–17884. doi: 10.1073/pnas.0708467104

Sasser, T. A., Chapman, S. E., Li, S., Hudson, C., Orton, S. P., Diener, J. M., et al. (2012). Segmentation and measurement of fat volumes in murine obesity models using X-ray computed tomography. *J. Vis. Exp.* 4, e3680. doi: 10.3791/3680

Sbarbati, A., Baldassarri, A. M., Zancanaro, C., Boicelli, A., and Osculati, F. (1991). In vivo morphometry and functional morphology of brown adipose tissue by magnetic resonance imaging. *Anat. Rec.* 231, 293–297. doi: 10.1002/ar.1092310302

Sbarbati, A., Cavallini, I., Marzola, P., Nicolato, E., and Osculati, F. (2006). Contrast-enhanced MRI of brown adipose tissue after pharmacological stimulation. *Magn. Reson. Med.* 55, 715–718. doi: 10.1002/mrm.20851

Sbarbati, A., Guerrini, U., Marzola, P., Asperio, R., and Osculati, F. (1997). Chemical shift imaging at 4.7 tesla of brown adipose tissue. *J. Lipid Res.* 38, 343–347.

Sbarbati, A., Leclercq, F., Osculati, F., and Gresser, I. (1995). Interferon alpha/beta-induced abnormalities in adipocytes of suckling mice. *Biol. Cell* 83, 163–167. doi: 10.1016/0248-4900(96)81304-9

Schade, K. N., Baranwal, A., Liang, C., Mirbolooki, M. R., and Mukherjee, J. (2015). Preliminary evaluation of β3-adrenoceptor agonist-induced 18F-FDG metabolic activity of brown adipose tissue in obese Zucker rat. *Nucl. Med. Biol.* 42, 691–694. doi: 10.1016/j.nucmedbio.2015.04.003

Schambach, S. J., Bag, S., Schilling, L., Groden, C., and Brockmann, M. A. (2010). Application of micro-CT in small animal imaging. *Methods* 50, 2–13. doi: 10.1016/j.ymeth.2009.08.007

Schoen, R. E., Evans, R. W., Sankey, S. S., Weissfeld, J. L., and Kuller, L. (1996). Does visceral adipose tissue differ from subcutaneous adipose tissue in fatty acid content? *Int. J. Obes. Relat. Metab. Disord.* 20, 346–352.

Shen, W., Wang, Z., Punyanita, M., Lei, J., Sinav, A., Kral, J. G., et al. (2003). Adipose tissue quantification by imaging methods: a proposed classification. *Obes. Res.* 11, 5–16. doi: 10.1038/oby.2003.3

Shulman, G. I. (2014). Ectopic fat in insulin resistance, dyslipidemia, and cardiometabolic disease. *N. Engl. J. Med.* 371, 1131–1141.

Sjögren, K., Hellberg, N., Bohlooly-Y, M., Savendahl, L., Johansson, M. S., Berglindh, T., et al. (2001). Body fat content can be predicted in vivo in mice using a modified dual-energy X-ray absorptiometry technique. *J. Nutr.* 131, 2963–2966.

Smith, D. L. Jr., Yang, Y., Hu, H. H., Zhai, G., and Nagy, T. R. (2013). Measurement of interscapular brown adipose tissue of mice in differentially housed temperatures by chemical-shift-encoded water-fat MRI. *J. Magn. Reson. Imaging* 38, 1425–1433. doi: 10.1002/jmri.24138

Smith, S. R., Lovejoy, J. C., Greenway, F., Ryan, D., deJonge, L., de la Bretonne, J., et al. (2001). Contributions of total body fat, abdominal subcutaneous adipose tissue compartments, and visceral adipose tissue to the metabolic complications of obesity. *Metabolism* 50, 425–435. doi: 10.1053/meta.2001.21693

Spinelli, A. E., and Boschi, F. (2015). Novel biomedical applications of Cerenkov radiation and radioluminescence imaging. *Phys. Med.* 31, 120–129. doi: 10.1016/j.ejmp.2014.12.003

Tchoukalova, Y. D., Sarr, M. G., and Jensen, M. D. (2004). Measuring committed preadipocytes in human adipose tissue from severely obese patients by using adipocyte fatty acid binding protein. *Am. J. Physiol. Regul. Integr. Comp. Physiol.* 287, R1132–R1140. doi: 10.1152/ajpregu.00337.2004

Toombs, R. J., Ducher, G., Shepherd, J. A., and De Souza, M. J. (2012). The impact of recent technological advances on the trueness and precision of DXA to assess body composition. *Obesity* 20, 30–39. doi: 10.1038/oby.2011.211

Tothill, P., Han, T. S., Avenell, A., McNeill, G., and Reid, D. M. (1996). Comparisons between fat measurements by dual-energy X-ray absorptiometry, underwater weighing and magnetic resonance imaging in healthy women. *Eur. J. Clin. Nutr.* 50, 747–752.

van der Veen, D. R., Shao, J., Chapman, S., Leevy, W. M., and Duffield, G. E. (2012). A diurnal rhythm in glucose uptake in brown adipose tissue revealed by in vivo PET-FDG imaging. *Obesity* 20, 1527–1529. doi: 10.1038/oby.2012.78

Vanderburgh, P. M. (1992). Fat distribution: its physiological significance, health implications, and its adaptation to exercise training. *Mil. Med.* 157, 189–192.

Varga, O., Harangi, M., Olsson, I. A., and Hansen, A. K. (2010). Contribution of animal models to the understanding of the metabolic syndrome: a systematic overview. *Obes. Rev.* 11, 792–807. doi: 10.1111/j.1467-789X.2009.00667.x

Vosselman, M. J., van Marken Lichtenbelt, W. D., and Schrauwen, P. (2013). Energy dissipation in brown adipose tissue: from mice to men. *Mol. Cell. Endocrinol.* 379, 43–50. doi: 10.1016/j.mce.2013.04.017

Wang, H., Chen, Y. E., and Eitzman, D. T. (2014). Imaging body fat: techniques and cardiometabolic implications. *Arterioscler. Thromb. Vasc. Biol.* 34, 2217–2223. doi: 10.1161/ATVBAHA.114.303036

Wang, X., Minze, L. J., and Shi, Z. Z. (2012). Functional imaging of brown fat in mice with [18 F]FDG micro-PET/CT. *J. Vis. Exp.* 69, 4060. doi: 10.3791/4060

Wang, Z. M., Pierson, R. N. Jr., and Heymsfield, S. B. (1992). The five level model: a new approach to organizing body composition research. *Am. J. Clin. Nutr.* 56, 19–28.

Wells, J. C., Ruto, A., and Treleaven, P. (2008). Whole-body three-dimensional photonic scanning: a new technique for obesity research and clinical practice. *Int. J. Obes.* 32, 232–238. doi: 10.1038/sj.ijo.0803727

Wu, C., Cheng, W., Sun, Y., Dang, Y., Gong, F., Zhu, H., et al. (2014). Activating brown adipose tissue for weight loss and lowering of blood glucose levels: a microPET study using obese and diabetic model mice. *PLoS ONE* 9:e113742. doi: 10.1371/journal.pone.0113742

Ye, Q., Danzer, C. F., Fuchs, A., Wolfrum, C., and Rudin, M. (2012). Hepatic lipid composition differs between ob/ob and ob/+ control mice as determined by using in vivo localized proton magnetic resonance spectroscopy. *MAGMA* 25, 381–389. doi: 10.1007/s10334-012-0310-2

Zhang, X., Kuo, C., Moore, A., and Ran, C. (2013). In vivo optical imaging of interscapular brown adipose tissue with 18F-FDG via Cerenkov luminescence imaging. *PLoS ONE* 8:e62007. doi: 10.1371/journal.pone.0062007

Conflict of Interest Statement: FM is employed in Bruker Italia s.r.l., and the other authors declare that the research was conducted in the absence of any commercial or financial relationships that could be construed as a potential conflict of interest.

7

Advances in Optical Imaging for Pharmacological Studies

Alicia Arranz [1]* *and Jorge Ripoll* [2,3]*

[1] *Department of Cell Biology and Immunology, Center for Molecular Biology "Severo Ochoa", Spanish National Research Council, Madrid, Spain,* [2] *Department of Bioengineering and Aerospace Engineering, Universidad Carlos III of Madrid, Madrid, Spain,* [3] *Experimental Medicine and Surgery Unit, Instituto de Investigación Sanitaria del Hospital Gregorio Marañón, Madrid, Spain*

Edited by:
Nicolau Beckmann,
Novartis Institutes for BioMedical
Research, Switzerland

Reviewed by:
Bastien Arnal,
Institut Langevin, France
Neal C. Burton,
iThera Medical, Germany

*Correspondence:
Alicia Arranz,
Department of Cell Biology
and Immunology, Center for Molecular
Biology "Severo Ochoa", Spanish
National Research Council, Nicolás
Cabrera 1, 28049 Madrid, Spain
alicia.arranz@cbm.csic.es;
Jorge Ripoll,
Department of Bioengineering
and Aerospace Engineering,
Universidad Carlos III of Madrid,
Avenida Universidad 30, Leganés,
28911 Madrid, Spain
jorge.ripoll@uc3m.es

Imaging approaches are an essential tool for following up over time representative parameters of *in vivo* models, providing useful information in pharmacological studies. Main advantages of optical imaging approaches compared to other imaging methods are their safety, straight-forward use and cost-effectiveness. A main drawback, however, is having to deal with the presence of high scattering and high absorption in living tissues. Depending on how these issues are addressed, three different modalities can be differentiated: planar imaging (including fluorescence and bioluminescence *in vivo* imaging), optical tomography, and optoacoustic approaches. In this review we describe the latest advances in optical *in vivo* imaging with pharmacological applications, with special focus on the development of new optical imaging probes in order to overcome the strong absorption introduced by different tissue components, especially hemoglobin, and the development of multimodal imaging systems in order to overcome the resolution limitations imposed by scattering.

Keywords: bioluminescence, planar fluorescence imaging, fluorescence molecular tomography, optoacoustics, multispectral optoacoustic tomography, multispectral imaging, hybrid systems, data processing

Introduction

Whole-body optical *in vivo* imaging approaches are valuable tools that enable the study of animal models of human diseases, reducing the number of animals required for experimentation and providing essential information in pharmacological studies. Depending on the physical principle providing image contrast, we find techniques based on light generation, such as bioluminescence or fluorescence imaging, or based on light absorption, such as optoacoustics. All these methodologies enable *in vivo* imaging of molecular and cellular processes with high sensitivity and have gained great popularity over the past decade mainly because of their safe and straightforward use due to the employment of non-ionizing wavelengths, and their cost-effectiveness compared with other imaging technologies (such as positron emission tomography, PET, or magnetic resonance imaging, MRI; Ntziachristos et al., 2007; Stuker et al., 2011b).

On the other hand, one of the main problems of optical *in vivo* technologies is dealing with the scattering and absorption properties of tissue (Boas et al., 2011; Ripoll, 2012): scattering is responsible for the loss of light directionality (and therefore a loss in resolution by consequently blurring the image), while the presence of high absorbers (such as melanin and blood) results in a reduction of light intensity (decreasing the signal to noise ratio dramatically in the visible range; Ripoll, 2012).

The most effective way to overcome the loss of signal intensity due to absorption is to employ excitation and emission wavelengths in the near-infrared optical imaging window (between 700 and 900 nm, approximately), where the main tissue constituents (hemoglobin, melanin, water, and lipids) absorb the least (Ntziachristos et al., 2005; Jacques, 2013). On the other hand, if one wishes to account for the effects of high scattering in light propagation within tissues in order to obtain a 3D image or quantitative information (note that location, probe concentration, and probe size are strongly interdependent), one needs to introduce a physical model of light propagation within complex media such as a living organism. Once this model is in place, a numerical inversion of this model (what is termed, "solving the inverse problem") is needed in order to obtain a 3D image providing the spatial distribution of probe concentration. Depending on the algorithm we use to reconstruct an image we will be able to recover probe size, position and concentration with varying accuracy. How this issue is addressed clearly distinguishes the different imaging approaches in optical *in vivo* imaging into the following three categories: (1) planar optical imaging, (2) optical tomography, and (3) optoacoustic tomography.

In this review we discuss the latest advances of optical *in vivo* imaging as a tool in pharmaceutical studies, addressing the different approaches that are being developed in order to overcome the strong absorption introduced by hemoglobin and the ill-posedness introduced by scattering, either through the use of multimodal imaging or photoacoustic tomography, or by developing new probes or proteins more adequate for *in vivo* imaging in deep tissues.

Planar Optical Imaging

Planar optical imaging techniques are by far the most common, mainly due to their simplicity of use and low cost. Two planar imaging modalities are available, depending on the light source generation: Bioluminescence and Fluorescence. In both cases a high sensitivity camera (CCD mainly) coupled to a high numerical aperture camera objective takes a single long exposure image, in the case of fluorescence using appropriate band-pass filters. In what follows we detail recent advances and applications in both modalities.

Bioluminescence *In Vivo* Imaging

Bioluminescence imaging is based on the oxidation of a substrate (luciferin) mediated by an enzyme (luciferase), being the most commonly used the luciferase originated from the North American firefly (*Photinus pyralis*). The firefly luciferase requires ATP and magnesium to catalyze the reaction that leads to the emission of light, which ranges from 530 to 640 nm, depending amongst other factors on the pH, polarity of the solvent, and the microenvironment of the enzyme (Li et al., 2013). Note how this emission falls within the portion of the visible spectrum where hemoglobin is strongly absorbing.

Since the firefly luciferase was cloned (de Wet et al., 1985), the *luc* gene has extensively been used in gene regulation studies. Bioluminescent probes have also been engineered in order to detect specific enzymatic activities. These probes are designed in such a way that the luciferin is "caged" and this conjugate has to be cleaved by an enzymatic activity (i.e., proteases such as caspases). Once cleaved, the luciferin can be oxidized by the luciferase and the signal is released (Li et al., 2013).

Techniques based on bioluminescence detection have largely been used for molecular biology assays in laboratories worldwide. Accordingly, bioluminescence has also been a reference method for *in vivo* imaging. Its main advantage is the absence of background signal (the commonly used cell or animal models do not express luciferase and therefore there is no "auto-bioluminescence"), which leads to a high specificity of the detected signals and an elevated signal-to-noise ratio. This has resulted in an impressive expansion of bioluminescence *in vivo* imaging applications for studies in cancer biology, inflammation, and infection, amongst others (Edinger et al., 2002; Andreu et al., 2010; Luker and Luker, 2011; Luwor et al., 2015). However, researchers using bioluminescence *in vivo* imaging have to deal with problems derived from the complexity of the luciferase-luciferin reaction and the effects of light propagation in living tissues. Regarding the luciferase-luciferin reaction, both substrate and co-factors (ATP, oxygen and magnesium) are required for the reaction to take place and therefore the limitation of any of them may result in altered readouts that are not a real representation of luciferase activity (Sadikot and Blackwell, 2005). There have also been significant efforts toward the development of bioluminescence tomography (BLT) approaches, requiring the prior knowledge of one of the parameters or the number of sources in order to produce a 3D image (Liu et al., 2010).

Fluorescence *In Vivo* Imaging

After a fluorescent agent is excited with a light source, fluorescence is emitted isotropically as a consequence of a radiative transition from an excited singlet state to a singlet state of lower energy (typically the ground state) following Stoke's Law (Sauer et al., 2011). Even though fluorescence has been extensively used in microscopy for over a century to study molecular and cellular processes (Masters, 2009), it has not been until this past decade that its use for *in vivo* small animal imaging became significant (Mahmood et al., 1999; Weissleder et al., 1999; Ntziachristos et al., 2005). The high sensitivity offered by this technique and the latest advances in fluorescence labeling have also promoted its relatively recent incursion in non-invasive *in vivo* imaging. Both planar and three-dimensional fluorescence imaging methods *in vivo* are now commonly used in pre-clinical research.

In order to acquire a fluorescence image, either as part of a tomographic data set or a single planar image, one requires an excitation source as close as possible to the excitation maximum of the fluorophore being used, if possible within the near infrared optical imaging window. The use of this excitation wavelength, however, will not only excite specifically the fluorophore but will generate non-specific fluorescence from several components present in tissue, generating what is termed "auto-fluorescence," reducing the signal to background ratio (i.e., the contrast in the image). One way to reduce this problem is performing several spectral measurements with different excitation/emission pairs and unmixing the specific signal of the fluorophore from the un-specific signal of the surrounding tissue (Xu and Rice, 2009).

With respect to recent pharmacological studies, Zhang et al. (2015b) make use of planar fluorescence molecular imaging to monitor therapy in murine models of Alzheimer's disease. In particular, the authors verify the feasibility of using CRANAD-3

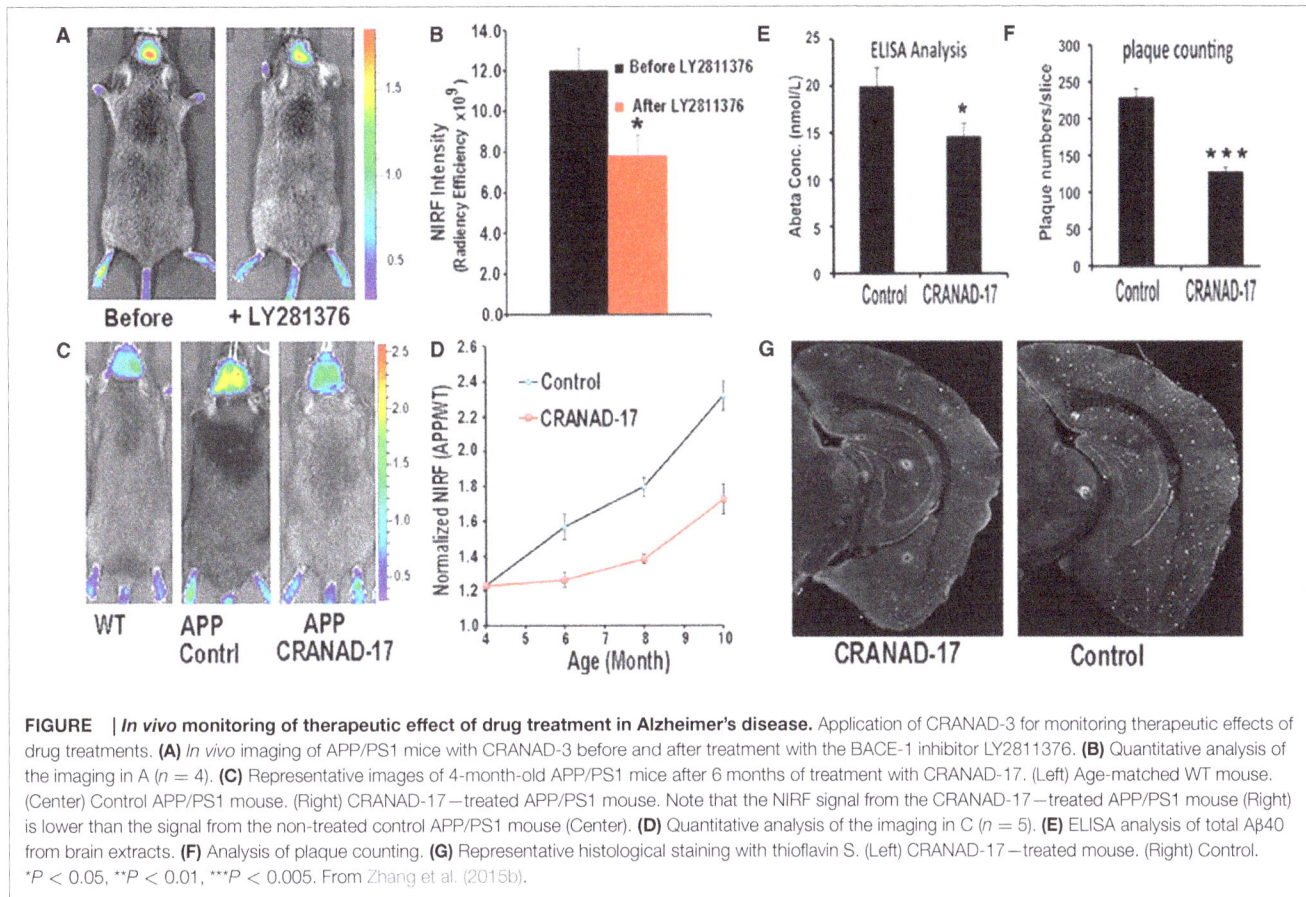

FIGURE | *In vivo* monitoring of therapeutic effect of drug treatment in Alzheimer's disease. Application of CRANAD-3 for monitoring therapeutic effects of drug treatments. **(A)** *In vivo* imaging of APP/PS1 mice with CRANAD-3 before and after treatment with the BACE-1 inhibitor LY2811376. **(B)** Quantitative analysis of the imaging in A ($n = 4$). **(C)** Representative images of 4-month-old APP/PS1 mice after 6 months of treatment with CRANAD-17. (Left) Age-matched WT mouse. (Center) Control APP/PS1 mouse. (Right) CRANAD-17—treated APP/PS1 mouse. Note that the NIRF signal from the CRANAD-17—treated APP/PS1 mouse (Right) is lower than the signal from the non-treated control APP/PS1 mouse (Center). **(D)** Quantitative analysis of the imaging in C ($n = 5$). **(E)** ELISA analysis of total Aβ40 from brain extracts. **(F)** Analysis of plaque counting. **(G)** Representative histological staining with thioflavin S. (Left) CRANAD-17—treated mouse. (Right) Control. *$P < 0.05$, **$P < 0.01$, ***$P < 0.005$. From Zhang et al. (2015b).

for monitoring therapy, and use it to monitor the therapeutic effect of CRANAD-17, a curcumin analog for inhibition of Aβ cross-linking (see **Figure**).

Diffuse Optical Tomography and Fluorescence Molecular Tomography

In order to account for the effect of scattering when imaging tissues with light, diffuse optical tomography (DOT) was developed, based on scanning a point source over the sample and measuring the intensity of the diffuse light either by fibers or with a camera focused onto the surface (see Arridge, 1999, for a review on this subject). With its first applications being targeted toward breast cancer (see, for example Ntziachristos et al., 2000) its use in small animal imaging came with the development of fluorescence molecular tomography, first published in 2002 (Ntziachristos et al., 2002), in the context of molecular imaging by employing an activatable probe to image protease activity in an *in vivo* mouse model of glioblastoma. Since this first publication in 2002 there have been several developments and applications, mainly in tumor biology (Ntziachristos et al., 2004; Deliolanis et al., 2006; Montet et al., 2007; Kossodo et al., 2010; Hensley et al., 2012) and inflammation studies (Martin et al., 2008; Kang et al., 2014; Thomas et al., 2015), amongst others.

Apart from suffering from auto-fluorescence in a manner similar to planar fluorescence imaging, DOT and FMT provide

no anatomical information and therefore benefit from its combination with measurements provided by other imaging systems such as X-ray computed tomography (CT) or MRI, issue which we will discuss at the end of this review. Additionally, the prior knowledge of anatomical features and optical properties significantly improves image quality and quantitation, as will be discussed later.

Optoacoustic *In Vivo* Imaging

Being based on the emission of sound after a transient increase in volume due to light absorption, the photoacoustic effect may be used to image in 3D the location and relative concentration of fluorescence probes using advanced acoustic transducers and light sources. Termed Optoacoustic or Photoacoustic imaging, it circumvents the "blurring" caused by scattering on the visible wavelengths by measuring the acoustic wave generated, which suffers several orders of magnitude less scattering, resulting in an increased penetration depth with no significant loss of signal to noise. In order for this approach to be implemented and transient volume changes generated, we need to use pulsed lasers and then record the ultrasound wave generated by the localized absorption of this pulse of light by the tissue. Recording this ultrasound wave at several locations simultaneously, we may make use of tomographic methods to recover a 3D image (Wang et al., 2003). When multispectral methods are used, such

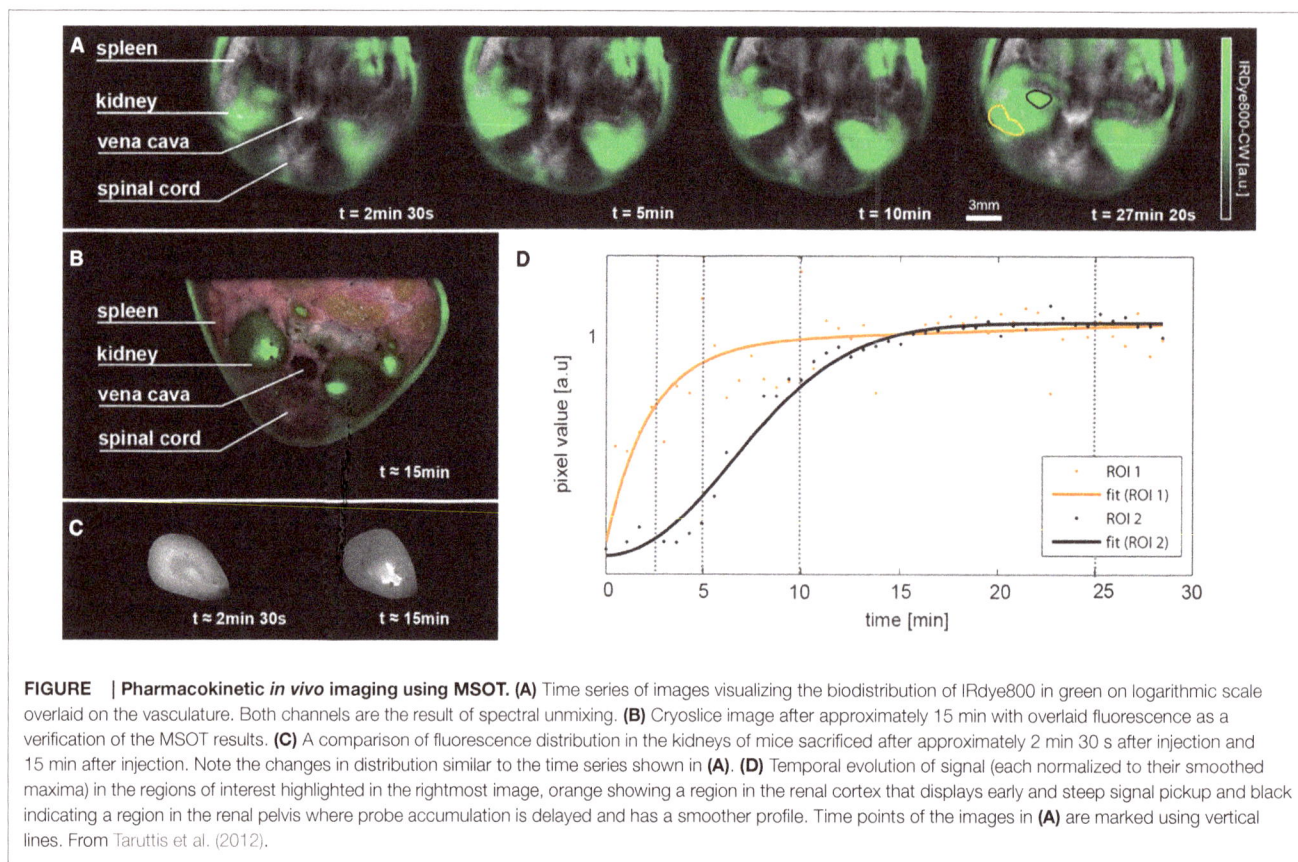

FIGURE | **Pharmacokinetic** *in vivo* **imaging using MSOT. (A)** Time series of images visualizing the biodistribution of IRdye800 in green on logarithmic scale overlaid on the vasculature. Both channels are the result of spectral unmixing. **(B)** Cryoslice image after approximately 15 min with overlaid fluorescence as a verification of the MSOT results. **(C)** A comparison of fluorescence distribution in the kidneys of mice sacrificed after approximately 2 min 30 s after injection and 15 min after injection. Note the changes in distribution similar to the time series shown in **(A)**. **(D)** Temporal evolution of signal (each normalized to their smoothed maxima) in the regions of interest highlighted in the rightmost image, orange showing a region in the renal cortex that displays early and steep signal pickup and black indicating a region in the renal pelvis where probe accumulation is delayed and has a smoother profile. Time points of the images in **(A)** are marked using vertical lines. From Taruttis et al. (2012).

as in multispectral optoacoustic tomography (MSOT), different fluorophores may be separated and their relative concentration quantified (Laufer et al., 2007; Ma et al., 2009; Tzoumas et al., 2014), underlying the use of MSOT for quantitative and highly specific *in vivo* imaging. Additionally, since hemoglobin is a strong absorber, optoacoustic tomography may also be used for resolving vascular structures and quantifying oxygen saturation and blood volume (Lao et al., 2008; Hu and Wang, 2010). The high resolution of MSOT—approximately ~100 µm and in some cases even better [~40 µm resolution was shown in Ma et al. (2009)], good anatomical information, and quantitative 3D images are the reason why this approach is becoming widespread in pharmacological studies.

One application of MSOT to pharmacological studies which show extremely high impact is the use of MSOT to follow pharmacokinetics *in vivo* (Kossodo et al., 2010; Razansky et al., 2011, 2012; Bednar and Ntziachristos, 2012; Taruttis et al., 2012). **Figure** shows an example of the potential of MSOT, where a time series of images visualizing *in vivo* the biodistribution of IRdye800 and vasculature are shown. This study shows how the spatially localized temporal evolution of drug delivery may be imaged in real time.

One of the drawbacks of optoacoustic tomography is its lower sensitivity when compared to pure fluorescence measurements and the difficulty of imaging in organs that present high acoustic contrast or high impedance mismatch, such as the lungs. Another drawback is that the signal generated is proportional to the light intensity that has been absorbed locally and thus decreases for

deeper tissues. Even though the lack of knowledge on the precise light distribution within the subject precludes this technique from being fully quantitative, the development of advanced inverse methods and imaging approaches are constantly improving the quantitative nature of MSOT (Razansky et al., 2011).

Latest Advances to Improve Quantification and Resolution

Once we have covered the main optical imaging approaches, we now will present the most recent advances to improve these imaging techniques either by changing the emission spectra of the probes or by including anatomical information and thus reducing the ill-posed nature of the inverse problem.

Avoiding Absorption in Living Tissues: Moving Toward the Near Infra-Red

As mentioned previously, working with wavelengths in the near infra-red (NIR), in particular in the 700–900 nm window, reduces the amount of light absorbed in tissues by ~3 orders of magnitude when compared to the visible spectrum. Due mainly to hemoglobin absorption and considering that the emission peak of the native firefly luciferase is in the range of ~562 nm, its detection is mainly limited to the surface. Great efforts have been focused on obtaining mutated versions of luciferase enzymes leading to red-shifted emission wavelengths, with emission peaks above 600 nm (Branchini et al., 2010a; Stepanyuk et al., 2010;

Mezzanotte et al., 2011; Wang et al., 2013). In order to obtain emitted light with longer-wavelengths, considerable effort has also been devoted to the development of analogs of the substrate (luciferin), such as aminoluciferins (Mofford et al., 2014) or selenium analogs (Conley et al., 2012). Other developments have been bioluminescence resonance energy transfer (BRET) conjugates, consisting on using the emitted bioluminescence light as excitation for fluorescent molecules. The use of these conjugates results in a final emitted light above 700 nm (Branchini et al., 2010b), although it has been discussed that they may alter the cellular uptake properties of the substrate (Conley et al., 2012).

In the case of fluorescence, an impressive development of new NIR fluorescent agents has taken place in recent years with excitation maxima above 650 nm, allowing the use of excitation sources and emission spectra within the optical window of the spectrum, where blood absorption is reduced to a minimum (Ntziachristos et al., 2005; Jacques, 2013). Researchers can now benefit from a wide portfolio of near infra-red fluorescent (NIRF) probes designed to be non-targeted (non-specific used for imaging of perfusion or vascular leakage), targeted (such as fluorescent-conjugated antibodies, which recognize and bind specific ligands), or activatable (the fluorescent signal is quenched unless a specific enzymatic activity cleaves the probe). Moreover, different approaches have been followed to obtain NIRF proteins, reaching excitation maxima above 670 nm (Shcherbo et al., 2007; Shu et al., 2009; Filonov et al., 2012). Constructs for the expression of these proteins and recently developed transgenic mice (Diéguez-Hurtado et al., 2011; Tran et al., 2014) provide an excellent tool for in vivo imaging applied to biomedical and pharmaceutical studies.

With respect to optoacoustics, all advances in fluorescent probes are directly compatible with this methodology, since probes with high quantum yield by definition present high absorption properties. Additionally, optoacoustic imaging methods are also benefiting from new engineered acoustic probes based on metallic nanoparticles (mainly gold) which exhibit high absorption profiles (Bao et al., 2013; Vonnemann et al., 2014).

Finally, a very interesting and promising new development is the use of Cherenkov excited luminescence imaging (CELSI) to improve resolution and partially avoid the effect of absorption while exciting the fluorophores (Zhang et al., 2012, 2013b, 2015a). This approach makes use of Cherenkov emitted NIR light from collimated ionizing radiation generated in a linear accelerator (LINAC), a technique which could potentially be applied for imaging fluorescent markers deep in tissue with high resolution.

Hybrid Systems

The combination of optical imaging modalities with structural imaging methods such as X-ray CT or MRI allows obtaining anatomical information that can be used as prior data on the reconstruction algorithm to improve both resolution and sensitivity (Ale et al., 2012).

For example, FMT-MRI hybrid systems have been developed and used to analyze protease activity and tumor morphology in mouse tumor models (Davis et al., 2010; Stuker et al., 2011a) or metalloproteinase activity in mouse models of atherosclerosis (Li et al., 2014). FMT-XCT hybrid systems are also examples

TABLE | Comparison of different imaging modalities.

Technique	Resolution	Throughput	Pharmacokinetics	3D Info
Bioluminescence	>5 mm*	High	No	No
Planar fluorescence	>5 mm*	High	No	No
FMT	1–2 mm	Medium	No	Yes
FMT/XCT	1 mm	Low	No	Yes
MSOT	0.1 mm	Low	Yes	Yes

*Resolution depends on depth location.

where we can make use of anatomical priors obtained from the geometric information provided by the XCT measurements in order to improve the 3D reconstruction of the fluorescence signal (Ale et al., 2012; Zhang et al., 2013a, 2014).

The technical complexity of these hybrid systems (for example, due to crosstalk between optical and MRI imaging) has led to the use of adapted animal holders which are compatible with different modality systems enabling sequential imaging (McCann et al., 2009).

Conclusions and Future Outlook

A wide range of optical imaging modalities are available for in vivo imaging in small animals, representing an essential tool in pharmacological studies. Each modality, however, presents its own drawbacks, mainly due to the effects of absorption and scattering of light propagation in living tissues. As shown in **Table**, the selection of a technique will depend on the model used and the information that we want to obtain. For example, if high-throughput imaging is required, planar imaging approaches will be useful, with the consequence that no quantitative information or depth location may be inferred (see **Table**). If quantitative imaging and probe location is important, tomography is needed and FMT and similar approaches are a good option, reaching their full potential when combined with an anatomical imaging modality such as MRI or X-ray CT. As a quickly growing modality, optoacoustic tomography and in particular MSOT shows great potential, so far offering the best imaging resolution, but with the problems associated with ultrasound imaging such as high impedance mismatch in some organs such as the lungs and the need for a matching gels.

We believe that as more specific near infrared fluorescent probes and proteins with distinct spectral features, and specific nanoparticles for high and specific optoacoustic signal generation are generated there will be further improvement of the performance of the technologies covered in this review, opening opportunities for new applications. The combination of several imaging modalities, specifically if they include optical imaging approaches, will ensure the sensitivity and specificity that optical probes uniquely offer may reach their full potential as imaging agents for 3D quantitative imaging in vivo.

Acknowledgments

JR acknowledges support from the EC FP7 CIG grant HIGH-THROUGHPUT TOMO, and MINECO grant FIS2013-41802-R MESO-IMAGING.

References

Ale, A., Ermolayev, V., Herzog, E., Cohrs, C., de Angelis, M. H., and Ntziachristos, V. (2012). FMT-XCT: *in vivo* animal studies with hybrid fluorescence molecular tomography-X-ray computed tomography. *Nat. Methods* 9, 615–620. doi: 10.1038/nmeth.2014

Andreu, N., Zelmer, A., Fletcher, T., Elkington, P. T., Ward, T. H., Ripoll, J., et al. (2010). Optimisation of bioluminescent reporters for use with mycobacteria. *PLoS ONE* 5:e10777. doi: 10.1371/journal.pone.0010777

Arridge, S. R. (1999). Optical tomography in medical imaging. *Inverse Probl.* 15, R41–R93. doi: 10.1088/0266-5611/15/2/022

Bao, C., Beziere, N., Del Pino, P., Pelaz, B., Estrada, G., Tian, F., et al. (2013). Gold nanoprisms as optoacoustic signal nanoamplifiers for *in vivo* bioimaging of gastrointestinal cancers. *Small* 9, 68–74. doi: 10.1002/smll.201201779

Bednar, B., and Ntziachristos, V. (2012). Opto-acoustic imaging of drug discovery biomarkers. *Curr. Pharm. Biotechnol.* 13, 2117–2127. doi: 10.2174/138920112802502079

Boas, D. A., Pitris, C., and Ramanujam, N. (eds). (2011). *Handbook of Biomedical Optics*. Boca Raton: CRC Press.

Branchini, B. R., Ablamsky, D. M., Davis, A. L., Southworth, T. L., Butler, B., Fan, F., et al. (2010a). Red-emitting luciferases for bioluminescence reporter and imaging applications. *Anal. Biochem.* 396, 290–297. doi: 10.1016/j.ab.2009.09.009

Branchini, B. R., Ablamsky, D. M., and Rosenberg, J. C. (2010b). Chemically modified firefly luciferase is an efficient source of near-infrared light. *Bioconjug. Chem.* 21, 2023–2030. doi: 10.1021/bc100256d

Conley, N. R., Dragulescu-Andrasi, A., Rao, J., and Moerner, W. E. (2012). A selenium analogue of firefly D-luciferin with red-shifted bioluminescence emission. *Angew. Chem. Int. Ed. Engl.* 51, 3350–3353. doi: 10.1002/anie.201105653

Davis, S. C., Samkoe, K. S., Hara, J. A. O., Gibbs, S. L., Payne, H. L., Hoopes, P. J., et al. (2010). MRI-coupled fluorescence tomography quantifies EGFR activity in brain tumors. *Acad. Radiol.* 17, 1–10. doi: 10.1016/j.acra.2009.11.001

Deliolanis, N., Lasser, T., Niedre, M., Soubret, A., and Ntziachristos, V. (2006). *In-vivo* lung cancer imaging in mice using 360° free-space fluorescence molecular tomography. *Conf. Proc. IEEE Eng. Med. Biol. Soc.* 1, 2370–2372. doi: 10.1109/IEMBS.2006.260683

de Wet, J. R., Wood, K. V., Helinski, D. R., and DeLuca, M. (1985). Cloning of firefly luciferase cDNA and the expression of active luciferase in *Escherichia coli*. *Proc. Natl. Acad. Sci. U.S.A.* 82, 7870–7873. doi: 10.1073/pnas.82.23.7870

Diéguez-Hurtado, R., Martín, J., Martínez-Corral, I., Martínez, M. D., Megías, D., Olmeda, D., et al. (2011). A Cre-reporter transgenic mouse expressing the far-red fluorescent protein Katushka. *Genesis* 49, 36–45. doi: 10.1002/dvg.20685

Edinger, M., Cao, Y. A., Hornig, Y. S., Jenkins, D. E., Verneris, M. R., Bachmann, M. H., et al. (2002). Advancing animal models of neoplasia through *in vivo* bioluminescence imaging. *Eur. J. Cancer* 38, 2128–2136. doi: 10.1016/S0959-8049(02)00410-0

Filonov, G., Piatkevich, K., Ting, L. M., Zhang, J., Kim, J., and Verkhusha, V. (2012). Bright and stable near infra-red fluorescent protein for *in vivo* imaging. *Nat. Biotechnol.* 29, 757–761. doi: 10.1038/nbt.1918

Hensley, H. H., Roder, N. A., Brien, S. W. O., Bickel, L. E., Xiao, F., Litwin, S., et al. (2012). Combined *in vivo* molecular and anatomic imaging for detection of ovarian carcinoma-associated protease activity and integrin expression in mice. *Neoplasia* 14, 451–462. doi: 10.1596/neo.12480

Hu, S., and Wang, L. V. (2010). Photoacoustic imaging and characterization of the microvasculature. *J. Biomed. Opt.* 15, 1–15. doi: 10.1117/1.3281673

Jacques, S. L. (2013). Optical properties of biological tissues: a review. *Phys. Med. Biol.* 58, 5007–5008. doi: 10.1088/0031-9155/58/14/5007

Kang, N.-Y., Park, S.-J., Ang, X. W. E., Samanta, A., Driessen, W. H. P., Ntziachristos, V., et al. (2014). A macrophage uptaking near-infrared chemical probe for *in vivo* imaging of inflammation. *Chem. Commun. (Camb.)* 50, 6589–6591. doi: 10.1039/c4cc02038c

Kossodo, S., Pickarski, M., Lin, S. A., Gleason, A., Gaspar, R., Buono, C., et al. (2010). Dual *in vivo* quantification of integrin-targeted and protease-activated agents in cancer using fluorescence molecular tomography (FMT). *Mol. Imaging Biol.* 12, 488–499. doi: 10.1007/s11307-009-0279-z

Lao, Y., Xing, D., Yang, S., and Xiang, L. (2008). Noninvasive photoacoustic imaging of the developing vasculature during early tumor growth. *Phys. Med. Biol.* 53, 4203–4212. doi: 10.1088/0031-9155/53/15/013

Laufer, J., Delpy, D., Elwell, C., and Beard, P. (2007). Quantitative spatially resolved measurement of tissue chromophore concentrations using photoacoustic spectroscopy: application to the measurement of blood oxygenation and haemoglobin concentration. *Phys. Med. Biol.* 52, 141–168. doi: 10.1088/0031-9155/52/1/010

Li, B., Maafi, F., Berti, R., Pouliot, P., Rhéaume, E., Tardif, J.-C., et al. (2014). Hybrid FMT-MRI applied to *in vivo* atherosclerosis imaging. *Biomed. Opt. Express* 5, 1664. doi: 10.1364/BOE.5.001664

Li, J., Chen, L., Du, L., and Li, M. (2013). Cage the firefly luciferin!—a strategy for developing bioluminescent probes. *Chem. Soc. Rev.* 42, 662–676. doi: 10.1039/C2CS35249D

Liu, J., Wang, Y., Qu, X., Li, X., Ma, X., Han, R., et al. (2010). *In vivo* quantitative bioluminescence tomography using heterogeneous and homogeneous mouse models. *Opt. Express* 18, 13102–13113. doi: 10.1364/OE.18.013102

Luker, K. E., and Luker, G. D. (2011). Bioluminescence imaging of reporter mice for studies of infection and inflammation. *Antiviral Res.* 86, 1–17. doi: 10.1016/j.antiviral.2010.02.002

Luwor, R. B., Stylli, S. S., and Kaye, A. H. (2015). Using bioluminescence imaging in glioma research. *J. Clin. Neurosci.* 22, 779–784. doi: 10.1016/j.jocn.2014.11.001

Ma, R., Taruttis, A., Ntziachristos, V., and Razansky, D. (2009). Multispectral optoacoustic tomography (MSOT) scanner for whole-body small animal imaging. *Opt. Express* 17, 21414–21426. doi: 10.1364/OE.17.021414

Mahmood, U., Tung, C. H., Bogdanov, A., and Weissleder, R. (1999). Near-infrared optical imaging of protease activity for tumor detection. *Radiology* 213, 866–870. doi: 10.1148/radiology.213.3.r99dc14866

Martin, A., Aguirre, J., Sarasa-Renedo, A., Tsoukatou, D., Garofalakis, A., Meyer, H., et al. (2008). Imaging changes in lymphoid organs *in vivo* after brain ischemia with three-dimensional fluorescence molecular tomography in transgenic mice expressing green fluorescent protein in T lymphocytes. *Mol. Imaging* 7, 157–167.

Masters, B. R. (2009). Encyclopedia of life sciences. West Sussex: John Wiley & Sons, 1–9. doi: 10.1002/9780470015902.a0022548

McCann, C. M., Waterman, P., Figueiredo, J. L., Aikawa, E., Weissleder, R., and Chen, J. W. (2009). Combined magnetic resonance and fluorescence imaging of the living mouse brain reveals glioma response to chemotherapy. *Neuroimage* 45, 360–369. doi: 10.1016/j.neuroimage.2008.12.022

Mezzanotte, L., Que, I., Kaijzel, E., Branchini, B., Roda, A., and Löwik, C. (2011). Sensitive dual color *in vivo* bioluminescence imaging using a new red codon optimized firefly luciferase and a green click beetle luciferase. *PLoS ONE* 6:e19277. doi: 10.1371/journal.pone.0019277

Mofford, D. M., Reddy, G. R., and Miller, S. C. (2014). Aminoluciferins extend firefly luciferase bioluminescence into the near-infrared and can be preferred substrates over D-luciferin. *J. Am. Chem. Soc.* 136, 13277–13282. doi: 10.1021/ja505795s

Montet, X., Figueiredo, J., Alencar, H., Ntziachristos, V., Mahmood, U., and Weissleder, R. (2007). Tomographic fluorescence imaging of tumor vascular volume in mice. *Radiology* 242, 751–758. doi: 10.1148/radiol.2423052065

Ntziachristos, V., Leroy-Willig, A., and Tavitian, B. (eds). (2007). *Textbook of In-Vivo Imaging in Vertebrates*. West Sussex: John Wiley & Sons.

Ntziachristos, V., Ripoll, J., Wang, L. V., and Weissleder, R. (2005). Looking and listening to light: the evolution of whole-body photonic imaging. *Nat. Biotechnol.* 23, 313–320. doi: 10.1038/nbt1074

Ntziachristos, V., Schellenberger, E. A., Ripoll, J., Yessayan, D., Graves, E., Bogdanov, A., et al. (2004). Visualization of antitumor treatment by means of fluorescence molecular tomography with an annexin V-Cy5.5 conjugate. *Proc. Natl. Acad. Sci. U.S.A.* 101, 12294–12299. doi: 10.1073/pnas.0401137101

Ntziachristos, V., Tung, C.-H., Bremer, C., and Weissleder, R. (2002). Fluorescence molecular tomography resolves protease activity *in vivo*. *Nat. Med.* 8, 757–760. doi: 10.1038/nm729

Ntziachristos, V., Yodh, A. G., Schnall, M., and Chance, B. (2000). Concurrent MRI and diffuse optical tomography of breast after indocyanine green enhancement. *Proc. Natl. Acad. Sci. U.S.A.* 97, 2767–2772. doi: 10.1073/pnas.040570597

Razansky, D., Buehler, A., and Ntziachristos, V. (2011). Volumetric real-time multispectral optoacoustic tomography of biomarkers. *Nat. Protoc.* 6, 1121–9. doi: 10.1038/nprot.2011.351

Razansky, D., Deliolanis, N. C., Vinegoni, C., and Ntziachristos, V. (2012). Deep tissue optical and optoacoustic molecular imaging technologies for pre-clinical research and drug discovery. *Curr. Pharm. Biotechnol.* 13, 504–522. doi: 10.2174/138920112799436258

Ripoll, J. (2012). *Principles of Diffuse Light Propagation*. Singapore: World Scientific.

Sadikot, R. T., and Blackwell, T. S. (2005). Bioluminescence imaging. *Proc. Am. Thorac Soc.* 2, 537–540, 511–512. doi: 10.1513/pats.200507-067DS

Sauer, M., Hofkens, J., and Enderlein, J. (eds). (2011). *Handbook of Fluorescence Spectroscopy and Imaging: From Ensemble to Single Molecules*. Weinheim: Wiley-VCH

Shcherbo, D., Merzlyak, E. M., Chepurnykh, T. V., Fradkov, A. F., Ermakova, G. V., Solovieva, E. A., et al. (2007). Bright far-red fluorescent protein for whole-body imaging. *Nat. Methods* 4, 741–746. doi: 10.1038/nmeth1083

Shu, X., Royant, A., Lin, M. Z., Aguilera, T. A., Lev-ram, V., Steinbach, A., et al. (2009). Mammalian expression of infrared fluorescent proteins engineered from a bacterial phytochrome. *Science* 324, 804–807. doi: 10.1126/science.1168683

Stepanyuk, G. a., Unch, J., Malikova, N. P., Markova, S. V., Lee, J., and Vysotski, E. S. (2010). Coelenterazine-v ligated to Ca^{2+}-triggered coelenterazine-binding protein is a stable and efficient substrate of the red-shifted mutant of *Renilla muelleri* luciferase. *Anal. Bioanal. Chem.* 398, 1809–1817. doi: 10.1007/s00216-010-4106-9

Stuker, F., Baltes, C., Dikaiou, K., Vats, D., Carrara, L., Charbon, E., et al. (2011a). Hybrid small animal imaging system combining magnetic resonance imaging with fluorescence tomography using single photon avalanche diode detectors. *IEEE Trans. Med. Imaging* 30, 1265–1273. doi: 10.1109/TMI.2011.2112669

Stuker, F., Ripoll, J., and Rudin, M. (2011b). Fluorescence molecular tomography: principles and potential for pharmaceutical research. *Pharmaceutics* 3, 229–274. doi: 10.3390/pharmaceutics3020229

Taruttis, A., Morscher, S., Burton, N. C., Razansky, D., and Ntziachristos, V. (2012). Fast multispectral optoacoustic tomography (MSOT) for dynamic imaging of pharmacokinetics and biodistribution in multiple organs. *PLoS ONE* 7:e30491. doi: 10.1371/journal.pone.0030491

Thomas, N., Li, P., Fleming, B. C., Chen, Q., Wei, X., Pan, X., et al. (2015). Attenuation of cartilage pathogenesis in post-traumatic osteoarthritis (PTOA) in mice by blocking the stromal derived factor 1 receptor (CXCR4) with the specific inhibitor, AMD3100. *J. Orthop. Res.* 33, 1071–1078. doi: 10.1002/jor.22862

Tran, M. T. N., Tanaka, J., Hamada, M., Sugiyama, Y., Sakaguchi, S., Nakamura, M., et al. (2014). *In vivo* image analysis using iRFP transgenic mice. *Exp. Anim.* 63, 311–9. doi: 10.1538/expanim.63.311

Tzoumas, S., Deliolanis, N., Morscher, S., and Ntziachristos, V. (2014). Unmixing molecular agents from absorbing tissue in multispectral optoacoustic tomography. *IEEE Trans. Med. Imaging* 33, 48–60. doi: 10.1109/TMI.2013.2279994

Vonnemann, J., Beziere, N., Böttcher, C., Riese, S. B., Kuehne, C., Dernedde, J., et al. (2014). Polyglycerolsulfate functionalized gold nanorods as optoacoustic signal nanoamplifiers for *in vivo* bioimaging of rheumatoid arthritis. *Theranostics* 4, 629–641. doi: 10.7150/thno.8518

Wang, X., Pang, Y., Ku, G., Xie, X., Stoica, G., and Wang, L. V. (2003). Noninvasive laser-induced photoacoustic tomography for structural and functional *in vivo* imaging of the brain. *Nat. Biotechnol.* 21, 803–806. doi: 10.1038/nbt839

Wang, Y., Akiyama, H., Terakado, K., and Nakatsu, T. (2013). Impact of site-directed mutant luciferase on quantitative green and orange/red emission intensities in firefly bioluminescence. *Sci. Rep.* 3, 2490. doi: 10.1038/srep02490

Weissleder, R., Tung, C. H., Mahmood, U., and Bogdanov, A. (1999). *In vivo* imaging of tumors with protease-activated near-infrared fluorescent probes. *Nat. Biotechnol.* 17, 375–378. doi: 10.1038/7933

Xu, H., and Rice, B. W. (2009). *In-vivo* fluorescence imaging with a multivariate curve resolution spectral unmixing technique. *J. Biomed. Opt.* 14, 064011. doi: 10.1117/1.3258838

Zhang, G., Liu, F., Pu, H., He, W., Luo, J., and Bai, J. (2014). A direct method with structural priors for imaging pharmacokinetic parameters in dynamic fluorescence molecular tomography. *IEEE Trans. Biomed. Eng.* 61, 986–990. doi: 10.1109/TBME.2013.2292714

Zhang, G., Liu, F., Zhang, B., He, Y., Luo, J., and Bai, J. (2013a). Imaging of pharmacokinetic rates of indocyanine green in mouse liver with a hybrid fluorescence molecular tomography/x-ray computed tomography system. *J. Biomed. Opt.* 18, 040505. doi: 10.1117/1.JBO.18.4.040505

Zhang, R., Davis, S. C., Demers, J.-L. H., Glaser, A. K., Gladstone, D. J., Esipova, T. V., et al. (2013b). Oxygen tomography by Čerenkov-excited phosphorescence during external beam irradiation. *J. Biomed. Opt.* 18, 50503. doi: 10.1117/1.JBO.18.5.050503

Zhang, R., D'Souza, A. V., Gunn, J. R., Esipova, T. V., Vinogradov, S. A., Glaser, A. K., et al. (2015a). Cherenkov-excited luminescence scanned imaging. *Opt. Lett.* 40, 827–830. doi: 10.1364/OL.40.000827

Zhang, X., Tian, Y., Zhang, C., Tian, X., Ross, A. W., Moir, R. D., et al. (2015b). Near-infrared fluorescence molecular imaging of amyloid beta species and monitoring therapy in animal models of Alzheimer's disease. *Proc. Natl. Acad. Sci. U.S.A.* 112, 9734–9739. doi: 10.1073/pnas.1505420112

Zhang, R., Glaser, A., Esipova, T. V, Kanick, S. C., Davis, S. C., Vinogradov, S., et al. (2012). Čerenkov radiation emission and excited luminescence (CREL) sensitivity during external beam radiation therapy: Monte Carlo and tissue oxygenation phantom studies. *Biomed. Opt. Express* 3, 2381–2394. doi: 10.1364/BOE.3.002381

Conflict of Interest Statement: The authors declare that the research was conducted in the absence of any commercial or financial relationships that could be construed as a potential conflict of interest.

8

Cardiovascular Imaging: What have we Learned from Animal Models?

Arnoldo Santos [1,2,3,4], Leticia Fernández-Friera [1,5], María Villalba [1], Beatriz López-Melgar [1,5], Samuel España [1,2,3], Jesús Mateo [1,2], Ruben A. Mota [1,6], Jesús Jiménez-Borreguero [1,7] and Jesús Ruiz-Cabello [1,2,8]*

[1] Centro Nacional de Investigaciones Cardiovasculares Carlos III, Madrid, Spain, [2] CIBER de Enfermedades Respiratorias (CIBERES), Madrid, Spain, [3] Madrid-MIT M+Visión Consortium, Madrid, Spain, [4] Department of Anesthesia, Massachusetts General Hospital, Harvard Medical School, Boston, MA, USA, [5] Hospital Universitario HM Montepríncipe, Madrid, Spain, [6] Charles River, Barcelona, Spain, [7] Cardiac Imaging Department, Hospital de La Princesa, Madrid, Spain, [8] Universidad Complutense de Madrid, Madrid, Spain

Edited by:
Nicolau Beckmann,
Novartis Institutes for BioMedical
Research, Switzerland

Reviewed by:
Beat M. Jucker,
GlaxoSmithKline, USA
Sebastian Kelle,
German Heart Institute Berlin,
Germany

*Correspondence:
Jesús Ruiz-Cabello
ruizcabe@cnic.es

Cardiovascular imaging has become an indispensable tool for patient diagnosis and follow up. Probably the wide clinical applications of imaging are due to the possibility of a detailed and high quality description and quantification of cardiovascular system structure and function. Also phenomena that involve complex physiological mechanisms and biochemical pathways, such as inflammation and ischemia, can be visualized in a non-destructive way. The widespread use and evolution of imaging would not have been possible without animal studies. Animal models have allowed for instance, (i) the technical development of different imaging tools, (ii) to test hypothesis generated from human studies and finally, (iii) to evaluate the translational relevance assessment of in vitro and ex-vivo results. In this review, we will critically describe the contribution of animal models to the use of biomedical imaging in cardiovascular medicine. We will discuss the characteristics of the most frequent models used in/for imaging studies. We will cover the major findings of animal studies focused in the cardiovascular use of the repeatedly used imaging techniques in clinical practice and experimental studies. We will also describe the physiological findings and/or learning processes for imaging applications coming from models of the most common cardiovascular diseases. In these diseases, imaging research using animals has allowed the study of aspects such as: ventricular size, shape, global function, and wall thickening, local myocardial function, myocardial perfusion, metabolism and energetic assessment, infarct quantification, vascular lesion characterization, myocardial fiber structure, and myocardial calcium uptake. Finally we will discuss the limitations and future of imaging research with animal models.

Keywords: animal models, biomedical imaging, heart failure, myocardial infarction, pulmonary hypertension, atherosclerosis

Introduction

Cardiovascular disease is the most important cause of mortality in the Western world. It is also responsible for a huge lost in years of healthy life and one of the principal reasons for hospitalizations and emergency room visits. Its epidemiological importance justifies the huge amount of both clinical and experimental research existing in this area. Such research has allowed outstanding therapeutic changes, with impact on patient outcomes. However, not only therapy has improved the outcomes of patients; diagnosis and monitoring tools have improved a lot in recent years. Between these diagnostic tools a special place is reserved for biomedical imaging. Diagnosis, monitoring, follow-up, and research in cardiovascular patients are possible using different imaging techniques.

Using imaging, anatomical, molecular, and functional evaluation is possible in a complete non-invasive way. The progress in cardiovascular patient care has benefited from a rapidly evolving imaging acquisition technique. In the same way imaging would not have developed without the use of animal models. Animal, *in vitro* and *ex-vivo* models are useful for testing hypotheses derived from the clinical setting. They also provide us a scenario in which to evaluate a new imaging tool or tracer. In this review we will discuss the principal animal models used in imaging studies of major cardiovascular diseases.

Characteristics of Animal Models For *in vivo* Cardiovascular Imaging Studies

Cardiovascular physiology and diseases are based on the interaction of multiple genes, metabolic processes and the environment, increasing significantly their complexity. These circumstances make highly complicated the full replacement of *in vivo* models by simulated *in vitro* or *in silico* ones. Therefore, animal models for cardiovascular research are pivotal for testing mechanistic hypothesis and for translational research, including the assessment of pharmacological interventions and the development of imaging technologies and surgical devices. In specific fields as drug development imaging techniques application allows to evaluate aspects as target validation, biodistribution, target interaction, pharmacodynamics, and toxicology. Non-invasive, imaging techniques allow multiple measurements to be obtained from a single animal in longitudinal studies. In this way imaging techniques generate significant outcomes using smaller and more efficient experimental designs. This can help to accomplish with the Reduce, Refine and Replace principles in preclinical development processes including experiments with animals. However, the animal model itself is important also in this regard. The selection of the adequate species and covering important aspects as animal manipulation are critical for preclinical drug development success.

Selection of the Adequate Animal Model

The correct selection of the animal model of cardiovascular research is a great challenge. Bibliography describes plenty of models that mimic the most frequent cardiovascular illnesses. However, in many cases, the authors do not perform a correct comparative anatomy study and the findings do not correlate in the same way that in humans. This issue is especially important for biomedical imaging in which the goal is to identify the aspects that directly interacts or modifies specific anatomical structures. The relative geometry of the heart of each species, the characteristic features of vasculature, muscle mass and conduction system are the main anatomical differences with humans (Hasenfuss, 1998; Hill and Iaizzo, 2009). The choice of the desired model should be made on grounds of etiological induction, animal availability, technological disposal

for the species, housing conditions, costs, biological level of study, quality, and quantity of the data, relevance for the human condition and ethical sensitivity (Power and Tonkin, 1999; Hearse and Sutherland, 2000).

Rodents and Other Small Mammals

The laboratory mouse is essential in the study of the cardiovascular system. The short gestation period and the low cost of breeding and housing are the main advantages of this species. The knowledge of its genome, the ability to modify it and the rapid data acquisition of genomic modification make attractive the use of mice for studying diverse mechanisms that are affected during the development of cardiovascular diseases (Doevendans et al., 1995, 1998; Bostick et al., 2011). Advances in laboratory animal technology have allowed the miniaturizing acquisition of murine cardiovascular physiology and diagnostic images that define, in a sequential way, the progress of the cardiac illness. However, the mouse shows some obstacles for extrapolation of any outcome of cardiac disease models. Other than animal size and beat (400–600), mouse heart differs from human by: (1) the direct drainage of persistent left superior cava vein into the right atrium; (2) a single opening of the pulmonary vein in the left atrium (Webb et al., 1996; Hoyt et al., 2006); (3) sinoatrial node localization above the junction of right atrium with the cava vein (Meijler, 1985; Hoyt et al., 2006); (4) helicoidal distribution of myocardial fibers (McLean and Prothero, 1992); (5); a large septal branch from the left coronary artery without a proper circumflex branch (still controversial); and (6) the blood support of internal mammary arteries to supply atria, flowing via cardiomediastinal arteries (Michael et al., 1995; Lutgens et al., 1999). Finally, it is important to consider that murine strains and mutations can alter additionally the structure, anatomy, pathology, and physiology of cells, in an unpredictable way and that may change with time (Chien, 1996; James et al., 1998; Kass et al., 1998).

Rat and mouse models show similar advantages, however rats are the classical choice for studying new drug targets in cardiovascular research. The larger physical dimension in rats allows an easier learning of surgical procedures and invasive hemodynamic assessments. The cardiac blood supply originates from both the coronary and extracoronary arteries (internal mammary and subclavian arteries), but the principal limitations are focused in myocardial function: a short action potential which normally lacks a plateau phase, and α-myosin heavy-chain isoform predominates with β-myosin isoform shift under hemodynamic load or hormonal condition (Swynghedauw, 1986; Hasenfuss, 1998; Bers, 2001).

Larger species as rabbits and dogs show a higher similarity with human heart and allow the study of the left ventricular function in models of heart failure. Like humans, in these two species, β-myosin heavy-chain predominates and excitation–contraction coupling processes seem to be analogous to those in the human myocardium (Lompre et al., 1981; Hasenfuss, 1998). However, canine heart presents a dense collateral coronary branching with a higher proportional relation of its size with respect of thoracic cavity. Besides, the proportion of heart to bodyweight is near the double of the human (Verdouw et al., 1998).

Large Animal Models

Direct translation from rodents to humans has to be taken with caution because of the species-related differences, such as contractility, architecture, heart rates (HRs), oxygen consumption, protein expression, etc... (Zaragoza et al., 2011). Instead, large animal models have a better translational bridge between preclinical and clinical studies because of their anatomical and physiological similarities (Fernández-Jiménez et al., 2015a). Predominately, swine species are the election in preclinical cardiovascular research. Their anatomical heart features resemble those described in humans: coronary arteries support a blood flow with a right-side dominant circulation to the conduction system from the posterior septal artery, and less subepicardical anastomosis than in other species such as the dog; the electrophysiological system is more neurogenic than myogenic with prominent Purkinje fibers; the aorta has a true vasa vasorum network like that of humans; and hemodynamic values that allow the extrapolation and translation of reliable experimental data (Verdouw et al., 1998; Unger, 2001; Laber et al., 2002; Swindle, 2007; Lelovas et al., 2014). On the contrary, pigs show a left azygous (hemiazygous) vein which drains the intercostal vessels into the coronary sinus instead of precava, and the endocardium and epicardium are activated simultaneously because of differences in distribution of the specialized conduction system in the ventricles (Swindle, 2007; Lelovas et al., 2014). The principal drawbacks of experimentation with pigs are the high cost of housing and care, especially in heart failure models. Also changes that occur during animal growth are particularly important for translational imaging research, specially the change in the proportional heart weight to bodyweight ratio. That ratio for a 25 Kg-farm pig is 5 gr/Kg (as human) and this proportion is kept in juvenile animals, and decreases significantly when the pig reaches the sexual maturity (Verdouw et al., 1998; Lelovas et al., 2014). Nowadays, the advent of miniature species like Yucatan, Hanford, Sinclair, and Göttingen minipigs has significantly solved both limitations (Bode et al., 2010).

Other species, like the sheep show morphologic similarities with humans in regard to adult heart size, venous drainage and physiological responses during the induction of cardiovascular diseases; thus, sheep allows an experimental scenario highly used and reliable in biomedical imaging studies. Among the differences with human anatomy, a left-dominance coronary artery support (but with a lack of preformed collateral circulation), the absence of intervalvar septum, the valvular "os cordis," aortic valves fragility and the left thoracic drainage of the azygous vein directly to coronary sinus, are the most noticeable. Nevertheless, the main limitations of ovine models are the risk of zoonotic diseases and their condition of ruminant, whose features of the stomach could interfere in some non-invasive image acquisitions (Walmsley, 1978; Dixon and Spinale, 2009; Hill and Iaizzo, 2009).

Methodological Considerations

The ideal scenario for any imaging acquisition conducted in cardiovascular disease animal models is the one performed with awake and cooperative animals. However, this requires acclimatization to restraint to reduce distress as confounding variable. Conversely, each model under normal sleep conditions is preconditioned by the type and doses of anesthesia and, in lesser extent, analgesia used in the experiments. The correct selection of the anesthetic protocol will determine the reliability and interpretation of the measured data. All the anesthetics induce a direct or indirect depression of hemodynamic values and cardiac functionality. Injectable drugs can create an adequate level of unconsciousness to perform the injury required in the model and permit a complete imaging study. But, the hemodynamic response to the same drugs is different between species which depends on their metabolic features. This can hinder an stable imaging acquisition. For example, rodents generally require 3–5 times the doses used for large animals. This is critical in those surgical models that imply an open-chest approach, which means a great impact in the animal thermoregulation and the size of the infarct area, anesthesia timing, cardiovascular depression, etc... Due to their minimal systemic metabolism and a short recovery phase, inhaled anesthetics offer more security for the development of the procedures; nevertheless, inhalation agents like sevofluorane or isofluorane protect the myocardium against the insult of the hypoxic states and diminish significantly the immune cellular transmigration on inflammatory injuries (Rao et al., 2008; Ge et al., 2010; Chappell et al., 2011).

During the imaging studies, anesthesia is crucial to maintain the animal within stable, well-defined physiologic parameters which is indispensable for detecting critical pathophysiologic responses associated to the cardiovascular disease model. Not only the primary affection that is provoked in the animal model but also variables related with the animal homeostasis in response to such affection should be taken into account. Also other indirect factors as risk of hypothermia (and the autonomic response to it) during surgical procedures can affect the results of cardiovascular imaging studies. Anesthesia affects the blood flow, blood oxygenation levels, and cardiac and respiratory functions, which should be correctly monitored, especially in those modalities involving long acquisition times. Inhaled agents are eliminated quicker via the lungs, whereas injectable agents need to be metabolized by the liver and excreted by the kidneys. Both sevofluorane and isofluorane are minimally metabolized by the liver and increase the efficiency of organ perfusion. This means a less toxic effect to the animal metabolism, rapid induction, minor impact on cardiovascular function and quick recovery, which make them in many cases the choice for imaging studies. Indeed, isofluorane has been described as the election for PET studies in experimental cardiology just for the improvement of cardiac radiotracer uptake vs. injectable anesthetics (Gargiulo et al., 2012a; Lee et al., 2012).

Another key point is the selection of a determined animal gender. It is has been described that males tend to develop an eccentric hypertrophy and left ventricular dilatation in certain cardiovascular disease, whilst females show a more concentric hypertrophy with a better preserved left ventricular function (Mahmoodzadeh et al., 2012). Several studies with rodents define a protective role of the female hormone 17-β-estradiol and its respective estrogen receptors mediating the cardiovascular responses to different pathophysiological situation. This steroid regulates the expression of a variety of dependent genes related to myocyte cytoskeletal proteins, cell-to-cell interaction, Ca^{2+} channels and apoptosis inhibition (Patten et al., 2004; Groten et al., 2005; Mahmoodzadeh et al., 2010, 2012). For that reason, females tended more easily to develop a ventricular hypertrophic response against extreme effort stimuli to preserve the heart outflow, and showed significantly smaller infarct area after ischemic myocardial conditions or even maintained the heart morphology and functionality under pressure overload stimuli (Wang et al., 2005; Johnson et al., 2006; Babiker et al., 2007; Patten et al., 2008; Foryst-Ludwig et al., 2011; Mahmoodzadeh et al., 2012).

Imaging in Myocardial Infarction and Coronary Artery Disease

Myocardial infarction (MI) may be the first manifestation of coronary artery disease (CAD) that is the number one cause of death among adults (Lloyd-Jones et al., 2010; Nichols et al., 2014). Myocardial tissue-specific biomarkers and high sensitive imaging techniques allow MI definition as any amount of myocardial injury or necrosis in the setting of myocardial ischemia (Thygesen et al., 2012). Animal models on MI are essential for the better understanding of CAD, for discovering risk biomarkers of MI, for studying early diagnostic test, and also for establishing beneficial effects of new therapies.

Small and Large Animal Models for MI Assessment: Mouse and Porcine Models

In small animals, including mice and rats, the left coronary artery ligation procedure developed by Pfeffer et al. (1979) is the most common method used to induce acute myocardial damage. The artery might be either permanently or temporary occluded to reproduce human ischemia/reperfusion injury. In respect to large animals, swine is the preferred animal model of heart damage, because of the absence of collateral coronary circulation, similar arterial anatomy compared to humans and the suitability to have clinically relevant imaging techniques to accurately quantify area at risk or infarcted tissue (Crick et al., 1998). One of the most widely used model of MI in pigs is the angioplasty balloon occlusion of the left anterior descending coronary artery (Ibanez et al., 2007). Moreover, the development of gene-engineered animals with the advent of molecular genetic techniques during the last years has allowed an explosion in the number of models resulting in a tremendous progress in the understanding of myocardial diseases.

Different Non-invasive Imaging Modalities to Assess Myocardial Structure and Function, Inflammation, and Viability in Animal Models of MI

Myocardial Structure and Function: Techniques and Current Evidence

Two-dimensional echocardiography is a well-established tool that has have been largely used for the assessment of cardiac function and structure using techniques and indices familiar from human echocardiography. It offers a rapid and low cost evaluation of heart anatomy, function and biomechanics (Richardson et al., 2013) and response to treatment (Bao et al., 2013; Matthews et al., 2013). But, its results depend on the body complexion, echographic window and the HR of the scanned animal. As a result, ultrasound based methods have been mostly limited to small-animal models these days. The advent of higher frame rates and smaller probes operating at higher frequencies equipment's have facilitated imaging of mice, a setting where CMR is still challenging. Basic measurements of LV systolic function, LV mass, and LV chamber dimensions are easy to achieve from a parasternal long and short-axis view of the heart. In the absence of wall motion abnormalities, M-mode is an accurate method for evaluating LV structure and function using the Teichholz method for fractional shortening (FS%) and ejection fraction (EF%) estimation (Tanaka et al., 1996). However, in mice models of MI, wall motion abnormalities and systolic function should be determined in 2D mode echocardiography with consecutive parasternal short-axis planes using the Simpson's rule (Gao et al., 2000). It is important to note that marked changes in echographic measurements occur when mice are anesthetized (Rottman et al., 2003). Anesthesia depresses HR, and the FS% is directly affected by cardiac frequency. Thus, it is important when protocols required consecutive measurements to perform all echoes under the same conditions. Regarding diastolic dysfunction, it is a critical condition where blood filling of the LV is impaired. It accompanies, and sometimes precedes many disease conditions like ischemic heart disease, but it is more difficult to define and to measure than systolic dysfunction. Moreover, its echographic measurement are highly affected by loading conditions, age and HR. Transmitral filling, alterations in the A-wave or the E/A ratio haven been used to define diastolic abnormalities. However, E and A waves are fused due to rapid HR in mice, so as, other indices like color M-mode flow propagation velocity (Schmidt et al., 2002), isovolumentric relaxation time, the A'-wave or the E'/A' ratio using tissular Doppler imaging (Schaefer et al., 2003, 2005), also the Tei index (Tei et al., 1995) that characterize global, systolic and diastolic left ventricular function after MI, have been used in mice. However, the accuracy with which these measurements quantify diastolic dysfunction is still open to discussion (Scherrer-Crosbie and Thibault, 2008).

Cardiac Magnetic Resonance (CMR) is up to date the preferred technique for the assessment of cardiac morphology and function in animal models (Stuckey et al., 2008; Makowski et al., 2010). CMR provides non-invasive high image quality tomographic views of the heart with sub-millimeter anatomical detail, high tissue contrast and excellent reproducibility, which can be used for accurate functional and structural assessment in coronary heart disease (Sinitsyn, 2001). They have been used to serially evaluate left and right ventricular dysfunction.

Medium-large animal models can be studied with conventional procedures established in the clinic for patients, but imaging small animal models with CMR is challenging due to their faster HR and smaller dimensions of the heart, and requires the use of high-field (>4.7T) scanners or substantial modifications of conventional protocols used in clinical 1.5 or 3T platforms (Gilson and Kraitchman, 2007; Bunck et al., 2009). Cine sequences in Magnetic Resonance Imaging (MRI) are used to study all relevant functional parameters of the left ventricle (LV) such as EF, ventricular volume, cardiac mass, and cardiac output with high accuracy (Franco et al., 1999). Several ECG-gated spin-echo and multiphase gradient-echo (cine MRI) have been developed for quantifying LV parameters in mice with similar reliability (Ruff et al., 1998; Slawson et al., 1998) becoming the gold standard for LV assessment in rodents (Slawson et al., 1998; Franco et al., 1999). Also, high in-plane resolution (0.1 × 0.1 mm) cine MRI has been developed to quantify right ventricular function in murine models (Wiesmann et al., 2002). Other techniques for quantitative wall-motion imaging like myocardial tagging (Epstein et al., 2002; Zhou et al., 2003) or velocity-encode phase-contrast imaging (Espe et al., 2015) have been optimized for animal studies. These approaches permit the tracking of regional myocardium and enable the quantification of principal strains and directions (radial, circumferential, and longitudinal) to depict the extent of the changes in contractility after MI (Young et al., 2006).

Myocardial ischemia also leads to a variety of changes in tissue structure. Myocardial fibrosis is the main structural damage after ischemia/reperfusion injury. Scar tissue can be evaluated with inversion recovery echo-pulse sequences for late gadolinium enhancement to differentiate between reversible damage and infarcted myocardium after MI (**Figure** ; Kim et al., 1999). Also, diffuse microfibrosis can be detected in the myocardium using recent T1-mapping sequences in animals (Stuckey et al., 2014; García-Álvarez et al., 2015). Nevertheless, efforts are still required to further improve and standardize protocols and to generate reference values for each animal model on cardiovascular disease.

Myocardial Inflammation: Area at Risk: Techniques and Current Evidence

The area at risk (AAR), defined as the hypoperfused myocardium during an acute coronary occlusion, is a major determinant of infarct size and clinical outcomes in MI. Additionally, accurate AAR quantification is important because it has been used as an end-point in clinical trials testing the efficacy of cardioprotective

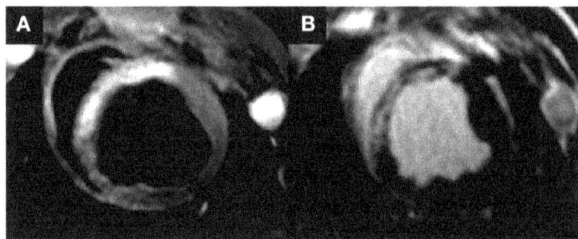

FIGURE | Cardiac magnetic resonance images of an anterior acute myocardial infarction in a pig model of ischemia/reperfusion injury. **(A)** Area at risk in T2-STIR sequence and hyperintense zone in anterior septum. **(B)** Necrotic zone in late enhancement sequence at the same zone. Published with publisher's permission. Original source: Fernández-Friera et al. (2013).

interventions (Feiring et al., 1987). Single-photon emission computed tomography (SPECT) is the traditional reference method for determining AAR by injection of technetium-based tracer before opening of the occluded vessel. However, CMR has been proposed as an alternative approach over the last years because of higher spatial resolution and the absence of tracer administration need or radiation exposure (Carlsson et al., 2009). In particular, T2-weighted (T2W) edema-sensitive sequences have enabled the identification of acutely ischemic myocardium by detecting increased signal intensity that reflects myocardial water content (Aletras et al., 2006; Friedrich et al., 2008). T2W imaging, however, is often limited by motion artifacts, incomplete blood suppression, low signal-to-noise ratio and coil sensitivity related-issues of surface coil. Newer quantitative CMR methods include: (1) T1 and T2 mapping imaging (**Figure**) that allow direct measurement of intrinsic tissue properties. These sequences are less dependent on confounders affecting signal intensity (Ugander et al., 2012) and their accuracy for AAR quantification is high compared to microsphere blood flow analysis in a dog model of ischemia/reperfusion injury (Fernandez-Jimenez et al., 2015b); (2) BOLD or modified blood oxygen level-dependent sequences which have been recently proposed to detect ischemic myocardium in a dog model of severe coronary stenosis (Tsaftaris et al., 2013); (3) Targeted microparticles of iron oxide, which shorten T2 and T2* relaxation times. By tracking up-regulated vascular cell and intercellular adhesion molecules, such as VCAM and ICAM, it is possible to detect and localize myocardial ischemia (Grieve et al., 2013); (4) Balanced steady-state free precession sequences with T2 preparation have also been proposed to detect myocardial edema in a porcine model and in patients with reperfused acute MI (Kellman et al., 2007).

In addition to CMR approaches, pre-reperfusion multidetector Computed Tomography (CT) imaging has also been described as a method to assess AAR size in a porcine acute MI model (Mewton et al., 2011).

Myocardial Perfusion and Viability by PET and MRI

Positron Emission Tomography (PET) currently plays an important role in clinical cardiology (Bengel et al., 2009). The basic principle of PET is the coincidence detection of the annihilation photons emitted after the emission of a positron by a beta+ radioisotope. The spatial resolution of PET images is currently in the range of 4–7 mm for clinical scanners and about 1 mm for small animal systems. Higher detection sensitivity allows measuring radiotracer at nano- to pico-molar concentrations. In addition, PET is a truly quantitative imaging tool that measures absolute concentrations of radioactivity in the body and allows for kinetic modeling of physiologic parameters such as absolute myocardial blood flow or glucose use. The data acquisition can be synchronized with an ECG or respiration signal and retrospectively used to obtain gated images. PET systems are nowadays combined with CT systems that offer fused anatomical and functional images. Combined PET and MRI systems have recently appeared as and attractive option but their use is still mostly limited to research studies (Nekolla et al., 2009).

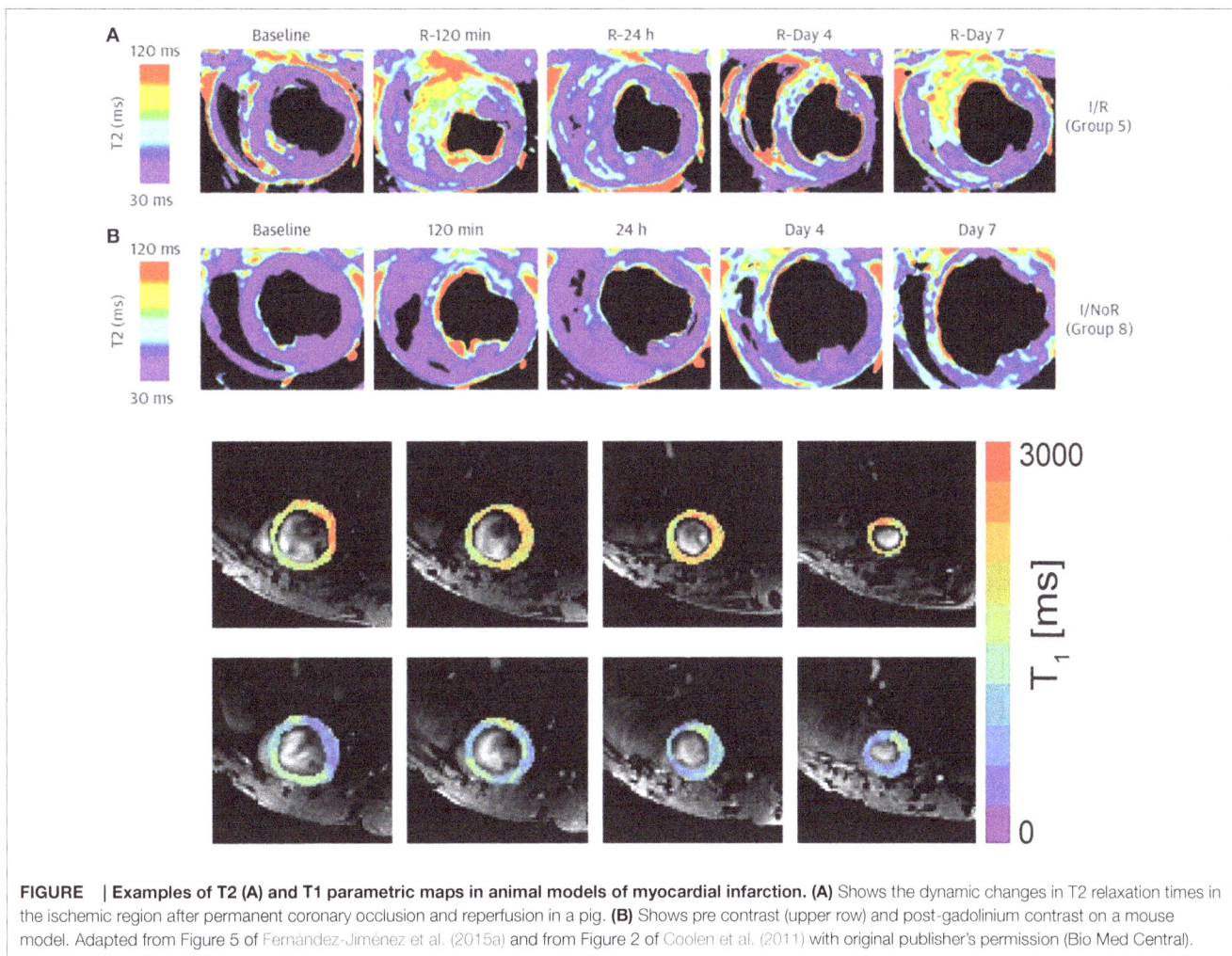

FIGURE | Examples of T2 (A) and T1 parametric maps in animal models of myocardial infarction. (A) Shows the dynamic changes in T2 relaxation times in the ischemic region after permanent coronary occlusion and reperfusion in a pig. (B) Shows pre contrast (upper row) and post-gadolinium contrast on a mouse model. Adapted from Figure 5 of Fernández-Jiménez et al. (2015a) and from Figure 2 of Coolen et al. (2011) with original publisher's permission (Bio Med Central).

Cardiac imaging in small animals is challenging due to the small ventricle volume and wall thickness and the high HR (Gargiulo et al., 2012b). Dedicated small animal PET systems with high spatial resolution and increased sensitivity have been developed (Levin and Zaidi, 2007). In the other hand, large animal models are typically imaged in clinical systems (Teramoto et al., 2011). In planning longitudinal PET studies with animals, many variables interfering with the accuracy of the experimental results must be taken into account (Adams et al., 2010; stress related to physical restraint, fasting, warming and anesthesia).

Myocardial Perfusion

Myocardial MRI based techniques are based (in large animal models and in humans) on regional differences in myocardial signal intensity during the first passage of an intravenously administered dual-bolus of gadolinium-based contrast agent, although quantitative approaches systemically underestimate myocardial reserve and require many manipulations and have limited inclusion in the clinical routine. For the successful application of these methods in mice, imaging technology requires the complete acquisition of imaging dataset at every single or every second heartbeat using non-conventional MRI pulse sequences. MRI offers the advantage by comparison with nuclear medicine-based techniques of high resolution and consequently betters assessment of transmural perfusion. MRI perfusion technology has also the advantage that can be integrated in routine CMR protocols of functional assessment and late gadolinium enhancement. Most of the semi-quantitative methods are based on the contrast enhancement ratios or upslope indexes, although these systematically underestimate myocardial perfusion. Finally, recent alternatives for absolute quantification included dual saturation strategies of single bolus acquisition, that will make easier to implement in clinical protocols (Sánchez-González et al., 2015).

Alternatively, other MRI based—Arterial Spin Labeling (ASL) perfusion methods does not use an exogenous contrast agent and has been used for single slices to measure and quantify myocardial perfusion also in small animals, although with long acquisition times (Kober et al., 2005). ASL uses the water of the blood as endogenous tracer and allows *in vivo* quantification of the absolute perfusion and the regional blood volume in the myocardium. These methods showed good agreement with standard *ex vivo* microspheres technique and is sensitive enough to detect and visualize regional alterations of the perfusion after MI (Streif et al., 2005).

Basic experiments based in nuclear medicine have provided complement or additional information to MRI based methods. Myocardial perfusion imaging with PET is a standard tool for detection of CAD, risk stratification of patients, and guidance of therapeutic interventions (Di Carli et al., 2007). Regional blood flow at rest may be normal until the stenosis is higher than 90%. However, autoregulation is incapable of preserving maximum blood flow during exercise or pharmacological stress test leading to reduced myocardial blood flow relative to demand and stress-induced ischemia. Thus, in a patient with coronary artery stenosis, when acute myocardial ischemia occurs, the initial abnormality is an imbalance in blood flow between the hypoperfused and normally perfused areas (Di Carli et al., 2007).

CT coronary angiography is considered the gold standard for evaluating the presence and the severity of coronary stenosis, which provides the anatomical extent of disease. However, perfusion imaging provides hemodynamic significance of epicardial stenosis. PET myocardial perfusion imaging combined with tracer-kinetic modeling can provide absolute quantification of regional myocardial blood flow of the LV. Tracer kinetic modeling requires dynamic imaging beginning briefly before the tracer injection and monitoring of tracer distribution in the myocardium for 2–30 min depending on the tracer and model. Rest and stress scans are typically performed sequentially and stress scans in animals are achieved by pharmacological stress by infusion of adenosine, dipyridamole, or dobutamine.

The available flow agents are characterized by a rapid myocardial extraction and by a cardiac uptake proportional to blood flow. PET radiotracers used for evaluation of myocardial blood flow include $^{13}NH_3$ (see **Figure**), ^{82}Rb, and $H_2^{15}O$. However, their short half-life limits their widespread clinical use, because of the need for nearby cyclotron (^{13}N and ^{15}O) or generator (^{82}Rb). Other agents based on ^{18}F as Flurpiridaz (Packard et al., 2014) shows potential to spread the use of PET for cardiac perfusion imaging, even with animal models, as it does not depend on onsite cyclotron or generator.

Myocardial Metabolic and Energetic Viability

Alterations in myocardial substrate metabolism are critical in the pathogenesis of many cardiovascular diseases. MI is associated with numerous biochemical and functional changes in the necrotic tissue, in the AAR, and in the remote myocardium.

^{18}F-fluorodeoxyglucose (FDG) is a glucose analog that is widely available due to its success as a metabolic imaging tracer in clinical oncology. FDG traces myocytic glucose uptake and can be used to quantify regional myocardial glucose metabolism (Dilsizian et al., 2009; see **Figure**). FDG is employed to determine the extent of myocardial viability or potentially reversible contractile dysfunction in response to revascularization as well as the extent of scar tissue or irreversible contractile dysfunction. Increased FDG uptake can be observed in ischemic tissue while significantly reduced or absent uptake indicates scar formation.

The diagnostic quality of the myocardial FDG image depends on the concentration of tracer in both myocardium and blood. Myocardial FDG uptake depends quantitatively on plasma concentrations of glucose and insulin, the rate of glucose utilization and the relationship between FDG and glucose defined by the lumped constant. High plasma concentrations of glucose lower the fractional utilization of FDG and thus degrade the quality of myocardial FDG uptake images. Myocardial glucose uptake also depends on myocardial work, plasma levels of free fatty acids, insulin, catecholamines, and oxygen supply. FDG uptake is heterogeneous in normal myocardium in the fasting state. Therefore, attempts have been made to standardize the metabolic environment for human myocardial FDG imaging (Knuuti et al., 1992), whereas procedures for animal imaging vary widely (Gargiulo et al., 2012b). In humans, patients are studied under fasting conditions following oral glucose loading or during hyper-insulinaemic-euglycaemic clamping to improve image quality and diagnostic accuracy.

Alternatively, Magnetic Resonance spectroscopy (MRS), primarily based in 31P and 1H provides an energetic profile (ATP, PCr, etc...) or lipid content, respectively that in are both connected to the possible change in myocardial substrate utilization from fatty acid toward glucose in the context of myocardial ischemia/reperfusion injury or provides useful insights into the effects of obesity on the heart. These methods have sometimes used to evaluate the improved cardiac energetic and function effect of novel drugs (Bao et al., 2011). 31P MRI is the only method available to provide non-invasive measures of endogenous quantitative concentration of these energetic metabolites and creatine kinase kinetics (Bottomley et al., 2009). Additionally, 13C in natural isotopic abundance is *per se* not very informative. However, possible hyperpolarization with an SNR increase in five orders of magnitude is the technique with

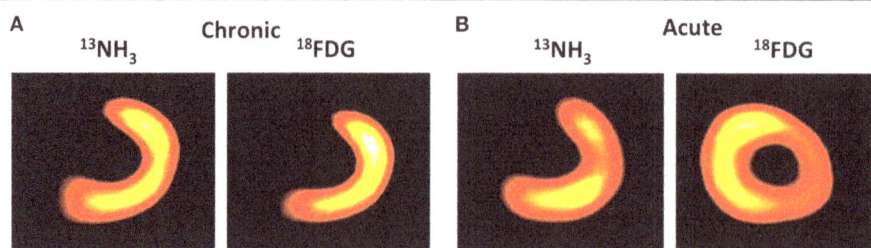

FIGURE | Representative midventricular short-axis slices PET myocardial perfusion at rest and PET myocardial metabolism using $^{13}NH_3$ and 18FDG tracers respectively in pigs studied in the chronic (A) and acute (B) phases after myocardial infarction. From Lautamäki et al. (2009) Figure . With permission.

promising future for enhanced 13C MRS studies, particularly of the glycolytic metabolism of the heart. There are some reports of 13C metabolic images of lactate, alanine, bicarbonate and pyruvate in a pig heart following coronary occlusion (Bottomley et al., 2009).

Heart Failure

A variety of animal models have been used to mimic the human disease with the highest interest in medical cardiology (**Table** ; Verdouw et al., 1998; Dixon and Spinale, 2009; Patten and Hall-Porter, 2009; Abarbanell et al., 2010; Houser et al., 2012). HF is caused by an unable heart to maintain oxygen level that vital organs demand deriving from an impaired blood filling and/or ejection (Houser et al., 2012). According to these two different causes, there are two phenotypes of HF, ones derived from the systolic dysfunction, where the EF decreases below 50%, called HF with reduced EF; and ones derived from a diastolic dysfunction, where the EF remains above 50%, called HF with preserved ejection EF. Valve diseases, hypertension, myocardial ischemia and genetic abnormalities that caused dilated and restrictive cardiomyopathies are the most common mechanisms used for creating experimental HF. Characterization of animal models of HF requires revealing an insufficient cardiac output, on one hand the left-, right-, or biventricular cardiac dysfunction, and o pulmonary findings compatibles with the course of HF (Houser et al., 2012).

Cardiac Hypertrophy

Several strategies have been described to induce an adaptive response to pressure overload, sarcomeric mutations or pulmonary/artery hypertension, to mimic the hypertrophic transformation of the heart: (1) hypertrophic growth where load exceeds heart output, (2) study of compensatory events to normalize workload/mass ratio and cardiac output, and (3) HF because of ventricular dilatation (Meerson, 1961). Aortic and pulmonary artery stenosis are the most common methods for stressing the heart for a pressure overload (Tarnavski et al., 2004). The critical feature is to establish a normalized constriction of the artery to observe the increased difference between the left ventricular and aortic pressures or the difference between right ventricle (RV) and pulmonary artery. In non-rodent models, the normalization of the injury is fairly easy due to the feasibility of previous imaging studies. The measurement of the artery determines the precise restriction desired. A recent publication of RV failure in rabbits details the constriction induction of the pulmonary artery by the inflation of a 5-mm surgically implanted band controlled by the echocardiographic measurement of the right ventricular end-systolic pressure (McKellar et al., 2015). Imaging technologies are used for hypertrophic progress evaluation for the development of new therapies. However, the main disadvantage of these models is the period required to observe each stage of the cardiomyopathy, involving 2–3 months. On the other hand, the rodent models display an abrupt and acute hemodynamic instability. Heart morphological alterations are quickly acquired with a certain grade of variability depending of proportional reduction of the arterial lumen (−70%). The

interest of the murine models is focused on the study of the compensatory events that occur after hypertrophic growth.

Other models that induce pressure overload without a required surgical expertise are: pulmonary hypertension (PH) by beads inoculation, genetic models of arterial hypertension and arrhythmogenic right ventricular cardiomyopathy. Murine genetic models and arrhythmogenic pathologies show a great advantage against other species. The spontaneous hypertension of rat (SH strains) or those induced in mutant mice are well characterized. However, the arrhythmogenic right ventricular cardiomyopathy of the Boxer and Hypertrophic Cardiomyopathy of MainCoon//Persian cats remain the best animal models for the study of both diseases regarding their similarities in genetic mutations etiologies and analogous mechanical-electrical dysfunctions (Kittleson et al., 1999; Basso et al., 2004; Palermo et al., 2011).

Dilated Cardiomyopathy

Animal models of dilated cardiomyopathy (DCM) should exhibit the structural and mechanical alterations observed in humans: LV dilatation, eccentric hypertrophy, wall thinning, reproducing cellular/molecular/neurohormonal features, depressed chamber output/flow, reduced ventricle contractility, and lusitropy, elevated filling pressure, and intolerance to stress situation due to a low functional reserve. Several strategies have been implemented (from rodent to large animal) to develop this disease phenotype.

The most used model is the myocardial ischemic injury, which can be performed with a permanent, temporary or progressive occlusion of the left coronary, just trying to mimic the atherosclerotic CAD. Depending on the animal species and surgical expertise, the technique can be performed in a closed or open-chest approach applying a surgical suture, beads microembolization, an intracoronary balloon-occlusion, or ameroid constriction. However, these experimental lesions are concentric contrary to the eccentric occlusion in human atherosclerosis (Bianco et al., 2009). Other strategies for the induction of congestive HF are: toxicological effect of doxorubicin or isoproterenol, pacing-induced tachycardia or genetic factors. In most of DCM animal models it is possible to observe a significant remodeling without severe clinical signs (Mann and Bristow, 2005). Asymptomatic LV dysfunction, reduced blood flow, elevated cardiac filling pressure, or other changes in hemodynamic could be absent while myocyte hypertrophy and fibrosis might be observed histologically. This is quite important to decide the experimental timing and the correlation with symptoms (Houser et al., 2012).

Imaging in Animals Models of HF

Current non-invasive imaging techniques developed in research allows longitudinal evaluation of HF. Echocardiography remains as the gold standard for assessment of cardiovascular structure and function in rodents (Ram et al., 2011). However, CMR and PET-CT have gained importance in small animal research for further cardiac evaluation in the context of heart disease, especially evaluating anatomy and metabolism. In particular CMR is becoming an useful tool in both, systolic and diastolic

TABLE | Schematic comparison of the different animal models used in cardiovascular imaging research.

Specie	Model	Failure etiology	Advantages	Disadvantages
CARDIAC HYPERTROPHY				
Mouse	Transverse aortic and pulmonary artery constriction	Acute and pressure overload	Easy use of GEM animals. Hypertrophy developed rapidly (2–3 weeks)	Surgical skills. Acute hypertension and expense of equipment for cardiovascular imaging and physiology assessment
Mouse	Isoproterenol infusion	Toxic injury of myocardium	Minimal surgery and good scenario for pharmacological or gene therapy	Hypertrophy is adjusted to dose and mouse strain
Rat	Spontaneous hypertensive rat and Dahl salt-sensitive rat	Chronic pressure overload	The onset of hypertension is gradual, being the heart failure in later stages. Genetic origin of hypertension. No surgery	Long experimental period (6–12 months)
Rat	Ascending aortic and pulmonary artery constriction	Gradual to quick onset pressure overload	Gradual to quick onset hypertension	Less GEM animals and similar cost of equipment for cardiovascular physiology assessment than mouse
Rat	Arteriovenous shunts	Overload of ventricular chambers	Progressive heart hypertrophy, more rapidly in the right ventricle. Well tolerate and it possible to reverse the volume-overload state	Greater surgical skills, with a grade of hypertrophy fistula localization-dependent
Guinea pig	Descending aortic constriction	Pressure overload and hypertension	Human mimicking alteration of sarcolemma calcium handling	Special and expensive requirements for husbandry
Rabbit	Aortic and pulmonary constriction	Gradual onset pressure overload	Imaging technology allows normalizing the grade of constriction. Possibility to reverse the pressure-overload situation	Thoracotomy surgery required
Rabbit	Doxorrubicin	Toxicological aggression	Myocyte function and structure modification	High risk of mortality dose dependent
Dog	Aortovenus shunt	Volume overload	Progressive heart hypertrophy, more rapidly in the right ventricle	Not so well tolerated than rats. Frequent arrhythmias, edema and quick health decrease
Dog	Arrhythmogenic right ventricular cardiomyopathy of Boxer	Desmosomes proteins mutation	Genetic origin which mimic the human disease	Social ethical considerations
Cat	Inherited Hypertrophic Cardiomyopathy of Maine Coon and Persian strains	Sarcomeric protein gene mutations	Genetic origin which mimic the human disease	Social ethical considerations
Pig	Descending aortic constriction	Pressure overload and hypertension	Progressive hypertrophy and animal well adapted (constriction grade progresses with animal growth)	Surgical skills and lateral thoracotomy
Pig	Pulmonary artery hypertension by microembolization	Increased vascular resistance	Progressive hypertrophy of right ventricle and final heart failure by dilated cardiomyopathy. No surgery	Great hypoxic vasoconstriction
Sheep	Ascending aortic constriction	Pressure overload and hypertension	Transition from compensated hypertrophy to left ventricular dysfunction	Zoonotic risk
Sheep	Pulmonary artery hypertension by microembolization	Increased vascular resistance	Progressive hypertrophy of right ventricle and final heart failure by dilated cardiomyopathy. No hypoxic vasoconstriction No surgery	Zoonotic risk
DILATED CARDIOPATHY				
Mouse	Genetic Engineering modified animals (GEM)	Dilated cardiomyopathy	Genetic modifications of structural and functionality of cardiomyocytes. No required surgery	Clinical reliability restricted to the molecule of study: e.g., TNF-α overexpression

TABLE | Continued

Specie	Model	Failure etiology	Advantages	Disadvantages
Rat	Isoproterenol toxicity	Toxicological aggression	Severe structural modification by necrosis and fibrosis of myocardium	Less GEM animals and similar cost of equipment for cardiovascular physiology assessment than mouse
Rabbit	Pacing Tachycardia	Congestive failure by low output	Mimic myocardial alteration of human edematous chronic low output	Limited imaging technology due to paced heart rate (400 beats/min)
Rabbit	Balloon occlusion of circumflex branch of left coronary artery	Myocardial infarction	Artery occlusion by catheterization	Great skill and specific material
Dog	Pacing Tachycardia	Congestive failure by low output	Mimic myocardial remodeling, neurohumoral activation and subcellular dysfunction	No hypertrophy
Dog	Coronary microembolization	Contractile dysfunction and a profound perfusion-contraction mismatch	No surgery requirements	Microspheres are chemically inert. Extensive arterial pattern of heart. Time consuming
Pig	Pacing Tachycardia	Congestive failure by low output	Mimic myocardial remodeling, neurohumoral activation and subcellular dysfunction	No hypertrophy nor fibrosis
Pig	Coronary microembolization	Contractile dysfunction and a profound perfusion-contraction mismatch	No surgery requirements	Microsphere are chemically inert
Pig	Hibernating myocardium	Progressive reduction of ventricle perfusion	Mimic human disease condition	Surgical technical experience and skill. There is a myocardial recovery in chronic studies
Sheep	Pacing Tachycardia	Congestive failure by low output	Mimic myocardial remodeling, neurohumoral activation and subcellular dysfunction	No hypertrophy nor fibrosis
Sheep	Coronary microembolization	Contractile dysfunction and a profound perfusion-contraction mismatch	No surgery requirements and resemble human condition than dog	Zoonotic risk. Microspheres are chemically inert. Extensive arterial pattern of heart. Time consuming
MYOCARDIAL INFARCTION				
Mouse	Left coronary ligation (total occlusion or ischemia/reperfusion)	Myocardial infarction	Easy use of GEM animals, low cost of husbandry and feasible cardiovascular assessment. Suitability for follow-up and survival studies.	Great surgical skill and expensive technological requirements. Limited sample collection (animal size)
Rat	Left coronary ligation (total occlusion or ischemia/reperfusion)	Myocardial infarction	Surgical procedure easier than in mouse and more volume of samples. Lower cost than large animals. Suitability for follow-up and survival studies.	Less GEM animals and similar cost of equipment for cardiovascular physiology assessment than mouse
Rabbit	Left coronary ligation (total occlusion or ischemia/reperfusion)	Myocardial infarction	Surgical procedure easier than in rodents and more volume of samples Lower cost than large animals.	Thoracotomy surgery required
Dog	Left coronary ligation (total occlusion or ischemia/reperfusion)	Myocardial infarction	Surgical procedure easier than in rodents and more volume of samples Lower cost than large animals.	High death incidence by arrhythmias
Pig	Angioplasty balloon occlusion of the left anterior descending coronary	Myocardial infarction	Anatomy and pathology closed to human. Good suitability to undergo imaging techniques. No surgery requirements.	Require skills for coronary catheterization and surgical specific material
Zebrafish	Myocardial criolesion	Myocardial infarction	Heart remodeling and regenerative model	Far of mammals biology

TABLE | Continued

Specie	Model	Failure etiology	Advantages	Disadvantages
VASCULAR DISEASE				
Mouse	APOE-deficiency and LDL Receptor deficiency	*Atherosclerosis*, Aortic root atherogenic lesions	Easy use of GEM animals, low cost of husbandry and feasible cardiovascular assessment. Great valuable data of molecular and cellular events.	Not mimic exactly the human chronic disease. The artery low size complicates the *in vivo* imaging acquisition
Rabbit	High-fat diet with/without balloon aortic injury	*Atherosclerosis*, Aortic arch and thoracic aorta lesions	Easy husbandry and feasible artery imaging acquisition.	Great skill for vessel damage, long term experimental induction of atherogenic lesions and no coronary affection
Rabbit	Watanabe WHHL (LDL Receptor deficiency)	*Atherosclerosis*, Aortic arch and thoracic aorta lesions	Easy husbandry and feasible artery imaging acquisition. Possible finding of coronary artery lesions. Not necessary high fat diet.	Unstable atherogenic plaque which could develop coronary occlusion and death
Pig	High-fat diet with/without angioplasty	*Atherosclerosis*, Aortic and coronary atherogenic lesions	Model closed to human disease	Long term experimental induction of atherogenic lesions. Skills for catheterism
PULMONARY HYPERTENSION				
Rat	Chronic Hypoxia	Increase in vascular tone	Repeatable maintained increase in pulmonary artery and RV pressure accompanied by RV remodeling	Minimal vascular remodeling. Suitable just for small animals
Rat	Chronic Hypoxia plus SU5416	Increase in vascular tone plus VEGFR-R blockade	Equal than chronic hypoxia more angiobliterative changes. More increase in RV pressure and more RV hypertrophy	Suitable just for small animals
Rat, dog, pig, sheep	Monocrotaline	Endothelial damage	Produces RV failure and vascular remodeling	No plexogenic arteriopathy
Dogs pig, sheep	Beads or clots injection	Decrease in total vessel area	Acute increase in pulmonary pressure RV remodeling	Decrease of the severity of vascular and RV changes with time. Hard to titrate the dose. High mortality in some reports
Pig, Rat	Aortocaval shunt	Increase in pulmonary artery flow	Resembles major features of human disease	Requires surgical skills. Complications related with surgery
Rodents, pig, sheep, dog	Vascular banding	Decrease in vascular compliance	Controllable and maintained increase in pulmonary artery pressure. RV remodeling	Requires surgical skills. Complications related with surgery

HF studies in murine models (Loganathan et al., 2006; Chung et al., 2013; Constantinides, 2013). Literature on advance imaging protocols and cardiac echocardiography and MRI mouse models of HF is very extensive, therefore only those aspects helpful in the assessment of HF in mice are described.

Impaired systolic function is the main characteristic of HF with reduced EF animal models. Main cardiac findings are reduced LV EF, dilated or overload LV and coronary flow disturbs. Furthermore, assessment of LV regional wall motion abnormalities and calculation of wall motion score index offers to investigators an interesting tool to complement systolic dysfunction characterization and a measurement of heart damage extension, especially in ischemic injury.

Models of HF with preserved EF have predominantly LV diastolic filling alterations. Therefore, in these studies evaluation of mitral inflow pattern, pulmonary vein flow and left atrium dimensions could be essential for evaluating this condition. An important consideration to mention is that diastolic impairment does not noticeable affect cardiac output, so atrial diameter enlargement and pulmonary changes related to congestion could be useful to determine the develop of HF.

Mice Transthoracic Echocardiography

Two-dimensional (2D), motion-mode (M-mode) and color and pulse wave Doppler (CD and PW, respectively) are the basic techniques used in research (Ram et al., 2011; Chen et al., 2012; Moran et al., 2013). Parasternal long axis view (PLAX) and parasternal short axis views (PSAX, at basal, medium, and apical) in 2D and M-mode allows entirely LV visualization, therefore LV function, regional wall motion as well as chamber and wall dimensions can be accurately determined (Zhang et al., 2007; Fayssoil and Tournoux, 2013). Apical four-chamber view is used to visualize both ventricles and as ultrasounds can be aligned with blood flow through mitral and PW Doppler is set in this plane to study mitral inflow pattern. Additional views or PLAX-angled views have also been described in mice to study coronary, pulmonary vein and pulmonary artery flows, which can be useful in the context of diastolic and systolic dysfunction (Wu et al., 2012; Cheng et al., 2014).

Conventional echocardiographic measures lack sensitivity for capturing subtle variations in global ventricular performance (Bauer et al., 2011). In this regard, novel echocardiographic techniques based on tracking tissue motion have emerged for clinical use and animal cardiac research to assess strain. These may provide quantitatively evaluation of myocardial function and early detection of ventricular performance alterations. Doppler tissue imaging (DTI) and speckle-tracking imaging (STI) based on strain analysis are the main echocardiographic tools described in human and small animal models in this regard, although current applications remain limited (Mor-Avi et al., 2011). In DTI, the same Doppler principles are used to identify signals of myocardial tissue motion. Peak myocardial velocities of early and late diastolic and systolic waves can be measured (also in mice) in the anterior/posterior LV wall for the radial component, and in the lateral free LV wall for the circumferential component on the PSAX view (Ho and Solomon, 2006; Mor-Avi et al., 2011; Ferferieva et al., 2013). STI based of strain analysis detects the gray scale "speckles" within the tissue on 2D ultrasound imaging and its movement during cardiac cycle and has been recently used for the estimation of the radial and circumferential strain in small animal models (Mor-Avi et al., 2011; Ferferieva et al., 2013).

In mice, assessment of deformation parameters through DTI or STI based on strain analysis correlated well with invasive hemodynamic measure of myocardial contractility and both techniques could be equally acceptable for assessing LV function (Ferferieva et al., 2013). However, these techniques are not yet routinely established in the echocardiography protocols of cardiac disease. The use of DTI and STI based on strain analysis to provide good cardiovascular phenotype in mice are of great interest but improvement of the analysis should be develop to make these new tools robust, reproducible and more user-friendly (Fayssoil and Tournoux, 2013).

In HF with reduced EF models, typically derived from systolic alterations, LV EF is the major parameter to determine this condition and can be determined from both, 2D and M-mode PLAX views. It is important to mention that in ischemic injury, M-mode echography cannot accurately estimate LV EF because the ventricle shape is abnormal, and geometric models and algorithms assumptions cannot be assumed. In these cases, EF is better estimated using the area-length formula in an 2D PLAX view; if additional 2D PSAX has been taken at basal, medium and apical, Simpson formula to calculate LV EF and regional wall motion can also be performed. LV dilatation or overload can be demonstrated obtained the end-diastolic volume of the LV, usually from 2D PLAX. Evaluation of coronary flow in murine models of HF with reduced EF could be essential in some cases as coronary disturbance could lead to abnormal myocardial perfusion and therefore could compromise systolic function. Hyperemic peak diastolic velocity and coronary flow reverse are the principal changes in coronary flow during ischemic injury and reduced EF (Wu et al., 2012).

Echocardiography evaluation of HF with preserved EF in mice, normally derived from diastolic alterations, can be challenging as small heart size and rapid ventricular rates make evaluation of diastolic function difficult (Chung et al., 2013). Variation in the mitral flow is the most consistent finding in these studies. Mitral inflow pattern can be achieve in the apical view, and common parameters altered are E wave-A wave ratio, isovolumetric relaxation time, E wave deceleration time and A wave time (Wichi et al., 2007; Ram et al., 2011; Fayssoil and Tournoux, 2013). Pulmonary vein flow changes are commonly used in human echography and could be a future marker of diastolic dysfunction in rodents but no consistent changes have been described. Pulmonary veins in these animals differ from human as venous confluence with a single orifice enters the left atrium in mice, thus, altering the pressures and, therefore, the wave patterns (Yuan et al., 2010).

Left atrial dilatation measured form 2D and M-mode long-axis has been described as a parameter indicating pulmonary congestion (Finsen et al., 2005), therefore, it could be used in both, reduced and preserved EF models, but could be especially useful in preserved EF where reduced cardiac output cannot be assessed. Pulmonary artery flow varies depending on lung abnormalities and mice have similar pattern to that observed in humans (Thibault et al., 2010). In both, HF with reduced or preserved EF, if there is a maintained pulmonary congestion, high pulmonary pressures can be achieved and typical pattern of hypertension can be visualized. Acceleration and total ejection time ratio is reduced in accordance with increase in pulmonary pressure in hypertension murine models (Thibault et al., 2010), whereas in some models of HF such as ischemic injury, the changes in arterial flow have not been very consistent with the presence or absence of pulmonary congestion (Finsen et al., 2005).

Mice Cardiac MRI

In vivo MRI provides excellent views of cardiac structures and allows high quality spatial resolution of the heart, and recently has emerged as an accurately instrument for functional cardiac evaluation as high temporal resolutions are also achieved (Yue et al., 2007; **Figure**). Cardiac gating is essential to reduce the level of motion artifacts and therefore, to obtain images of sufficient quality (Cassidy et al., 2004). Assessment of cardiac anatomy, regional wall motion, myocardial perfusion, myocardial viability plus cardiac chamber quantification, and cardiac function are applications described in mice (Pohlmann et al., 2011). Conventional views in mice are similar to those used in human cardiac MRI. Long-axis, two and four-chamber views as well as a multi-slice short-axis view from base to apex are commonly used in bright-blood and black-blood spin-echo.

CMR in HF with reduced EF models is becoming progressively more used as it allows precisely data of LV volumes with no need of making geometric assumptions regarding ventricular shape, which is especially important in ischemic injury models. In these models, MRI also allows measuring the total infarcted area as the scar can be well visualized. Besides, the high anatomical resolution and improvements achieved in temporal resolution make MRI a powerful tool to assess cardiac

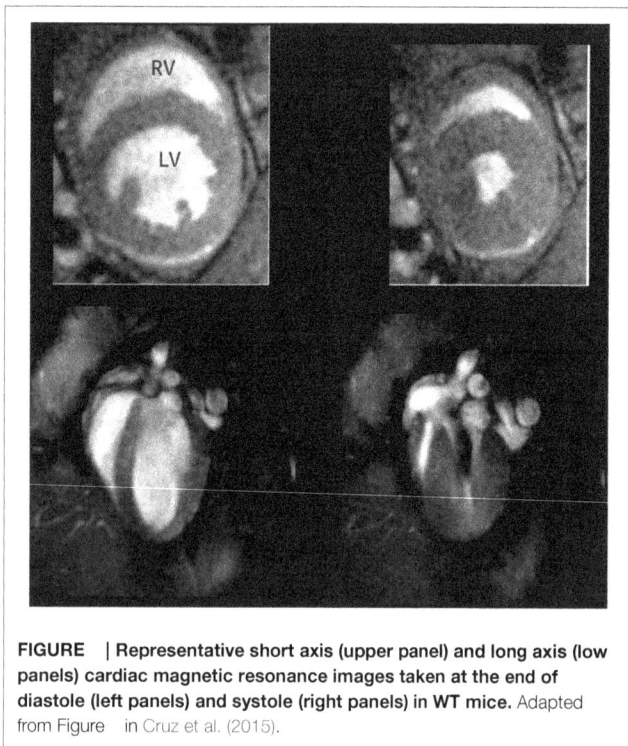

FIGURE | Representative short axis (upper panel) and long axis (low panels) cardiac magnetic resonance images taken at the end of diastole (left panels) and systole (right panels) in WT mice. Adapted from Figure   in Cruz et al. (2015).

systolic dysfunction and wall motion, not only in LV but also in the RV. Normally, LV and RV EF as well as volumes are calculated after obtaining planimetry of each short-axis slice in end-systole and end-diastole.

As it has been describe previously in this report, non-invasively imaging evaluation of diastolic dysfunction in rodents is limited because of the short diastolic period. As most of the HF with preserved EF models are characterized by diffuse myocardial fibrosis and structural alterations, MRI has become an important imaging technique to describe cardiac mass, tissue changes, and interstitial fibrosis through special analysis as pixel intensity values (Loganathan et al., 2006). Furthermore, evaluation of LV filling rate calculated from slopes of the volume-time curves can also provide relaxation information useful for determining diastolic dysfunction in these models (Yu et al., 2007). Finally, CMR can be simultaneously used to assess the progression of ventricular dysfunction with lung congestion. This non-invasive technology is especially applicable to serial studies and in drug discovery programs exploring the use of novel pharmacological or molecular agents for treatment of heart failure and/or pulmonary congestion (Alsaid et al., 2012).

New Challenge in Heart Failure Imaging
One of the ultimate goals of HF treatment is aimed to cardiac repair by the regeneration of the myocardium after injury. The mammalian heart is one of the least regenerative organs in the body, although postnatal hearts undergo some degree of cardiomyocyte renewal during normal aging and disease. Together with mouse, zebrafish has proven to be a particularly useful model, given its amenability to genetic manipulation and its tissue regenerative capacity (Poss et al., 2002). Zebrafish

models are directed to observe the cardiomyocyte proliferation after heart ablation or myocardium crioinjury. Significantly, the principal limitations of this model is the handling and HF procedure performing in an aquatic species, the anatomical differences of cardiovascular system with mammals and the setting up of imaging techniques for hemodynamic measurements (González-Rosa et al., 2014). However, the interspecies jump is too high to conclude the evidence acquired in zebrafish cardiovascular studies for human or mammal cardiac diseases. For that purpose, heart regeneration models have been established in mouse neonates. Obviously, the cardiac repair differs from zebrafish, but the cardiac insult is quite similar. Crioinjury infarct and apex ablation are basically the preference model in this field. Surgical expertise and special handling are crucial for the success of the technique. The main point in the surgical part is the promptness to open the chest and damage the myocardium. The anesthetic regimen is based on the immobility by cold, which should be recovered as soon as possible. Later, the most important *tour de force* is the reinstatement to the mother due to the easy induction to cannibalism by the extremely sensitive olfactory and visual sense (Laflamme and Murry, 2011). While a number of imaging methods and applications have been shown mainly using optical microscopy, MRI can be adapted and can provide additional *in vivo* information (**Figure**).

Atherosclerosis and Vascular Lesion Characterization

Atherosclerosis is a chronic inflammatory disease, affecting the medium and large arteries, characterized by the progressive accumulation of lipid deposits and different cell types in the subendothelial space (mainly immune cells and vascular smooth muscle cells) to form the atherosclerotic plaques. The major clinical manifestations of atherosclerosis are CAD, leading to acute MI (see Section Imaging in Myocardial Infarction and Coronary Artery Disease); cerebrovascular disease, leading to stroke; and peripheral arterial disease, leading to ischemic limbs and viscera (Libby, 2002). Traditionally, diagnosis of atherosclerosis was only possible at advanced stages of disease, either by directly revealing the narrowing of the arterial lumen (stenosis) or by evaluating the effect of arterial stenosis on organ perfusion. However, it is now well recognized that the atherosclerotic plaques responsible for thrombus formation are not necessarily those that impinge most on the lumen of the vessel. New imaging approaches allow the assessment not only of the morphology of blood vessels but also of the composition of the vessel walls, enabling atherosclerosis-associated abnormalities in the arteries to be observed, down to the cellular and molecular level in some cases. Some of these approaches are now in clinical use or are being tested in clinical trials, whereas others are better suited for basic and translational research (Sanz and Fayad, 2008; Owen et al., 2011).

Animal Models of Atherosclerosis
Experimental models of atherosclerosis are required to understand the natural history of the disease and the factors leading to plaque progression and rupture. Thus, ideally,

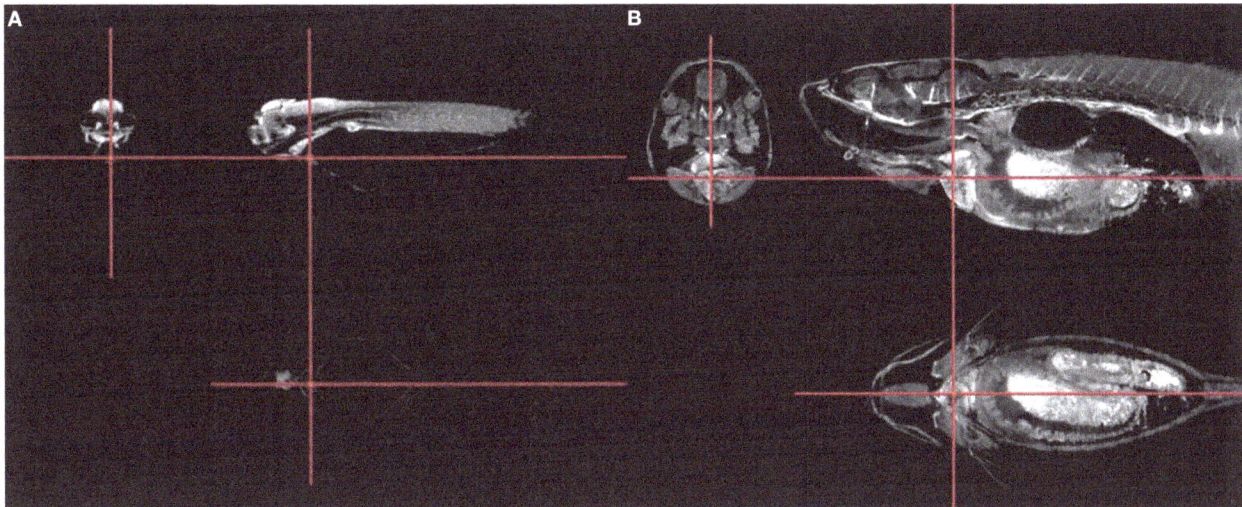

FIGURE | Representative high resolution MRI sections to visualize the normal heart structure of zebrafish embryo (A) and an adult fish (B). From Bryson-Richardson et al. (2007) Figure with original publisher's permission (Bio Med Central).

animal models of atherosclerosis should present a progressive development of arterial lesions throughout life, from initial fatty streak to advanced complicated lesions (ulceration, thrombus, etc...), with shared histological features and clinical events (MI, stroke) similar to humans (Russell and Proctor, 2006; Fuster et al., 2012).

Animal models of atherosclerosis started emerging in the literature at the beginning of the twentieth century with rabbits being the first animal species to be described (Ignatowski, 1908). Since then, a wide variety of animal models, including mice, rats, guinea pigs, hamsters, avian, swine, and non-human primates, have provided valuable information about diagnostic and therapeutic strategies for atherosclerosis (Xiangdong et al., 2011; Fuster et al., 2012). Currently, mice, rabbits, and pigs dominate this field of research. Susceptibility to atherosclerosis varies not only between animal species but also between genetic strains within the same species.

The mouse is the most frequently used animal species in atherosclerosis research. Some of the reasons include low costs, availability, rapid development of plaque, well-known genome, possibility of genetic manipulations, and easy usability. But mice are highly resistant to atherosclerosis as compared to humans, due in part to a markedly different lipid profile. Therefore, genetic variants that do develop the disease have been created either by spontaneous mutations or by gene manipulation methods. The majority of mouse models are based on disturbance of lipid metabolism through genetic manipulation of the C57BL/6 strain. Among those, the apolipoprotein E-deficient mouse (apoE-KO) is the most distributed worldwide. Arterial lesions observed in apoE-KO are relatively similar to lesions found in humans: from foam cell-rich fatty streaks to atherosclerotic lesions with large necrotic core, and fibro-fatty nodules. In mice, the most advanced lesions have been described to occur in the aortic root, aortic arch, and innominate artery

(brachiocephalic trunk), whereas in humans the lesions are more frequent in the coronary arteries, carotids, and peripheral vessels, such as the iliac artery (Nakashima et al., 1994). In addition, most murine models do not manifest the unstable atherosclerotic plaque with overlying thrombosis, the lesion most often associated with clinically significant acute cardiovascular episodes. This is due to a spontaneous high fibrinolytic activity in the mouse (Zhu et al., 1999). Moreover, the size of the arteries makes it extremely difficult to image with sufficient resolution in clinical scanners used for humans, precluding the efficient translation of techniques from animal model to human scanning.

When the size becomes more important, small animal models need to be complemented by larger animal models in which vessel characteristics are more similar to human arteries. Rabbits develop atherosclerotic lesions on a high cholesterol diet, and have been used extensively in atherosclerosis research (Yanni, 2004). The most widely used, the New Zealand white rabbit, develops fatty streaks and intimal thickening when fed a high cholesterol diet, with most of the lipids localized within the profuse macrophage-derived foam cells. Lesions are preferentially localized in the aortic arch and the thoracic aorta. More advanced lesions can be induced by performing a balloon injury of the aorta or the carotid artery and further fed with high fat diet. This combined protocol accelerates the formation of atherosclerotic lesions and produces plaques that exhibit a lipid core surrounded by a fibrous cap due to increased proliferation of vascular smooth muscle cells, thus resembling more closely human advanced plaques (Badimon, 2001). Like mice, some rabbit strains carry genetic mutations that lead to hyperlipidemia and atherosclerosis, with the Watanabe heritable hyperlipidemic rabbit being the most commonly used; these animals spontaneously develop lesions due to an inactivating mutation in the gene encoding the LDL receptor (Watanabe,

1980). In these animals the atherosclerosis progresses with age even with a cholesterol-free diet.

One major advantage of the rabbit model is the relatively small animal size, which makes it easy to care, handle and feed, and therefore inexpensive, but large enough to monitor physiological changes and use clinical scanners. Rabbits are favored when imaging arteries; the diameter of the rabbit aorta is 2–4 mm, comparable to the size of human coronary arteries. Imaging techniques such as ultrasound or MRI can be effectively applied to determine the plaque composition and its vulnerability (Helft et al., 2002; Wetterholm et al., 2007; Phinikaridou et al., 2010). The major disadvantage of this model is the relatively slow progression of the pathological condition and the required length of the studies.

However, when trying to obtain close-to-clinical models, pigs and minipigs seem to be the most representative ones. Pigs have a highly comparable anatomy and physiology of the coronary system with humans (White et al., 1986), as well as a very similar lipoprotein profile and metabolism (Dixon et al., 1999). Unlike mice and rabbits, pigs develop spontaneous atherosclerosis during aging, and the development of plaques can be induced by diet, hyperglycemia and by introducing vascular injury, usually by angioplasty. In addition, with use of toxin-mediated pancreatic damage and a high fat diet, human diabetes mellitus-like metabolic alterations will develop, followed by coronary lesions resembling the human condition closely, with even some characteristics of vulnerable plaque (Gerrity et al., 2001). Also, porcine models of familial hypercholesterolemia based on delayed LDL clearance have been shown to develop complex atherosclerotic lesions. The lesions are preferentially localized in the aorta, coronary and iliac arteries, and are characterized by necrotic cores, calcification, neovascularization and intraplaque hemorrhage, closely mimicking advanced human plaques (Prescott et al., 1991). However, the size and composition of the LDL differ in the high-fat diet fed pigs and the familial hypercholesterolemic pigs (Checovich et al., 1988). Although pigs are an excellent model for studying the basic mechanisms, pathophysiology, and progression of atherosclerosis, their high cost of maintenance and longer diet-induction time limit the use of pigs in research of atherosclerosis on a large scale.

The Imaging Modality of Choice for Atherosclerosis Assessment

Different non-invasive imaging modalities can provide information about plaque anatomy and composition. Nonetheless, post-mortem histological analysis of atherosclerotic lesions in experimental animal models (and human autopsies) is fundamental to validate the model and the technique and remains the gold standard.

Ultrasound imaging can be used for plaque detection and analysis in animal models of atherosclerosis (e.g., rabbit, monkey), typically by measuring carotid or aortic wall thickness using high-frequency ultrasound transducers (Zeng et al., 2015). Determination of plaque composition with ultrasound is based on tissue echogenicity: hypoechoic heterogeneous plaque is associated with both intraplaque hemorrhage and lipids, whereas hyperechoic homogeneous plaque is mostly fibrous; however, precise plaque characterization (lipid core, intraplaque hemorrhage, or fibrous cap rupture) is not possible using non-invasive ultrasound measurements and image acquisition is complex and operator dependent. Notably, recent advances with contrast-enhanced ultrasound based on microbubbles have allowed detection of plaque neovascularization and disease progression monitoring (Giannarelli et al., 2010; Nitta-Seko et al., 2010; Tian et al., 2013).

CT is also well suited for studying atherosclerosis non-invasively in all vascular regions, although it requires the use of ionizing radiation and contrast agents. The main advantages of CT include its high spatial resolution and the short scan times, but its major disadvantage for atherosclerotic plaque characterization is the limited discrimination of soft tissue. Although vascular calcification is the main target of this imaging modality, CT can also provide reasonably accurate quantification of plaque size and crude characterization of plaque composition on the basis of lipid-rich tissue attenuating X-rays to a smaller extent than fibrous tissue (Viles-Gonzalez et al., 2004; Cordeiro and Lima, 2006). The development of micro- and nano-CT has allowed higher spatial resolution, enabling in vivo and ex vivo studies in small animal models (Awan et al., 2011). CT imaging can also be merged with positron emission tomographic (PET) modalities, most prominently with ^{18}F-fluorodeoxyglucose (^{18}F-FDG), to study the metabolic state of the vascular lesion in addition to its anatomical features (Vucic et al., 2011).

MRI can provide information on both plaque burden and composition in multiple arterial territories. Compared with other imaging modalities, MRI appears to have the greatest potential for plaque characterization. Based on differences in the biophysical and biochemical properties of the different components of the plaque, it is possible to determine the anatomy and composition of the lesions (lipid-rich necrotic core, fibrous cap, calcification, fibrosis) by combining multiple contrast sequences (T1, T2, and proton-density weightings; Corti and Fuster, 2011). Vulnerability criteria such as ulceration, cap rupture and intraplaque hemorrhage are also easily identifiable. The main advantages of MRI include its high spatial resolution, great soft-tissue contrast, lack of radiation exposure and good clinical translatability. Several studies have validated the feasibility of high resolution MRI to quantify atherosclerosis progression/regression and to determine composition of atherosclerotic lesions in animal models, including mouse (Fayad et al., 1998), rabbit (Helft et al., 2001; Ibanez et al., 2012), and pig (Worthley et al., 2000). **Figure** shows an example of in vivo MRI plaque characterization of rabbit abdominal aorta. Furthermore, use of contrast agents such as gadolinium (Koktzoglou et al., 2006) or ultrasmall paramagnetic iron-oxide particles (Millon et al., 2013) and the possibility of combination with PET (Davies et al., 2005; Millon et al., 2013) can provide information on the inflammatory activity and the presence of macrophages in the plaque. Thus, MRI is an excellent imaging modality to monitor atherosclerotic plaque formation and destabilization in preclinical animal models. Multimodal molecular imaging approaches such as PET/CT, PET/MRI,

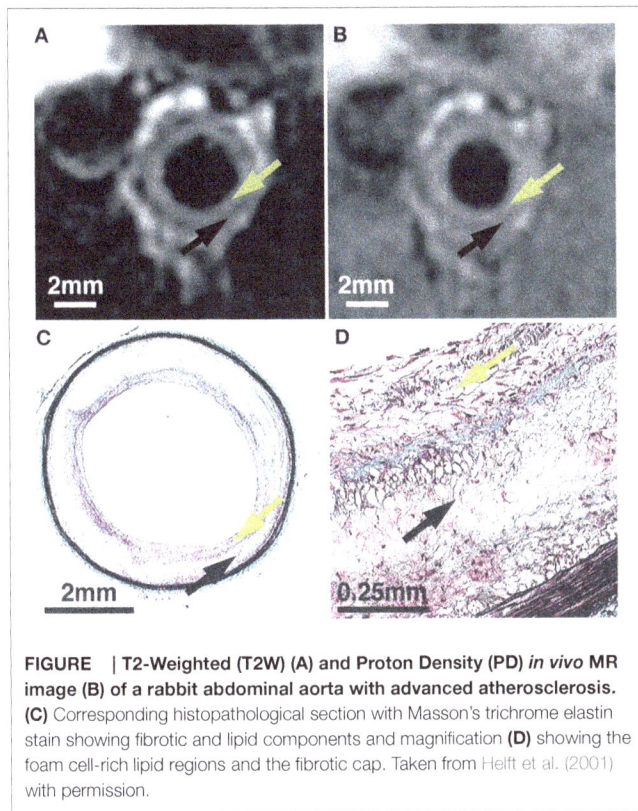

FIGURE | T2-Weighted (T2W) (A) and Proton Density (PD) *in vivo* MR image (B) of a rabbit abdominal aorta with advanced atherosclerosis. (C) Corresponding histopathological section with Masson's trichrome elastin stain showing fibrotic and lipid components and magnification (D) showing the foam cell-rich lipid regions and the fibrotic cap. Taken from Helft et al. (2001) with permission.

MRI-optical, and PET-optical focuses in identifying cellular and molecular targets (e.g., dysfunctional endothelium, mineral deposition, enzymatic activity, inflammation, neovascularization, thrombosis, extracellular matrix production, etc...), and is playing a role in understanding these key biological processes of atherogenesis *in vivo*. The use of coordination chemistry (including various chelates depending on the final application) or colloidal chemistry including metallic nanoparticles or nanosystems such as biocompatible polymers or liposomes, modified or coated with peptides, proteins or antibodies for increasing *in vivo* specificity and target specific molecules. One very recurrent demonstration is the imaging of the vascular cell adhesion molecule (VCAM-1) for what different radiolabeled ligands (Nahrendorf et al., 2009) or nanoparticles functionalized with different molecules have been tested (Kelly et al., 2005; Nahrendorf et al., 2006; Broisat et al., 2012; Michalska et al., 2012). In the road for translation, it is especially relevant the role of different animal models. There are many examples in the bibliography and excellent reviews are continuously covering these new aspects (Nahrendorf et al., 2009; Mulder et al., 2014). These advances are also relevant in other cardiovascular conditions, but for the sake of simplicity we are not covering them.

In addition to the aforementioned non-invasive techniques, optical coherence tomography (OCT), a novel invasive catheter-based technology, has gained much interest as a preclinical tool for plaque characterization. OCT is analogous to ultrasound, measuring the back-reflection of infrared light rather than sound. OCT generates high-resolution (5–20 μm) three-dimensional images with high data acquisition rates and small and inexpensive guidewires/catheters. Its main drawback is the limited tissue penetration (1–3 mm; Stamper et al., 2006).

Animal Models for Pulmonary Hypertension Image Studies

Animal models are indispensable for the advance of imaging in PH. In this disease imaging tools have helped to the mechanistic understanding of PH evaluating pulmonary vasculature and RV function and allowing identification of innovative biomarkers. It is important to recognize that PH accomplish different conditions that finally share a common finding, the chronic increase in pulmonary artery pressure. The conditions that lead to the development of PH are grouped according to the Nice Classification (Simonneau et al., 2013). At the time we need to choose an animal model, this should fit: (a) the primary change that is related with the specific PH that we want to study and (b) the functional and structural changes that occurs in cardiovascular system as consequence of the disease.

Special attention deserves the RV as this is the major determinant of functional state and prognosis in PH (Ryan and Archer, 2014). Usually when RV failure is late diagnosed, patient mortality in a short term and worsening quality of life are increased. In this way, implementation of imaging tools in animal models can be used for detection of early changes in RV and pulmonary vessel function that could be modified preventing worsening and failure.

Echocardiography is probably the most extendedly used imaging tool in PH in both, clinical practice and animal studies. An estimation of the pulmonary artery pressure can be done using a modified Bernoulli equation. Doppler echocardiography provides a non-invasive assessment of the RV structure and function, and it is used to monitor progression and response to therapy. The interval between the onset of flow and peak flow of the pulmonary artery (pulmonary artery acceleration time) is inversely related with pulmonary artery pressure and can be used to estimate the severity of PH (**Figure**).

MRI is becoming the gold standard in the study of patients with PH and also its application in animal studies is increasing. MRI facilitates a well-detailed anatomical description of RV. Using MRI important advances have been done in the description of flow in 2D and 3D (4D) bringing new insights related with functional hemodynamic changes during PH. MRI allows the simultaneous measurement of pulmonary artery area and flow velocity allowing complex hemodynamic assessment. This assessment includes the calculus of wave speed and the evaluation of wave reflection phenomena. Also, PA distensibility can be estimated by area changes in PA.

CT can be a diagnostic and also a complimentary tool in PH. It is nowadays the reference tool for diagnosis of pulmonary embolism, which is involved in the etiology of chronic thromboembolic PH. CT provides unbeaten structural information of the lungs which is essential to reveal the direct relation between lung parenchyma and pulmonary vessels.

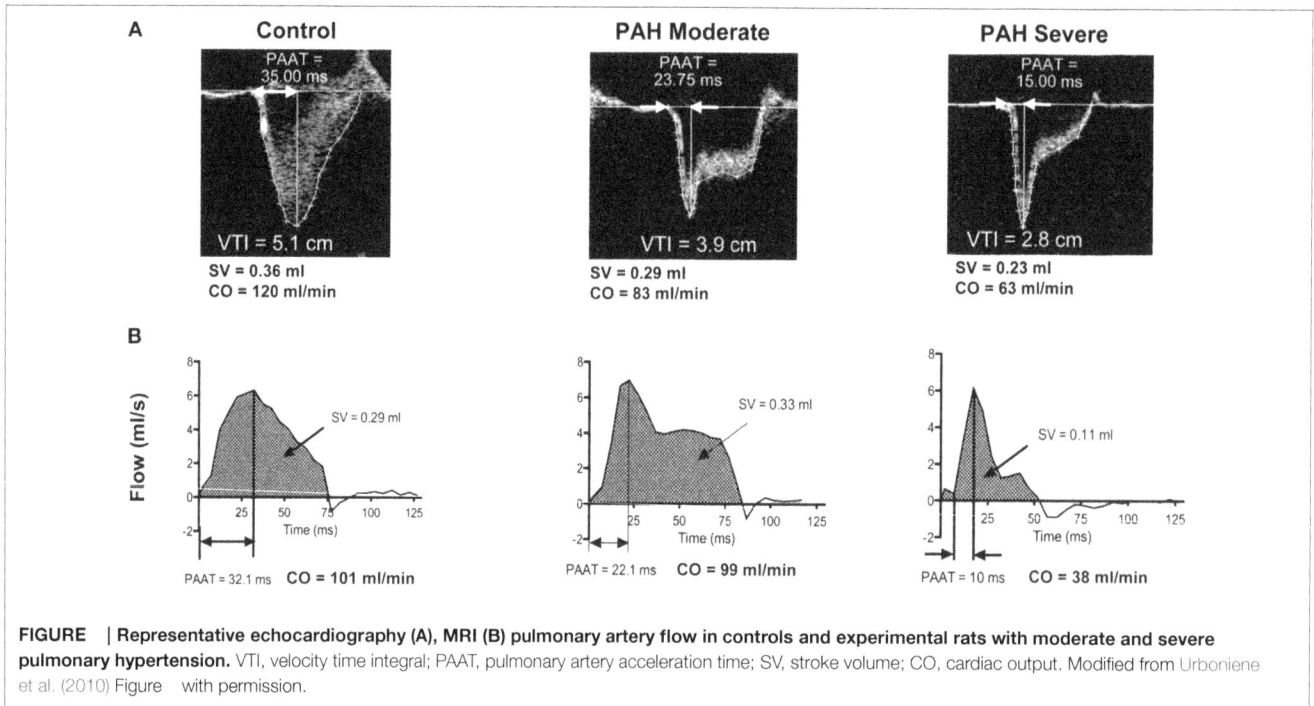

FIGURE | Representative echocardiography (A), MRI (B) pulmonary artery flow in controls and experimental rats with moderate and severe pulmonary hypertension. VTI, velocity time integral; PAAT, pulmonary artery acceleration time; SV, stroke volume; CO, cardiac output. Modified from Urboniene et al. (2010) Figure with permission.

PET is less used in clinical practice and is not a routine tool for the evaluation of PH patients. However, new mechanistic insides are described due to its ability of tracking complex process such as cellular proliferation, metabolic pathways, inflammation, and ventilation/perfusion distribution. These processes can be critical in the understanding of PH physiopathology and can also be used in the near future for patient follow-up and therapeutic targeting. All this has made PET a promising field for new animal and clinical studies.

No animal model is perfect in any of the PH types. This is due to the complex changes related with vessel remodeling, which involve different molecular and cellular pathways and depend on multiple variables. Models that combine multiple insults yield more severe PH with better hemodynamic and histological fidelity to human pathology. However, animal models can represent specific changes that can be studied. Given this, we can describe the different animal models used in PH as follows:

- An increase in the pulmonary vasomotor tone caused by hypoxia. This model resembles pulmonary arterial hypertension (Group 1 of the Nice classification). Hypoxia can be created in a normobaric or hypobaric environment. This model is used in small animal, as the animal should be enclosed in the hypoxic environment. Rats exposed to this model show a decrease in blood flow velocity measured by dynamic MRI (de La Roque et al., 2011). Novel experimental treatments for PH have been tested using this model. For example, treatment with dehydroepiandrosterone improves the right ventricular systolic and diastolic functions assessed by Doppler echocardiography (Dumas de La Roque et al., 2012).

Although causing an elevation in pulmonary artery pressure, chronic hypoxia is associated with minimal vascular remodeling,

which limits its use (Ciuclan et al., 2011). More recently, vascular endothelial growth factor receptor (VEGF-R) blockade with the tyrosine kinase inhibitor SU5416 have been introduced and the SU5416 plus chronic hypoxia model is now being extensively used (de Raaf et al., 2014). This model features angio-obliterative PH resembling human pulmonary arterial hypertension and also increases RV pressure and RV hypertrophy comparing to mice just submitted to chronic hypoxia (Ciuclan et al., 2011). Dehydroepiandrosterone was also tested in this model. Echocardiography data showed that this drug significantly reduced RV internal diameter during diastole and restored the normal position and orientation of the interventricular septum, which had been otherwise flattened (Alzoubi et al., 2013).

- Endothelial damage produced by monocrotaline. This model also resembles Group 1 of the Nice Classification. Monocrotaline elicits pulmonary arterial endothelial cells dysfunction on multiple levels but is characterized by pulmonary artery arterial medial hypertrophy and not by endothelial cell-mediated angioobliteration (the last is present in the human disease and in the SU5416/hypoxia model). Monocrotaline has been well described to produce RV failure, however is criticized because it does not produce plexogenic arteriopathy, but produces left and RV myocarditis (Gomez-Arroyo et al., 2012). Using FDG PET authors have shown an increase in glucose uptake during compensated RV hypertrophy, which was reversed during decompensated RV hypertrophy (Sutendra et al., 2013). This behavior was paralleled by activated hypoxia-inducible factor 1 α (HIF1α) and angiogenesis evaluated by means of lectin imaging in vivo (Sutendra et al., 2013). Several proposed treatments have been evaluated in this model. Using echocardiography, sildenafil, pimobendam (a calcium sensitizer and phosphodiesterase inhibitor) and nicorandil (a vasodilator) were tested. The 2D mode in echocardiography and tissue Doppler imaging data indicated improved cardiac morphology and function in all treatment groups (Nakata et al., 2015). Authors showed that Carvedilol improves fibrosis and hemodynamic behavior despite persistent RV increased afterload. Carvedilol improved tricuspid annular displacement and global LV radial and RV longitudinal strain (Okumura et al., 2015). Other investigators tested Macitentan therapy showing an increase in pulmonary artery acceleration time and a decreased deceleration time and decreased RV wall thickness with this therapy (Temple et al., 2014).

- Decrease in the total vessel area produced by clots or beads injection. These models resemble chronic thromboembolic PH (Group 4 of the Nice classification). An increase in pulmonary artery pressure and resistance as well as signs of RV remodeling have been described after repeated injections of beads. Different protocols of injection has been tested to find an important increase in pulmonary artery pressure and resistance without causing death of the animal. Using microbeads injection in dogs authors have demonstrated that both magnitude and flow-sensitive data from a single 4D flow CMR acquisition permit simultaneous quantification of cardiac function and cardiopulmonary hemodynamic parameters important in the assessment of PH (Roldán-Alzate et al., 2014). The same authors demonstrated the benefit of using the same sequence for measuring cardiac chamber volumes and flow resulting in an overall shortened examination acquisition time (Roldán-Alzate et al., 2014).

- Increase in the pulmonary artery flow produced by shunt. The mechanisms of PH with left-to-right shunt are different from those of hypoxia and inflammation. Possible inciting factors of the former are mechanical stretch and shear stress. MRI was evaluated in rats with aortocaval shunt to reliably produce right ventricular volume overload and secondary PH. Due to a combination of left ventricular dysfunction and pulmonary overflow, the PH produced show features similar to those found in patients with chronic atrial-level shunt. The RV end-diastolic area and the thickness of the RV free wall increased significantly and a mesosystolic notch was demonstrated in the Doppler wave profile of the pulmonary flow after 20 weeks of shunt (Linardi et al., 2014).

- Pulmonary vessels (artery or vein) decrease in compliance and increase in resistance produced by banding. These models resemble PH due to left heart disease (Group 2 of the Nice Classification). Selecting artery or vein a model of pre or post-capillary PH can be developed. A porcine model of postcapillary PH by non-restrictive banding of the confluent of both inferior pulmonary veins was developed and evaluated (Pereda et al., 2014). All banded animals developed PH. Ventricular remodeling produced progressive increase in end diastolic and systolic volumes of the RV, an increase in its mass, and an EF decrease. Also this model consistently reproduced most pathology changes usually seen on pulmonary arterial circulation, including intimal fibrosis (Pereda et al., 2014). In a precapillary PH model by pulmonary artery banding, early

compensatory mechanisms of the RA and RV response to RV pressure overload were investigated (Voeller et al., 2011). In this study, MRI with tissue tagging was used to measure circumferential and minimum principle strain. The resulting data revealed that early RV pressure overload, without chamber enlargement, has a measurable effect on RA function and RV strain patterns when overload is severe. With a 2.5-fold rise in RV afterload, RV filling became more dependent on RA conduit than reservoir function, which likely reflects loss of RV diastolic compliance and consequent stiffening of the RA and RV walls (Voeller et al., 2011).

- In some studies, authors have combined different models of PH. For example, using the monocrotaline plus pulmonary artery banding, the inhibition of pyruvate dehydrogenase kinase by dichloroacetate on RV hypertrophy was evaluated (Piao et al., 2010). The rationale for combining two models was that in the monocrotaline model, there is an intrinsic coupling between severity of RV hypertrophy and severity of the pulmonary vascular disease, while pulmonary artery banding results in RV hypertrophy secondary to pure pressure overload. The study was performed by echocardiography and PET. FDG uptake in RV and the RV/LV FDG was increased in monocrotaline and pulmonary artery banded rats. Dichloroacetate tended to reduce FDG uptake ratio and also improved the pulmonary artery acceleration time (Piao et al., 2010).

A recent report includes three different models (one acute and two chronic) of PH and one vasodilator testing to validate a CMR estimation of pulmonary vascular resistance (García-Álvarez et al., 2013). Acute and chronic beads embolization and pulmonary vein banding were used as models of PH. They showed that changes in pulmonary artery velocity inversely correlate with pulmonary vascular resistance and that MRI can be used to track acute and chronic in PVR (García-Álvarez et al., 2013).

Cardiovascular Imaging for Translational Research

Nowadays, we have the possibility of using in animal research the same cardiovascular imaging technology used for human diagnosis to establish the severity and prognosis of diseases. Imaging systems and methods previously described provide a common link between humans and experimental animal models for identifying common phenotypes of cardiovascular diseases in their functional and morphological aspects. Tissue characterization by MRI in the evaluation of necrosis, fibrosis, fat, perfusion, flow, and myocardial edema and in the evaluation of cardiovascular pathologies is one of the vanguard tools for clinical and translational research. Nuclear medicine based techniques for molecular imaging using PET or SPECT for myocardial metabolic and perfusion characterization have been used for years. PET is currently used for human atherosclerosis and FDG PET has recently gained a role in the assessment of patients with PH. Due to the high sensitivity of these nuclear medicine based protocols, applications are surely in a prominent position to investigate novel metabolic and cellular targets in animal models with potential human translation. Similar or alternative molecular procedures for MRI are based in Gadolinium, Fluorine, iron oxide nanoparticles, and recently in hyperpolarization procedures (Schroeder et al., 2008; Bhattacharya et al., 2009; Rider and Tyler, 2013). Despite the many examples targeting multiple molecular and cellular pathways in animal models, the reduced sensitivity of MRI probably hampers its further development on translational research. However, cardiovascular hybrid imaging including MRI technology are leading tools for new translational research, since they provide simultaneous or sequential acquisitions covering molecular, functional, cellular and tissue characterization of different cardiovascular disease phenotypes.

Conclusions

Imaging technologies for the study of cardiovascular diseases are in constant progress and their relevance in the guidance of patients will probably expand in the next years. Specific structural, functional and molecular changes will be surely be observed by imaging technologies. In this process, the discovery of new pathophysiological pathways will bring new approaches for both diagnostic and therapeutics targets. This growth will also generate new hypotheses and original research lines will consequently emerge. During this phase, any innovative imaging technology will require to be tested in specific disease mimicking malignant conditions and new imaging tracers to study particular molecular and physiological changes will also be evaluated using imaging methodologies. All these examples will always require the optimization of animal models trying to find a better approach to the human disease.

Author Contributions

AS, LF, MV, BL, SE, JM, RM, JJ, and JR participated in the conception, design and draft of this review and agree to be accountable for all aspects of the work in ensuring that questions related to the accuracy or integrity of any part of the work are appropriately investigated and resolved.

Funding

AS and SE are M+Visión COFUND Advanced Fellows and have received funding from Consejería de Educación, Juventud y Deporte of Comunidad de Madrid and the People Programme (Marie Curie Actions) of the European Union's Seventh Framework Programme (FP7/2007-2013) under REA grant agreement n° 291820.

Acknowledgments

Figure use a figure from Coolen et al. (2011). Figure was taken from Bryson-Richardson et al. (2007).

References

Abarbanell, A. M., Herrmann, J. L., Weil, B. R., Wang, Y., Tan, J., Moberly, S. P., et al. (2010). Animal models of myocardial and vascular injury. *J. Surg. Res.* 162, 239–249. doi: 10.1016/j.jss.2009.06.021

Adams, M. C., Turkington, T. G., Wilson, J. M., and Wong, T. Z. (2010). A systematic review of the factors affecting accuracy of SUV measurements. *AJR Am. J. Roentgenol.* 195, 310–320. doi: 10.2214/AJR.10.4923

Aletras, A. H., Tilak, G. S., Natanzon, A., Hsu, L. Y., Gonzalez, F. M., Hoyt, R. F. Jr., et al. (2006). Retrospective determination of the area at risk for reperfused acute myocardial infarction with T2-weighted cardiac magnetic resonance imaging: histopathological and displacement encoding with stimulated echoes (DENSE) functional validations. *Circulation* 113, 1865–1870. doi: 10.1161/CIRCULATIONAHA.105.576025

Alsaid, H., Bao, W., Rambo, M. V., Logan, G. A., Figueroa, D. J., Lenhard, S. C., et al. (2012). Serial MRI characterization of the functional and morphological changes in mouse lung in response to cardiac remodeling following myocardial infarction. *Magn. Reson. Med.* 67, 191–200. doi: 10.1002/mrm.22973

Alzoubi, A., Toba, M., Abe, K., O'Neill, K. D., Rocic, P., Fagan, K. A., et al. (2013). Dehydroepiandrosterone restores right ventricular structure and function in rats with severe pulmonary arterial hypertension. *Am. J. Physiol. Heart Circ. Physiol.* 304, H1708–H1718. doi: 10.1152/ajpheart.00746.2012

Awan, Z., Denis, M., Bailey, D., Giaid, A., Prat, A., Goltzman, D., et al. (2011). The LDLR deficient mouse as a model for aortic calcification and quantification by micro-computed tomography. *Atherosclerosis* 219, 455–462. doi: 10.1016/j.atherosclerosis.2011.08.035

Babiker, F. A., Lips, D. J., Delvaux, E., Zandberg, P., Janssen, B. J., Prinzen, F., et al. (2007). Oestrogen modulates cardiac ischaemic remodelling through oestrogen receptor-specific mechanisms. *Acta Physiol. (Oxf).* 189, 23–31. doi: 10.1111/j.1748-1716.2006.01633.x

Badimon, L. (2001). Atherosclerosis and thrombosis: lessons from animal models. *Thromb. Haemost.* 86, 356–365.

Bao, W., Aravindhan, K., Alsaid, H., Chendrimada, T., Szapacs, M., Citerone, D. R., et al. (2011). Albiglutide, a long lasting glucagon-like peptide-1 analog, protects the rat heart against ischemia/reperfusion injury: evidence for improving cardiac metabolic efficiency. *PLoS ONE* 6:e23570. doi: 10.1371/journal.pone.0023570

Bao, W., Ballard, V. L., Needle, S., Hoang, B., Lenhard, S. C., Tunstead, J. R., et al. (2013). Cardioprotection by systemic dosing of thymosin beta four following ischemic myocardial injury. *Front. Pharmacol.* 4:149. doi: 10.3389/fphar.2013.00149

Basso, C., Fox, P. R., Meurs, K. M., Towbin, J. A., Spier, A. W., Calabrese, F., et al. (2004). Arrhythmogenic right ventricular cardiomyopathy causing sudden cardiac death in boxer dogs: a new animal model of human disease. *Circulation* 109, 1180–1185. doi: 10.1161/01.CIR.0000118494.07530.65

Bauer, M., Cheng, S., Jain, M., Ngoy, S., Theodoropoulos, C., Trujillo, A., et al. (2011). Echocardiographic speckle-tracking based strain imaging for rapid cardiovascular phenotyping in mice. *Circ. Res.* 108, 908–916. doi: 10.1161/CIRCRESAHA.110.239574

Bengel, F. M., Higuchi, T., Javadi, M. S., and Lautamäki, R. (2009). Cardiac positron emission tomography. *J. Am. Coll. Cardiol.* 54, 1–15. doi: 10.1016/j.jacc.2009.02.065

Bers, D. M. (2001). "Control of cardiac contraction by SR and sarcolemmal Ca fluxes," in *Excitation-Contraction Coupling and Cardiac Contractile Force*, Vol. 237 (Dordrecht: Springer), 245–272.

Bhattacharya, P., Ross, B. D., and Bünger, R. (2009). Cardiovascular applications of hyperpolarized contrast media and metabolic tracers. *Exp. Biol. Med. (Maywood).* 234, 1395–1416. doi: 10.3181/0904-MR-135

Bianco, R. W., Gallegos, R. P., Rivard, A. L., Voight, J., and Dalmasso, A. P. (2009). "Animal models for cardiac research," in *Handbook of Cardiac Anatomy,*

Physiology, and Devices, 2nd Edn, ed P. A. Iaizzo (Minneapolis, MN: Springer Science + Business Media), 393–410.

Bode, G., Clausing, P., Gervais, F., Loegsted, J., Luft, J., Nogues, V., et al. (2010). The utility of the minipig as an animal model in regulatory toxicology. *J. Pharmacol. Toxicol. Methods* 62, 196–220. doi: 10.1016/j.vascn.2010.05.009

Bostick, B., Yue, Y., and Duan, D. (2011). Phenotyping cardiac gene therapy in mice. *Methods Mol. Biol.* 709, 91–104. doi: 10.1007/978-1-61737-982-6_6

Bottomley, P. A., Wu, K. C., Gerstenblith, G., Schulman, S. P., Steinberg, A., and Weiss, R. G. (2009). Reduced myocardial creatine kinase flux in human myocardial infarction: an *in vivo* phosphorus magnetic resonance spectroscopy study. *Circulation* 119, 1918–1924. doi: 10.1161/CIRCULATIONAHA.108.823187

Broisat, A., Hernot, S., Toczek, J., De Vos, J., Riou, L. M., Martin, S., et al. (2012). Nanobodies targeting mouse/human VCAM1 for the nuclear imaging of atherosclerotic lesions. *Circ. Res.* 110, 927–937. doi: 10.1161/CIRCRESAHA.112.265140

Bryson-Richardson, R. J., Berger, S., Schilling, T. F., Hall, T. E., Cole, N. J., Gibson, A. J., et al. (2007). FishNet: an online database of zebrafish anatomy. *BMC Biol.* 5:34. doi: 10.1186/1741-7007-5-34

Bunck, A. C., Engelen, M. A., Schnackenburg, B., Furkert, J., Bremer, C., Heindel, W., et al. (2009). Feasibility of functional cardiac MR imaging in mice using a clinical 3 Tesla whole body scanner. *Invest. Radiol.* 44, 749–756. doi: 10.1097/RLI.0b013e3181b2c135

Carlsson, M., Ubachs, J. F., Hedström, E., Heiberg, E., Jovinge, S., and Arheden, H. (2009). Myocardium at risk after acute infarction in humans on cardiac magnetic resonance: quantitative assessment during follow-up and validation with single-photon emission computed tomography. *JACC Cardiovasc. Imaging* 2, 569–576. doi: 10.1016/j.jcmg.2008.11.018

Cassidy, P. J., Schneider, J. E., Grieve, S. M., Lygate, C., Neubauer, S., and Clarke, K. (2004). Assessment of motion gating strategies for mouse magnetic resonance at high magnetic fields. *J. Magn. Resonance Imaging* 19, 229–237. doi: 10.1002/jmri.10454

Ciuclan, L., Bonneau, O., Hussey, M., Duggan, N., Holmes, A. M., Good, R., et al. (2011). A novel murine model of severe pulmonary arterial hypertension. *Am. J. Respir. Crit. Care Med.* 184, 1171–1182. doi: 10.1164/rccm.201103-0412OC

Constantinides, C. (2013). "Study of the murine cardiac mechanical function using magnetic resonance imaging: the current status, challenges, and future perspectives," in *Practical Applications in Biomedical Engineering*, eds A. A. P. A. O. Andrade, E. L. M. Naves, and A. B. Soares (Rijeka: InTech). doi: 10.5772/51364

Coolen, B. F., Geelen, T., Paulis, L. E., Nicolay, K., and Strijkers, G. J. (2011). Regional contrast agent quantification in a mouse model of myocardial infarction using 3D cardiac T1 mapping. *J. Cardiovasc. Magn. Reson.* 13:56. doi: 10.1186/1532-429X-13-56

Cordeiro, M. A. S., and Lima, J. A. C. (2006). Atherosclerotic plaque characterization by multidetector row computed tomography angiography. *J. Am. Coll. Cardiol.* 47(8 Suppl.), C40–C47. doi: 10.1016/j.jacc.2005.09.076

Corti, R., and Fuster, V. (2011). Imaging of atherosclerosis: magnetic resonance imaging. *Eur. Heart J.* 32, 1709b–1719b. doi: 10.1093/eurheartj/ehr068

Crick, S. J., Sheppard, M. N., Ho, S. Y., Gebstein, L., and Anderson, R. H. (1998). Anatomy of the pig heart: comparisons with normal human cardiac structure. *J. Anat.* 193(Pt 1), 105–119. doi: 10.1046/j.1469-7580.1998.19310105.x

Cruz, F. M., Sanz-Rosa, D., Roche-Molina, M., García-Prieto, J., García-Ruiz, J. M., Pizarro, G., et al. (2015). Exercise triggers ARVC phenotype in mice expressing a disease-causing mutated version of human plakophilin-2. *J. Am. Coll. Cardiol.* 65, 1438–1450. doi: 10.1016/j.jacc.2015.01.045

Chappell, D., Heindl, B., Jacob, M., Annecke, T., Chen, C., Rehm, M., et al. (2011). Sevoflurane reduces leukocyte and platelet adhesion after ischemia-reperfusion by protecting the endothelial glycocalyx. *Anesthesiology* 115, 483–491. doi: 10.1097/ALN.0b013e3182289988

Checovich, W. J., Fitch, W. L., Krauss, R. M., Smith, M. P., Rapacz, J., Smith, C. L., et al. (1988). Defective catabolism and abnormal composition of low-density lipoproteins from mutant pigs with hypercholesterolemia. *Biochemistry* 27, 1934–1941. doi: 10.1021/bi00406a020

Chen, G., Li, Y., Tian, J., Zhang, L., Jean-Charles, P., Gobara, N., et al. (2012). Application of echocardiography on transgenic mice with cardiomyopathies. *Biochem. Res. Int.* 2012, 715197–715199. doi: 10.1155/2012/715197

Cheng, H.-W., Fisch, S., Cheng, S., Bauer, M., Ngoy, S., Qiu, Y., et al. (2014). Assessment of right ventricular structure and function in mouse model of pulmonary artery constriction by transthoracic echocardiography. *J. Vis. Exp.* 84:e51041. doi: 10.3791/51041

Chien, K. R. (1996). Genes and physiology: molecular physiology in genetically engineered animals. *J. Clin. Invest.* 97, 901–909. doi: 10.1172/JCI118512

Chung, J., Liu, H., Jeong, E.-M., Gu, L., Gladstein, S., Farzaneh-Far, A., et al. (2013). *In vivo* validation of an ultra-high field, high temporal resolution myocardial tagging technique for assessment of diastolic function in mice. *J. Cardiovasc. Magn. Reson.* 15(Suppl. 1), P129. doi: 10.1186/1532-429X-15-S1-P129

Davies, J. R., Rudd, J. H. F., Fryer, T. D., Graves, M. J., Clark, J. C., Kirkpatrick, P. J., et al. (2005). Identification of culprit lesions after transient ischemic attack by combined 18F fluorodeoxyglucose positron-emission tomography and high-resolution magnetic resonance imaging. *Stroke* 36, 2642–2647. doi: 10.1161/01.STR.0000190896.67743.b1

de La Roque, E. D., Thiaudière, E., Ducret, T., Marthan, R., Franconi, J. M., Guibert, C., et al. (2011). Effect of chronic hypoxia on pulmonary artery blood velocity in rats as assessed by electrocardiography-triggered three-dimensional time-resolved MR angiography. *NMR Biomed.* 24, 225–230. doi: 10.1002/nbm.1574

de Raaf, M. A., Schalij, I., Gomez-Arroyo, J., Rol, N., Happé, C., de Man, F. S., et al. (2014). SuHx rat model: partly reversible pulmonary hypertension and progressive intima obstruction. *Eur. Respir. J.* 44, 160–168. doi: 10.1183/09031936.00204813

Di Carli, M. F., Dorbala, S., Meserve, J., El Fakhri, G., Sitek, A., and Moore, S. C. (2007). Clinical myocardial perfusion PET/CT. *J. Nucl. Med.* 48, 783–793. doi: 10.2967/jnumed.106.032789

Dilsizian, V., Bacharach, S. L., Beanlands, R. S., Bergmann, S. R., Delbeke, D., Gropler, R. J., et al. (2009). PET myocardial perfusion and metabolism clinical imaging. *J. Nucl. Cardiol.* 16, 651–651. doi: 10.1007/s12350-009-9094-9

Dixon, J. A., and Spinale, F. G. (2009). Large animal models of heart failure: a critical link in the translation of basic science to clinical practice. *Circ. Heart Fail.* 2, 262–271. doi: 10.1161/CIRCHEARTFAILURE.108.814459

Dixon, J. L., Stoops, J. D., Parker, J. L., Laughlin, M. H., Weisman, G. A., and Sturek, M. (1999). Dyslipidemia and vascular dysfunction in diabetic pigs fed an atherogenic diet. *Arterioscler. Thromb. Vasc. Biol.* 19, 2981–2992. doi: 10.1161/01.ATV.19.12.2981

Doevendans, P. A., Daemen, M. J., de Muinck, E. D., and Smits, J. F. (1998). Cardiovascular phenotyping in mice. *Cardiovasc. Res.* 39, 34–49. doi: 10.1016/S0008-6363(98)00073-X

Doevendans, P. A., Hunter, J. J., Lembo, G., and Wollert, K. C. (1995). "Strategies for studying cardiovascular diseases in transgenic mice and gene-targeted mice," in *Transgenic Animal Science*, ed R. J. Monastersky (Washington, DC: American Socity of Microbiology), 107–144.

Dumas de La Roque, E., Bellance, N., Rossignol, R., Begueret, H., Billaud, M., dos Santos, P., et al. (2012). Dehydroepiandrosterone reverses chronic hypoxia/reoxygenation-induced right ventricular dysfunction in rats. *Eur. Respir. J.* 40, 1420–1429. doi: 10.1183/09031936.00011511

Epstein, F. H., Yang, Z., Gilson, W. D., Berr, S. S., Kramer, C. M., and French, B. A. (2002). MR tagging early after myocardial infarction in mice demonstrates contractile dysfunction in adjacent and remote regions. *Magn. Reson. Med.* 48, 399–403. doi: 10.1002/mrm.10210

Espe, E. K., Aronsen, J. M., Eriksen, G. S., Zhang, L., Smiseth, O. A., Edvardsen, T., et al. (2015). Assessment of regional myocardial work in rats. *Circ. Cardiovasc. Imaging* 8:e002695. doi: 10.1161/CIRCIMAGING.114.002695

Fayad, Z. A., Fallon, J. T., Shinnar, M., Wehrli, S., Dansky, H. M., Poon, M., et al. (1998). Noninvasive *in vivo* high-resolution magnetic resonance imaging of atherosclerotic lesions in genetically engineered mice. *Circulation* 98, 1541–1547. doi: 10.1161/01.CIR.98.15.1541

Fayssoil, A., and Tournoux, F. (2013). Analyzing left ventricular function in mice with Doppler echocardiography. *Heart Fail. Rev.* 18, 511–516. doi: 10.1007/s10741-012-9345-8

Feiring, A. J., Johnson, M. R., Kioschos, J. M., Kirchner, P. T., Marcus, M. L., and White, C. W. (1987). The importance of the determination of the myocardial area at risk in the evaluation of the outcome of acute myocardial infarction in patients. *Circulation* 75, 980–987. doi: 10.1161/01.CIR.75.5.980

Ferferieva, V., Van den Bergh, A., Claus, P., Jasaityte, R., La Gerche, A., Rademakers, F., et al. (2013). Assessment of strain and strain rate by two-dimensional speckle tracking in mice: comparison with tissue Doppler echocardiography and conductance catheter measurements. *Eur. Heart J. Cardiovasc. Imaging* 14, 765–773. doi: 10.1093/ehjci/jes274

Fernández-Friera, L., García-Álvarez, A., and Ibáñez, B. (2013). Imaginando el futuro del diagnóstico por imagen. *Rev. Esp. Cardiol.* 66, 134–143. doi: 10.1016/j.recesp.2012.10.012

Fernández-Jiménez, R., García-Prieto, J., Sánchez-González, J., Agüero, J., López-Martín, G. J., Galán-Arriola, C., et al. (2015a). Pathophysiology Underlying the Bimodal Edema Phenomenon After Myocardial Ischemia/Reperfusion. *J. Am. Coll. Cardiol.* 66, 816–828. doi: 10.1016/j.jacc.2015.06.023

Fernandez-Jimenez, R., Sanchez-Gonzalez, J., Aguero, J., Garcia-Prieto, J., Lopez-Martin, G. J., Garcia-Ruiz, J. M., et al. (2015b). Myocardial edema after ischemia/reperfusion is not stable and follows a bimodal pattern: imaging and histological tissue characterization. *J. Am. Coll. Cardiol.* 65, 315–323. doi: 10.1016/j.jacc.2014.11.004

Finsen, A. V., Christensen, G., and Sjaastad, I. (2005). Echocardiographic parameters discriminating myocardial infarction with pulmonary congestion from myocardial infarction without congestion in the mouse. *J. Appl. Physiol.* 98, 680–689. doi: 10.1152/japplphysiol.00924.2004

Foryst-Ludwig, A., Kreissl, M. C., Sprang, C., Thalke, B., Böhm, C., Benz, V., et al. (2011). Sex differences in physiological cardiac hypertrophy are associated with exercise-mediated changes in energy substrate availability. *Am. J. Physiol. Heart Circ. Physiol.* 301, H115–H122. doi: 10.1152/ajpheart. 01222.2010

Franco, F., Thomas, G. D., Giroir, B., Bryant, D., Bullock, M. C., Chwialkowski, M. C., et al. (1999). Magnetic resonance imaging and invasive evaluation of development of heart failure in transgenic mice with myocardial expression of tumor necrosis factor-alpha. *Circulation* 99, 448–454. doi: 10.1161/01.CIR.99.3.448

Friedrich, M. G., Abdel-Aty, H., Taylor, A., Schulz-Menger, J., Messroghli, D., and Dietz, R. (2008). The salvaged area at risk in reperfused acute myocardial infarction as visualized by cardiovascular magnetic resonance. *J. Am. Coll. Cardiol.* 51, 1581–1587. doi: 10.1016/j.jacc.2008.01.019

Fuster, J. J., Castillo, A. I., Zaragoza, C., Ibáñez, B., and Andrés, V. (2012). Animal models of atherosclerosis. *Prog. Mol. Biol. Transl. Sci.* 105, 1–23. doi: 10.1016/B978-0-12-394596-9.00001-9

Gao, X. M., Dart, A. M., Dewar, E., Jennings, G., and Du, X. J. (2000). Serial echocardiographic assessment of left ventricular dimensions and function after myocardial infarction in mice. *Cardiovasc. Res.* 45, 330–338. doi: 10.1016/S0008-6363(99)00274-6

García-Álvarez, A., Fernández-Friera, L., García-Ruiz, J. M., Nuño-Ayala, M., Pereda, D., Fernández-Jiménez, R., et al. (2013). Noninvasive monitoring of serial changes in pulmonary vascular resistance and acute vasodilator testing using cardiac magnetic resonance. *J. Am. Coll. Cardiol.* 62, 1621–1631. doi: 10.1016/j.jacc.2013.07.037

García-Álvarez, A., García-Lunar, I., Pereda, D., Fernández-Jimenez, R., Sánchez-González, J., Mirelis, J. G., et al. (2015). Association of myocardial T1-mapping CMR with hemodynamics and RV performance in pulmonary hypertension. *JACC Cardiovasc. Imaging* 8, 76–82. doi: 10.1016/j.jcmg.2014.08.012

Gargiulo, S., Greco, A., Gramanzini, M., Esposito, S., Affuso, A., Brunetti, A., et al. (2012a). Mice anesthesia, analgesia, and care, Part II: anesthetic considerations in preclinical imaging studies. *ILAR J.* 53, E70–E81. doi: 10.1093/ilar.53.1.70

Gargiulo, S., Greco, A., Gramanzini, M., Petretta, M. P., Ferro, A., Larobina, M., et al. (2012b). PET/CT imaging in mouse models of myocardial ischemia. *J. Biomed. Biotechnol.* 2012, 541872–541812. doi: 10.1155/2012/541872

Ge, Z. D., Pravdic, D., Bienengraeber, M., Pratt, P. F. Jr., Auchampach, J. A., Gross, G. J., et al. (2010). Isoflurane postconditioning protects against reperfusion injury by preventing mitochondrial permeability transition by an endothelial nitric oxide synthase-dependent mechanism. *Anesthesiology* 112, 73–85. doi: 10.1097/ALN.0b013e3181c4a607

Gerrity, R. G., Natarajan, R., Nadler, J. L., and Kimsey, T. (2001). Diabetes-induced accelerated atherosclerosis in swine. *Diabetes* 50, 1654–1665. doi: 10.2337/diabetes.50.7.1654

Giannarelli, C., Ibanez, B., Cimmino, G., Garcia Ruiz, J. M., Faita, F., Bianchini, E., et al. (2010). Contrast-enhanced ultrasound imaging detects intraplaque neovascularization in an experimental model of atherosclerosis. *JACC Cardiovasc. Imaging* 3, 1256–1264. doi: 10.1016/j.jcmg.2010. 09.017

Gilson, W. D., and Kraitchman, D. L. (2007). Cardiac magnetic resonance imaging in small rodents using clinical 1.5 T and 3.0 T scanners. *Methods* 43, 35–45. doi: 10.1016/j.ymeth.2007.03.012

Gomez-Arroyo, J. G., Farkas, L., Alhussaini, A. A., Farkas, D., Kraskauskas, D., Voelkel, N. F., et al. (2012). The monocrotaline model of pulmonary hypertension in perspective. *Am. J. Physiol. Lung Cell. Mol. Physiol.* 302, L363–L369. doi: 10.1152/ajplung.00212.2011

González-Rosa, J. M., Guzmán-Martínez, G., Marques, I. J., Sánchez-Iranzo, H., Jiménez-Borreguero, L. J., and Mercader, N. (2014). Use of echocardiography reveals reestablishment of ventricular pumping efficiency and partial ventricular wall motion recovery upon ventricular cryoinjury in the zebrafish. *PLoS ONE* 9:e115604. doi: 10.1371/journal.pone.0115604

Grieve, S. M., Lønborg, J., Mazhar, J., Tan, T. C., Ho, E., Liu, C. C., et al. (2013). Cardiac magnetic resonance imaging of rapid VCAM-1 up-regulation in myocardial ischemia-reperfusion injury. *Eur. Biophys. J.* 42, 61–70. doi: 10.1007/s00249-012-0857-x

Groten, T., Pierce, A. A., Huen, A. C., and Schnaper, H. W. (2005). 17 β-estradiol transiently disrupts adherens junctions in endothelial cells. *FASEB J* 19, 1368–1370. doi: 10.1096/fj.04-2558fje

Hasenfuss, G. (1998). Animal models of human cardiovascular disease, heart failure and hypertrophy. *Cardiovasc. Res.* 39, 60–76. doi: 10.1016/S0008-6363(98)00110-2

Hearse, D. J., and Sutherland, F. J. (2000). Experimental models for the study of cardiovascular function and disease. *Pharmacol. Res.* 41, 597–603. doi: 10.1006/phrs.1999.0651

Helft, G., Worthley, S. G., Fuster, V., Fayad, Z. A., Zaman, A. G., Corti, R., et al. (2002). Progression and regression of atherosclerotic lesions: monitoring with serial noninvasive magnetic resonance imaging. *Circulation* 105, 993–998. doi: 10.1161/hc0802.104325

Helft, G., Worthley, S. G., Fuster, V., Zaman, A. G., Schechter, C., Osende, J. I., et al. (2001). Atherosclerotic aortic component quantification by noninvasive magnetic resonance imaging: an in vivo study in rabbits. *J. Am. Coll. Cardiol.* 37, 1149–1154. doi: 10.1016/S0735-1097(01)01141-X

Hill, J. A., and Iaizzo, P. A. (2009). "Comparative cardiac anatomy," in *Handbook of Cardiac Anatomy, Physiology, and Devices*, ed P. A. Iaizzo (Totowa, NJ: Springer Science & Business Media), 87–108. doi: 10.1007/978-1-60327-372-5_6

Ho, C. Y., and Solomon, S. D. (2006). A clinician's guide to tissue Doppler imaging. *Circulation* 113, e396–e398. doi: 10.1161/CIRCULATIONAHA.105. 579268

Houser, S. R., Margulies, K. B., Murphy, A. M., Spinale, F. G., Francis, G. S., Prabhu, S. D., et al. (2012). Animal models of heart failure: a scientific statement from the American Heart Association. *Circ. Res.* 111, 131–150. doi: 10.1161/RES.0b013e3182582523

Hoyt, R. E., Hawkins, J. V., St Clair, M. B., and Kennett, M. J. (2006). "Mouse physiology," in *The Mouse in Biomedical Research*, eds J. G. Fox, M. T. Davisson, F. W. Quimby, S. W. Barthold, C. E. Newcomer, and A. L. Smith (Burlington, MA: Academic Press. III), 23–90.

Ibanez, B., Giannarelli, C., Cimmino, G., Santos-Gallego, C. G., Alique, M., Pinero, A., et al. (2012). Recombinant HDL(Milano) exerts greater anti-inflammatory and plaque stabilizing properties than HDL(wild-type). *Atherosclerosis* 220, 72–77. doi: 10.1016/j.atherosclerosis.2011.10.006

Ibanez, B., Prat-González, S., Speidl, W. S., Vilahur, G., Pinero, A., Cimmino, G., et al. (2007). Early metoprolol administration before coronary reperfusion results in increased myocardial salvage: analysis of ischemic myocardium at risk using cardiac magnetic resonance. *Circulation* 115, 2909–2916. doi: 10.1161/CIRCULATIONAHA.106.679639

Ignatowski, A. (1908). Changes in parenchymatous organs and in the aorta of rabbits under the influence of animal protein. *Izvestia Imperatorskoi Voenno-Medicinskoi Akademii* 18, 231–244.

James, J. F., Hewett, T. E., and Robbins, J. (1998). Cardiac physiology in transgenic mice. *Circ. Res.* 82, 407–415. doi: 10.1161/01.RES.82.4.407

Johnson, M. S., Moore, R. L., and Brown, D. A. (2006). Sex differences in myocardial infarct size are abolished by sarcolemmal KATP channel blockade in rat. *Am. J. Physiol. Heart Circ. Physiol.* 290, H2644–H2647. doi: 10.1152/ajpheart.01291.2005

Kass, D. A., Hare, J. M., and Georgakopoulos, D. (1998). Murine cardiac function: a cautionary tail. *Circ. Res.* 82, 519–522. doi: 10.1161/01.RES.82.4.519

Kellman, P., Aletras, A. H., Mancini, C., McVeigh, E. R., and Arai, A. E. (2007). T2-prepared SSFP improves diagnostic confidence in edema imaging in acute myocardial infarction compared to turbo spin echo. *Magn. Reson. Med.* 57, 891–897. doi: 10.1002/mrm.21215

Kelly, K. A., Allport, J. R., Tsourkas, A., Shinde-Patil, V. R., Josephson, L., and Weissleder, R. (2005). Detection of vascular adhesion molecule-1 expression using a novel multimodal nanoparticle. *Circ. Res.* 96, 327–336. doi: 10.1161/01.RES.0000155722.17881.dd

Kim, R. J., Fieno, D. S., Parrish, T. B., Harris, K., Chen, E. L., Simonetti, O., et al. (1999). Relationship of MRI delayed contrast enhancement to irreversible injury, infarct age, and contractile function. *Circulation* 100, 1992–2002. doi: 10.1161/01.CIR.100.19.1992

Kittleson, M. D., Meurs, K. M., Munro, M. J., Kittleson, J. A., Liu, S. K., Pion, P. D., et al. (1999). Familial hypertrophic cardiomyopathy in maine coon cats: an animal model of human disease. *Circulation* 99, 3172–3180. doi: 10.1161/01.CIR.99.24.3172

Knuuti, M. J., Nuutila, P., Ruotsalainen, U., Saraste, M., Harkonen, R., Ahonen, A., et al. (1992). Euglycemic hyperinsulinemic clamp and oral glucose load in stimulating myocardial glucose utilization during positron emission tomography. *J. Nucl. Med.* 33, 1255–1262.

Kober, F., Iltis, I., Cozzone, P. J., and Bernard, M. (2005). Myocardial blood flow mapping in mice using high-resolution spin labeling magnetic resonance imaging: influence of ketamine/xylazine and isoflurane anesthesia. *Magn. Reson. Med.* 53, 601–606. doi: 10.1002/mrm.20373

Koktzoglou, I., Harris, K. R., Tang, R., Kane, B. J., Misselwitz, B., Weinmann, H.-J., et al. (2006). Gadofluorine-enhanced magnetic resonance imaging of carotid atherosclerosis in Yucatan miniswine. *Invest. Radiol.* 41, 299–304. doi: 10.1097/01.rli.0000188362.12555.62

Laber, K. E., Whary, M. T., and Bingel, S. A. (2002). "Biology and diseases of swine," *Biology and Diseases of Swine*, eds J. G. Fox, L. C. Anderson, F. M. Loew, and F. W. Quimby (Waltham, MA: Laboratory Animal), 616–665. doi: 10.1016/b978-012263951-7/50018-1

Laflamme, M. A., and Murry, C. E. (2011). Heart regeneration. *Nature* 473, 326–335. doi: 10.1038/nature10147

Lautamäki, R., Schuleri, K. H., Sasano, T., Javadi, M. S., Youssef, A., Merrill, J., et al. (2009). Integration of infarct size, tissue perfusion, and metabolism by hybrid cardiac positron emission tomography/computed tomography: evaluation in a porcine model of myocardial infarction. *Circ. Cardiovasc. Imaging* 2, 299–305. doi: 10.1161/CIRCIMAGING.108.846253

Lee, Y. A., Kim, J. I., Lee, J. W., Cho, Y. J., Lee, B. H., Chung, H. W., et al. (2012). Effects of various anesthetic protocols on 18F-flurodeoxyglucose uptake into the brains and hearts of normal miniature pigs (Sus scrofa domestica). *J. Am. Assoc. Lab. Anim. Sci.* 51, 246–252.

Lelovas, P. P., Kostomitsopoulos, N. G., and Xanthos, T. T. (2014). A comparative anatomic and physiologic overview of the porcine heart. *J. Am. Assoc. Lab. Anim. Sci.* 53, 432–438.

Levin, C. S., and Zaidi, H. (2007). Current Trends in Preclinical PET System Design. *PET Clin.* 2, 125–160. doi: 10.1016/j.cpet.2007.12.001

Libby, P. (2002). Inflammation in atherosclerosis. *Nature* 420, 868–874. doi: 10.1038/nature01323

Linardi, D., Rungatscher, A., Morjan, M., Marino, P., Luciani, G. B., Mazzucco, A., et al. (2014). Ventricular and pulmonary vascular remodeling induced by pulmonary overflow in a chronic model of pretricuspid shunt. *J. Thorac. Cardiovasc. Surg.* 148, 2609–2617. doi: 10.1016/j.jtcvs.2014.04.044

Loganathan, R., Bilgen, M., Al-Hafez, B., Alenezy, M. D., and Smirnova, I. V. (2006). Cardiac dysfunction in the diabetic rat: quantitative evaluation using high resolution magnetic resonance imaging. *Cardiovasc. Diabetol.* 5:7. doi: 10.1186/1475-2840-5-7

Lompre, A. M., Mercadier, J. J., Wisnewsky, C., Bouveret, P., Pantaloni, C., D'Albis, A., et al. (1981). Species- and age-dependent changes in the relative amounts of cardiac myosin isoenzymes in mammals. *Dev. Biol.* 84, 286–290. doi: 10.1016/0012-1606(81)90396-1

Lutgens, E., Daemen, M. J., de Muinck, E. D., Debets, J., Leenders, P., and Smits, J. F. (1999). Chronic myocardial infarction in the mouse: cardiac structural and functional changes. *Cardiovasc. Res.* 41, 586–593. doi: 10.1016/S0008-6363(98)00216-8

Lloyd-Jones, D., Adams, R. J., Brown, T. M., Carnethon, M., Dai, S., De Simone, G., et al. (2010). Executive summary: heart disease and stroke statistics–2010 update: a report from the American Heart Association. *Circulation* 121, 948–954. doi: 10.1161/CIRCULATIONAHA.109.192666

Mahmoodzadeh, S., Dworatzek, E., Fritschka, S., Pham, T. H., and Regitz-Zagrosek, V. (2010). 17beta-Estradiol inhibits matrix metalloproteinase-2 transcription via MAP kinase in fibroblasts. *Cardiovasc. Res.* 85, 719–728. doi: 10.1093/cvr/cvp350

Mahmoodzadeh, S., Fliegner, D., and Dworatzek, E. (2012). Sex differences in animal models for cardiovascular diseases and the role of estrogen. *Handb. Exp. Pharmacol.* 214, 23–48. doi: 10.1007/978-3-642-30726-3_2

Makowski, M. R., Wiethoff, A. J., Jansen, C. H., and Botnar, R. M. (2010). Cardiovascular MRI in small animals. *Expert Rev. Cardiovasc. Ther.* 8, 35–47. doi: 10.1586/erc.09.126

Mann, D. L., and Bristow, M. R. (2005). Mechanisms and models in heart failure: the biomechanical model and beyond. *Circulation* 111, 2837–2849. doi: 10.1161/CIRCULATIONAHA.104.500546

Matthews, P. M., Coatney, R., Alsaid, H., Jucker, B., Ashworth, S., Parker, C., et al. (2013). Technologies: preclinical imaging for drug development. *Drug Discov. Today Technol.* 10, e343–e350. doi: 10.1016/j.ddtec.2012.04.004

McKellar, S. H., Javan, H., Bowen, M. E., Liu, X., Schaaf, C. L., Briggs, C. M., et al. (2015). Animal model of reversible, right ventricular failure. *J. Surg. Res.* 194, 327–333. doi: 10.1016/j.jss.2014.11.006

McLean, M., and Prothero, J. (1992). Determination of relative fiber orientation in heart muscle: methodological problems. *Anat. Rec.* 232, 459–465. doi: 10.1002/ar.1092320402

Meerson, F. Z. (1961). On the mechanism of compensatory hyperfunction and insufficiency of the heart. *Cor Vasa* 3, 161–177.

Meijler, F. L. (1985). Atrioventricular conduction versus heart size from mouse to whale. *J. Am. Coll. Cardiol.* 5(2 Pt 1), 363–365. doi: 10.1016/s0735-1097(85)80060-7

Mewton, N., Rapacchi, S., Augeul, L., Ferrera, R., Loufouat, J., Boussel, L., et al. (2011). Determination of the myocardial area at risk with pre- versus post-reperfusion imaging techniques in the pig model. *Basic Res. Cardiol.* 106, 1247–1257. doi: 10.1007/s00395-011-0214-8

Michael, L. H., Entman, M. L., Hartley, C. J., Youker, K. A., Zhu, J., Hall, S. R., et al. (1995). Myocardial ischemia and reperfusion: a murine model. *Am. J. Physiol.* 269(6 Pt 2), H2147–H2154.

Michalska, M., Machtoub, L., Manthey, H. D., Bauer, E., Herold, V., Krohne, G., et al. (2012). Visualization of vascular inflammation in the atherosclerotic mouse by ultrasmall superparamagnetic iron oxide vascular cell adhesion molecule-1-specific nanoparticles. *Arterioscler. Thromb. Vasc. Biol.* 32, 2350–2357. doi: 10.1161/ATVBAHA.112.255224

Millon, A., Dickson, S. D., Klink, A., Izquierdo-Garcia, D., Bini, J., Lancelot, E., et al. (2013). Monitoring plaque inflammation in atherosclerotic rabbits with an iron oxide (P904) and (18)F-FDG using a combined PET/MR scanner. *Atherosclerosis* 228, 339–345. doi: 10.1016/j.atherosclerosis.2013.03.019

Mor-Avi, V., Lang, R. M., Badano, L. P., Belohlavek, M., Cardim, N. M., Derumeaux, G., et al. (2011). Current and evolving echocardiographic techniques for the quantitative evaluation of cardiac mechanics: ASE/EAE consensus statement on methodology and indications endorsed by the Japanese Society of Echocardiography. *Eur. J. Echocardiogr.* 12, 167–205. doi: 10.1093/ejechocard/jer021

Moran, C. M., Thomson, A. J. W., Rog-Zielinska, E., and Gray, G. A. (2013). High-resolution echocardiography in the assessment of cardiac physiology and disease in preclinical models. *Exp. Physiol.* 98, 629–644. doi: 10.1113/expphysiol.2012.068577

Mulder, W. J., Jaffer, F. A., Fayad, Z. A., and Nahrendorf, M. (2014). Imaging and nanomedicine in inflammatory atherosclerosis. *Sci. Transl. Med.* 6, 239sr231. doi: 10.1126/scitranslmed.3005101

Nahrendorf, M., Jaffer, F. A., Kelly, K. A., Sosnovik, D. E., Aikawa, E., Libby, P., et al. (2006). Noninvasive vascular cell adhesion molecule-1 imaging identifies inflammatory activation of cells in atherosclerosis. *Circulation* 114, 1504–1511. doi: 10.1161/CIRCULATIONAHA.106.646380

Nahrendorf, M., Keliher, E., Panizzi, P., Zhang, H., Hembrador, S., Figueiredo, J. L., et al. (2009). 18F-4V for PET-CT imaging of VCAM-1 expression in atherosclerosis. *JACC Cardiovasc. Imaging* 2, 1213–1222. doi: 10.1016/j.jcmg.2009.04.016

Nakashima, Y., Plump, A. S., Raines, E. W., Breslow, J. L., and Ross, R. (1994). ApoE-deficient mice develop lesions of all phases of atherosclerosis throughout the arterial tree. *Arterioscler. Thromb.* 14, 133–140. doi: 10.1161/01.ATV.14.1.133

Nakata, T. M., Tanaka, R., Yoshiyuki, R., Fukayama, T., Goya, S., and Fukushima, R. (2015). Effects of single drug and combined short-term administration of sildenafil, pimobendan, and nicorandil on right ventricular function in rats with monocrotaline-induced pulmonary hypertension. *J. Cardiovasc. Pharmacol.* 65, 640–648. doi: 10.1097/FJC.0000000000000236

Nekolla, S. G., Martinez-Moeller, A., and Saraste, A. (2009). PET and MRI in cardiac imaging: from validation studies to integrated applications. *Eur. J. Nucl. Med. Mol. Imaging* 36 (Suppl. 1), S121–S130. doi: 10.1007/s00259-008-0980-1

Nichols, M., Townsend, N., Scarborough, P., and Rayner, M. (2014). Cardiovascular disease in Europe 2014: epidemiological update. *Eur. Heart J.* 35, 2950–2959. doi: 10.1093/eurheartj/ehu299

Nitta-Seko, A., Nitta, N., Shiomi, M., Sonoda, A., Ota, S., Tsuchiya, K., et al. (2010). Utility of contrast-enhanced ultrasonography for qualitative imaging of atherosclerosis in Watanabe heritable hyperlipidemic rabbits: initial experimental study. *Jpn. J. Radiol.* 28, 656–662. doi: 10.1007/s11604-010-0487-0

Okumura, K., Kato, H., Honjo, O., Breitling, S., Kuebler, W. M., Sun, M., et al. (2015). Carvedilol improves biventricular fibrosis and function in experimental pulmonary hypertension. *J. Mol. Med.* 93, 663–674. doi: 10.1007/s00109-015-1251-9

Owen, D. R., Lindsay, A. C., Choudhury, R. P., and Fayad, Z. A. (2011). Imaging of atherosclerosis. *Annu. Rev. Med.* 62, 25–40. doi: 10.1146/annurev-med-041709-133809

Packard, R. R. S., Huang, S.-C., Dahlbom, M., Czernin, J., and Maddahi, J. (2014). Absolute quantitation of myocardial blood flow in human subjects with or without myocardial ischemia using dynamic flurpiridaz F 18 PET. *J. Nucl. Med.* 55, 1438–1444. doi: 10.2967/jnumed.114.141093

Palermo, V., Stafford Johnson, M. J., Sala, E., Brambilla, P. G., and Martin, M. W. (2011). Cardiomyopathy in Boxer dogs: a retrospective study of the clinical presentation, diagnostic findings and survival. *J. Vet. Cardiol.* 13, 45–55. doi: 10.1016/j.jvc.2010.06.005

Patten, R. D., and Hall-Porter, M. R. (2009). Small animal models of heart failure: development of novel therapies, past and present. *Circ. Heart Fail.* 2, 138–144. doi: 10.1161/CIRCHEARTFAILURE.108.839761

Patten, R. D., Pourati, I., Aronovitz, M. J., Alsheikh-Ali, A., Eder, S., Force, T., et al. (2008). 17 Beta-estradiol differentially affects left ventricular and cardiomyocyte hypertrophy following myocardial infarction and pressure overload. *J. Card. Fail.* 14, 245–253. doi: 10.1016/j.cardfail.2007. 10.024

Patten, R. D., Pourati, I., Aronovitz, M. J., Baur, J., Celestin, F., Chen, X., et al. (2004). 17beta-estradiol reduces cardiomyocyte apoptosis *in vivo* and *in vitro* via activation of phospho-inositide-3 kinase/Akt signaling. *Circ. Res.* 95, 692–699. doi: 10.1161/01.RES.0000144126.57786.89

Pereda, D., García-Alvarez, A., Sánchez-Quintana, D., Nuño, M., Fernández-Friera, L., Fernández-Jiménez, R., et al. (2014). Swine model of chronic postcapillary pulmonary hypertension with right ventricular remodeling: long-term characterization by cardiac catheterization, magnetic resonance, and pathology. *J. Cardiovasc. Transl. Res.* 7, 494–506. doi: 10.1007/s12265-014-9564-6

Pfeffer, M. A., Pfeffer, J. M., Fishbein, M. C., Fletcher, P. J., Spadaro, J., Kloner, R., A., et al. (1979). Myocardial infarct size and ventricular function in rats. *Circ. Res.* 44, 503–512. doi: 10.1161/01.RES.44.4.503

Phinikaridou, A., Ruberg, F. L., Hallock, K. J., Qiao, Y., Hua, N., Viereck, J., et al. (2010). *In vivo* detection of vulnerable atherosclerotic plaque by MRI in a rabbit model. *Circ. Cardiovasc. Imaging* 3, 323–332. doi: 10.1161/CIRCIMAGING.109.918524

Piao, L., Fang, Y. H., Cadete, V. J., Wietholt, C., Urboniene, D., Toth, P. T., et al. (2010). The inhibition of pyruvate dehydrogenase kinase improves impaired cardiac function and electrical remodeling in two models of right ventricular hypertrophy: resuscitating the hibernating right ventricle. *J. Mol. Med. (Berl).* 88, 47–60. doi: 10.1007/s00109-009-0524-6

Pohlmann, A., Boye, P., Wagenhaus, B., Muller, D., Kolanczyk, M., Kohle, S., et al. (2011). *Cardiac MR Imaging in Mice: Morphometry and Functional Assessment.* Billerica, MA: Bruker.

Poss, K. D., Wilson, L. G., and Keating, M. T. (2002). Heart regeneration in zebrafish. *Science* 298, 2188–2190. doi: 10.1126/science.1077857

Power, J. M., and Tonkin, A. M. (1999). Large animal models of heart failure. *Aust. N.Z. J. Med.* 29, 395–402. doi: 10.1111/j.1445-5994.1999.tb00734.x

Prescott, M. F., McBride, C. H., Hasler-Rapacz, J., Von Linden, J., and Rapacz, J. (1991). Development of complex atherosclerotic lesions in pigs with inherited hyper-LDL cholesterolemia bearing mutant alleles for apolipoprotein B. *Am. J. Pathol.* 139, 139–147.

Ram, R., Mickelsen, D. M., Theodoropoulos, C., and Blaxall, B. C. (2011). New approaches in small animal echocardiography: imaging the sounds of silence. *Am. J. Physiol. Heart Circ. Physiol.* 301, H1765–H1780. doi: 10.1152/ajpheart.00559.2011

Rao, Y., Wang, Y. L., Zhang, W. S., and Liu, J. (2008). Emulsified isoflurane produces cardiac protection after ischemia-reperfusion injury in rabbits. *Anesth. Analg.* 106, 1353–1359. doi: 10.1213/ane.0b013e3181679347

Richardson, J. D., Bertaso, A. G., Frost, L., Psaltis, P. J., Carbone, A., Koschade, B., et al. (2013). Cardiac magnetic resonance, transthoracic and transoesophageal echocardiography: a comparison of *in vivo* assessment of ventricular function in rats. *Lab. Anim.* 47, 291–300. doi: 10.1177/0023677213494373

Rider, O. J., and Tyler, D. J. (2013). Clinical implications of cardiac hyperpolarized magnetic resonance imaging. *J. Cardiovasc. Magn. Reson.* 15:93. doi: 10.1186/1532-429X-15-93

Roldán-Alzate, A., Frydrychowicz, A., Johnson, K. M., Kellihan, H., Chesler, N. C., Wieben, O., et al. (2014). Non-invasive assessment of cardiac function and pulmonary vascular resistance in an canine model of acute thromboembolic pulmonary hypertension using 4D flow cardiovascular magnetic resonance. *J. Cardiovasc. Magn. Reson.* 16:23. doi: 10.1186/1532-429X-16-23

Rottman, J. N., Ni, G., Khoo, M., Wang, Z., Zhang, W., Anderson, M. E., et al. (2003). Temporal changes in ventricular function assessed echocardiographically in conscious and anesthetized mice. *J. Am. Soc. Echocardiogr.* 16, 1150–1157. doi: 10.1067/S0894-7317(03)00471-1

Ruff, J., Wiesmann, F., Hiller, K. H., Voll, S., von Kienlin, M., Bauer, W. R., et al. (1998). Magnetic resonance microimaging for noninvasive quantification of myocardial function and mass in the mouse. *Magn. Reson. Med.* 40, 43–48. doi: 10.1002/mrm.1910400106

Russell, J. C., and Proctor, S. D. (2006). Small animal models of cardiovascular disease: tools for the study of the roles of metabolic syndrome, dyslipidemia, and atherosclerosis. *Cardiovasc. Pathol.* 15, 318–330. doi: 10.1016/j.carpath.2006.09.001

Ryan, J. J., and Archer, S. L. (2014). The right ventricle in pulmonary arterial hypertension: disorders of metabolism, angiogenesis and adrenergic signaling in right ventricular failure. *Circ. Res.* 115, 176–188. doi: 10.1161/CIRCRESAHA.113.301129

Sánchez-González, J., Fernandez-Jiménez, R., Nothnagel, N. D., López-Martín, G., Fuster, V., and Ibañez, B. (2015). Optimization of dual-saturation single bolus acquisition for quantitative cardiac perfusion and myocardial blood flow maps. *J. Cardiovasc. Magn. Reson.* 17:21. doi: 10.1186/s12968-015-0116-2

Sanz, J., and Fayad, Z. A. (2008). Imaging of atherosclerotic cardiovascular disease. *Nature* 451, 953–957. doi: 10.1038/nature06803

Schaefer, A., Klein, G., Brand, B., Lippolt, P., Drexler, H., Meyer, G. P. (2003). Evaluation of left ventricular diastolic function by pulsed Doppler tissue imaging in mice. *J. Am. Soc. Echocardiogr.* 16, 1144–1149. doi: 10.1067/S0894-7317(03)00679-5

Schaefer, A., Meyer, G. P., Hilfiker-Kleiner, D., Brand, B., Drexler, H., and Klein, G. (2005). Evaluation of Tissue Doppler Tei index for global left ventricular function in mice after myocardial infarction: comparison with Pulsed Doppler Tei index. *Eur. J. Echocardiogr.* 6, 367–375. doi: 10.1016/j.euje.2005. 01.007

Scherrer-Crosbie, M., and Thibault, H. B. (2008). Echocardiography in translational research: of mice and men. *J. Am. Soc. Echocardiogr.* 21, 1083–1092. doi: 10.1016/j.echo.2008.07.001

Schmidt, A. G., Gerst, M., Zhai, J., Carr, A. N., Pater, L., Kranias, E. G., et al. (2002). Evaluation of left ventricular diastolic function from spectral and color M-mode Doppler in genetically altered mice. *J. Am. Soc. Echocardiogr.* 15, 1065–1073. doi: 10.1067/mje.2002.121863

Schroeder, M. A., Cochlin, L. E., Heather, L. C., Clarke, K., Radda, G. K., and Tyler, D. J. (2008). *In vivo* assessment of pyruvate dehydrogenase flux in the heart using hyperpolarized carbon-13 magnetic resonance. *Proc. Natl. Acad. Sci. U.S.A.* 105, 12051–12056. doi: 10.1073/pnas.0805953105

Simonneau, G., Gatzoulis, M. A., Adatia, I., Celermajer, D., Denton, C., Ghofrani, A., et al. (2013). Updated clinical classification of pulmonary hypertension. *J. Am. Coll. Cardiol.* 62(25 Suppl.), D34–D41. doi: 10.1016/j.jacc.2013.10.029

Sinitsyn, V. (2001). Magnetic resonance imaging in coronary heart disease. *Eur. J. Radiol.* 38, 191–199. doi: 10.1016/S0720-048X(01)00307-2

Slawson, S. E., Roman, B. B., Williams, D. S., and Koretsky, A. P. (1998). Cardiac MRI of the normal and hypertrophied mouse heart. *Magn. Reson. Med.* 39, 980–987. doi: 10.1002/mrm.1910390616

Stamper, D., Weissman, N. J., and Brezinski, M. (2006). Plaque characterization with optical coherence tomography. *J. Am. Coll. Cardiol.* 47(8 Suppl.), C69–C79. doi: 10.1016/j.jacc.2005.10.067

Streif, J. U., Nahrendorf, M., Hiller, K. H., Waller, C., Wiesmann, F., Rommel, E., et al. (2005). *In vivo* assessment of absolute perfusion and intracapillary blood volume in the murine myocardium by spin labeling magnetic resonance imaging. *Magn. Reson. Med.* 53, 584–592. doi: 10.1002/mrm.20327

Stuckey, D. J., Carr, C. A., Tyler, D. J., and Clarke, K. (2008). Cine-MRI versus two-dimensional echocardiography to measure *in vivo* left ventricular function in rat heart. *NMR Biomed.* 21, 765–772. doi: 10.1002/nbm.1268

Stuckey, D. J., McSweeney, S. J., Thin, M. Z., Habib, J., Price, A. N., Fiedler, L. R., et al. (2014). T(1) mapping detects pharmacological retardation of diffuse cardiac fibrosis in mouse pressure-overload hypertrophy. *Circ. Cardiovasc. Imaging* 7, 240–249. doi: 10.1161/CIRCIMAGING.113.000993

Sutendra, G., Dromparis, P., Paulin, R., Zervopoulos, S., Haromy, A., Nagendran, J., et al. (2013). A metabolic remodeling in right ventricular hypertrophy is associated with decreased angiogenesis and a transition from a compensated to a decompensated state in pulmonary hypertension. *J. Mol. Med. (Berl)* 91, 1315–1327. doi: 10.1007/s00109-013-1059-4

Swindle, M. M. (2007). "Cardiothoracic and vascular surgery/chronic intravascular catheterization," in *Swine in the Laboratory: Surgery, Anesthesia, Imaging, and Experimental Techniques*, ed M. M. Swindle (Boca Raton, FL: CRC Press), 195–260. doi: 10.1201/9781420009156.ch9

Swynghedauw, B. (1986). Developmental and functional adaptation of contractile proteins in cardiac and skeletal muscles. *Physiol. Rev.* 66, 710–771.

Tanaka, N., Dalton, N., Mao, L., Rockman, H. A., Peterson, K. L., Gottshall, K. R., et al. (1996). Transthoracic echocardiography in models of cardiac disease in the mouse. *Circulation* 94, 1109–1117. doi: 10.1161/01.CIR.94.5.1109

Tarnavski, O., McMullen, J. R., Schinke, M., Nie, Q., Kong, S., and Izumo, S. (2004). Mouse cardiac surgery: comprehensive techniques for the generation of mouse models of human diseases and their application for genomic studies. *Physiol. Genomics* 16, 349–360. doi: 10.1152/physiolgenomics.00041.2003

Tei, C., Ling, L. H., Hodge, D. O., Bailey, K. R., Oh, J. K., Rodeheffer, R. J., et al. (1995). New index of combined systolic and diastolic myocardial performance: a simple and reproducible measure of cardiac function–a study in normals and dilated cardiomyopathy. *J. Cardiol.* 26, 357–366.

Temple, I. P., Monfredi, O., Quigley, G., Schneider, H., Zi, M., Cartwright, E. J., et al. (2014). Macitentan treatment retards the progression of established pulmonary arterial hypertension in an animal model. *Int. J. Cardiol.* 177, 423–428. doi: 10.1016/j.ijcard.2014.09.005

Teramoto, N., Koshino, K., Yokoyama, I., Miyagawa, S., Zeniya, T., Hirano, Y., et al. (2011). Experimental pig model of old myocardial infarction with long survival leading to chronic left ventricular dysfunction and remodeling as evaluated by PET. *J. Nucl. Med.* 52, 761–768. doi: 10.2967/jnumed.110.084848

Thibault, H. B., Kurtz, B., Raher, M. J., Shaik, R. S., Waxman, A., Derumeaux, G., et al. (2010). Noninvasive assessment of murine pulmonary arterial pressure: validation and application to models of pulmonary hypertension. *Circ. Cardiovasc. Imaging* 3, 157–163. doi: 10.1161/circimaging.109.887109

Thygesen, K., Alpert, J. S., Jaffe, A. S., Simoons, M. L., Chaitman, B. R., White, H. D., et al. (2012). Third universal definition of myocardial infarction. *J. Am. Coll. Cardiol.* 60, 1581–1598. doi: 10.1016/j.jacc.2012.08.001

Tian, J., Hu, S., Sun, Y., Yu, H., Han, X., Cheng, W., et al. (2013). Vasa vasorum and plaque progression, and responses to atorvastatin in a rabbit model of atherosclerosis: contrast-enhanced ultrasound imaging and intravascular ultrasound study. *Heart* 99, 48–54. doi: 10.1136/heartjnl-2012-302775

Tsaftaris, S. A., Zhou, X., Tang, R., Li, D., and Dharmakumar, R. (2013). Detecting myocardial ischemia at rest with cardiac phase-resolved blood oxygen level-dependent cardiovascular magnetic resonance. *Circ. Cardiovasc. Imaging* 6, 311–319. doi: 10.1161/CIRCIMAGING.112.976076

Ugander, M., Bagi, P. S., Oki, A. J., Chen, B., Hsu, L. Y., Aletras, A. H., et al. (2012). Myocardial edema as detected by pre-contrast T1 and T2 CMR delineates area at risk associated with acute myocardial infarction. *JACC Cardiovasc. Imaging* 5, 596–603. doi: 10.1016/j.jcmg.2012.01.016

Unger, E. F. (2001). Experimental evaluation of coronary collateral development. *Cardiovasc. Res.* 49, 497–506. doi: 10.1016/S0008-6363(00)00285-6

Urboniene, D., Haber, I., Fang, Y. H., Thenappan, T., and Archer, S. L. (2010). Validation of high-resolution echocardiography and magnetic resonance imaging vs. high-fidelity catheterization in experimental pulmonary hypertension. *Am. J. Physiol. Lung Cell Mol. Physiol.* 299, L401–L412. doi: 10.1152/ajplung.00114.2010

Verdouw, P. D., van den Doel, M. A., de Zeeuw, S., and Duncker, D. J. (1998). Animal models in the study of myocardial ischaemia and ischaemic syndromes. *Cardiovasc. Res.* 39, 121–135. doi: 10.1016/S0008-6363(98)00069-8

Viles-Gonzalez, J. F., Poon, M., Sanz, J., Rius, T., Nikolaou, K., Fayad, Z. A., et al. (2004). *In vivo* 16-slice, multidetector-row computed tomography for the assessment of experimental atherosclerosis: comparison with magnetic resonance imaging and histopathology. *Circulation* 110, 1467–1472. doi: 10.1161/01.CIR.0000141732.28175.2A

Voeller, R. K., Aziz, A., Maniar, H. S., Ufere, N. N., Taggar, A. K., Bernabe, N. J. Jr., et al. (2011). Differential modulation of right ventricular strain and right atrial mechanics in mild vs. severe pressure overload. *Am. J. Physiol. Heart Circ. Physiol.* 301, H2362–H2371. doi: 10.1152/ajpheart.00138.2011

Vucic, E., Dickson, S. D., Calcagno, C., Rudd, J. H. F., Moshier, E., Hayashi, K., et al. (2011). Pioglitazone modulates vascular inflammation in atherosclerotic rabbits noninvasive assessment with FDG-PET-CT and dynamic contrast-enhanced MR imaging. *JACC Cardiovasc. Imaging* 4, 1100–1109. doi: 10.1016/j.jcmg.2011.04.020

Walmsley, R. (1978). Anatomy of human mitral valve in adult cadaver and comparative anatomy of the valve. *Br. Heart J.* 40, 351–366. doi: 10.1136/hrt.40.4.351

Wang, M., Baker, L., Tsai, B. M., Meldrum, K. K., and Meldrum, D. R. (2005). Sex differences in the myocardial inflammatory response to ischemia-reperfusion injury. *Am. J. Physiol. Endocrinol. Metab.* 288, E321–E326. doi: 10.1152/ajpendo.00278.2004

Watanabe, Y. (1980). Serial inbreeding of rabbits with hereditary hyperlipidemia (WHHL-rabbit). *Atherosclerosis* 36, 261–268. doi: 10.1016/0021-9150(80)90234-8

Webb, S., Brown, N. A., and Anderson, R. H. (1996). The structure of the mouse heart in late fetal stages. *Anat. Embryol.* 194, 37–47. doi: 10.1007/BF00196313

Wetterholm, R., Caidahl, K., Volkmann, R., Brandt-Eliasson, U., Fritsche-Danielson, R., and Gan, L. M. (2007). Imaging of atherosclerosis in WHHL rabbits using high-resolution ultrasound. *Ultrasound Med. Biol.* 33, 720–726. doi: 10.1016/j.ultrasmedbio.2006.11.012

White, F. C., Roth, D. M., and Bloor, C. M. (1986). The pig as a model for myocardial ischemia and exercise. *Lab. Anim. Sci.* 36, 351–356.

Wichi, R., Malfitano, C., Rosa, K., De Souza, S. B., Salemi, V., Mostarda, C., et al. (2007). Noninvasive and invasive evaluation of cardiac dysfunction in experimental diabetes in rodents. *Cardiovasc. Diabetol.* 6:14. doi: 10.1186/1475-2840-6-14

Wiesmann, F., Frydrychowicz, A., Rautenberg, J., Illinger, R., Rommel, E., Haase, A., et al. (2002). Analysis of right ventricular function in healthy mice and a murine model of heart failure by *in vivo* MRI. *Am. J. Physiol. Heart Circ. Physiol.* 283, H1065–H1071. doi: 10.1152/ajpheart.00802.2001

Worthley, S. G., Helft, G., Fuster, V., Fayad, Z. A., Rodriguez, O. J., Zaman, A. G., et al. (2000). Noninvasive *in vivo* magnetic resonance imaging of experimental coronary artery lesions in a porcine model. *Circulation* 101, 2956–2961. doi: 10.1161/01.CIR.101.25.2956

Wu, J., You, J., Jiang, G., Li, L., Guan, A., Ye, Y., et al. (2012). Noninvasive estimation of infarct size in a mouse model of myocardial infarction by echocardiographic coronary perfusion. *J. Ultrasound Med.* 31, 1111–1121. doi: 10.1136/heartjnl-2012-302920c.1

Xiangdong, L., Yuanwu, L., Hua, Z., Liming, R., Qiuyan, L., and Ning, L. (2011). Animal models for the atherosclerosis research: a review. *Protein Cell.* 2, 189–201. doi: 10.1007/s13238-011-1016-3

Yanni, A. E. (2004). The laboratory rabbit: an animal model of atherosclerosis research. *Lab. Anim.* 38, 246–256. doi: 10.1258/002367704323133628

Young, A. A., French, B. A., Yang, Z., Cowan, B. R., Gilson, W. D., Berr, S. S., et al. (2006). Reperfused myocardial infarction in mice: 3D mapping of late gadolinium enhancement and strain. *J. Cardiovasc. Magn. Reson.* 8, 685–692. doi: 10.1080/10976640600721767

Yu, X., Tesiram, Y. A., Towner, R. A., Abbott, A., Patterson, E., Huang, S., et al. (2007). Early myocardial dysfunction in streptozotocin-induced diabetic mice: a study using *in vivo* magnetic resonance imaging (MRI). *Cardiovasc. Diabetol.* 6:6. doi: 10.1186/1475-2840-6-6

Yuan, L., Wang, T., Liu, F., Cohen, E. D., and Patel, V. V. (2010). An evaluation of transmitral and pulmonary venous Doppler indices for assessing murine left ventricular diastolic function. *J. Am. Soc. Echocardiogr.* 23, 887–897. doi: 10.1016/j.echo.2010.05.017

Yue, P., Arai, T., Terashima, M., Sheikh, A. Y., Cao, F., Charo, D., et al. (2007). Magnetic resonance imaging of progressive cardiomyopathic changes in the db/db mouse. *Am. J. Physiol. Heart Circ. Physiol.* 292, H2106–H2118. doi: 10.1152/ajpheart.00856.2006

Zaragoza, C., Gomez-Guerrero, C., Martin-Ventura, J. L., Blanco-Colio, L., Lavin, B., Mallavia, B., et al. (2011). Animal models of cardiovascular diseases. *J. Biomed. Biotechnol.* 2011:497841. doi: 10.1155/2011/497841

Zeng, W., Wen, X., Gong, L., Sun, J., Yang, J., Liao, J., et al. (2015). Establishment and ultrasound characteristics of atherosclerosis in rhesus monkey. *Biomed. Eng. Online* 14(Suppl. 1):S13. doi: 10.1186/1475-925X-14-S1-S13

Zhang, Y., Takagawa, J., Sievers, R. E., Khan, M. F., Viswanathan, M. N., Springer, M. L., et al. (2007). Validation of the wall motion score and myocardial performance indexes as novel techniques to assess cardiac function in mice after myocardial infarction. *Am. J. Physiol. Heart Circ. Physiol.* 292, H1187–H1192. doi: 10.1152/ajpheart.00895.2006

Zhou, R., Pickup, S., Glickson, J. D., Scott, C. H., and Ferrari, V. A. (2003). Assessment of global and regional myocardial function in the mouse using cine and tagged MRI. *Magn. Reson. Med.* 49, 760–764. doi: 10.1002/mrm.10423

Zhu, Y., Carmeliet, P., and Fay, W. P. (1999). Plasminogen activator inhibitor-1 is a major determinant of arterial thrombolysis resistance. *Circulation* 99, 3050–3055. doi: 10.1161/01.CIR.99.23.3050

Conflict of Interest Statement: The authors declare that the research was conducted in the absence of any commercial or financial relationships that could be construed as a potential conflict of interest.

9

Sonochemotherapy: From Bench to Bedside

Bart H. A. Lammertink[1]*, Clemens Bos[1], Roel Deckers[1], Gert Storm[2,3], Chrit T. W. Moonen[1] and Jean-Michel Escoffre[1]*

[1] *Image Guided Therapy, Imaging Division, University Medical Center Utrecht, Utrecht, Netherlands,* [2] *Department of Pharmaceutical Sciences, Faculty of Science, Utrecht University, Utrecht, Netherlands,* [3] *Targeted Therapeutics, MIRA Institute for Biomedical Technology and Technical Medicine, University of Twente, Enschede, Netherlands*

Edited by:
Nicolau Beckmann,
Novartis Institutes for BioMedical
Research, Switzerland

Reviewed by:
Maja Cemazar,
Institute of Oncology Ljubljana,
Slovenia
Twan Lammers,
Rheinisch-Westfälische Technische
Hochschule Aachen University,
Germany

*Correspondence:
Bart H. A. Lammertink
and Jean-Michel Escoffre,
Image Guided Therapy, Imaging
Division, University Medical Center
Utrecht, Heidelberglaan 100,
P.O. Box 85500, 3508 GA, Utrecht,
Netherlands
b.h.a.lammertink@umcutrecht.nl;
jean-michel.escoffre@univ.tours.fr

The combination of microbubbles and ultrasound has emerged as a promising method for local drug delivery. Microbubbles can be locally activated by a targeted ultrasound beam, which can result in several bio-effects. For drug delivery, microbubble-assisted ultrasound is used to increase vascular- and plasma membrane permeability for facilitating drug extravasation and the cellular uptake of drugs in the treated region, respectively. In the case of drug-loaded microbubbles, these two mechanisms can be combined with local release of the drug following destruction of the microbubble. The use of microbubble-assisted ultrasound to deliver chemotherapeutic agents is also referred to as sonochemotherapy. In this review, the basic principles of sonochemotherapy are discussed, including aspects such as the type of (drug-loaded) microbubbles used, the routes of administration used *in vivo*, ultrasound devices and parameters, treatment schedules and safety issues. Finally, the clinical translation of sonochemotherapy is discussed, including the first clinical study using sonochemotherapy.

Keywords: ultrasound, microbubble, sonoporation, chemotherapeutic drug, drug delivery, sonochemotherapy

Introduction

Cancer presents the second leading cause of death in the European Union with 3.45 million new cases of cancer and 1.75 million deaths from cancer in 2012 (Ferlay et al., 2013). Although a lot of progress has been made in the treatment of several cancers, many types of cancer are still lacking effective treatment options. Surgery, radiotherapy, and chemotherapy are the standard treatment possibilities and they are often combined to improve patient outcome.

While for most advanced cancers, chemotherapy remains the treatment of choice, it is rarely curative for solid tumors (Qin et al., 2015). To be successful, sufficient quantities of chemotherapeutic drugs have to reach the interior of tumor cells. Most small molecular weight chemotherapeutics (<4 kDa) are rapidly cleared from the circulation (e.g., $t_{1/2}$ < 15 min for 5-fluorouracil, 5-FU), which is a limiting factor for drug accumulation in the tumor. In addition to challenges related to the physicochemical properties of drugs, tumors also possess physiological barriers (Jain, 2001). Contrary to healthy tissues, tumor tissues have a high interstitial fluid pressure (IFP), which is related to the lack of functional lymphatics and the leaky tumor vasculature (Boucher et al., 1990). These high pressures establish an outward fluid motion from the core of the solid tumor to the periphery and reduce fluid infiltration across the vascular wall. Thus, even if the leaky vasculature permits drug extravasation, diffusion-driven drug penetration deeper into the tumor tissue is severely restricted due to the high IFP. The increase in mean distance between vessels and tumor cells following tumor growth is another constraint for sufficient delivery of drugs. High tumor cell proliferation results in tumor cells forcing vessels apart, leading to a decrease in vascular density and a limitation in the access of drugs to distant tumor cells (Minchinton and Tannock, 2006). In addition, the presence of high levels of extracellular matrix limits the interstitial transport of drugs (Weinberg, 2014). Altogether these barriers oppose sufficient and uniform distribution of drugs in solid tumors, thereby limiting the therapeutic success of chemotherapy.

In addition, reaching the target site is not a guarantee that a drug will be effective. As most chemotherapeutic drugs need to enter the cell to become active, they need to pass the cell membrane. For several hydrophilic and charged drugs, e.g., bleomycin, this is a serious challenge and requires active uptake through plasma membrane transporters, which are not always present in the target cells (Pron et al., 1999).

In order to improve the efficiency of anti-cancer chemotherapeutics, physical methods including electroporation, laser, and magnetic fields have been developed (Sersa et al., 2008; Podaru et al., 2014; Sklar et al., 2014). The general principle of physical methods is based on the transient disruption of endothelial barrier and tumor cell membrane in order to facilitate the drug extravasation and the drug uptake into the endothelial and tumor cells. In recent years, research in the field of microbubble-assisted ultrasound (also known as sonoporation) aimed at delivering therapeutic molecules *in vitro* and *in vivo* has grown rapidly (Aryal et al., 2014; Azagury et al., 2014; Kiessling et al., 2014; Rychak and Klibanov, 2014; Unga and Hashida, 2014; Unger et al., 2014). Microbubble-assisted ultrasound transiently increases the permeability of biological barriers, such as blood vessel walls (i.e., drug extravasation) and cellular membranes (i.e., cellular uptake of drugs), thus enhancing the local delivery of therapeutic molecules across these barriers in the targeted region (Lentacker et al., 2014). Nowadays, the great potential of this modality for cancer therapy is clearly shown in an increasing number of publications on *in vitro* and *in vivo* drug delivery using microbubble-assisted ultrasound (**Tables** respectively). This method is a non-invasive, easy to apply, and cost-effective treatment modality, that can be used to deliver a wide range of anticancer molecules including low molecular weight chemotherapeutic agents (sonochemotherapy), nucleic acids and monoclonal antibodies to a target site, e.g., tumor (Escoffre et al., 2013c; Ibsen et al., 2013; Unga and Hashida, 2014). In addition, this method offers the possibility to treat superficial (e.g., skin) as well as deep organs (e.g., brain, liver, prostate), under the guidance of medical imaging modalities (magnetic resonance imaging, ultrasound imaging; Kinoshita et al., 2006; Deckers and Moonen, 2010; Lammers et al., 2015).

This review first focuses on the biological effects of microbubble-assisted ultrasound (i.e., increasing plasma membrane- and vascular endothelium permeability) and subsequently on *in vitro* and *in vivo* chemotherapeutic drug delivery studies using microbubble-assisted ultrasound for cancer treatment. The limitations and future developments of sonochemotherapy will be further discussed.

TABLE | *In vitro* sonochemotherapy.

Reference	Cell line	Drug (free vs. MB-loaded)	Microbubble	Frequency	Intensity	Duty cycle	Time	Outcome vs. drug alone
Iwanaga et al. (2007)	Ca9-22	Free bleomycin	Optison	1 MHz	1.0 W/cm²	10%	20 s	2.5-fold increase in apoptosis
Heath et al. (2012)	SCC-1, SCC-5, Cal27	Free cisplatin	Definity	1 MHz	0.5 MI	20%	5 min	≈50% increase in apoptosis
Escoffre et al. (2011)	U87MG, MDA-231	Free doxorubicin (DOX)	Vevo, BR14, SonoVue	1 MHz	400-800 kPa	40%	30 s	30-40% decrease in viability, depending on cell line
Sorace et al. (2012)	2LMP	Free paclitaxel (PTX)	Definity	1 MHz	1.0 MPa PNP	20%	5 min	50% increase in cell death
Hu et al. (2012)	BEL-7402	Free 10-HCPT (free)	Polymer	3.5 MHz	22.57 mW/cm²	ND	10 min	20-30% decrease in viability
Ren et al. (2013)	DLD-1	Docetaxel-loaded MB	Lipid	800 kHz	2.56 W/cm²	50%	10 min	40% increase in inhibition rate
Tinkov et al. (2010)	295/KDR	DOX-loaded MB	Lipid	1 MHz	1 W/cm²	50%	20 s	40% decrease in cell viability
Yan et al. (2013)	4T1	PTX-liposome loaded MB	Lipid	1 MHz	1.0 MPa	50%	1 min	20-30% decrease in viability
Deng et al. (2014)	MCF7/ADR	DOX-liposome loaded MB	Lipid	1 MHz	1.65 W/cm²	20%	15 s	Increased cellular accumulation and retention, 30% decrease in viability

10-HCPT, 10-hydroxycamptothecin; ND, non-defined; PNP, peak-negative-pressure.

TABLE | In vivo sonochemotherapy.

Reference	Tumor (site, animal)	Drug	Microbubble	Administration route	US parameters Frequency	Intensity	Duty cycle	Time	Outcome vs drug alone
Yan et al. (2013)	4T1 (s.c., mouse)	PTX-liposome loaded MB	Lipid	intravenous (i.v.)	2.25 MHz	1.9 MPa	1%	10 min	Fourfold increase it PTX accumulation, 2.5-fold decrease in tumor volume compared to PTX-loaded MB alone
Burke et al. (2014)	C6 (s.c., rat)	5FU-NPs loaded MB	Albumin	i.v.	1 MHz	1.2 MPa (PNP)	ND	Every 5 s for 60 min	Twofold decrease in tumor volume, increase in median survival (34 days vs. 26 days) compared to free 5FU
Fan et al. (2013)	C6 (i.c., rat)	VEGFR2-BCNU-loaded MB	Lipid	i.v. (infusion)	1 MHz	0.7 MPa	5%	1 min / sonication site	1.86-fold increase in it BCNU accumulation, threefold decrease in liver BCNU accumulation, 1.75-fold decrease in tumor volume, increase in median survival (>75 days vs. <40 days) compared to untargeted BCNU-loaded MB
Iwanaga et al. (2007)	Caco-9 (s.c., mouse)	Free Bleomycin	Optison	Intratumoral (i.t.; co-injection)	1 MHz	2 W/cm²	50%	2 min	Twofold decrease in tumor volume compared to free BLM
Kang et al. (2010)	VX2 (liver, rabbit)	Docetaxel-loaded MB	Lipid	i.v. (infusion)	0.3 MHz	2 W/cm²	50%	6 min	Threefold increase tumor inhibition, twofold increase in apoptosis, twofold decrease in proliferation compared to free Docetaxel
Li et al. (2012)	H22 (s.c., mouse)	10-HCPT loaded MB	Lipid	i.v.	1 MHz	2 W/cm²	50%	6 min	Sixfold increase in it 10-HCPT accumulation, twofold decrease in tumor volume compared to free 10-HCPT
Pu et al. (2014)	A2780/DDP (i.p. mouse)	LHRHa-PTX loaded MB	Lipid	intraperitoneal (i.p.)	0.3 MHz	1 W/cm²	50%	3 min	Twofold decrease in apoptotic index, twofold decrease in vessel number, twofold decrease in VEGF expression, 1.7-fold increase in caspase-3 expression, increase in survival median (>50 days vs. <40 days) compared to free PTX
Sonoda et al. (2007)	B16 (s.c., mouse)	Free BLM	Optison	i.t. (co-injection)	1 MHz	2 W/cm²	50%	4 min	Tumor eradication compared to free BLM
Treat et al. (2012)	9L (i.c., rat)	Free Doxil	Definity	i.v.	1.7 MHz	1.2 MPa	1%	1–2 min	1.5-fold decrease in tumor volume and median survival compared to free Doxil
Escoffre et al. (2013b)	U-87 MG (s.c., mouse)	Free Irinotecan	MM1	i.v.	1 MHz	0.4 MPa (PNP)	40%	3 min	Threefold decrease in tumor volume, twofold decrease in tumor perfusion, threefold increase necrosis, 35% decrease in mitosis index, no acute liver toxicity compared to free irinotecan
Ting et al. (2012)	C6 (i.c., rat)	BCNU-loaded MB	Lipid	i.v.	1 MHz	0.5–0.7 MPa	5%	1 min / sonication site	Fivefold increase in circulatory half-life of BCNU, fivefold decrease in liver accumulation, 13-fold decrease in tumor volume, 12% increase in median survival compared to free BCNU
Tinkov et al. (2010)	DSL6A (s.c., rat)	DOX-loaded MB	Lipid	i.v (perfusion)	1.3 MHz	1.2 MPa	ND	Four ultrasound frames every four cardiac cycles	10-fold i.t. DOX accumulation, twofold decrease in tumor volume compared to DOX-loaded MB treatment alone

s.c., subcutaneous; i.c., intracerebral; 10-HCPT, 10-hydroxycamptothecin; BLM, bleomycin; DOX, doxorubicin; ND, non-defined; PNP, peak-negative-pressure.

Microbubble-Assisted Ultrasound

The combination of high frequency ultrasound (1–10 MHz) and ultrasound contrast agents (i.e., consisting of gas microbubbles) was introduced as a promising method in improving the therapeutic efficacy of drugs by increasing local delivery, while minimizing side effects to healthy tissues (Price et al., 1998). In this paper, we refer to this combination as microbubble-assisted ultrasound. The first generation of microbubbles was composed of air encapsulated by albumin (Albunex®) or galactose/palmitic acid (Levovist®) shells. However, such air-filled microbubbles dissolve in the bloodstream within a few seconds after intravenous (i.v.) administration because of the high solubility of air in blood and their low resistance to arterial pressure gradients. To overcome these issues, a second generation of microbubbles was developed, which were filled with heavy-weight hydrophobic gas (e.g., perfluorocarbon, sulfur hexafluoride) encapsulated by a biocompatible shell (e.g., lipids, polymer; Hernot and Klibanov, 2008; Sirsi and Borden, 2014; **Figure**). In studies on drug delivery by microbubble-assisted ultrasound, the bubbles are mixed with cells in vitro or injected in vivo intravascularly or directly into the tissue of interest. Microbubble behavior in an ultrasound field has been widely studied, which led to more understanding and subsequent control of the induced bio-effects that can be used for drug delivery (Kooiman et al., 2014). The response of a microbubble to ultrasound waves depends on the acoustic parameters used, such as frequency, pressure levels, and pulse duration. In short, microbubbles stably oscillate over time upon exposure to a low acoustic pressure, a process termed stable cavitation (**Figures**). These oscillations generate fluid flows

surrounding the bubble, known as acoustic micro-streaming, and when in close contact with cells, result in shear stress on the cell membrane, leading to cellular uptake of drugs (Leighton, 1994; Wu, 2002; Doinikov and Bouakaz, 2010). At higher acoustic pressures, microbubbles oscillate more rigorously, leading to their violent collapse and destruction, i.e., inertial cavitation (**Figure**). Microbubble disruption can be accompanied by generation of shock waves in the medium close to the microbubbles (Junge et al., 2003; Ohl and Wolfrum, 2003). The ultrasound-induced collapse of the microbubble can be asymmetrical, leading to the formation of high velocity jets (Postema et al., 2005; Ohl et al., 2006). While shock waves induce shear stress to cells in close proximity, resulting in membrane permeability, the high velocity jets can pierce the cell membrane, and thereby create permeability. Stable and inertial cavitation are both exploited to transiently increase the permeability of biological barriers, including the vascular endothelium and plasma membrane, and therefore enhance the extravasation and the cellular uptake of drugs (Lentacker et al., 2014; **Figure**).

Extravasation of Drugs

Microbubbles are intravascular contrast agents, which do not cross the vascular endothelium (Wilson and Burns, 2010). Cavitating microbubbles close to the endothelial wall can result in several bio-effects including vascular disruption, vasoconstriction, or even shutdown of the vessels (Goertz, 2015). Several studies observed that microbubble-assisted ultrasound increased (model-) drug extravasation by stimulating paracellular (i.e., disruption of tight junctions) and transcellular pathways (i.e., transcytosis), both in vitro as well as in vivo (;

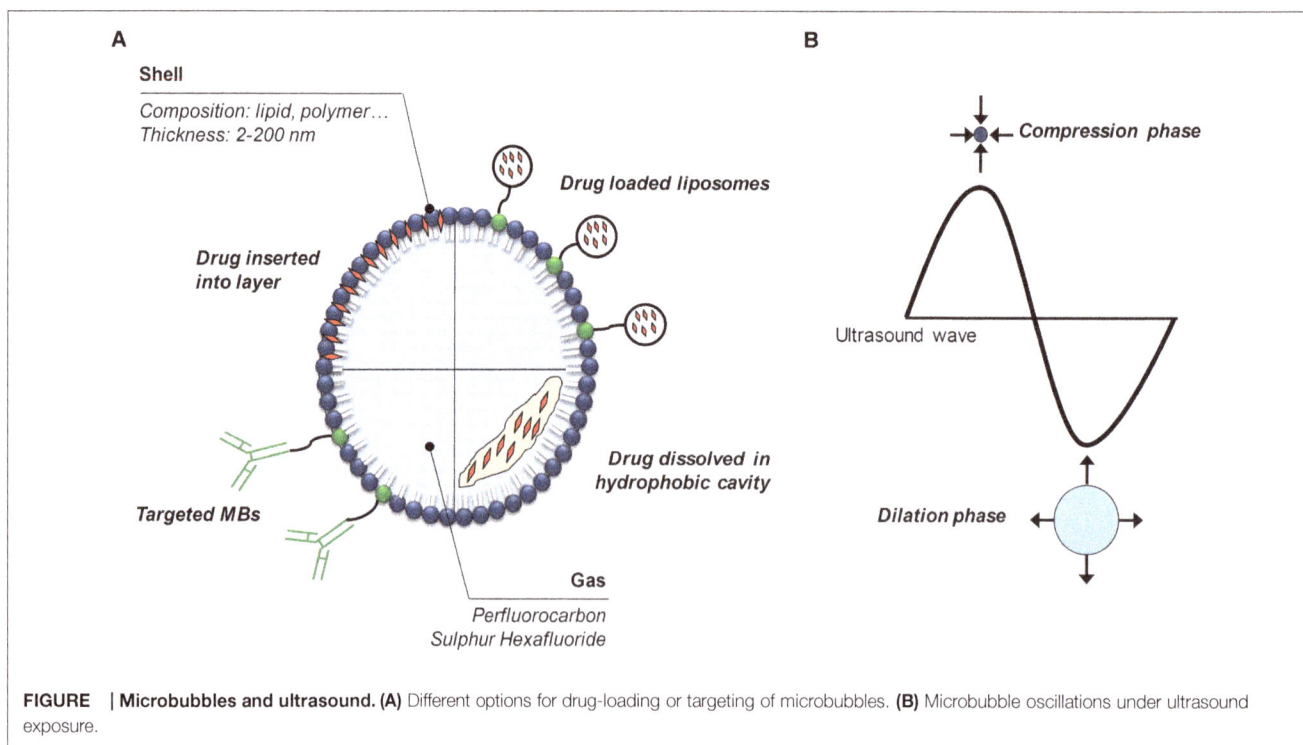

FIGURE | **Microbubbles and ultrasound. (A)** Different options for drug-loading or targeting of microbubbles. **(B)** Microbubble oscillations under ultrasound exposure.

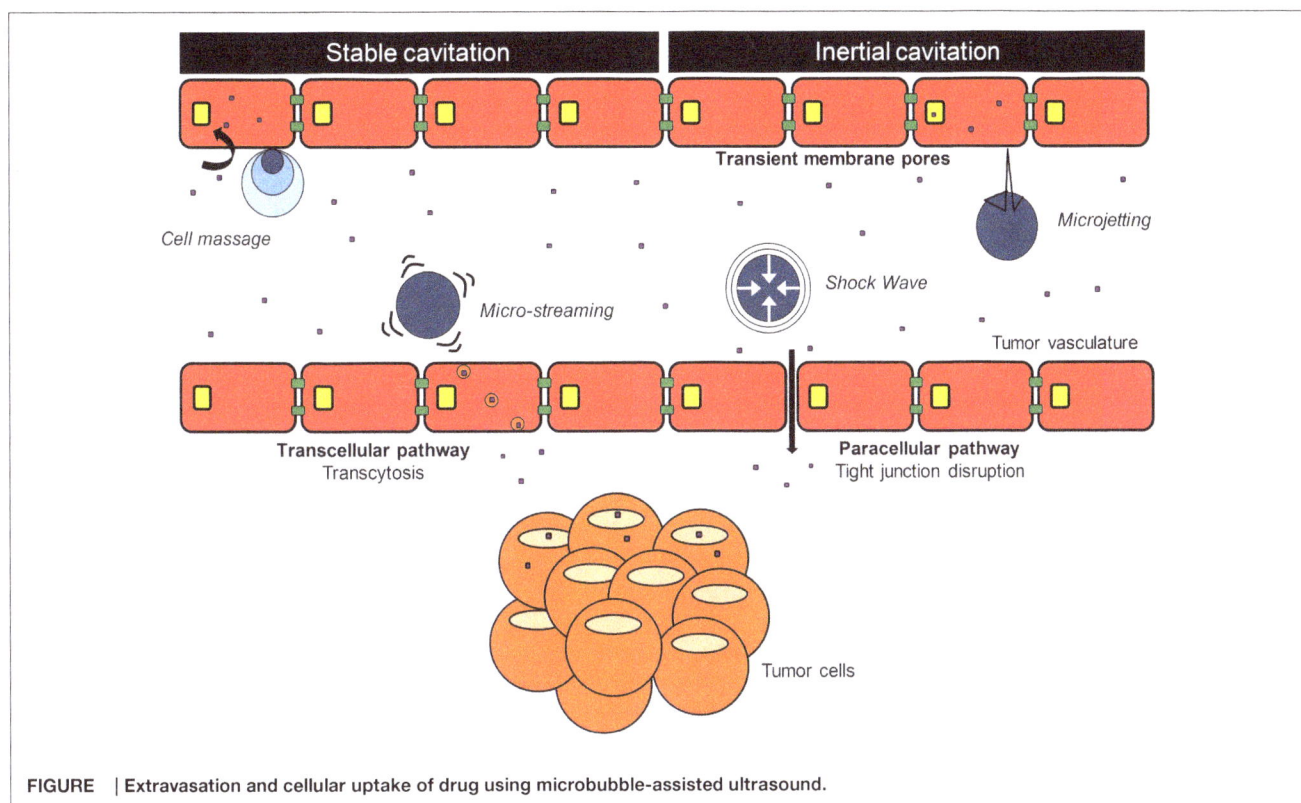

FIGURE | **Extravasation and cellular uptake of drug using microbubble-assisted ultrasound.**

Price et al., 1998; Sheikov et al., 2008; Juffermans et al., 2009; Kooiman et al., 2010). In an *in vitro* endothelial barrier model, Kooiman et al. (2010) showed that microbubble-assisted ultrasound induced a 40% decrease in transendothelial electric resistance showing a loss of endothelial barrier integrity. In addition, Juffermans et al. (2009) showed that microbubble-assisted ultrasound significantly affected the integrity of *in vitro* endothelial monolayers by the destabilization of the tight junctions. At low acoustic pressures (1 MHz, 0.1 MPa), the integrity of the *in vitro* endothelial barrier was restored within 30 min. *In vivo*, an acoustical pressure threshold ranging from 0.1 to 0.75 MPa was required to enhance the extravasation of intravascular agents (e.g., red blood cells, imaging tracers, fluorescent dyes, or drugs) in skeletal muscle (Price et al., 1998), brain (Raymond et al., 2007; Sheikov et al., 2008), liver (Gao et al., 2012), and tumor (Bohmer et al., 2010; Hu et al., 2012) tissues. This extravasation occurs through tight junctions between endothelial cells (0.2–200 μm; Price et al., 1998; Song et al., 2002; Stieger et al., 2007). *In vivo,* the integrity of the blood–brain barrier was restored within 1–4 h following ultrasound exposure (Sheikov et al., 2008; Ting et al., 2012). However, Marty et al. (2012) showed that the duration of extravasation after ultrasound exposure depends on the particle size. The microbubble-assisted ultrasound enhanced transcellular pathways (e.g., transcytosis) have been mainly investigated on the brain vasculature (Raymond et al., 2007; Sheikov et al., 2008; Deng et al., 2012). They reported that low (1 MHz, 0.2 MPa) and high (1.63 MHz, 1-3 MPa) acoustic pressures increased the number of transcytotic vesicles on both the luminal and

abluminal surface of the endothelium. Sheikov et al. (2004) hypothesized that the transient vasoconstriction constitutes a potential cause for the increased transcytosis *in vivo*. In addition, Hu et al. (2012) showed that the destruction of microbubbles with a high acoustic pressure (5 MHz, 2 MPa) decreased the tumor blood flow for 30 min before it returned back to normal, without an increase in hemorrhage. Whereas it was demonstrated that the extravasation of fluorescent dextrans was enhanced during this period, the authors did not investigate whether transcytosis was involved. Transient vasoconstriction has been only reported in mice, which exhibit higher vasomotor excitability than other rodents and animal species.

Heating and Acoustic Radiation Force

Besides cavitation, ultrasound can also induce heating and acoustic radiation force (ARF) to improve the extravasation of drugs (Deckers and Moonen, 2010). Heating can result from the absorbance of acoustic energy as the ultrasound beam propagates through tissue. Mild heating of a tumor (41 – 43°C for 10 – 60 min) may improve the therapeutic efficacy of drugs by acting on tumor hemodynamics (**Figure**): (i) by increasing tumor perfusion, thus enhancing drug bioavailability in tumor tissue (Song, 1984); (ii) by increasing vascular permeability (Lefor et al., 1985; Kong et al., 2001) and reducing tumor interstitial pressure (Vaupel and Kelleher, 2012), leading to better drug penetration within tumor tissue. In addition, local heating can act as an external trigger for drug release from a carrier, e.g., thermosensitive nanoparticles (Yatvin et al., 1978; Lindner et al., 2004; Manzoor et al., 2012; Hijnen et al., 2014; Al Sabbagh

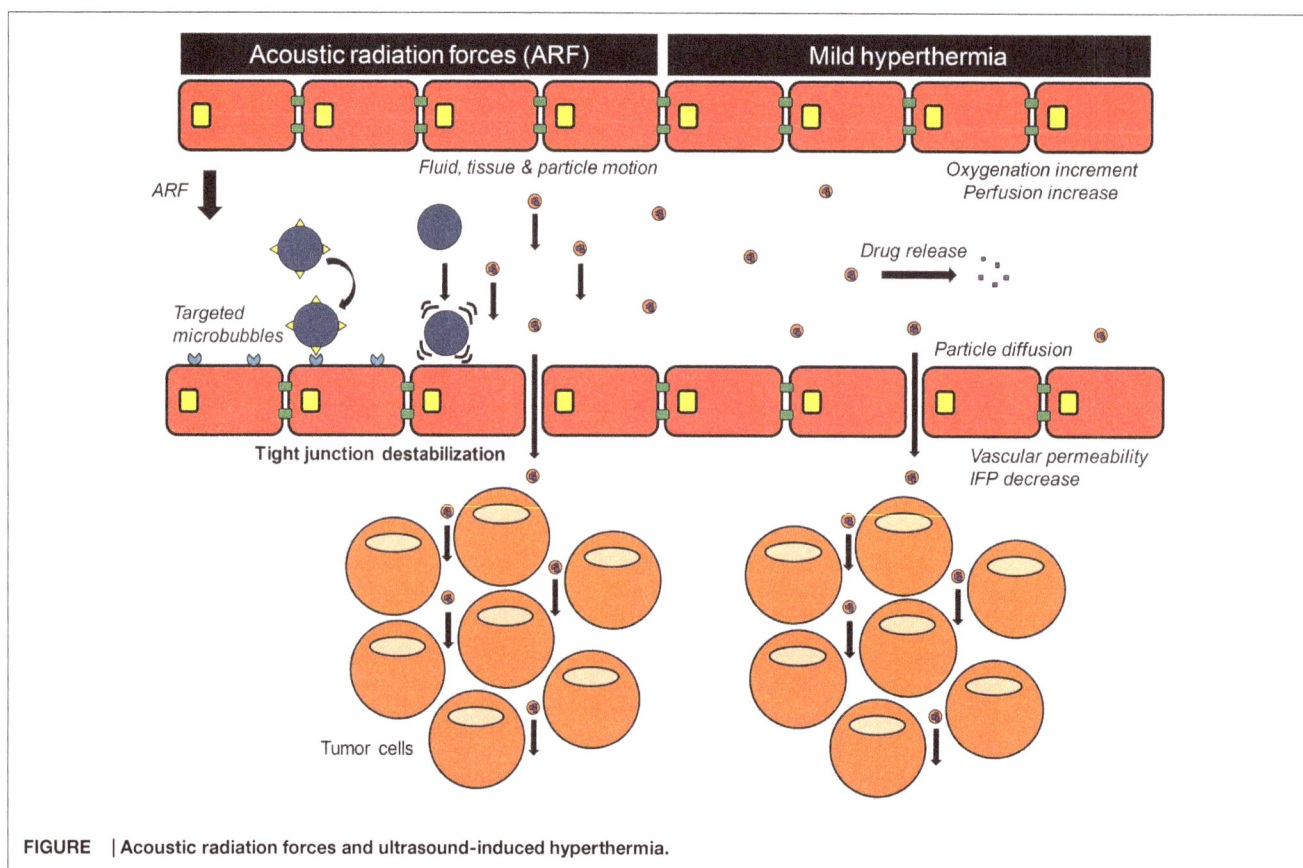

FIGURE | Acoustic radiation forces and ultrasound-induced hyperthermia.

et al., 2015). Ultrasound can also generate directional ARF on molecules along its propagation path (Sarvazyan et al., 2010; **Figure**). This enhances the extravasation of free drug or drug-loaded nanoparticles into tumor tissue by causing tissue shear stress and opening of endothelial tight junctions (Seidl et al., 1994; Mesiwala et al., 2002). ARF induces fluid streaming through the interstitium, thus improving biodistribution of intravascular dyes and drugs in the target tissue (Lum et al., 2006; Hancock et al., 2009). Using optical imaging, Shortencarier et al. (2004) showed that the application of ARF induced visible aggregates of fluorescent dye-loaded gas liposheres in the direction of the beam on the far vessel wall. The liposheres disappeared when the ARF pulses were turned off (Shortencarier et al., 2004). In addition to liposheres, ARFs can push circulating microbubbles toward the endothelial wall, thereby improving microbubble–cell contact, which might enhance cavitation-mediated extravasation of intravascular compounds (Rychak et al., 2005; Wang et al., 2014). Using ultrasound imaging, Frinking et al. (2012) reported that ARF (38 kPa PNP, 95% DC) induced a sevenfold increase in the binding of VEGFR2-targeted microbubbles (also known as BR-55) on the endothelial wall in a prostate adenocarcinoma rat model compared with the binding without ARF.

Cellular Uptake of Drugs

Cavitating microbubbles in the vicinity of the plasma membrane can result in cell permeabilization by creating membrane pores and stimulating the endocytosis pathways, thereby facilitating intracellular drug uptake. Based on the uptake or release of non-permeant dyes (Meijering et al., 2009; Kaddur et al., 2010) and by measuring changes in membrane electrophysiology (Tran et al., 2007; Juffermans et al., 2008), previous studies showed that microbubble-assisted ultrasound induced a transient increase in membrane permeability through the generation of transient hydrophilic pores. The intracellular delivery of molecules through membrane pores is likely governed by passive diffusion or by ultrasound-mediated propulsion (i.e., microstreaming, ARF; Shortencarier et al., 2004; Lum et al., 2006). The size of these ultrasound induced pores depend on the acoustic parameters used, ranging from 1 to 94 nm at 0.19 MPa PSP and from 2 to 4 µm at 0.48 MPa PSP (Yang et al., 2008).

In addition to hydrophilic pore formation, enhancement of endocytosis has also been demonstrated following microbubble-assisted ultrasound exposure (Meijering et al., 2009). Electrophysiological studies reported that microbubble-assisted ultrasound induced an influx of Ca^{2+}, followed by an activation of BK_{Ca} channels that results in local hyperpolarization of the cell membrane (Tran et al., 2007; Juffermans et al., 2008). At moderate ultrasound conditions (1 MHz, 0.15–0.3 MPa), the membrane hyperpolarization facilitates the molecular uptake through endocytosis and macropinocytosis. Similar to pore formation, the contribution of endocytosis processes depends strongly on the marker size and the acoustic pressures.

Meijering et al. (2009) reported that low acoustic pressures (1 MHz, 0.22 MPa PNP) resulted in the cellular uptake of 4.4 and 70 kDa fluorescent dextrans through membrane pores while the entrance of 155 and 500 kDa fluorescent dextrans is dominated by endocytosis pathways. It should be mentioned that little is known about the faith of the agents in the endocytic vesicles, if they are degraded in the lysosome or escape from the endosome. However, De Cock et al. (2015) showed that increasing the acoustic pressures (1 MHz, 0.5 MPa, PNP) induced the intracellular delivery of large fluorescent dextrans (2 MDa) to shift from uptake by endocytosis to uptake via the membrane pores. Regardless of the mechanism of uptake, the duration of microbubble-assisted ultrasound-mediated uptake is dependent on the plasma membrane recovery time, which is a few seconds to a few hours (van Wamel et al., 2006; Lammertink et al., 2015). The different kinetics depends on the ultrasound conditions, the model drug size and the cell physiology.

Anti-Cancer Drug Delivery Protocols

As any drug delivery technique, microbubble-assisted ultrasound treatments aim to deliver optimal quantities of chemotherapeutic drugs in targeted tumor cells and tissues. The efficiency of this delivery method depends on (i) sufficient accumulation of microbubbles and drugs near tumor cells or tissues, which is directly influenced by the properties of microbubbles, drugs (i.e., plasma circulation lifetime), and tumor (i.e., vascularization, localization), as well as administration routes (i.e., intratumoral, intravenous, intraperitoneal); (ii) the acoustic conditions including ultrasound parameters (i.e., central frequency, acoustic pressure, exposure time, etc.) and devices (i.e., home-made, commercial, medical systems); (iii) treatment schedule including the time interval between the drug and/or microbubbles administration and ultrasound treatment as well as the number of microbubble-assisted ultrasound drug delivery treatments and the time interval between them. Over the past decade, the influence of these factors on drug delivery efficiency has been investigated in order to enhance the intratumoral (i.t.) accumulation of drug, thereby increasing the treatment effect, while minimizing side effects to healthy tissues. This review shows that the drug delivery efficacy varied between the tumor models used in vivo. It is commonly known in the field that the tumor type is an important determinant for successful drug delivery. This is due to the specific properties of each tumor tissue, such as differences in tissue organization, extracellular matrix, presence of necrosis and hypoxia, cell density, and the endothelial lining of the tumor vasculature (Chauhan et al., 2011). To the best of our knowledge, no comparative study between tumor tissues with different properties has been reported using microbubble-assisted ultrasound for drug delivery. However, unlike many other drug delivery strategies, sonochemotherapy does not depend on the enhanced permeability and retention (EPR) effect, which is very heterogeneous between or within tumors, and often overestimated (Lammers et al., 2012). Interestingly, you

could argue that the largest effect of sonochemotherapy can be expected in tissues with 'non-leaky' vessels, such as the brain (Ting et al., 2012), since the potential of increasing extravasation is highest. An overview of different drug delivery protocols and outcomes in vitro and in vivo are shown in **Tables** , respectively. It should be noted that this is not a complete overview, but rather a selection of different drug delivery protocols.

Microbubbles

In most studies, clinically approved microbubbles (i.e., SonoVue®, Definity®) for ultrasound imaging are employed for drug delivery. The use of these microbubbles may facilitate the clinical translation of sonochemotherapy, but any undesired side effect might have a negative impact on the use of these microbubbles in ultrasound-based diagnostics. Modification of these microbubbles (e.g., drug-loaded microbubbles) for therapeutic applications will delay clinical translation, requiring new authorization from the regulatory and health authorities.

Coadministration of Microbubbles and Drug

The simplest method for drug delivery using microbubble-assisted ultrasound is to use coadministration (Heath et al., 2012; Unga and Hashida, 2014). This approach includes drugs that are administered in patients anyway in current clinical practice, with the addition of an injection of (clinically approved) microbubbles. Microbubbles and drugs can be mixed in solution in vitro and the mixture is then injected in vivo. This strategy offers two main advantages: (i) both constituents can be handled completely separately until in vitro or in vivo administration; (ii) instead of mixing microbubbles and drug before injection, two separate injections of the constituents can also be performed, thus allowing drugs to reach plasma peak levels before injecting microbubbles (Escoffre et al., 2013b). Microbubbles have a short circulation time and therefore need to be exposed to ultrasound within minutes after injection, otherwise they will be degraded and unable to induce bio-effects. The coadministration approach seems to be the best strategy for in vitro purposes (Escoffre et al., 2011; Sorace et al., 2012) or, in vivo, i.t. injection of the mixture (Sasaki et al., 2014), where similar spatio-temporal distribution of both components will be ensured. Iwanaga et al. (2007) showed that the in vitro delivery of bleomycin using microbubble-assisted ultrasound induced twofold decrease in cell viability compared to the bleomycin treatment alone (**Table**). In vivo, they reported that the exposure of a tumor to ultrasound following the i.t. co-injection of microbubbles and bleomycin also resulted in a twofold decrease in tumor volume (Iwanaga et al., 2007). Kotopoulis et al. (2014) coadministered commercially available microbubbles and gemcitabine i.v. in a pancreatic cancer model in mice. They showed that ultrasound exposure (1 MHz, 0.2 MPa PNP) decreased the tumor volume twofold compared to gemcitabine alone (Kotopoulis et al., 2014). Opposed to the advantages of coadministration using clinically approved microbubbles and drugs that allow clinical translation, there are also disadvantages. The main limitations of the i.v.

injection of microbubble/drug mixture compared to drug-loaded microbubbles are: (i) differential distribution of both constituents because of their physicochemical properties; (ii) fast degradation of free drugs and microbubbles; (iii) unspecific accumulation of free drugs in the healthy tissues.

Drug-Loaded Microbubbles

To overcome these limitations of i.v. coadministration, microbubbles have been modified to function not only as cavitation nuclei, but also as drug delivery carriers. For example, lipophilic drugs can be incorporated into the lipid monolayer shell of microbubbles or dissolved in an oil pocket between the gas core and the microbubble's shell (Ibsen et al., 2013). By applying this approach, Burke et al. (2014) found that the application of ultrasound (1 MHz, 1.2 MPa, every 5 s for 60 min) on subcutaneous C6 glioma tumor following the i.v. injection of 5-FU-loaded microbubbles (1×10^5 microbubbles/g body weight) led to twofold decrease in tumor volume compared to 5-FU treatment alone (Burke et al., 2014). While these approaches seem to be promising, the low drug loading capacity of microbubbles is a major drawback. Consequently, the use of drug-loaded microbubbles requires either enhancement of the drug loading efficiency, administration of high dose of drug-loaded microbubbles, or application of consecutive treatments.

The small size of microbubbles and their gaseous lumen restricts the space for drug loading. Recent publications reported that the binding of drug-loaded nanoparticles on the microbubble's surface could increase the amount of loaded drug (Geers et al., 2011). The loading efficiency can be further improved by applying multiple layers of drug-loaded nanoparticles around the microbubble shell. The binding of drug-loaded nanoparticles on microbubbles may not be necessary for polymer-based microbubbles, as significant amounts of (model) drug can be loaded into the polymer-based shell (Fokong et al., 2012). Cochran et al. (2011) showed that the loading capacity is higher for hydrophobic drugs compared to hydrophilic drugs, and that the acoustic properties of the microbubbles were unaffected (Cochran et al., 2011).

Based on current studies, a high dose of drug-loaded microbubbles, i.e., $>10^{10}$ microbubbles, must be intravenously injected to reach a therapeutic dose similar to the one used in clinical chemotherapy. However, the recommended diagnostic doses of microbubbles currently approved for contrast-enhanced ultrasound imaging (e.g., SonoVue®, Definity®) are between 10^9 and 10^{10} microbubbles for an 80-kg adult (Wilson and Burns, 2010). Nevertheless, preclinical and clinical studies have reported a good tolerance with 100- and 1000-fold higher doses of these microbubbles in non-human primates and patients (Grauer et al., 1996; Bokor et al., 2001). Consequently, the injection of a high dose of drug-loaded microbubbles may not be a limitation for clinical use, but further preclinical studies might be necessary to identify any potential toxicity of high concentrations of liposome and shell's components (i.e., lipid, polymer, and albumin).

Finally, several preclinical studies reported the use of repeated sonochemotherapy treatments (Kang et al., 2010; Tinkov et al.,

2010; Li et al., 2012; Ting et al., 2012). For example, Li et al. (2012) reported that the repetitive treatment (i.e., once a day for seven consecutive days) of subcutaneous hepatic tumor using 10-hydroxycamptothecin-loaded microbubbles (4 mg/kg) induced twofold stronger decrease in tumor volume in a subcutaneous hepatic tumor model (1 MHz, 2 W/cm^2, 6 min) compared to the 10-hydroxycamptothecin-based chemotherapy alone (Li et al., 2012).

Targeted Microbubbles

Microbubbles can be modified to target specific overexpressed markers on tumor cells (i.e., PSMA, prostate specific membrane antigen; LHR, luteinizing hormone receptor) or tumor microvasculature (VEGF-R2, vascular endothelial growth factor receptor -2) through attachment of targeting ligands or antibodies onto the microbubble's shell (Kiessling et al., 2012, 2014; Novell et al., 2013). This may lead to enhanced accumulation of the microbubbles in the target tumor cells or tissues. For example, Fan et al. (2013) designed targeted BCNU-loaded microbubbles, which bind the VEGF-R2 overexpressed on tumor microvasculature (VEGFR2-BCNU-loaded microbubbles; **Figure**). The exposure of orthotopic glioma to ultrasound (1 MHz, 0.7 MPa, 1 min/sonication site) following i.v. injection of VEGFR2-BCNU-loaded microbubbles (1.25 mg BCNU) resulted in 1.75-fold decrease in tumor volume compared to the untargeted BCNU-loaded microbubbles (**Figure** ; Fan et al., 2013). The use of microbubbles targeting overexpressed markers on the tumor cells themselves is limited to *in vitro* drug delivery, i.t. or intraperitoneal (i.p.) injection of microbubbles and drugs, primarily because the microbubbles, when administered intravenously, cannot extravasate due to the size (Cavalieri et al., 2010). For imaging, several groups have reported on the *in vivo* accumulation of targeted microbubbles in the tumor microvasculature by binding inflammation markers overexpressed on tumor endothelial cells (Deshpande et al., 2010). Although these microbubbles were designed as ultrasound contrast agents for molecular imaging, it might be possible to develop optimal tissue- or organ-selective drug delivery agents by combining targeting capacities and drug loading of microbubbles (Kiessling et al., 2012). However, no evidence of their use for drug delivery has been reported yet.

To summarize, the coadministration of drugs/microbubbles and drug-loaded microbubbles can both be used for drug delivery. The coadministration approach is likely to be the fastest way into the clinic, as it combines clinically approved drugs and microbubbles. However, the drug-loaded microbubbles may hold the greatest therapeutic potential, as it locally releases the drug upon ultrasound exposure. Since this approach represents new therapeutic entities, such 'therapeutic microbubbles' require extensive testing for safety and efficacy before they can be approved for clinical use. To the best of our knowledge, no study has been published that directly compares drug-loaded microbubbles with coadministration of free drugs and microbubbles at equal dosing schemes.

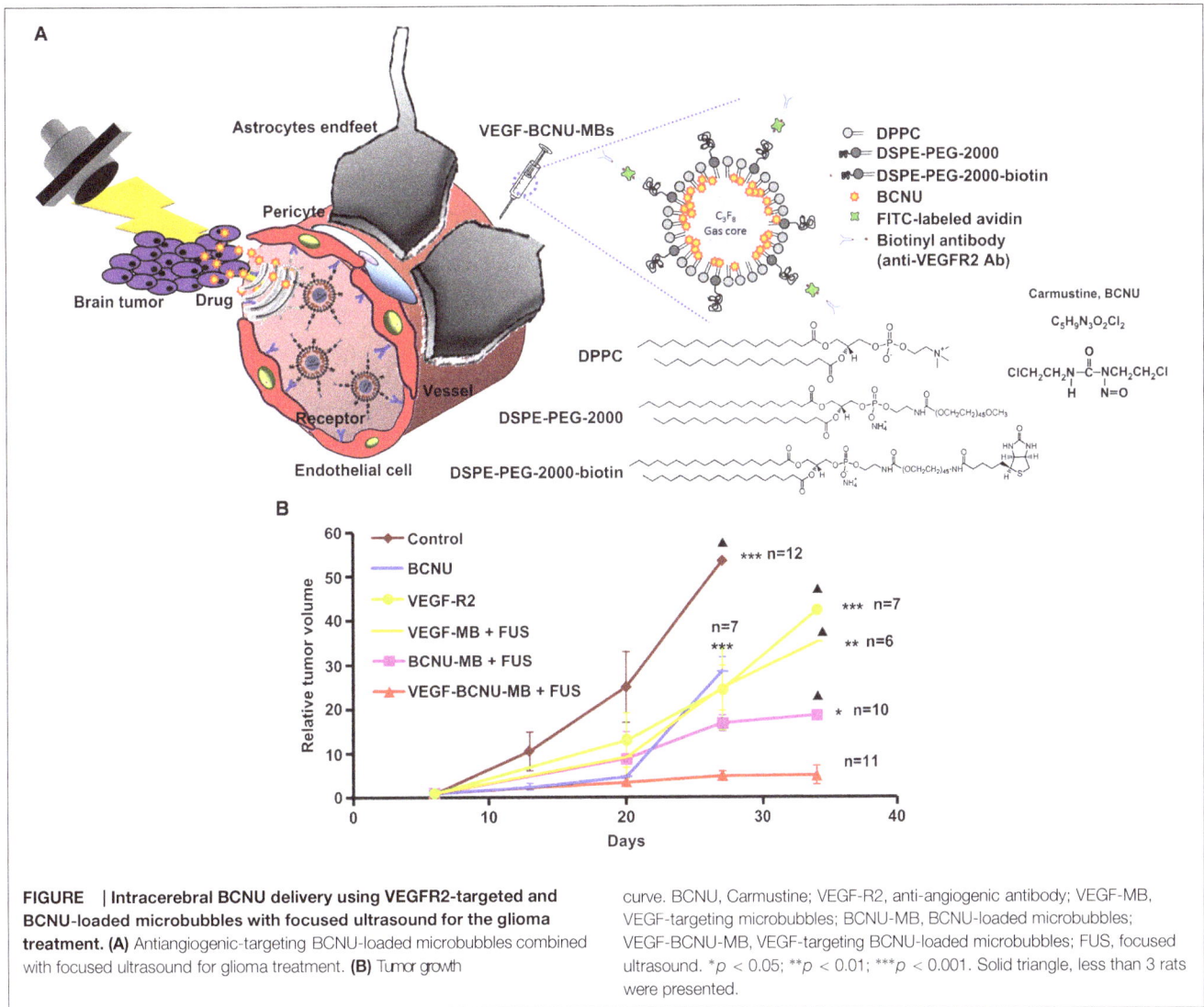

FIGURE | Intracerebral BCNU delivery using VEGFR2-targeted and BCNU-loaded microbubbles with focused ultrasound for the glioma treatment. **(A)** Antiangiogenic-targeting BCNU-loaded microbubbles combined with focused ultrasound for glioma treatment. **(B)** Tumor growth curve. BCNU, Carmustine; VEGF-R2, anti-angiogenic antibody; VEGF-MB, VEGF-targeting microbubbles; BCNU-MB, BCNU-loaded microbubbles; VEGF-BCNU-MB, VEGF-targeting BCNU-loaded microbubbles; FUS, focused ultrasound. $*p < 0.05$; $**p < 0.01$; $***p < 0.001$. Solid triangle, less than 3 rats were presented.

Administration Routes

The most direct administration route for drug delivery is i.t. injection (Sonoda et al., 2007; Sasaki et al., 2014). The advantages of i.t. administration over systemic injection include the circumvention of the transvascular barrier and the generation of transient interstitial pressure gradients. The latter can induce convection and tissue deformation, which can decrease the connectedness of the extracellular matrix and size of pores in the tumor interstitial space (Frenkel, 2008). By using i.t. administration, a high drug dose can be directly delivered into the target tumor while minimizing its side effects toward healthy tissues. This administration route overcomes the drawback related to the short plasma half-life of drugs and microbubbles after i.v. injection. In addition, this route is most interesting for hydrophilic small chemotherapeutic drugs that have difficulties to enter tumor cells. By applying i.t. injection, microbubbles and drugs are distributed within the tumor by diffusion and convection, and subsequent US exposure will result in drug uptake in tumor cells. However, in i.t injection, there are some limitations such as the injected volume and the accessibility of the tumor site, which restrict the application of microbubble-assisted ultrasound to superficial tumors such as melanoma, and cutaneous and subcutaneous tumors.

For deep-seated tumors, most protocols recommend injection of drugs and microbubbles via blood flow, providing better access to deeper tumors (Treat et al., 2012; Yan et al., 2013; Burke et al., 2014). The i.v. route is a relatively easy and safe way to be used in the clinic for the administration of therapeutics and microbubbles. As previously described, the main limitation of this administration route is the rapid clearance of drug from plasma and the unspecific accumulation of this drug in healthy tissues. Therefore, drugs can be loaded on microbubbles to overcome these shortcomings (Ting et al., 2012; Sirsi and Borden, 2014). The success of i.v. drug delivery relies on sufficient tumor vascularization, thus restricting the application of this administration route to hypervascularized tumors. Next to extravasation, microbubble-assisted ultrasound can also increase the penetration of drugs into the tissue.

In addition, it can "homogenize" drug uptake, since drug distribution tends to be very heterogeneous throughout the tumor. Since microbubble-assisted ultrasound will mostly affect the vascular endothelium, the i.v. route is most suitable for drugs that can benefit from ultrasound-induced extravasation and penetration or intracellular delivery in endothelial cells.

Recent studies reported that the i.p. injection may be useful for drug delivery using microbubble-assisted ultrasound for the treatments of primary peritoneal cancers or cancers with i.p. metastases. Pu et al. (2014) investigated the i.p. delivery of paclitaxel (PTX) for the treatment of ovarian cancer using luteinizing hormone-releasing hormone analog (LHRHa) - targeted and PTX-loaded microbubbles (20 mg/kg PTX) and ultrasound (0.3 MHz, 1 W/cm^2, 3 min). This therapeutic protocol led to a twofold increase in apoptotic index and a 2.5-fold decrease in vessel number compared to the single injection of free PTX or PTX delivery using ultrasound alone (Pu et al., 2014). Due to the microbubble size, penetration of the microbubbles by convection throughout the tumor is hindered, thereby limiting the tumor cell binding to the peripheral rim of the tumor. Nevertheless, the targeted microbubbles in this study showed superior efficacy compared to the untargeted bubbles.

Ultrasound Devices, Transducer, and Parameters

Several investigations showed extensive optimization of the acoustic parameters to result in an efficient and safe *in vitro* and *in vivo* drug delivery. Among these studies, clinical ultrasound scanners have been used to deliver drugs using microbubble-assisted ultrasound (Tinkov et al., 2010; Sasaki et al., 2014), which has the advantage of enabling both imaging of- and drug delivery to the targeted tumor. However, the ultrasound settings that are allowed on such equipment are limited for safety reasons. Specific ultrasound parameters [low cycles and mechanical index (MI) 0.5 < MI < 1.9] are used to destroy microbubbles during a diagnostic tissue perfusion study (Szabo, 2013). However, such parameters might not be efficient for drug delivery. In addition, clinical ultrasound probes are unfocused and thus the ultrasound energy will have substantial effects in the regions surrounding the target tissue. Clinical ultrasound scanners are "black-boxes" which do not allow controlling all ultrasound parameters. Hence, home-made and commercial therapeutic ultrasound devices have been designed to control many ultrasound parameters, which can subsequently be optimized for drug delivery (Zhao et al., 2011; Lin et al., 2012; Escoffre et al., 2013a). Ultrasound transducers used in the literature can be focused or unfocused (Sanches et al., 2011). Focused beams are created using spherically curved transducers, which greatly increase the ultrasound intensity in a small region of interest, e.g., a tumor. Due to a lack of standardized calibration methods concerning the applied ultrasound parameters and the heterogeneity in equipment used, it is not straightforward to compare the results of most studies directly (ter Haar et al., 2011).

The transmission center frequency used for *in vivo* drug delivery studies listed in **Table** ranges from 0.3 to 2.25 MHz. The choice of frequency to be used can depend on the microbubble's size and its resonance frequency, but also on the depth of the tissue to be reached, as higher frequencies suffer from increased attenuation. The resonance frequency of microbubble decreases as their size increases (Minnaert, 1933). When using a low frequency range, the acoustic pressure threshold to initiate microbubble cavitation can be reduced, thereby limiting putative tissue damage. In most of the reported investigations, 1 MHz was used as a frequency to achieve drug delivery using microbubble-assisted ultrasound (**Tables**).

The ultrasound dose is usually expressed in different units depending on whether a medical ultrasound scanner, commercial or laboratory-made device is used for drug delivery (**Table**). With home-made or commercial therapeutic ultrasound devices, ultrasound exposure is usually expressed either in acoustic pressure amplitude (kPa) or in intensity (W/cm^2) while for medical ultrasound scanners, the dose is usually expressed in the terms of MI (expressed as the ratio of the peak negative pressure in MPa to the square root of the frequency in MHz). Among the published studies, it is not clearly stated whether ultrasound intensity are spatial averaged, temporal averaged intensity (I_{SATA}) or spatial peak, temporal averaged intensity (I_{SPTA}). I_{SATA} is frequently used when non-focused transducer is employed for drug delivery. Ultrasound intensities ranging from 0.064 to 3 W/cm^2 (n.b., I_{SPTA} 0.0003 – 0.9 W/cm^2 for ultrasound-based diagnostics) have been applied in recent studies to deliver drugs in tumor tissue without injuries (Kang et al., 2010; Lu et al., 2011). The MI used for *in vivo* drug delivery ranges from 0.2 to 2 (n.b., MI threshold for clinical diagnosis is 1.9). Drug delivery requires a minimum MI known as the permeabilization threshold, which is typically lower than 1 (Choi et al., 2007). Exposure of tumor tissues above, but near the cavitation threshold has so far yielded the most promising results of drug delivery without significant side effects. Increasing the ultrasound dose further enhanced drug delivery in the target tissue but was also accompanied by hemorrhage and tissue injuries (Kang et al., 2010; Lu et al., 2011).

The duty cycle is the percentage of time that an ultrasound device is transmitting acoustic waves. The duty cycle ranges from 0.25 to 50% for drug delivery into tumors (**Table**). To prevent thermal tissue damage, low duty cycles are used when high ultrasound intensities are applied and vice versa (Lin et al., 2012; Wei et al., 2013).

Ultrasound exposure time plays a major role in drug delivery using microbubble-assisted ultrasound. During this time, ultrasound pulses are emitted repeatedly at a pulsing interval to induce the complete destruction of microbubbles in the targeted tumor. Ultrasound exposure times from 2 s to 10 min have been reported (**Table**). However, exposure times of 1–5 min are recommended to prevent tissue injuries (e.g., hemorrhages; Mei et al., 2009; Yan et al., 2013).

Treatment Schedule

The therapeutic protocol depends on the duration of microbubble-assisted ultrasound-mediated permeability of tumor tissues and the pharmacokinetics of chemotherapeutic drugs. Some studies reported drug administration at different time points following the exposure of tumor to microbubble-assisted ultrasound to assess the duration of enhanced permeability (few seconds – few hours, depending on the particle size; Marty et al., 2012; Tzu-Yin et al., 2014; Lammertink et al., 2015). Other investigations recommend waiting for the peak concentration of drug in the blood before the administration of microbubbles and the subsequent exposure of tumors to ultrasound. For example, Escoffre et al. (2013b) succeeded to optimize therapeutic efficacy of irinotecan using microbubble-assisted ultrasound in subcutaneous glioblastoma. In this study, the protocol consisted of an i.v. injection of irinotecan followed 1 h later by an i.v. administration of microbubbles (Escoffre et al., 2013b). This delay is required to reach the maximal systemic concentration of SN-38, the active metabolite of irinotecan, in the blood. This strategy induced a twofold decrease in tumor volume and perfusion compared to irinotecan without subsequent ultrasound exposure.

In most therapeutic protocols using the coadministration approach or drug-loaded microbubbles, ultrasound was applied to the tumors immediately (5–10 s) after microbubble injection (Sonoda et al., 2007; Matsuo et al., 2011). This strategy supposes that drugs and microbubbles are sufficiently accumulated in the target tissue during the few seconds following their administration. However, no real evidence has been reported whether this is actually the case. In addition, monitoring of microbubble arrival at the target tissue using contrast-enhanced ultrasound prior to ultrasound therapy is rarely performed. At present, all investigations show that at least several consecutive treatments (2–20 times) at optimal time intervals (1 day – 1 week) are required to achieve significant decrease in tumor growth or even tumor eradication (Table).

Therapeutic Efficacy vs. Safety: from *In Vitro* to Preclinical Studies

As described above, the therapeutic benefit of drug delivery using microbubble-assisted ultrasound relies on enhancing accumulation of drugs in tumor cells or tissues and on decreasing their deposition in healthy tissues, thus reducing their side effects (Tinkov et al., 2010; Li et al., 2012; Fan

et al., 2013; Burke et al., 2014). Using the coadministration approach or drug-loaded microbubbles, microbubble-assisted ultrasound enhances *in vitro* the therapeutic efficacy of clinically approved chemotherapeutics including doxorubicin (Dox), cisplatin, bleomycin, PTX, and docetaxel (Table). Most *in vitro* studies only monitor drug effectiveness with or without microbubble-assisted ultrasound. However, some studies also investigated the underlying mechanism. For example, Deng et al. (2014) showed enhanced intracellular Dox levels (Figure) and increased retention due to a down-regulation of P-glycoprotein following ultrasound exposure in the presence of Dox-liposome loaded microbubbles. This resulted in a significant increase of double-stranded DNA breaks and reduced cell viability (Figure). The exposure of tumor cells to microbubble-assisted ultrasound without any drugs had no or few effects on cell viability (>85% cell viability).

In *in vivo* studies it was clearly observed that microbubble-assisted ultrasound improves the therapeutic efficacy of drugs for different tumor animal models. However, most studies only monitor outcomes like survival and tumor size. Unfortunately, i.t. drug accumulation and distribution is often not investigated. Regardless of the administration route, only 40% of preclinical studies showed that an enhanced therapeutic efficacy could be attributed to increased i.t. drug levels. For example, Tinkov et al. (2010) demonstrated that the exposure of pancreas carcinoma in rats to ultrasound (1.3 MHz, 1.2 MPa PNP, four frames of ultrasound every four cardiac cycles) after i.v. injection of DOX-loaded microbubbles (140 µg – 3.14×10^9 microbubbles) induced a 10-fold increase in i.t. DOX accumulation compared to DOX-loaded microbubble injection alone (Tinkov et al., 2010). This therapeutic protocol led to a twofold decrease in tumor volume.

Next to increased drug concentration in the target tissue, one of the expected consequences of i.t. drug delivery using microbubble-assisted ultrasound is the reduction of drug deposition in healthy tissues. However, this effect is expected to be only significant for local release from drug-loaded microbubbles compared to the coadministration approach,

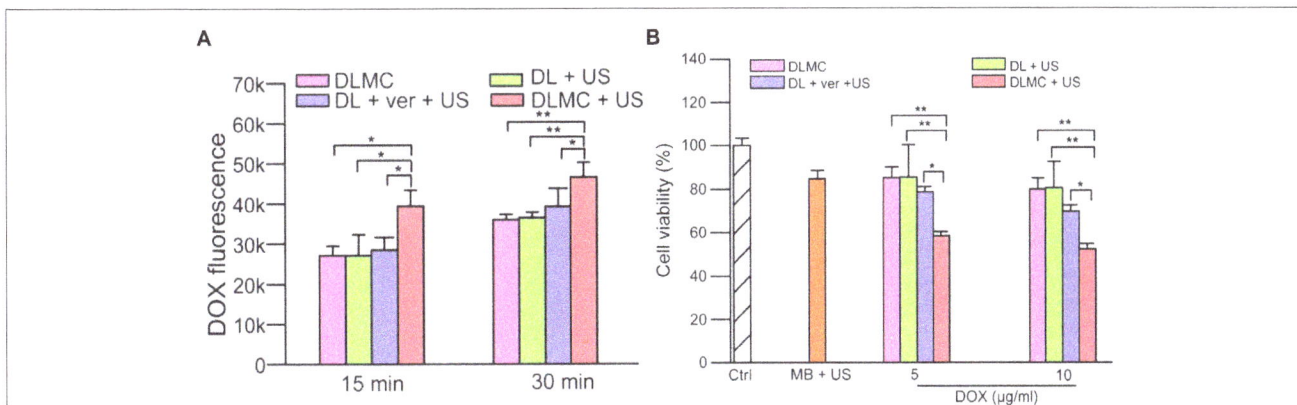

FIGURE | (A) Intracellular doxorubicin (DOX) concentration in MCF-7/ADR cells 15 and 30 min post treatment. (B) Cell cytotoxicity after several treatments with or without US. DLMC, DOX-liposome-microbubble complexes; DL, DOX-liposomes; ver, verapamil; US, Ultrasound. $*p < 0.05$, $**p < 0.01$.

where free drugs can enter healthy tissue anyway, without ultrasound exposure. Less than 10% of preclinical studies reported on drug distribution toward healthy tissues. Among the studies that do measure this, Yan et al. (2013) reported that the application of ultrasound (2.25 MHz, 1.9 MPa, 10 min, three treatments: one treatment every 3 days) on subcutaneous breast tumor following the i.v. injection of PTX-loaded microbubbles (120 μg – 1 × 10^9 microbubbles) resulted in fourfold increase in i.t. accumulation of PTX (**Figure**) and 2.5-fold decrease in tumor volume compared to PTX-loaded microbubbles treatment alone (**Figure**). The authors also investigated the drug biodistribution in healthy organs including heart, liver, spleen, lung, and kidney 1 h after i.v. administration of the PTX-loaded microbubbles and ultrasound exposure (Yan et al., 2013). The PTX biodistribution in heart, spleen, and lung was not significantly different between mice that received PTX-loaded microbubbles treatment alone or combined with ultrasound (**Figure**). However, the PTX delivery using microbubble-assisted ultrasound led to a slight but significant decrease in PTX concentration in liver and kidney compared to PTX-loaded microbubbles injection alone (**Figure**). No significant loss of body weight and other adverse effects were observed during the therapeutic procedure. Moreover, Ting et al. (2012) designed a therapeutic protocol based on BCNU-loaded microbubbles (0.8 mg – 1 × 10^{10}) with focused ultrasound (1 MHz, 0.5–0.7 MPa, 2 sonications, 1 min/sonication) to improve BCNU-based chemotherapy for glioblastoma treatment. They showed that the encapsulation of BCNU in microbubbles prolonged its circulatory half-life fivefold and intrahepatic accumulation of BCNU was reduced fivefold due to the slow reticuloendothelial system uptake of BCNU-loaded microbubbles (Ting et al., 2012). These microbubbles alone or in combination with focused ultrasound were associated with lower levels of aspartate- and alanine-aminotransferases

compared to free BCNU, suggesting that these microbubbles may effectively reduce liver toxicity and damage. In glioblastoma-bearing rats, BCNU-loaded microbubbles with ultrasound led to 13-fold decrease in tumor volume. However, median survival was extended by only 12% compared to BCNU and control.

However, for all microbubble-based ultrasound therapies, the effect on the vasculature should be closely monitored. There is a 'fine line' between stimulating vascular permeability and inducing vascular damage, which can result in inhibition of tumor perfusion. Although this may be a desired effect in some studies, for drug delivery from the vasculature, a reduced tumor perfusion might limit the i.t. drug supply. For example, Burke et al. (2011) demonstrated that the mechanical effect of low duty cycle ultrasound (1 MHz, 1 MPa PNP) in combination with microbubbles could inhibit glioma growth by blocking tumor perfusion. The anti-vascular action of microbubble-assisted ultrasound (1 MHz, 1.6 MPa PNP) was also adopted by Todorova et al. (2013) who subsequently injected an anti-angiogenic agent to prevent the formation of new vessels. In the light of these results, animal studies conducted with ultrasound pressures >1.0 MPa should always include a control group with microbubble-assisted ultrasound only, and preferably monitor the perfusion of the exposed tissue (e.g., by Doppler or contrast-enhanced ultrasound imaging).

To summarize, a growing number of preclinical investigations show promising results for future clinical applications. Future studies will have to confirm that the increase in therapeutic efficacy of sonochemotherapy is correlated with enhanced i.t. accumulation and penetration of drugs. To demonstrate the safety of this method, drug biodistribution toward healthy organs and tissues should be monitored and physiological functions of healthy organs should be examined using imaging, histological analysis, and blood biochemistry analysis. Information on *in vivo* biodistribution and pharmacokinetics of intact and destroyed

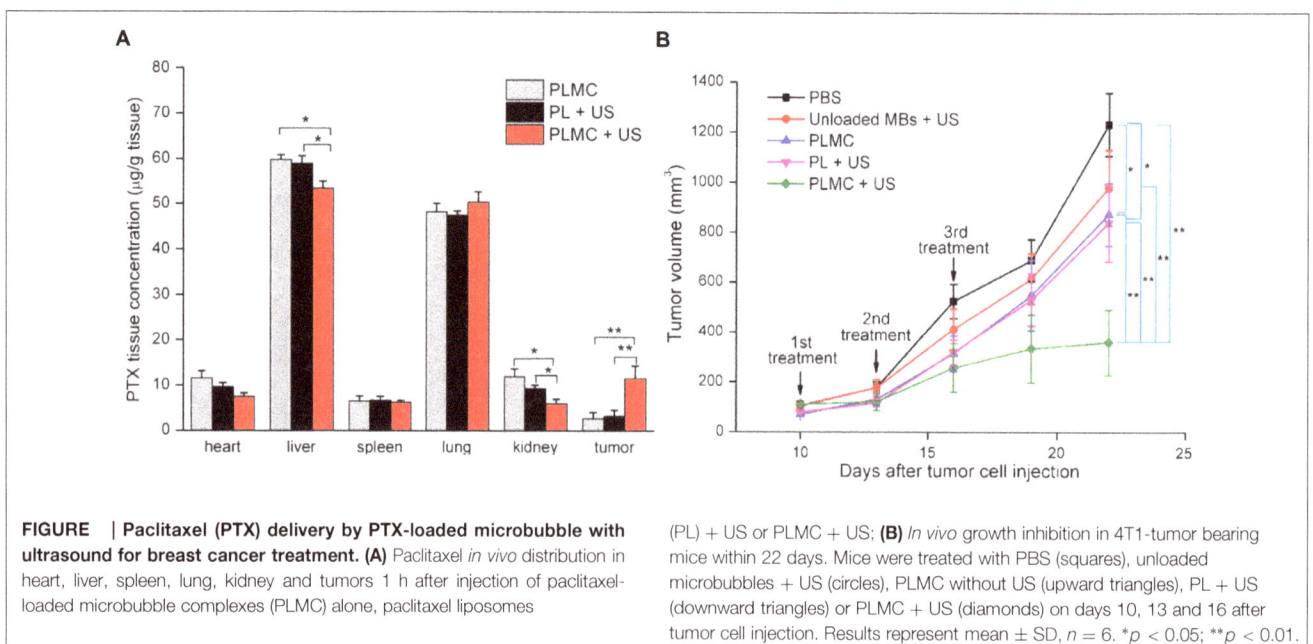

FIGURE | Paclitaxel (PTX) delivery by PTX-loaded microbubble with ultrasound for breast cancer treatment. (A) Paclitaxel *in vivo* distribution in heart, liver, spleen, lung, kidney and tumors 1 h after injection of paclitaxel-loaded microbubble complexes (PLMC) alone, paclitaxel liposomes

(PL) + US or PLMC + US; **(B)** *In vivo* growth inhibition in 4T1-tumor bearing mice within 22 days. Mice were treated with PBS (squares), unloaded microbubbles + US (circles), PLMC without US (upward triangles), PL + US (downward triangles) or PLMC + US (diamonds) on days 10, 13 and 16 after tumor cell injection. Results represent mean ± SD, $n = 6$. *$p < 0.05$; **$p < 0.01$.

microbubbles as well as an evaluation of their systemic side effects are still absent in most available publications. These aspects need to be integrated in future studies. It must be noted that the sonochemotherapy approach has mainly been evaluated in small animals. Studies in large animals are still lacking and might face challenging and unexpected physical (e.g., ultrasound penetration depth, ultrasound attenuation) and biological (e.g., plasma life time of drug and microbubbles) limitations.

Translation to the Clinics

Despite the novelty of the field of ultrasound-mediated drug delivery, a first clinical case study has been conducted in five patients with locally advanced pancreatic cancer (Kotopoulis et al., 2013, 2015). In this study, gemcitabine was administered by i.v. infusion at a dose of 1000 mg/m^2 over 30 min (**Figure**). During the last 10 min of chemotherapy, ultrasound imaging was performed in standard abdominal imaging mode to locate the position of the tumor (**Figure**). At the end of gemcitabine infusion, when drug plasma level peaked, 0.5 mL of clinically approved SonoVue® contrast agents followed by 5 mL saline were intravenously injected every 3.5 min to ensure their presence throughout the whole treatment. Tumors were exposed to ultrasound (1.9 MHz, 0.49 MI, 1% DC) using an ultrasound diagnostic scanner. The cumulative ultrasound exposure was only 18.9 s (**Figure**). All five patients tolerated an increased

number of treatment cycles compared to gemcitabine treatment without ultrasound (16 ± 7 vs. 9 ± 6 cycles), reflecting an improved physical state as well as an increased survival. In two out of five patients, the maximum tumor diameter was either transiently or permanently reduced, while the other patients exhibited reduced tumor growth compared to a historical control group of 80 patients (**Figure** ; Kotopoulis et al., 2013). Compared to this historical data, survival increased with 60% (Kotopoulis et al., 2015). The authors did not report side effects related to this therapeutic protocol. Nevertheless, the true clinical benefit was not clearly established because of the low number of patients studied. The therapeutic protocol (i.e., ultrasound parameters, doses of drug, type and concentrations of microbubbles) should be optimized and long-term safety aspects have to be addressed in future investigations in a larger number of patients.

Moreover, we are referring to a safety study of combining ultrasound microbubbles and chemotherapy to treat liver metastases from gastrointestinal tumors and pancreatic carcinoma conducted by the Profs. K. Yan and L. Shen at Beijing Cancer Hospital (Yan and Shen, 2014). This study is currently recruiting patients. In this clinical trial, gemcitabine will be intravenously injected to patients with pancreatic carcinoma while oxaliplatin and taxol based chemotherapy will be administered by i.v. perfusion to patients with liver metastases. Thirty min after chemotherapy, 1 mL of SonoVue® contrast agents will be intravenously injected during six times

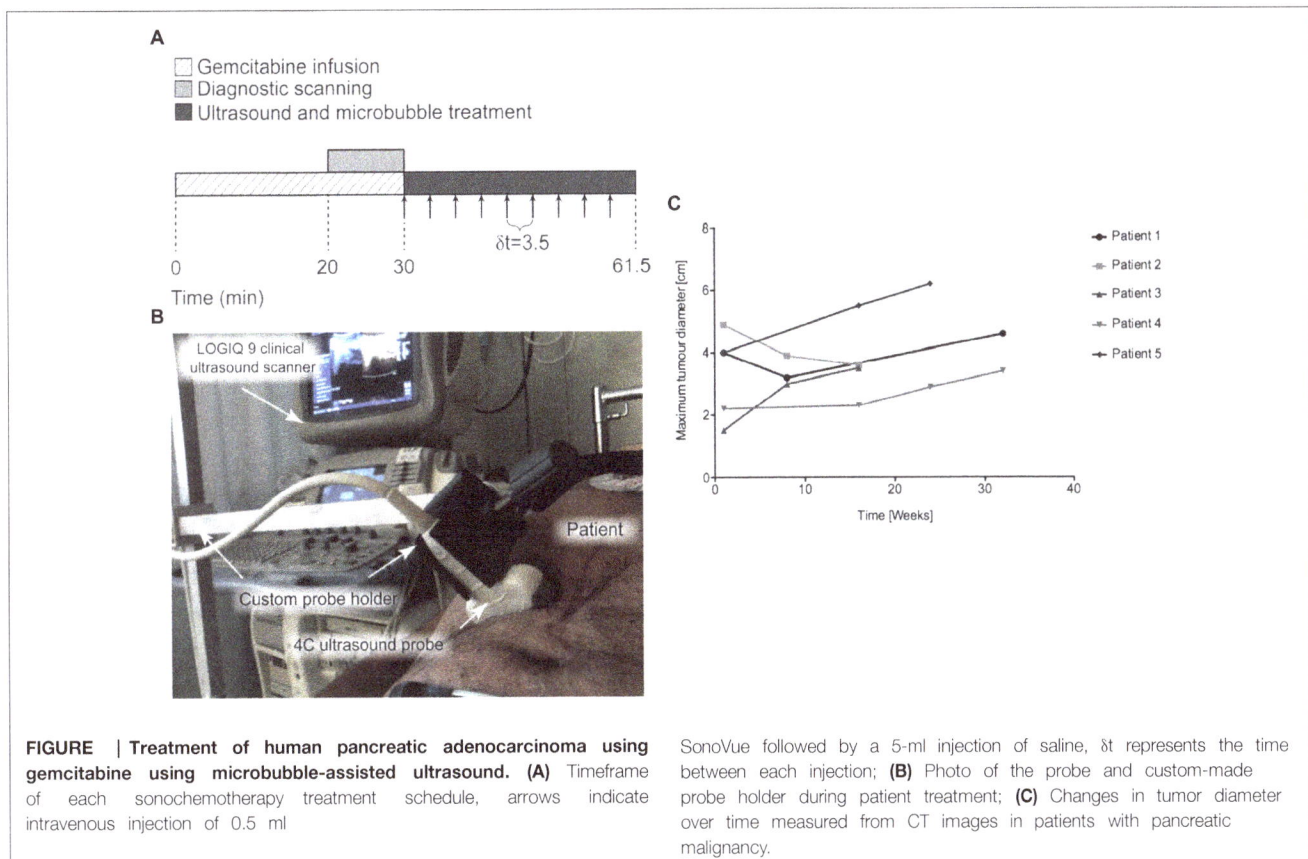

FIGURE | Treatment of human pancreatic adenocarcinoma using gemcitabine using microbubble-assisted ultrasound. (A) Timeframe of each sonochemotherapy treatment schedule, arrows indicate intravenous injection of 0.5 ml SonoVue followed by a 5-ml injection of saline, δt represents the time between each injection; **(B)** Photo of the probe and custom-made probe holder during patient treatment; **(C)** Changes in tumor diameter over time measured from CT images in patients with pancreatic malignancy.

in 20 min. In addition to the safety of the therapeutic protocol, the authors will explore the largest MI and ultrasound treatment time patients can tolerate. The secondary objectives of this clinical trial are to observe the tumor clinical benefit rate and to evaluate the preliminary effects including time to failure and time to death.

Conclusion

Targeted drug delivery using microbubble-assisted ultrasound has the potential to become a clinically accepted way of improving local anticancer chemotherapy. Although the co-administration approach, using clinically approved microbubbles and free chemotherapeutic drugs, can be seen as the fast-track toward the clinic, the greatest therapeutic potential may lie in the custom-made drug-loaded microbubbles. The latter combines the enhanced vascular permeability and cellular uptake following microbubble-assisted ultrasound with a local release of the drug. However, this implies that new therapeutic particles are to be developed, which require thorough

pre-clinical testing for efficacy and safety. A growing number of preclinical experiments have successfully reported the therapeutic benefits of microbubble-assisted ultrasound in the delivery of (anti-cancer) drugs in several animal models. Clinical translation of this method requires further improvements on: (i) the design, characterization, and GMP production of therapeutic microbubbles with prolonged plasma half-life and high drug-loading capacity; (ii) the optimization and standardization of ultrasound parameters used in the field; (iii) the insertion of a medical imaging modality (MRI, ultrasound) to monitor the *in vivo* effects of ultrasound and (iv) the evaluation of drug biodistribution, therapeutic efficacy, and side effects in orthotopic tumor models in small and large animals.

Acknowledgment

This work was supported by Advanced ERC grant Sound Pharma – 268906 (CM).

References

Al Sabbagh, C., Tsapis, N., Novell, A., Calleja-Gonzalez, P., Escoffre, J. M., Bouakaz, A., et al. (2015). Formulation and pharmacokinetics of thermosensitive stealth(R) liposomes encapsulating 5-Fluorouracil. *Pharm. Res.* 32, 1585–1603. doi: 10.1007/s11095-014-1559-0

Aryal, M., Arvanitis, C. D., Alexander, P. M., and Mcdannold, N. (2014). Ultrasound-mediated blood-brain barrier disruption for targeted drug delivery in the central nervous system. *Adv. Drug Deliv. Rev.* 72, 94–109. doi: 10.1016/j.addr.2014.01.008

Azagury, A., Khoury, L., Enden, G., and Kost, J. (2014). Ultrasound mediated transdermal drug delivery. *Adv. Drug Deliv. Rev.* 72, 127–143. doi: 10.1016/j.addr.2014.01.007

Bohmer, M. R., Chlon, C. H., Raju, B. I., Chin, C. T., Shevchenko, T., and Klibanov, A. L. (2010). Focused ultrasound and microbubbles for enhanced extravasation. *J. Control. Release* 148, 18–24. doi: 10.1016/j.jconrel.2010.06.012

Bokor, D., Chambers, J. B., Rees, P. J., Mant, T. G., Luzzani, F., and Spinazzi, A. (2001). Clinical safety of SonoVue, a new contrast agent for ultrasound imaging, in healthy volunteers and in patients with chronic obstructive pulmonary disease. *Invest. Radiol.* 36, 104–109. doi: 10.1097/00004424-200102000-00006

Boucher, Y., Baxter, L. T., and Jain, R. K. (1990). Interstitial pressure gradients in tissue-isolated and subcutaneous tumors: implications for therapy. *Cancer Res.* 50, 4478–4484.

Burke, C. W., Alexander, E. T., Timbie, K., Kilbanov, A. L., and Price, R. J. (2014). Ultrasound-activated agents comprised of 5FU-bearing nanoparticles bonded to microbubbles inhibit solid tumor growth and improve survival. *Mol. Ther.* 22, 321–328. doi: 10.1038/mt.2013.259

Burke, C. W., Klibanov, A. L., Sheehan, J. P., and Price, R. J. (2011). Inhibition of glioma growth by microbubble activation in a subcutaneous model using low duty cycle ultrasound without significant heating. *J. Neurosurg.* 114, 1654–1661. doi: 10.3171/2010.11.JNS101201

Cavalieri, F., Zhou, M., and Ashokkumar, M. (2010). The design of multifunctional microbubbles for ultrasound image-guided cancer therapy. *Curr. Top. Med. Chem.* 10, 1198–1210. doi: 10.2174/156802610791384180

Chauhan, V. P., Stylianopoulos, T., Boucher, Y., and Jain, R. K. (2011). Delivery of molecular and nanoscale medicine to tumors: transport barriers and strategies. *Annu. Rev. Chem. Biomol. Eng.* 2, 281–298. doi: 10.1146/annurev-chembioeng-061010-114300

Choi, J. J., Pernot, M., Brown, T. R., Small, S. A., and Konofagou, E. E. (2007). Spatio-temporal analysis of molecular delivery through the blood-brain barrier using focused ultrasound. *Phys. Med. Biol.* 52, 5509–5530. doi: 10.1088/0031-9155/52/18/004

Cochran, M. C., Eisenbrey, J., Ouma, R. O., Soulen, M., and Wheatley, M. A. (2011). Doxorubicin and paclitaxel loaded microbubbles for ultrasound triggered drug delivery. *Int. J. Pharm.* 414, 161–170. doi: 10.1016/j.ijpharm.2011.05.030

De Cock, I., Zagato, E., Braeckmans, K., Luan, Y., de Jong, N., De Smedt, S. C., et al. (2015). Ultrasound and microbubble mediated drug delivery: acoustic pressure as determinant for uptake via membrane pores or endocytosis. *J. Control. Release* 197, 20–28. doi:10.1016/j.jconrel.2014.10.031

Deckers, R., and Moonen, C. T. (2010). Ultrasound triggered, image guided, local drug delivery. *J. Control. Release* 148, 25–33. doi: 10.1016/j.jconrel.2010.07.117

Deng, J., Huang, Q., Wang, F., Liu, Y., Wang, Z., Wang, Z., et al. (2012). The role of caveolin-1 in blood-brain barrier disruption induced by focused ultrasound combined with microbubbles. *J. Mol. Neurosci.* 46, 677–687. doi: 10.1007/s12031-011-9629-9

Deng, Z., Yan, F., Jin, Q., Li, F., Wu, J., Liu, X., et al. (2014). Reversal of multidrug resistance phenotype in human breast cancer cells using doxorubicin-liposome-microbubble complexes assisted by ultrasound. *J. Control. Release* 174, 109–116. doi: 10.1016/j.jconrel.2013.11.018

Deshpande, N., Needles, A., and Willmann, J. K. (2010). Molecular ultrasound imaging: current status and future directions. *Clin. Radiol.* 65, 567–581. doi: 10.1016/j.crad.2010.02.013

Doinikov, A. A., and Bouakaz, A. (2010). Acoustic microstreaming around an encapsulated particle. *J. Acoust. Soc. Am.* 127, 1218–1227. doi: 10.1121/1.3290997

Escoffre, J. M., Mannaris, C., Geers, B., Novell, A., Lentacker, I., Averkiou, M., et al. (2013a). Doxorubicin liposome-loaded microbubbles for contrast imaging and ultrasound-triggered drug delivery. *IEEE Trans. Ultrason. Ferroelectr. Freq. Control* 60, 78–87. doi: 10.1109/TUFFC.2013.2539

Escoffre, J. M., Novell, A., Serriere, S., Lecomte, T., and Bouakaz, A. (2013b). Irinotecan delivery by microbubble-assisted ultrasound: in vitro validation and a pilot preclinical study. *Mol. Pharm.* 10, 2667–2675. doi: 10.1021/mp400081b

Escoffre, J. M., Zeghimi, A., Novell, A., and Bouakaz, A. (2013c). In-vivo gene delivery by sonoporation: recent progress and prospects. *Curr. Gene Ther.* 13, 2–14. doi: 10.2174/156652313804806606

Escoffre, J. M., Piron, J., Novell, A., and Bouakaz, A. (2011). Doxorubicin delivery into tumor cells with ultrasound and microbubbles. *Mol. Pharm.* 8, 799–806. doi: 10.1021/mp100397p

Fan, C. H., Ting, C. Y., Liu, H. L., Huang, C. Y., Hsieh, H. Y., Yen, T. C., et al. (2013). Antiangiogenic-targeting drug-loaded microbubbles combined with focused ultrasound for glioma treatment. *Biomaterials* 34, 2142–2155. doi: 10.1016/j.biomaterials.2012.11.048

Ferlay, J., Steliarova-Foucher, E., Lortet-Tieulent, J., Rosso, S., Coebergh, J. W., Comber, H., et al. (2013). Cancer incidence and mortality patterns in Europe:

estimates for 40 countries in 2012. *Eur. J. Cancer* 49, 1374–1403. doi: 10.1016/j.ejca.2012.12.027

Fokong, S., Theek, B., Wu, Z., Koczera, P., Appold, L., Jorge, S., et al. (2012). Image-guided, targeted and triggered drug delivery to tumors using polymer-based microbubbles. *J. Control. Release* 163, 75–81. doi: 10.1016/j.jconrel.2012.05.007

Frenkel, V. (2008). Ultrasound mediated delivery of drugs and genes to solid tumors. *Adv. Drug Deliv. Rev.* 60, 1193–1208. doi: 10.1016/j.addr.2008.03.007

Frinking, P. J., Tardy, I., Theraulaz, M., Arditi, M., Powers, J., Pochon, S., et al. (2012). Effects of acoustic radiation force on the binding efficiency of BR55, a VEGFR2-specific ultrasound contrast agent. *Ultrasound Med. Biol.* 38, 1460–1469. doi: 10.1016/j.ultrasmedbio.2012.03.018

Gao, Y., Gao, S., Zhao, B., Zhao, Y., Hua, X., Tan, K., et al. (2012). Vascular effects of microbubble-enhanced, pulsed, focused ultrasound on liver blood perfusion. *Ultrasound Med. Biol.* 38, 91–98. doi: 10.1016/j.ultrasmedbio.2011.09.018

Geers, B., Lentacker, I., Sanders, N. N., Demeester, J., Meairs, S., and De Smedt, S. C. (2011). Self-assembled liposome-loaded microbubbles: the missing link for safe and efficient ultrasound triggered drug-delivery. *J. Control. Release* 152, 249–256. doi: 10.1016/j.jconrel.2011.02.024

Goertz, D. E. (2015). An overview of the influence of therapeutic ultrasound exposures on the vasculature: high intensity ultrasound and microbubble-mediated bioeffects. *Int. J. Hyperthermia* 31, 134–144. doi: 10.3109/02656736.2015.1009179

Grauer, S. E., Sutherland, G., and Fritz, T. (1996). "Safety and echo contrast efficacy of multiple doses of Aerosomes MRX-115 in a phase I clinical trial," in *Proceedings of the AHA, 69th Scientific Sessions, Circulation*, New Orleans, LA, I316–I319.

Hancock, H. A., Smith, L. H., Cuesta, J., Durrani, A. K., Angstadt, M., Palmeri, M. L., et al. (2009). Investigations into pulsed high-intensity focused ultrasound-enhanced delivery: preliminary evidence for a novel mechanism. *Ultrasound Med. Biol.* 35, 1722–1736. doi: 10.1016/j.ultrasmedbio.2009.04.020

Heath, C. H., Sorace, A., Knowles, J., Rosenthal, E., and Hoyt, K. (2012). Microbubble therapy enhances anti-tumor properties of cisplatin and cetuximab in vitro and in vivo. *Otolaryngol. Head Neck Surg.* 146, 938–945. doi: 10.1177/0194599812436648

Hernot, S., and Klibanov, A. L. (2008). Microbubbles in ultrasound-triggered drug and gene delivery. *Adv. Drug Deliv. Rev.* 60, 1153–1166. doi: 10.1016/j.addr.2008.03.005

Hijnen, N., Langereis, S., and Grull, H. (2014). Magnetic resonance guided high-intensity focused ultrasound for image-guided temperature-induced drug delivery. *Adv. Drug Deliv. Rev.* 72, 65–81. doi: 10.1016/j.addr.2014.01.006

Hu, X., Kheirolomoom, A., Mahakian, L. M., Beegle, J. R., Kruse, D. E., Lam, K. S., et al. (2012). Insonation of targeted microbubbles produces regions of reduced blood flow within tumor vasculature. *Invest. Radiol.* 47, 398–405. doi: 10.1097/RLI.0b013e31824bd237

Ibsen, S., Schutt, C. E., and Esener, S. (2013). Microbubble-mediated ultrasound therapy: a review of its potential in cancer treatment. *Drug Des. Devel. Ther.* 7, 375–388. doi: 10.2147/DDDT.S31564

Iwanaga, K., Tominaga, K., Yamamoto, K., Habu, M., Maeda, H., Akifusa, S., et al. (2007). Local delivery system of cytotoxic agents to tumors by focused sonoporation. *Cancer Gene Ther.* 14, 354–363. doi: 10.1038/sj.cgt.7701026

Jain, R. K. (2001). Delivery of molecular and cellular medicine to solid tumors. *Adv. Drug Deliv. Rev.* 46, 149–168. doi: 10.1016/S0169-409X(00)00131-9

Juffermans, L. J., Kamp, O., Dijkmans, P. A., Visser, C. A., and Musters, R. J. (2008). Low-intensity ultrasound-exposed microbubbles provoke local hyperpolarization of the cell membrane via activation of BK(Ca) channels. *Ultrasound Med. Biol.* 34, 502–508. doi: 10.1016/j.ultrasmedbio.2007.09.010

Juffermans, L. J., Van Dijk, A., Jongenelen, C. A., Drukarch, B., Reijerkerk, A., De Vries, H. E., et al. (2009). Ultrasound and microbubble-induced intra- and intercellular bioeffects in primary endothelial cells. *Ultrasound Med. Biol.* 35, 1917–1927. doi: 10.1016/j.ultrasmedbio.2009.06.1091

Junge, L., Ohl, C. D., Wolfrum, B., Arora, M., and Ikink, R. (2003). Cell detachment method using shock-wave-induced cavitation. *Ultrasound Med. Biol.* 29, 1769–1776. doi: 10.1016/j.ultrasmedbio.2003.08.010

Kaddur, K., Lebegue, L., Tranquart, F., Midoux, P., Pichon, C., and Bouakaz, A. (2010). Transient transmembrane release of green fluorescent proteins with sonoporation. *IEEE Trans. Ultrason. Ferroelectr. Freq. Control* 57, 1558–1567. doi: 10.1109/TUFFC.2010.1586

Kang, J., Wu, X., Wang, Z., Ran, H., Xu, C., Wu, J., et al. (2010). Antitumor effect of docetaxel-loaded lipid microbubbles combined with ultrasound-targeted microbubble activation on VX2 rabbit liver tumors. *J. Ultrasound Med.* 29, 61–70.

Kiessling, F., Fokong, S., Bzyl, J., Lederle, W., Palmowski, M., and Lammers, T. (2014). Recent advances in molecular, multimodal and theranostic ultrasound imaging. *Adv. Drug Deliv. Rev.* 72, 15–27. doi: 10.1016/j.addr.2013.11.013

Kiessling, F., Fokong, S., Koczera, P., Lederle, W., and Lammers, T. (2012). Ultrasound microbubbles for molecular diagnosis, therapy, and theranostics. *J. Nucl. Med.* 53, 345–348. doi: 10.2967/jnumed.111.099754

Kinoshita, M., Mcdannold, N., Jolesz, F. A., and Hynynen, K. (2006). Noninvasive localized delivery of Herceptin to the mouse brain by MRI-guided focused ultrasound-induced blood-brain barrier disruption. *Proc. Natl. Acad. Sci. U.S.A.* 103, 11719–11723. doi: 10.1073/pnas.0604318103

Kong, G., Braun, R. D., and Dewhirst, M. W. (2001). Characterization of the effect of hyperthermia on nanoparticle extravasation from tumor vasculature. *Cancer Res.* 61, 3027–3032.

Kooiman, K., Emmer, M., Foppen-Harteveld, M., Van Wamel, A., and De Jong, N. (2010). Increasing the endothelial layer permeability through ultrasound-activated microbubbles. *IEEE Trans. Biomed. Eng.* 57, 29–32. doi: 10.1109/TBME.2009.2030335

Kooiman, K., Vos, H. J., Versluis, M., and De Jong, N. (2014). Acoustic behavior of microbubbles and implications for drug delivery. *Adv. Drug Deliv. Rev.* 72, 28–48. doi: 10.1016/j.addr.2014.03.003

Kotopoulis, S., Delalande, A., Popa, M., Mamaeva, V., Dimcevski, G., Gilja, O. H., et al. (2014). Sonoporation-enhanced chemotherapy significantly reduces primary tumour burden in an orthotopic pancreatic cancer xenograft. *Mol. Imaging Biol.* 16, 53–62. doi: 10.1007/s11307-013-0672-5

Kotopoulis, S., Dimcevski, G., Gilja, O. H., Hoem, D., and Postema, M. (2013). Treatment of human pancreatic cancer using combined ultrasound, microbubbles, and gemcitabine: a clinical case study. *Med. Phys.* 40, 072902. doi: 10.1118/1.4808149

Kotopoulis, S., Dimcevski, G., Hoem, D., Postema, M., and Gilja, O. H. (2015). "Therapeutic ultrasound in pancreatic adenocarcinoma - Oral communication," in *Proceedings of the 20th European Symposium on Ultrasound Contrast Imaging*, Rotterdam.

Lammers, T., Kiessling, F., Hennink, W. E., and Storm, G. (2012). Drug targeting to tumors: principles, pitfalls and (pre-) clinical progress. *J. Control. Release* 161, 175–187. doi: 10.1016/j.jconrel.2011.09.063

Lammers, T., Koczera, P., Fokong, S., Gremse, F., Ehling, J., Vogt, M., et al. (2015). Theranostic USPIO-loaded microbubbles for mediating and monitoring blood-brain barrier permeation. *Adv. Funct. Mater.* 25, 36–43. doi: 10.1002/adfm.201401199

Lammertink, B., Deckers, R., Storm, G., Moonen, C., and Bos, C. (2015). Duration of ultrasound-mediated enhanced plasma membrane permeability. *Int. J. Pharm.* 482, 92–98. doi: 10.1016/j.ijpharm.2014.12.013

Lefor, A. T., Makohon, S., and Ackerman, N. B. (1985). The effects of hyperthermia on vascular permeability in experimental liver metastasis. *J. Surg. Oncol.* 28, 297–300. doi: 10.1002/jso.2930280412

Leighton, T. G. (1994). *The Acoustic Bubble*. London: Elsevier.

Lentacker, I., De Cock, I., Deckers, R., De Smedt, S. C., and Moonen, C. T. (2014). Understanding ultrasound induced sonoporation: definitions and underlying mechanisms. *Adv. Drug Deliv. Rev.* 72, 49–64. doi: 10.1016/j.addr.2013.11.008

Li, P., Zheng, Y., Ran, H., Tan, J., Lin, Y., Zhang, Q., et al. (2012). Ultrasound triggered drug release from 10-hydroxycamptothecin-loaded phospholipid microbubbles for targeted tumor therapy in mice. *J. Control. Release* 162, 349–354. doi: 10.1016/j.jconrel.2012.07.009

Lin, C. Y., Tseng, H. C., Shiu, H. R., Wu, M. F., Chou, C. Y., and Lin, W. L. (2012). Ultrasound sonication with microbubbles disrupts blood vessels and enhances tumor treatments of anticancer nanodrug. *Int. J. Nanomedicine* 7, 2143–2152. doi: 10.2147/IJN.S29514

Lindner, L. H., Eichhorn, M. E., Eibl, H., Teichert, N., Schmitt-Sody, M., Issels, R. D., et al. (2004). Novel temperature-sensitive liposomes with prolonged circulation time. *Clin. Cancer Res.* 10, 2168–2178. doi: 10.1158/1078-0432.CCR-03-0035

Lu, C. T., Zhao, Y. Z., Wu, Y., Tian, X. Q., Li, W. F., Huang, P. T., et al. (2011). Experiment on enhancing antitumor effect of intravenous epirubicin hydrochloride by acoustic cavitation in situ combined with phospholipid-based microbubbles. *Cancer Chemother. Pharmacol.* 68, 343–348. doi: 10.1007/s00280-010-1489-4

Lum, A. F., Borden, M. A., Dayton, P. A., Kruse, D. E., Simon, S. I., and Ferrara, K. W. (2006). Ultrasound radiation force enables targeted deposition of model drug carriers loaded on microbubbles. *J. Control. Release* 111, 128–134. doi: 10.1016/j.jconrel.2005.11.006

Manzoor, A. A., Lindner, L. H., Landon, C. D., Park, J. Y., Simnick, A. J., Dreher, M. R., et al. (2012). Overcoming limitations in nanoparticle drug delivery: triggered, intravascular release to improve drug penetration into tumors. *Cancer Res.* 72, 5566–5575. doi: 10.1158/0008-5472.CAN-12-1683

Marty, B., Larrat, B., Van Landeghem, M., Robic, C., Robert, P., Port, M., et al. (2012). Dynamic study of blood-brain barrier closure after its disruption using ultrasound: a quantitative analysis. *J. Cereb. Blood Flow Metab.* 32, 1948–1958. doi: 10.1038/jcbfm.2012.100

Matsuo, M., Yamaguchi, K., Feril, L. B. Jr., Endo, H., Ogawa, K., Tachibana, K., et al. (2011). Synergistic inhibition of malignant melanoma proliferation by melphalan combined with ultrasound and microbubbles. *Ultrason. Sonochem.* 18, 1218–1224. doi: 10.1016/j.ultsonch.2011.03.005

Mei, J., Cheng, Y., Song, Y., Yang, Y., Wang, F., Liu, Y., et al. (2009). Experimental study on targeted methotrexate delivery to the rabbit brain via magnetic resonance imaging-guided focused ultrasound. *J. Ultrasound Med.* 28, 871–880.

Meijering, B. D., Juffermans, L. J., Van Wamel, A., Henning, R. H., Zuhorn, I. S., Emmer, M., et al. (2009). Ultrasound and microbubble-targeted delivery of macromolecules is regulated by induction of endocytosis and pore formation. *Circ. Res.* 104, 679–687. doi: 10.1161/CIRCRESAHA.108.183806

Mesiwala, A. H., Farrell, L., Wenzel, H. J., Silbergeld, D. L., Crum, L. A., Winn, H. R., et al. (2002). High-intensity focused ultrasound selectively disrupts the blood-brain barrier in vivo. *Ultrasound Med. Biol.* 28, 389–400. doi: 10.1016/S0301-5629(01)00521-X

Minchinton, A. I., and Tannock, I. F. (2006). Drug penetration in solid tumours. *Nat. Rev. Cancer* 6, 583–592. doi: 10.1038/nrc1893

Minnaert, M. (1933). On musical air-bubbles and the sounds of running water. *Philos. Mag.* 16, 235–249. doi: 10.1080/14786443309462277

Novell, A., Escoffre, J. M., and Bouakaz, A. (2013). Ultrasound contrast imaging in Cancer - Technical aspects and prospects. *Curr. Mol. Imaging* 2, 77–88. doi: 10.2174/2211555211302010009

Ohl, C. D., Arora, M., Ikink, R., De Jong, N., Versluis, M., Delius, M., et al. (2006). Sonoporation from jetting cavitation bubbles. *Biophys. J.* 91, 4285–4295. doi: 10.1529/biophysj.105.075366

Ohl, C. D., and Wolfrum, B. (2003). Detachment and sonoporation of adherent HeLa-cells by shock wave-induced cavitation. *Biochim. Biophys. Acta* 1624, 131–138. doi: 10.1016/j.bbagen.2003.10.005

Podaru, G., Ogden, S., Baxter, A., Shrestha, T., Ren, S., Thapa, P., et al. (2014). Pulsed magnetic field induced fast drug release from magneto liposomes via ultrasound generation. *J. Phys. Chem. B* 118, 11715–11722. doi: 10.1021/jp5022278

Postema, M., Van Wamel, A., Ten Cate, F. J., and De Jong, N. (2005). High-speed photography during ultrasound illustrates potential therapeutic applications of microbubbles. *Med. Phys.* 32, 3707–3711. doi: 10.1118/1.2133718

Price, R. J., Skyba, D. M., Kaul, S., and Skalak, T. C. (1998). Delivery of colloidal particles and red blood cells to tissue through microvessel ruptures created by targeted microbubble destruction with ultrasound. *Circulation* 98, 1264–1267. doi: 10.1161/01.CIR.98.13.1264

Pron, G., Mahrour, N., Orlowski, S., Tounekti, O., Poddevin, B., Belehradek, J., et al. (1999). Internalisation of the bleomycin molecules responsible for bleomycin toxicity: a receptor-mediated endocytosis mechanism. *Biochem. Pharmacol.* 57, 45–56. doi: 10.1016/S0006-2952(98)00282-2

Pu, C., Chang, S., Sun, J., Zhu, S., Liu, H., Zhu, Y., et al. (2014). Ultrasound-mediated destruction of LHRHa-targeted and paclitaxel-loaded lipid microbubbles for the treatment of intraperitoneal ovarian cancer xenografts. *Mol. Pharm.* 11, 49–58. doi: 10.1021/mp400523h

Qin, J., Wang, T. Y., and Willman, J. K. (2015). "Sonoporation: applications for cancer therapy," in *Therapeutic Ultrasound*, eds J. M. Escoffre and A. Bouakaz (Berlin: Springer).

Raymond, S. B., Skoch, J., Hynynen, K., and Bacskai, B. J. (2007). Multiphoton imaging of ultrasound/Optison mediated cerebrovascular effects in vivo. *J. Cereb. Blood Flow Metab.* 27, 393–403. doi: 10.1038/sj.jcbfm.9600336

Ren, S. T., Liao, Y. R., Kang, X. N., Li, Y. P., Zhang, H., Ai, H., et al. (2013). The antitumor effect of a new docetaxel-loaded microbubble combined with low-frequency ultrasound in vitro: preparation and parameter analysis. *Pharm. Res.* 30, 1574–1585. doi: 10.1007/s11095-013-0996-5

Rychak, J. J., and Klibanov, A. L. (2014). Nucleic acid delivery with microbubbles and ultrasound. *Adv. Drug Deliv. Rev.* 72, 82–93. doi: 10.1016/j.addr.2014.01.009

Rychak, J. J., Klibanov, A. L., and Hossack, J. A. (2005). Acoustic radiation force enhances targeted delivery of ultrasound contrast microbubbles: in vitro verification. *IEEE Trans. Ultrason. Ferroelectr. Freq. Control* 52, 421–433. doi: 10.1109/TUFFC.2005.1417264

Sanches, P. G., Grull, H., and Steinbach, O. C. (2011). See, reach, treat: ultrasound-triggered image-guided drug delivery. *Ther. Deliv.* 2, 919–934. doi: 10.4155/tde.11.63

Sarvazyan, A. P., Rudenko, O. V., and Nyborg, W. L. (2010). Biomedical applications of radiation force of ultrasound: historical roots and physical basis. *Ultrasound Med. Biol.* 36, 1379–1394. doi: 10.1016/j.ultrasmedbio.2010.05.015

Sasaki, N., Kudo, N., Nakamura, K., Lim, S., et al. (2014). Ultrasound image-guided therapy enhances antitumor effect of cisplatin. *J. Med. Ultrasonics* 41, 11–21. doi: 10.1007/s10396-013-0475-y

Seidl, M., Steinbach, P., Worle, K., and Hofstadter, F. (1994). Induction of stress fibres and intercellular gaps in human vascular endothelium by shock-waves. *Ultrasonics* 32, 397–400. doi: 10.1016/0041-624X(94)90111-2

Sersa, G., Miklavcic, D., Cemazar, M., Rudolf, Z., Pucihar, G., and Snoj, M. (2008). Electrochemotherapy in treatment of tumours. *Eur. J. Surg. Oncol.* 34, 232–240. doi: 10.1016/j.ejso.2007.05.016

Sheikov, N., Mcdannold, N., Sharma, S., and Hynynen, K. (2008). Effect of focused ultrasound applied with an ultrasound contrast agent on the tight junctional integrity of the brain microvascular endothelium. *Ultrasound Med. Biol.* 34, 1093–1104. doi: 10.1016/j.ultrasmedbio.2007.12.015

Sheikov, N., Mcdannold, N., Vykhodtseva, N., Jolesz, F., and Hynynen, K. (2004). Cellular mechanisms of the blood-brain barrier opening induced by ultrasound in presence of microbubbles. *Ultrasound Med. Biol.* 30, 979–989. doi: 10.1016/j.ultrasmedbio.2004.04.010

Shortencarier, M. J., Dayton, P. A., Bloch, S. H., Schumann, P. A., Matsunaga, T. O., and Ferrara, K. W. (2004). A method for radiation-force localized drug delivery using gas-filled liposheres. *IEEE Trans. Ultrason. Ferroelectr. Freq. Control* 51, 822–831. doi: 10.1109/TUFFC.2004.1320741

Sirsi, S. R., and Borden, M. A. (2014). State-of-the-art materials for ultrasound-triggered drug delivery. *Adv. Drug Deliv. Rev.* 72, 3–14. doi: 10.1016/j.addr.2013.12.010

Sklar, L. R., Burnett, C. T., Waibel, J. S., Moy, R. L., and Ozog, D. M. (2014). Laser assisted drug delivery: a review of an evolving technology. *Lasers Surg. Med.* 46, 249–262. doi: 10.1002/lsm.22227

Song, C. W. (1984). Effect of local hyperthermia on blood flow and microenvironment: a review. *Cancer Res.* 44, 4721s–4730s.

Song, J., Chappell, J. C., Qi, M., Vangieson, E. J., Kaul, S., and Price, R. J. (2002). Influence of injection site, microvascular pressure and ultrasound variables on microbubble-mediated delivery of microspheres to muscle. *J. Am. Coll. Cardiol.* 39, 726–731. doi: 10.1016/S0735-1097(01)01793-4

Sonoda, S., Tachibana, K., Uchino, E., Yamashita, T., Sakoda, K., Sonoda, K. H., et al. (2007). Inhibition of melanoma by ultrasound-microbubble-aided drug delivery suggests membrane permeabilization. *Cancer Biol. Ther.* 6, 1276–1283. doi: 10.4161/cbt.6.8.4485

Sorace, A. G., Warram, J. M., Umphrey, H., and Hoyt, K. (2012). Microbubble-mediated ultrasonic techniques for improved chemotherapeutic delivery in cancer. *J. Drug Target.* 20, 43–54. doi: 10.3109/1061186X.2011.622397

Stieger, S. M., Caskey, C. F., Adamson, R. H., Qin, S., Curry, F. R., Wisner, E. R., et al. (2007). Enhancement of vascular permeability with low-frequency contrast-enhanced ultrasound in the chorioallantoic membrane model. *Radiology* 243, 112–121. doi: 10.1148/radiol.2431060167

Szabo, T. L. (2013). *Diagnostic Ultrasound Imaging: Inside Out.* Waltham, MA: Academic Press.

ter Haar, G., Shaw, A., Pye, S., Ward, B., Bottomley, F., Nolan, R., et al. (2011). Guidance on reporting ultrasound exposure conditions for bio-effects studies. *Ultrasound Med. Biol.* 37, 177–183. doi: 10.1016/j.ultrasmedbio.2010.10.021

Ting, C. Y., Fan, C. H., Liu, H. L., Huang, C. Y., Hsieh, H. Y., Yen, T. C., et al. (2012). Concurrent blood-brain barrier opening and local drug delivery using drug-carrying microbubbles and focused ultrasound for brain glioma treatment. *Biomaterials* 33, 704–712. doi: 10.1016/j.biomaterials.2011.09.096

Tinkov, S., Coester, C., Serba, S., Geis, N. A., Katus, H. A., Winter, G., et al. (2010). New doxorubicin-loaded phospholipid microbubbles for targeted tumor therapy: in-vivo characterization. *J. Control. Release* 148, 368–372. doi: 10.1016/j.jconrel.2010.09.004

Todorova, M., Agache, V., Mortazavi, O., Chen, B., Karshafian, R., Hynynen, K., et al. (2013). Antitumor effects of combining metronomic chemotherapy with the antivascular action of ultrasound stimulated microbubbles. *Int. J. Cancer* 132, 2956–2966. doi: 10.1002/ijc.27977

Tran, T. A., Roger, S., Le Guennec, J. Y., Tranquart, F., and Bouakaz, A. (2007). Effect of ultrasound-activated microbubbles on the cell electrophysiological properties. *Ultrasound Med. Biol.* 33, 158–163. doi: 10.1016/j.ultrasmedbio.2006.07.029

Treat, L. H., Mcdannold, N., Zhang, Y., Vykhodtseva, N., and Hynynen, K. (2012). Improved anti-tumor effect of liposomal doxorubicin after targeted blood-brain barrier disruption by MRI-guided focused ultrasound in rat glioma. *Ultrasound Med. Biol.* 38, 1716–1725. doi: 10.1016/j.ultrasmedbio.2012.04.015

Tzu-Yin, W., Wilson, K. E., Machtaler, S., and Willman, J. K. (2014). Ultrasound and microbubble guided drug delivery: mechanistic understanding and clinical implications. *Curr. Pharm. Biotechnol.* 14, 743–752. doi: 10.2174/1389201014666131226114611

Unga, J., and Hashida, M. (2014). Ultrasound induced cancer immunotherapy. *Adv. Drug Deliv. Rev.* 72, 144–153. doi: 10.1016/j.addr.2014.03.004

Unger, E., Porter, T., Lindner, J., and Grayburn, P. (2014). Cardiovascular drug delivery with ultrasound and microbubbles. *Adv. Drug Deliv. Rev.* 72, 110–126. doi: 10.1016/j.addr.2014.01.012

van Wamel, A., Kooiman, K., Harteveld, M., Emmer, M., Ten Cate, F. J., Versluis, M., et al. (2006). Vibrating microbubbles poking individual cells: drug transfer into cells via sonoporation. *J. Control. Release* 112, 149–155. doi: 10.1016/j.jconrel.2006.02.007

Vaupel, P. W., and Kelleher, D. K. (2012). Blood flow and associated pathophysiology of uterine cervix cancers: characterisation and relevance for localised hyperthermia. *Int. J. Hyperthermia* 28, 518–527. doi: 10.3109/02656736.2012.699134

Wang, S., Hossack, J. A., Klibanov, A. L., and Mauldin, F. W. Jr. (2014). Binding dynamics of targeted microbubbles in response to modulated acoustic radiation force. *Phys. Med. Biol.* 59, 465–484. doi: 10.1088/0031-9155/59/2/465

Wei, K. C., Chu, P. C., Wang, H. Y., Huang, C. Y., Chen, P. Y., Tsai, H. C., et al. (2013). Focused ultrasound-induced blood-brain barrier opening to enhance temozolomide delivery for glioblastoma treatment: a preclinical study. *PLoS ONE* 8:e58995. doi: 10.1371/journal.pone.0058995

Weinberg, R. A. (2014). *The Biology of Cancer.* New York, NY: Garland Science.

Wilson, S. R., and Burns, P. N. (2010). Microbubble-enhanced US in body imaging: what role? *Radiology* 257, 24–39. doi: 10.1148/radiol.10091210

Wu, J. (2002). Theoretical study on shear stress generated by microstreaming surrounding contrast agents attached to living cells. *Ultrasound Med. Biol.* 28, 125–129. doi: 10.1016/S0301-5629(01)00497-5

Yan, F., Li, L., Deng, Z., Jin, Q., Chen, J., Yang, W., et al. (2013). Paclitaxel-liposome-microbubble complexes as ultrasound-triggered therapeutic drug delivery carriers. *J. Control. Release* 166, 246–255. doi: 10.1016/j.jconrel.2012.12.025

Yan, K., and Shen, L. (2014). *Safety Study of Combining Ultrasound Microbubbles and Chemotherapy to Treat Malignant Neoplasms of Digestive System.* Available at: https://clinicaltrials.gov/ct2/show/study/NCT02233205

Yang, F., Gu, N., Chen, D., Xi, X., Zhang, D., Li, Y., et al. (2008). Experimental study on cell self-sealing during sonoporation. *J. Control. Release* 131, 205–210. doi: 10.1016/j.jconrel.2008.07.038

Yatvin, M. B., Weinstein, J. N., Dennis, W. H., and Blumenthal, R. (1978). Design of liposomes for enhanced local release of drugs by hyperthermia. *Science* 202, 1290–1293. doi: 10.1126/science.364652

Zhao, Y. Z., Lu, C. T., Zhou, Z. C., Jin, Z., Zhang, L., Sun, C. Z., et al. (2011). Enhancing chemotherapeutic drug inhibition on tumor growth by ultrasound: an in vivo experiment. *J. Drug Target.* 19, 154–160. doi: 10.3109/10611861003801834

Conflict of Interest Statement: The authors declare that the research was conducted in the absence of any commercial or financial relationships that could be construed as a potential conflict of interest.

10

The Power of using Functional fMRI on Small Rodents to Study Brain Pharmacology and Disease

Elisabeth Jonckers, Disha Shah, Julie Hamaide, Marleen Verhoye and
Annemie Van der Linden*

Bio-Imaging Lab, Department of Biomedical Sciences, University of Antwerp, Antwerp, Belgium

Edited by:
Nicolau Beckmann,
Novartis Institutes for BioMedical
Research, Switzerland

Reviewed by:
Pasquina Marzola,
University of Verona, Italy
Aileen Schroeter,
ETH Zurich, Switzerland

*Correspondence:
Annemie Van der Linden
annemie.vanderlinden@uantwerpen.be

Functional magnetic resonance imaging (fMRI) is an excellent tool to study the effect of pharmacological modulations on brain function in a non-invasive and longitudinal manner. We introduce several blood oxygenation level dependent (BOLD) fMRI techniques, including resting state (rsfMRI), stimulus-evoked (st-fMRI), and pharmacological MRI (phMRI). Respectively, these techniques permit the assessment of functional connectivity during rest as well as brain activation triggered by sensory stimulation and/or a pharmacological challenge. The first part of this review describes the physiological basis of BOLD fMRI and the hemodynamic response on which the MRI contrast is based. Specific emphasis goes to possible effects of anesthesia and the animal's physiological conditions on neural activity and the hemodynamic response. The second part of this review describes applications of the aforementioned techniques in pharmacologically induced, as well as in traumatic and transgenic disease models and illustrates how multiple fMRI methods can be applied successfully to evaluate different aspects of a specific disorder. For example, fMRI techniques can be used to pinpoint the neural substrate of a disease beyond previously defined hypothesis-driven regions-of-interest. In addition, fMRI techniques allow one to dissect how specific modifications (e.g., treatment, lesion etc.) modulate the functioning of specific brain areas (st-fMRI, phMRI) and how functional connectivity (rsfMRI) between several brain regions is affected, both in acute and extended time frames. Furthermore, fMRI techniques can be used to assess/explore the efficacy of novel treatments in depth, both in fundamental research as well as in preclinical settings. In conclusion, by describing several exemplary studies, we aim to highlight the advantages of functional MRI in exploring the acute and long-term effects of pharmacological substances and/or pathology on brain functioning along with several methodological considerations.

Keywords: fMRI, rsfMRI, phMRI, BOLD, rodents

Abbreviations: 5-HT, serotonin; 5-HT1A-R, serotonin 1A receptor; AD, Alzheimer's disease; ALFF, amplitude of low frequency fluctuations; ASL, arterial spin labeling; BOLD, blood oxygenation level dependent; CBF, cerebral blood flow; CBV, cerebral blood volume; CMRO2, cerebral metabolic rate of oxygen consumption; CT, computed tomography; DCE, dynamic contrast enhanced; DSC, dynamic susceptibility contrast; EEG, electroencephalography; EPI, echo planar imaging; FC, functional connectivity; FDG, fluoro-deoxy-glucose; fMRI, functional MRI; FSL, FMRIB software library; GABA, gamma amino-butyric acid; GRASE, gradient- and spin-echo; GS, global signal; HD, Huntington's disease; HDR, hemodynamic response; ICA, independent component analysis; LFP, local field potential; mAChR, muscarinic Acetylcholine receptor; MEG, magnetoencephalography; MRI, magnetic resonance imaging; NIRS, near-infrared spectroscopy; NMDA, N-methyl-D-aspartate; ofMRI, optogenetic fMRI; pCO2, partial pressure of CO2; PD, Parkinson's disease; PET, positron emission tomography; phMRI, pharmacological MRI; ROI, region-of-interest; rsfMRI, resting state fMRI; SPM, statistical parametric mapping; st-fMRI, stimulus-evoked fMRI; SSRI, selective serotonin re-uptake inhibitors.

INTRODUCTION

Magnetic resonance imaging tools are widely used to evaluate brain structure and function even in a single experiment. The major advantage of MRI techniques is that they are non-invasive, do not use radioactive agents (as opposed to PET) and do not rely on hazardous ionizing radiation (as opposed to CT), rendering MRI a safe imaging tool appropriate for longitudinal follow up. MRI is based on a magnetic field and radiofrequency pulses and most of the MRI applications use the intrinsic tissue contrast relying on different features of ^{1}H protons in tissue water without the need of injecting contrast agents.

In short, the technique provides excellent soft tissue contrast, rendering it very appropriate to investigate the brain. Apart from giving anatomical information, MRI allows studying other specific properties of brain tissue using Diffusion-weighted, Diffusion Tensor, and Diffusion Kurtosis Imaging. Additionally, metabolic information can be obtained using Magnetic Resonance Spectroscopy or Chemical Exchange Saturation Transfer. Moreover brain function can be assessed by measuring cerebral perfusion, blood flow (ASL, DSC MRI, and DCE MRI) and brain activity (Functional MRI, rsfMRI, phMRI; [for review see for example (Denic et al., 2011)].

These different techniques can be applied within a single scanning session. After co-registration of the different images, multi-parameter information can be obtained on voxel level or from specific brain regions of interest. Although anatomical and diffusion information allows assessing structural changes induced by neurological disorders, functional changes might occur even much earlier and are of great interest for early diagnosis.

The focus of this review is to describe the use of fMRI to evaluate the effects of pharmacological agents on neuronal activity in small animals using different fMRI techniques. Since its introduction over 20 years ago (Ogawa et al., 1990; Kwong et al., 1992), fMRI has gained immense popularity to study brain activation and brain activity patterns in health (Di Salle et al., 1999; Logothetis, 2008; Bandettini, 2012) and disease (Iannetti and Wise, 2007), both in humans and animal models (Van Der Linden et al., 2007). These methods are especially useful to document the neuro-modulatory actions of pharmacologically active compounds. fMRI allows to determine and localize the target area, that is, the area with the appropriate receptors for the neuromodulator (phMRI). At the same time the technique can estimate the effect on the targeted brain circuitry and potentially beyond (st-fMRI) and rsfMRI. Furthermore, longitudinal fMRI allows to unravel the effect of pharmacological agents upon acute and chronic treatment and one can investigate the interaction between the neuromodulator, the brain and the resulting behavior in the same animal over time.

In this review we try to give an overview of the vast amount of information that can be obtained with small rodent fMRI in pharmacology completed with an overview of specific applications in different animal disease models and their translation to the clinic.

fMRI METHODOLOGY

Physiological Basis of fMRI

A variety of MRI pulse sequences exist which exploit different features of water protons in tissue. The most widely used MRI contrasts are found in T1-, T2-, T2*- and proton density weighted images. The resulting images provide superior anatomical contrast allowing qualitative and quantitative assessment of overall brain anatomy. To study brain functioning the sequence is adapted to acquire the BOLD contrast which is based on the differential magnetic properties of oxygenated (diamagnetic) and deoxygenated (paramagnetic) hemoglobin. Upon neural activation, changes in local CBF, CBV, and CMRO2, i.e., the hemodynamic response leads to a locally increased ratio of oxygenated over deoxygenated hemoglobin, resulting in an enhancement in T2$^{(*)}$-weighted signal intensity (cfr. **Figure**). BOLD fMRI is thus an indirect measure of neuronal activity. For a more detailed description please consult (Buxton and Frank, 1997; Logothetis and Wandell, 2004).

The hemodynamic response, is markedly slower (in the order of seconds) than the actual neural activity elicited by neurons, which is in the order of milliseconds (Logothetis et al., 2001; Logothetis and Wandell, 2004). Although over recent years, numerous variations to the well-established EPI and GRASE pulse sequences have been developed enabling a repetition time up to 0.500 s [for review of recently implemented fast and high-resolution fMRI sequences (Feinberg and Yacoub, 2012)] this strongly contrasts to other functional imaging measurements such as EEG, MEG, NIRS which provide more direct information and require a substantially higher temporal resolution (sampling frequency in the range of kHz). Despite its relatively low temporal resolution, fMRI provides the best three dimensional spatial resolution covering the entire brain in comparison to the other techniques mentioned above.

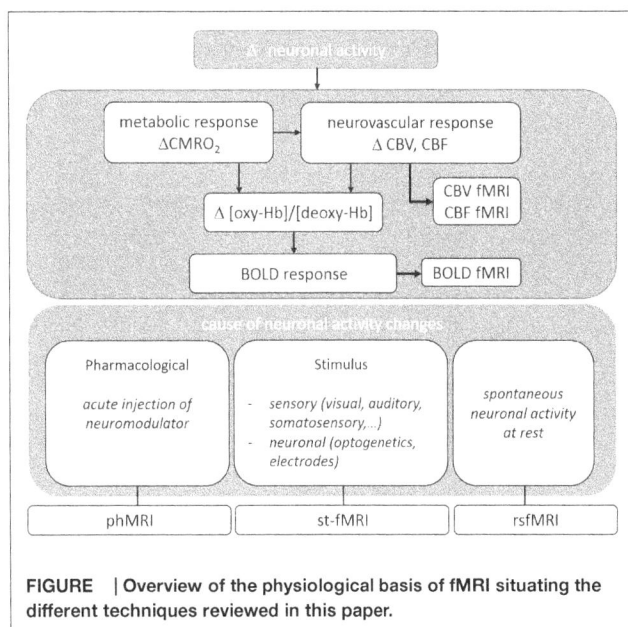

FIGURE | Overview of the physiological basis of fMRI situating the different techniques reviewed in this paper.

Magnetic resonance imaging also allows to detect brain activity based on local changes in CBF or CBV and specific methods exist to assess these changes. One of these methods is ASL, in which the inflowing water proton spins in the arterial blood are magnetically tagged (inverted) serving as endogenous tracer to observe the effects of inversion on the contrast of brain MRI which can then be used to measure stimulus-evoked changes in CBF (Williams et al., 1992; Detre and Wang, 2002).

In CBV-weighted fMRI (Mandeville et al., 1998; Smirnakis et al., 2007; Ciris et al., 2014), injection of exogenous intravascular contrast agent (e.g., iron oxide particles) is required to monitor brain activity changes represented by signal intensity changes induced by local CBV alterations (Mandeville, 2012).

Within this review we opted to describe BOLD based fMRI techniques and applications while methods using labeling methods or contrast injections -which are also applied in pharmacological research (Borsook and Becerra, 2011; Jenkins, 2012)- were considered beyond the current scope.

Different fMRI Methods

Different applications of BOLD fMRI allow for the study of neuronal activity after imposing a certain task or stimulus (**st-fMRI**), during rest (**rsfMRI**), or as response to acute drug challenges (**phMRI**). In the following sections, each of these techniques will be discussed in detail (For an overview cfr. **Figure**).

Stimulus-evoked fMRI allows for the investigation of neural activity as a response to a specific stimulus or task. In most rodent st-fMRI studies externally applied sensory-motor stimuli are used while in human st-fMRI studies also cognitive task can be applied. The most commonly used stimulus presentation designs for fMRI experiments are (i) a block design and (ii) an event-related design (Amaro and Barker, 2006). In a block design, two or more different conditions are alternated in order to determine the differences between the two conditions. A control or rest situation may be included in the presentation occurring between the two conditions. In event related designs the time in between stimuli can vary while also much shorter stimuli are used. Although preclinical studies most often implement block designs, event-related designs are becoming more and more established (Schlegel et al., 2015).

Instead of using sensory or cognitive stimuli, BOLD fMRI can be used to study the direct effect of pharmacological modulations on neuronal activity (**phMRI**). In this case the acute injection of a compound during the fMRI scan evokes changes in the BOLD response in brain areas that express specific receptors for the injected compound and also in their projection areas. In phMRI the experimental design is dependent on the pharmacokinetic and pharmacodynamic profile of the drug. The inability to control, or even to know the timing and amplitude of the stimulus renders this method considerably more challenging than conventional st-fMRI studies where the timing depends on the predefined paradigm (Jenkins, 2012).

Both techniques, fMRI and phMRI, can be combined when investigating the modulatory effects of a pharmaceutical compound on a conventional st-fMRI read-out, such as the effects of dopaminergic drugs on cognitive tasks (Dodds et al.,

2009). Moreover, repeated phMRI studies after chronic drug application could provide insights in the resulting adaptations of the brain such as changes in receptor density or sensitivity. However, additional measures (such as CBV and CBF) are required in case the used pharmacological compound has concomitant vaso-active properties.

Functional imaging can also be used to study FC by monitoring BOLD signals at rest (**rsfMRI**). During rest, it was shown that the BOLD signal shows spontaneous fluctuations over time. Functional connectivity is defined as the temporal correlation of low frequency (0.01–0.1 Hz) fluctuations of the BOLD signal between spatially distinct brain regions (Lowe et al., 2000). Consequently, the spontaneous low frequency fluctuations of the BOLD signal are used as indirect marker to depict the functional architecture of the brain.

Several applications of rsfMRI have demonstrated that the healthy brain is organized into functional networks and that these networks can be affected by neurological disorders. In humans, and to some extent also in rodents, large scale 'resting state networks' can be detected that include brain regions involved in auditory processing, motor function, visual processing, memory, and executive functioning (Damoiseaux et al., 2006; Jonckers et al., 2011). Moreover networks anatomically homologous to the so-called human 'default-mode network' (DMN), which is activated during rest and deactivated during goal-directed tasks (Fransson, 2005; Upadhyay et al., 2011; Lu et al., 2012; Sierakowiak et al., 2015) and its anti-correlated 'salience network' (SN) are also detected in rodents (Sforazzini et al., 2014).

fMRI Data Processing and Presentation

Although most fMRI processing software so far was optimized for human data, processing strategies are usually similar in humans and rodents. Also, an increasing number of analysis packages are being tailored to fMRI studies of rodents (Sawiak et al., 2009; Chavarrias et al., 2015).

Functional MRI data (fMRI, rsfMRI, and phMRI) are typically pre-processed before the actual data analysis. The most commonly used software packages are SPM[1] and FSL[2]. Pre-processing includes (1) slice timing correction and realignment over time, (2) spatial normalization to a standardized stereotactic space, and (3) smoothing (James et al., 2014). An important difference between human and rodent fMRI processing is the way group data are handled. The Montreal Neurological institute (MNI) defined a standard brain from a large series of MRI scans of normal controls (Evans et al., 1992). For instance, this template is automatically provided in SPM, one of the commonly used fMRI processing toolboxes. Although the same toolbox can be used for rodent fMRI, the rodent data has to be normalized to a study-specific template such as the mean of all control animals. Alternatively, an atlas can be developed from in-house measurements or obtained from a publically available source [e.g., (mice)[3]; (mice, rats, etc.[4]).

---

[1] http://www.fil.ion.ucl.ac.uk/spm/software/spm8
[2] http://www.fmrib.ox.ac.uk/fsl
[3] http://brainatlas.mbi.ufl.edu/
[4] http://scalablebrainatlas.incf.org/

Resting state fMRI data pre-processing might include extra steps such as GS regression, and temporal filtering. GS regression serves to remove global fluctuations that mask circuit-level organization, to remove global physiological artifacts, and to enhance the reliability of the experimental results (Fox et al., 2009). Temporal filtering may be included to restrict to fluctuations between 0.01 and 0.1 Hz, which are of interest in rsfMRI research. Nevertheless, recently an increasing number of studies explored correlations in BOLD fluctuations beyond this frequency band. The resulting data suggested that long-distance connections peak at low frequency bands, whereas short-distance connections are distributed in a relatively wider frequency range. Moreover, the dominance of different frequencies seems to characterize different brain networks. (Wu et al., 2008; Boubela et al., 2013).

After pre-processing, st-fMRI and phMRI data can be processed by different methods. Typically, a voxel-based approach is adopted. After pre-processing, the BOLD signal is modeled (e.g., general linear model) as the convolution of the applied stimulation design (block or event-related design) with the hemodynamic response function (HRF) in order to have a better estimation of the true design-related BOLD signal (Lindquist et al., 2009).

Finally, statistics can be performed on the model estimates (i.e., stimulus specific BOLD responses) via parametric or non-parametric methods resulting in statistical maps indicating areas of activation. These maps are first created on the single subject level (first level analysis) after which they are used in second level analyses to perform group statistics. To define brain regions activated by acute compound injection (phMRI) also a voxel based approach can be applied by statistical comparison of the repetitions before injection (baseline) with those after injection.

The aforementioned analyses techniques do not take into account the temporal dynamics of the BOLD-signal after sensory or pharmacological stimulation. Upcoming analysis methods apply spectral analysis to the BOLD time series to obtain information on the temporal behavior of the BOLD response function [for more details see (Muller et al., 2001)]. **Figure** shows examples of typical time courses for the different techniques and how they are related to the applied stimulus.

Both rsfMRI and event related st-fMRI need fast MRI sequences (e.g., TR = 2 s, i.e., one image in 2 s) to be able to acquire BOLD fluctuations and responses to the fast consecutive stimuli, respectively. A typical rsfMRI acquisition lasts 5–12 min. In a block design the length of the different blocks in the paradigm determines the required acquisition speed. Moreover the total scan-length is dependent on the complexity of the paradigm, increasing the number of scans needed when more stimuli are introduced or the differences between stimuli are more subtle. For phMRI the timing is dependent on the pharmacokinetics of the injected compound.

For processing of **rsfMRI** data, various software packages exist, supporting different processing strategies (Margulies et al., 2010). The most widely used methods in FC analysis of resting state data are ROI-based (Biswal et al., 1995), seed-based and model-free, data-driven approaches such as ICA (Calhoun et al., 2001; Beckmann and Smith, 2004). Other data-driven techniques are clustering approaches and graph analysis [for methodological review: (Margulies et al., 2010)] (see **Figure**). Finally alternative processing techniques are available to map the directionality of the connectivity, such as dynamic causal modeling (Friston et al., 2003) and Granger causality analysis (Roebroeck et al., 2005) which can also be applied on activity-induced fMRI data to define regions that drive the activation. Apart from FC analysis, also the low frequency fluctuation themselves can be affected during disease conditions and studied using ALFF analysis. ALFF is defined as the total power within the frequency range between 0.01 and 0.1 Hz, and thus indexes the strength or intensity of Low Frequency Fluctuations. Measurements of ALFF are more often applied in humans but some rodent students already report changes in ALFF in animal models (Li et al., 2012; Yao et al., 2012).

Important Considerations when Planning fMRI Experiments in Rodents

Rodent fMRI studies have great potentials and can provide an immense contribution to pharmacological research, but it must be underscored that attention and expertise is necessary when rodent fMRI experiments are designed and performed. The functional status of the brain is highly

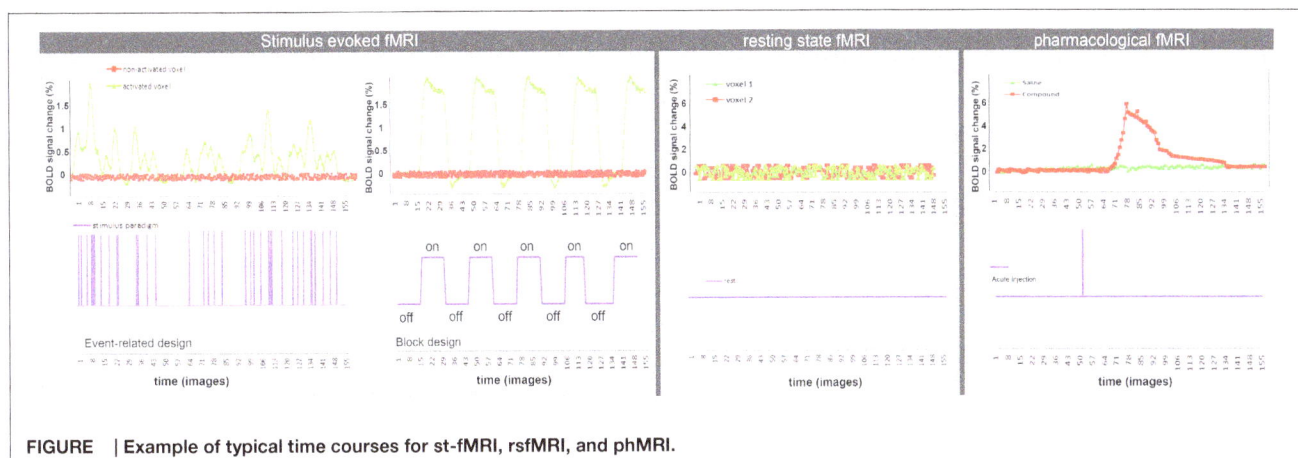

FIGURE | Example of typical time courses for st-fMRI, rsfMRI, and phMRI.

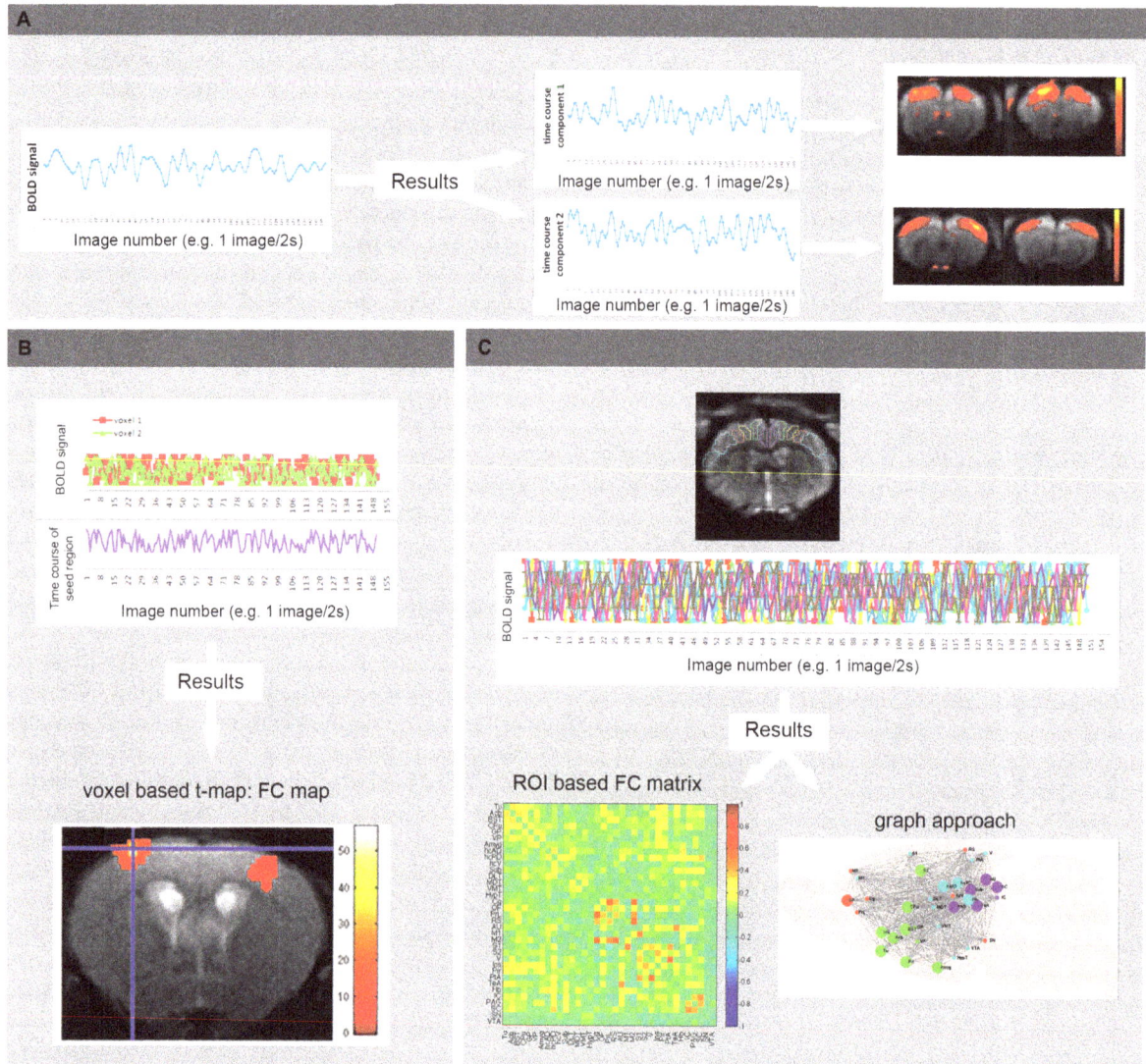

FIGURE | Basic principles of rsfMRI Analysis. (A) Independent Component Analysis divides the BOLD signal of all brain-voxels in different spatially confined independent sources, or components. Each ICA component consists of brain regions with correlated BOLD time courses. In other words, voxels of one component represent regions that are functionally connected. **(B)** In voxel-based analyses, the mean BOLD signal time course of a specific seed region is extracted from a series of EPI images. This time course is compared to the time course of all other voxels in the brain, resulting in a functional connectivity map (voxel based processing). **(C)** In an ROI based approach, the mean BOLD signal time courses of multiple brain regions are compared, resulting in FC matrices showing the strength of connectivity between each pair of brain regions (warmer colors indicate stronger functional connectivity, colder colors represent anti-correlation). These matrices can then be used to visualize brain networks as nodes (brain regions) and edges (connections). Moreover, the brain network can be divided into modules that represent brain circuits where similar time courses are displayed by different colors (graph approach). (Adopted from Jonckers et al., 2013b).

dependent on the physiology of the animal. Much more than for anatomical imaging, monitoring and controlling for this physiology is essential during rodent fMRI studies. Accounting for physiological changes is especially important in rodent studies since typically animals need to be anesthetized.

Moreover optimized protocols of the imaging set-up and processing tools for rats can not always simply be duplicated for mice since there are important differences between these rodent species, which we outline below.

First of all, it is important to mention that most of the reported fMRI work in rodents is performed in rats, despite the existence of a wide array of mouse models mimicking neurological disorders. One of the reasons behind this is the fact that it is very challenging to acquire reproducible brain activation upon stimulation in mice. Since the introduction of rsfMRI, more studies use mice as an animal model but most of the basic research, (i.e., optimization of analysis and unraveling the underlying mechanisms) is still performed in rats. Nevertheless, it is very important to take into account that conclusions drawn in rats are not necessarily applicable in mice. Moreover, recent advances such as the development of cryo-coils have dramatically improved mouse fMRI (Ratering et al., 2008).

When studying functional connectivity using rsfMRI, one should also consider the impact of hormones and age-related hormonal changes on brain connectivity as was demonstrated in human studies. In a recent review, the association between functional connectivity and endogenous sex hormone fluctuations across the menstrual cycle in humans was described (Weis et al., 2011). When endogenous estradiol and progesterone levels are high, functional communication between both hemispheres is enhanced. Also gender and overall hormonal status throughout the lifespan of an individual has a major impact on the functional connectivity of the brain. Specifically, ovarian hormones (estradiol and progesterone) may enhance both cortico-cortical and subcortico-cortical functional connectivity, whereas androgens (testosterone) may decrease subcortico-cortical functional connectivity but increase functional connectivity between subcortical brain areas. Similar investigations using rsfMRI in rodents have not been reported yet but human studies suggest that caution is required when examining healthy brain development and aging or when investigating possible biological mechanisms of 'brain connectivity' diseases. Therefore, the contribution of sex steroids should not be ignored (Peper et al., 2011).

Effects of Anesthesia on the st-fMRI and phMRI Outcome

Magnetic resonance imaging studies in rodents require the use of anesthetic agents to minimize stress and to prevent motion artifacts during the scans. Several anesthetics are optimized for MRI acquisitions, but for fMRI it is utterly important to take into account how the anesthesia affects neuronal activity and the hemodynamic response. Moreover, distinct levels of consciousness could result in different fMRI outcome. Finally, when a pharmacological agent is used in phMRI, possible interactions between the pharmacological compound and the applied anesthetic have to be taken into account as well (Hodkinson et al., 2012). On the other hand phMRI protocols can be used to assess the time-dependent effects of anesthetics on the BOLD signal. **Figure** shows the T2* signal intensity changes over time induced by a single bolus of medetomidine (Shah et al., 2015a). These changes over time underscore the need for a highly optimized anesthesia protocol applied in exactly the same manner to every animal within the study (Magnuson et al., 2014). Moreover stable conditions can be obtained by combining bolus injections to induce anesthesia followed by continuous infusion.

A robust and reproducible BOLD response can be observed in rats and mice anesthetized with commonly used anesthetics for MRI, such as medetomidine, isoflurane, α-chloralose and urethane (Austin et al., 2005; Adamczak et al., 2010). Nevertheless, under anesthesia, more intense stimuli must be presented to evoke a BOLD response in comparison to awake conditions. The cerebral hemodynamic response upon sensory stimulation shows an anesthesia-specific modulation which can be largely explained by the effects of the anesthetics on animal physiology. Strikingly, independent of the anesthetic used, fMRI responses may additionally be influenced by stimulus-induced cardiovascular changes, which may mask specific fMRI signals associated to the stimulus (Schroeter et al., 2014).

The anesthetic agent α-**chloralose** is a GABA-A agonist that binds to a site on the GABA-A receptor complex distinct from the benzodiazepine neurosteroid and barbiturate sites (Garrett and Gan, 1998). It has long been considered the gold standard for fMRI due to its minor effects on cardiovascular function, and is presumed to only minimally suppress neuronal activation. When using α-chloralose, strong neuronal activation is induced even with very subtle stimuli such as whisker deflection. Nevertheless, due to its toxicity -mainly for the liver- it has been considered as a terminal drug and its use was abandoned.

However, it was recently demonstrated that using a new formulation in a careful application scheme this anesthetic allows for repeated fMRI studies on the same rat (Alonso Bde et al., 2011).

Medetomidine, which results in sedation rather than deep anesthesia, is the anesthetic of choice for longitudinal functional imaging studies in rats (Fukuda et al., 2013). Medetomidine is an α2 agonist predominantly acting on presynaptic receptors in the locus coeruleus, resulting in decreased noradrenaline release. Medetomidine typically induces cerebral vasoconstriction mediated by direct agonist binding to receptors on the cerebral vessels resulting in reduced baseline CBV and CBF (Nakai et al., 1986). The degree of vasoconstriction depends on the dose and delivery method (topical vs. systemic). The effects of medetomidine can easily be reverted with Atipamezole (Scheinin et al., 1987).

Inhalation anesthetics (e.g., **isoflurane**) are preferred for longitudinal fMRI experiments (Kim et al., 2010) due to fast recovery and low mortality rates. Isoflurane acts on γ-amino butyric acid type A (GABA-A) receptors through depression of excitatory synaptic transmission (Larsen and Langmoen, 1998). Importantly, most inhalation anesthetics evoke vasodilation in a dose-dependent manner, which might obscure the actual experimental outcome since changes in vascular properties are very likely to affect the BOLD signal. Therefore, functional experiments are typically performed under lower doses (1–1.5%) as compared to structural MRI studies (2%). The dose used can even be lowered by combining isoflurane with medetomidine. This combination protocol has the additional advantage that the epileptic activity, seen when medetomidine is infused for longer than 120 min, is prevented, enabling longer experiments with equally fast recovery than for medetomidine alone (Fukuda et al., 2013).

Finally, **propofol and urethane** anesthesia, which both enhance GABAergic transmission, are occasionally used for fMRI experiments, in comparison to other previously described anesthetics, the induced fMRI activation is lower under the same stimulus intensity which impedes the detection of very subtle functional alterations (Lahti et al., 1999; Huttunen et al., 2008).

Effect of Anesthesia on Functional Connectivity as Assessed by rsfMRI

Apart from affecting the BOLD response post-stimulus, anesthetic agents could influence the correlations in intrinsic activity used to estimate functional connectivity. Moreover, these effects are different for rats and mice.

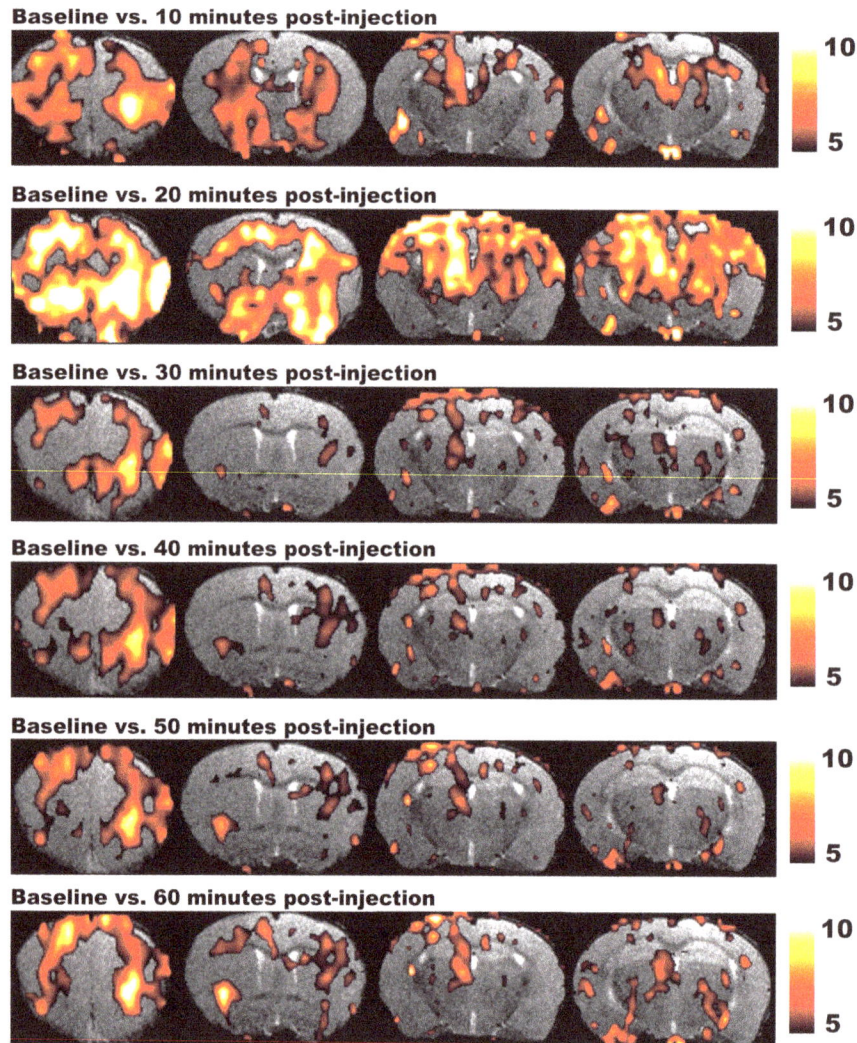

FIGURE | Results of phMRI with a single bolus of medetomidine. This figure shows four consecutive slices of the statistical difference maps of the BOLD signal at 10, 20, 30, 40, 50, and 60 min post-injection (medetomidine, 0.3 mg/kg, s.c.) vs. baseline. The statistical maps are shown on a T2-weighted anatomical MRI template. The color scale at the right indicates the *T*-value (i.e., the strength of the T2* signal intensity decrease induced by medetomidine vs. baseline in all conditions). Medetomidine induces T2* signal changes at 10 min post-injection vs. baseline, mainly in frontal regions and the striatum. At 20 min post-injection, the T2* signal changes increase and include additional regions such as the sensory cortex, hippocampus and thalamus. Starting from 30 min post-injection, medetomidine-induced T2* signal changes start to decrease and stabilize until 60 min post-injection (Shah et al., 2015a).

Medetomidine is considered as the gold standard for FC mapping in rats based on its reliable and spatially specific outcome (Kalthoff et al., 2013). In mice, however, medetomidine induces decreased inter-hemispheric FC (Jonckers et al., 2011) resulting in the need of other anesthesia protocols in these animals (Jonckers et al., 2013a). Important dosage effects showing decreased inter-hemispheric connectivity in the rat brain at high dose might explain the decreased inter-hemispheric FC in mice, which require a relatively higher dose compared to rats (Nasrallah et al., 2014).

Rats anesthetized with **isoflurane** show less localized clusters of high FC unless a low dose of 1% is used (Williams et al., 2010). In mice, however, it is not straightforward to gain consistent results using the same dose of isoflurane as in rats creating the need for adapted protocols (Jonckers et al., 2013a). Interestingly, combining a low dose of medetomidine with a low dose of isoflurane seems to give the required results (Grandjean et al., 2014a).

α-chloralose and urethane also allow robust detection of FC in rats (Hutchison et al., 2010; Williams et al., 2010; Jonckers et al., 2011) suggesting that the strongest connections are preserved even during deeper states of anesthesia (Bettinardi et al., 2015). Besides physiological confounds, changes in resting-state networks may reflect a functional reorganization of the brain at different anesthesia levels or brain states related to the level of consciousness (Liu et al., 2013). For example **Propofol** shows a dose-dependent decrease of thalamo-cortical FC (Tu et al., 2011; Liu et al., 2013).

Although the sensori-motor networks are detected with the different anesthesia regimes mentioned above, lower doses seem to be needed to preserve the DMN-like and SN. This effect may infer that these networks support higher level consciousness since these networks are well defined in awake rats (Upadhyay et al., 2011). Using a low dose of isoflurane, both the DMN-like and SNs could be detected in mice (Sforazzini et al., 2014; Liska et al., 2015). The long range anterior–posterior connections in the DMN-like network seem to be disturbed after medetomidine injection but restored when the level of anesthesia is lowering over time (Shah et al., 2015b).

The aforementioned effects of anesthesia on fMRI results yielded several attempts to optimize awake imaging protocols (Ferris et al., 2011). Moreover, weak functional connections are more likely to be picked up in awake animals (Liang et al., 2012). The drawback to awake imaging, however, is that the brain may be in different functional states depending on how well the conscious animals are acclimatized to the MRI scanner environment (Upadhyay et al., 2011) and this variance in consciousness will contribute to an increased variability in the fMRI outcome.

Nevertheless, several groups succeeded in optimizing training protocols, showing that rats can adapt to the scanner environment (King et al., 2005) resulting in reliable fMRI results (Febo, 2011) and robust reproducible resting state networks (Zhang et al., 2010; Becerra et al., 2011).

Mice, however, seem to be more difficult to train for these types of experiments (Jonckers et al., 2013a). The labor intensive effort of training protocols is not always suitable in experiments with high numbers of animals (e.g., when different groups are compared) or when following animals over time, especially starting from a very young age. Therefore, the application of awake imaging in models of neurological disease will remain limited.

The Need for Monitoring and Controlling Physiological Parameters

Since fMRI measures signals related to the hemodynamic response, a stable physiology of the animal during fMRI acquisitions is of uttermost importance to enable accurate and reproducible measurements. Therefore, physiological parameters need to be monitored and if possible continuously adjusted.

Partial pressure of CO_2 (pCO_2) must be monitored during the fMRI measurements for two major reasons. First, increased pCO_2 leads to vasodilatation and thus an increased CBV. Increased CBV results in a reduced stimulus-induced hemodynamic response. Second, increased pCO_2 leads to a decreased oxygen affinity of Hb (the so-called Bohr effect), changing the ratio of oxygenated over deoxygenated hemoglobin. Both phenomena affect the BOLD signal without any underlying neuronal origin. In the past, pCO_2 monitoring was achieved through repetitive blood sampling. Currently, continuous and non-invasive recordings of transcutaneous pCO_2 (Mueggler et al., 2001) or end-tidal pCO_2 values with MRI-compatible capnometry are used (Silverman and Muir, 1993; Van Camp et al., 2005) for which linear correlations with arterial pCO_2 have been established (Zhang et al., 1997).

Body temperature is the second major modulator, as the BOLD signal shows a strong negative correlation with body temperature due to a decreased oxygen affinity of Hb with increasing temperature (Hyder et al., 1994).

Moreover, the brain's metabolism is also affected by the body temperature of the animal. Consequently, temperature changes can mask the true contribution of neuronal activity (Vanhoutte et al., 2006). Since the body temperature gradually lowers in anesthetized rodents, a feed-back mechanism with hot air or warm water circuit is vital to keep the temperature at $\pm 37°C$.

Apart from the aforementioned parameters, follow-up of **blood pressure, heart rate,** and **breathing rate** are essential as a read-out of the animal's sedative state and will affect the hemodynamic response. Typical values for the different parameters are highly dependent on the anesthesia protocol and differ between rats and mice. For example the heart rate in awake rats is about 400 beats per minute in comparison to 600 beats per minute in mice. Also breathing rate is typically lower in rats (± 85 breaths per minute) than in mice (± 150 breaths per minute) making mouse fMRI more dependent on motion artifacts due to breathing. Especially during the fMRI acquisition it is essential to gain a stable physiology to induce as less variation as possible. (Bernstein, 1966; Baker et al., 1979).

A better control of blood gas parameters and breathing rate can be obtained by mechanical ventilation. Gated imaging, in which the imaging sequence is triggered by the respiratory cycle, can then be used to reduce motion artifacts caused by breathing (Cassidy et al., 2004). New methods have been suggested that allow recognition of artifacts and subsequent removal from the fMRI data (Salimi-Khorshidi et al., 2014).

Finally, when acute drug effects are investigated, it is important to take into account the systemic effect of the drug on the physiology of the animal which in turn could influence the BOLD signal. For example, pharmacological induction of vasodilation with acetazolamide attenuates the activity-induced BOLD response resulting from an increase in CBF (Bruhn et al., 1994).

The Advantage of Hybrid Systems: Simultaneous PET/MRI and MRI/Electrophysiology

Apart from fMRI, PET studies can be used to assess brain activation using the short half-life tracer [(15)O]H_2O as a marker for CBF or the radiotracer FDG [(18)F]FDG which estimates glucose metabolism. Higher sensitivity of PET, combined with a better contrast-to-noise ratio and spatial resolution for BOLD fMRI underlies the rationale for combining both techniques.

Interestingly, resting state networks can be defined using both PET and rsfMRI. Consequently, simultaneous PET/MRI systems are gaining more and more interest (Wehrl et al., 2014), since simultaneous studies can reveal/provide comprehensive and complementary information to further decode brain function and brain networks (Wehrl et al., 2013).

Combining electrophysiology with fMRI allows for the correlation of indirect BOLD signals with the underlying neurological ones (Logothetis, 2002; Logothetis and Wandell, 2004; Sloan et al., 2010; Sumiyoshi et al., 2012). Evoked LFP measured simultaneously with the BOLD response (Huttunen et al., 2011) show the neuronal origin of the spontaneous BOLD signal measured during rest. The low frequency fluctuations in the BOLD signal are significantly correlated with infra-slow LFP signals as well as with the slow power modulations of higher-frequency LFPs (1–100Hz) at a delay comparable to the hemodynamic response time under anesthesia (Pan et al., 2013). Nevertheless, the combination of MRI and electrical recording is technically challenging because the electrodes used for recording need to be MRI compatible and the MRI acquisition induces noise in the electrical recording. To minimize the mutual interference of the two modalities, glass rather than metal microelectrodes can be used and noise removal algorithms are implemented to analyze electrophysiology data (Pan et al., 2010).

fMRI APPLICATIONS WITH RELEVANCE FOR PHARMACOLOGICAL RESEARCH

The non-invasive nature and possibility to translate preclinical findings to the clinic render the multiple fMRI techniques outlined in this review into attractive methods for a wide variety of pharmacological applications. Indeed, phMRI can be used to unravel underlying neurobiological mechanisms of drug action and neurotransmitter-related disorders (Canese et al., 2011). Moreover, phMRI enables the investigation of a specific neurotransmitter system after administering known compounds, e.g., investigation of dopamine D2 transmission after dopamine reuptake inhibition (Squillace et al., 2014).

A very specific approach was proposed by Schwarz et al. (2007a,b) based on a combination of phMRI and FC analysis of rsfMRI data. The outcome convincingly identified connectivity patterns underlying the central effects of the injected compound. This approach can be extended by modulating the FC in an antagonist–agonist framework. First, a certain connectivity pattern is induced by acute injection of a first known compound during the scanning session. Next, the second compound of interest is also injected during the same scanning session inducing a modulation of this known connectivity pattern (Schwarz et al., 2007c; Shah et al., 2015b).

The added value of fMRI depends on the pathological phenotype of the disorder and the most prevalent pathologies will be discussed in detail below. The following sections will discuss how different fMRI techniques have led to important insights into several of the most prevalent pathologies. For example, in neurodegenerative disorders changes in brain function potentially precede structural degradation. Both st-fMRI and rsfMRI can be used to study neurological changes on a functional level, which might be of interest in terms of early diagnosis and drug intervention before the occurrence of irreversible damage. During and after therapeutic interventions the same techniques can be used to determine the efficacy of a treatment (both acutely and longitudinally) and assess recovery of functional networks (see **Figure** for an overview).

(rs)fMRI Studies in Pharmacologically Induced Models

Based on the NMDA depletion theory in **schizophrenia**, NMDA receptor antagonists (e.g., memantine) are used to mimic this disorder in rodents. Typically, behavioral assessments are generally accepted as a reliable read-out and display locomotor hyperactivity after NMDA receptor antagonist administration. Multimodal MRI extends the characterization of this model showing dose-dependent pharmacological activation in the prelimbic cortex after acute memantine administration. Sub-chronic memantine injection revealed significant effects in the hippocampus, cingulate, prelimbic, and retrosplenial cortices. These are potentially vulnerable regions in schizophrenia and are known to be involved in the mediation of specific cognitive functions affected in schizophrenia (Tamminga, 2006).

Interestingly, FC as well as ultra-structural features, defined with diffusion imaging, were significantly decreased in the same regions (Sekar et al., 2010). Similar FC results were reported in a genetic model for schizophrenia (Song et al., 2015).

Additionally, the effects of new antipsychotic drugs can be tested using the same read-outs, enabling target validation and early assessment of drugs (Sekar et al., 2010; Bifone and Gozzi, 2012; Song et al., 2015).

Seizures are due to abnormal, excessive, or synchronous neuronal activity in the brain. They can be pharmacologically induced in rats by increasing neuronal excitation, for example by excessively activating glutamate receptors (kainic acid) or acetylcholine receptors (pilocarpine) or by decreasing inhibition with antagonizing GABA-A (bicuculline; Fritsch et al., 2014).

For example systemic kainic acid injection induces limbic seizures originating from the hippocampus (Ben-Ari et al., 1981) which can be monitored with st-fMRI (Airaksinen et al., 2010; DeSalvo et al., 2010; see **Figure**). Moreover, BOLD activation as a response to electrical stimulation is modulated upon consecutive seizures (Vuong et al., 2011).

Simultaneous BOLD and electrophysiological recordings show potential decoupling of the BOLD response from neuronal activity in a small number of seizures defined with electrophysiology. This may relate to a development of recurrent seizure activity (*status epilepticus*), which associates with remarkably increased cerebral metabolic rate of CMRO2. If CMRO2 reaches the limit of the compensatory capacity of CBF, no positive BOLD response can be detected which has implications for the interpretation of st-fMRI data obtained during prolonged epileptiform activity (Airaksinen et al., 2012). RsfMRI can be used to explore how seizures modulate the affected brain circuitry. This rsfMRI functionality was shown in (WAG/Rij) rats –a model for human absence seizures– where researchers reported increased cortico-cortical correlations in rest in comparison to non-epileptic controls. This finding is indicative of augmented FC between brain regions which are most intensely involved in seizures (Mishra et al., 2013).

Similar to Major Depression Disorder (MDD) in humans, and using rsfMRI, the inbred Wistar Kyoto More Immobile rat, an accepted model for depression, shows functional

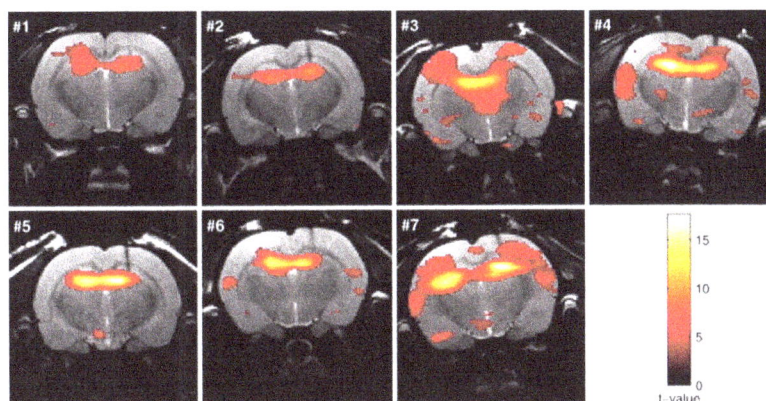

FIGURE | Activation maps (rats no. 1–7) in response to kainic acid–induced seizures superimposed on the anatomic images. The threshold for statistical significance was set at $p < 0.05$ (FWE corrected). Rats were sedated with medetomidine (figure reproduced with permission of John Wiley and Sons; Airaksinen et al., 2010).

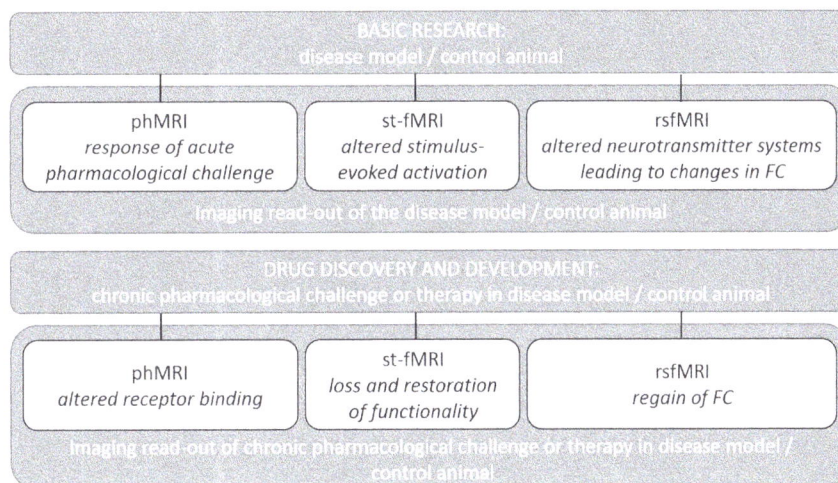

FIGURE | Overview of the applications of fMRI methods in research explaining the outcome for each type of fMRI acquisition. Detailed examples are given in the text.

connectivity anomalies between hippocampus, cortical, and subcortical regions (Williams et al., 2014). Serotonin 1A receptor (5-HT1A-R) knockout mice or healthy mice administered a specific 5-HT1A-R antagonist have been used to mimic brain serotonin depletion in **depression.** Both show reduced FC of the serotonergic system (Razoux et al., 2013). Moreover, st-fMRI can be used to assess the neural substrate of typical MDD behavioral characteristics. Changed BOLD responses to fear stimuli in the cortico-amygdalar network as well as the insular cortex may be the basis for fear and aversion in depression (Huang et al., 2011).

Treatment of depression disorders consists of increasing the level of 5HT, for example with SSRI. The resulting acute activation of the 5-HT system can be picked up with phMRI (Sekar et al., 2011a,b; Klomp et al., 2012a). Interestingly, phMRI studies show that the response to acute SSRI challenge changes in chronically SSRI treated adult animals (Klomp et al., 2012b).

The cholinergic system is important for learning and memory processes. Muscarinic cholinergic receptors (mAChR) are widely affected in AD, which might be tightly correlated with cognitive disabilities observed in those patients (Schneider et al., 2014). Pharmacological inhibition of cholinergic functioning with the mAChR antagonist scopolamine leads to cognitive impairments that are similar to the behavioral characteristics observed in **dementia** (Klinkenberg and Blokland, 2010). The possibility of non-invasively detecting alterations of the cholinergic system in mice might greatly improve early diagnosis and treatment strategies in AD mouse models and eventually in the clinic. A recent study showed how phMRI and rsfMRI can be used as tools to detect alterations in the cholinergic system (Shah et al., 2015a). This study showed that scopolamine induced a dose-dependent effect on FC in brain regions with abundant mAChRs and are known to be involved in cognitive functions (**Figure**). Moreover, some FC deficits elicited by

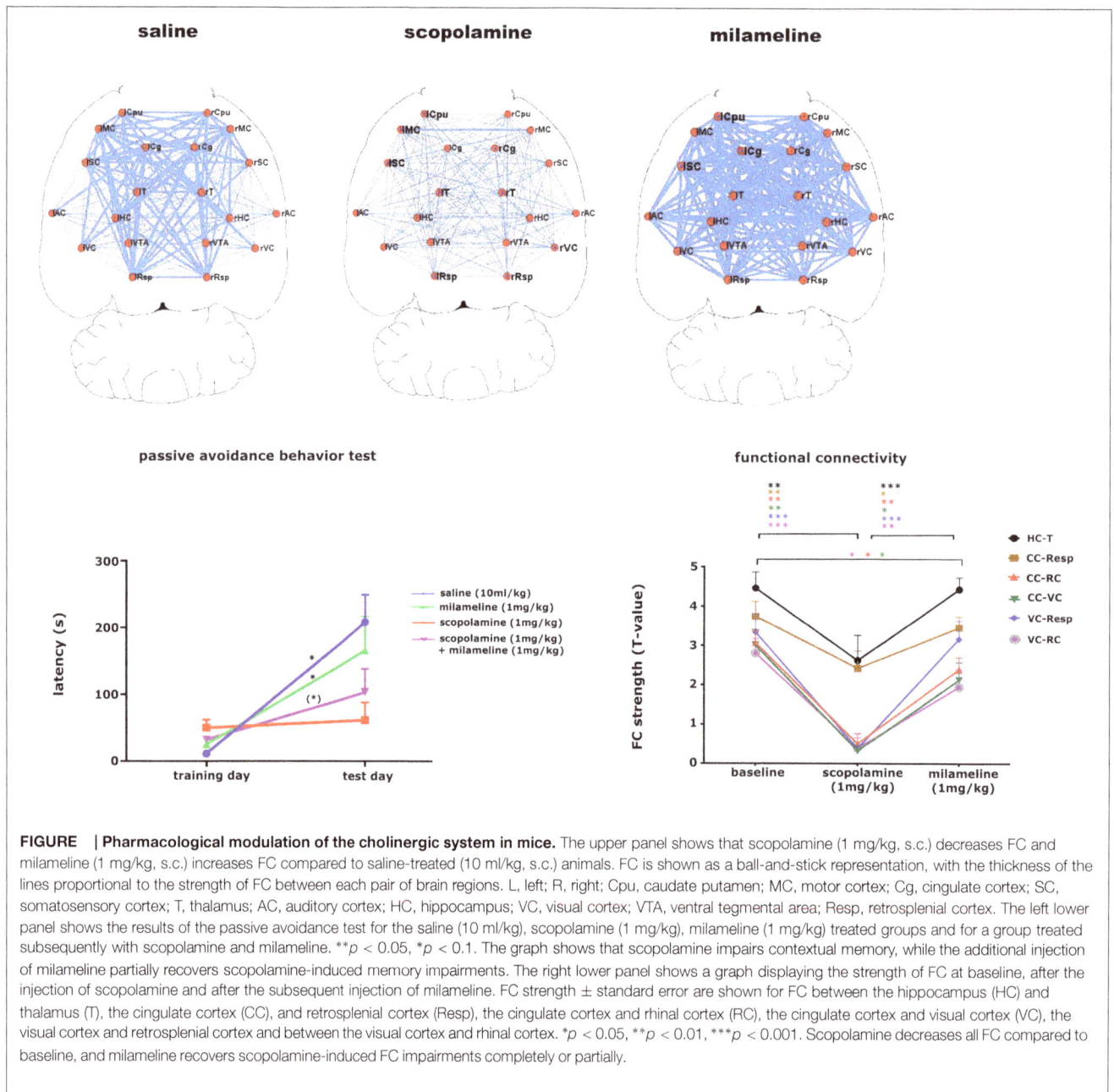

FIGURE | Pharmacological modulation of the cholinergic system in mice. The upper panel shows that scopolamine (1 mg/kg, s.c.) decreases FC and milameline (1 mg/kg, s.c.) increases FC compared to saline-treated (10 ml/kg, s.c.) animals. FC is shown as a ball-and-stick representation, with the thickness of the lines proportional to the strength of FC between each pair of brain regions. L, left; R, right; Cpu, caudate putamen; MC, motor cortex; Cg, cingulate cortex; SC, somatosensory cortex; T, thalamus; AC, auditory cortex; HC, hippocampus; VC, visual cortex; VTA, ventral tegmental area; Resp, retrosplenial cortex. The left lower panel shows the results of the passive avoidance test for the saline (10 ml/kg), scopolamine (1 mg/kg), milameline (1 mg/kg) treated groups and for a group treated subsequently with scopolamine and milameline. $^{**}p < 0.05$, $^*p < 0.1$. The graph shows that scopolamine impairs contextual memory, while the additional injection of milameline partially recovers scopolamine-induced memory impairments. The right lower panel shows a graph displaying the strength of FC at baseline, after the injection of scopolamine and after the subsequent injection of milameline. FC strength ± standard error are shown for FC between the hippocampus (HC) and thalamus (T), the cingulate cortex (CC), and retrosplenial cortex (Resp), the cingulate cortex and rhinal cortex (RC), the cingulate cortex and visual cortex (VC), the visual cortex and retrosplenial cortex and between the visual cortex and rhinal cortex. $^*p < 0.05$, $^{**}p < 0.01$, $^{***}p < 0.001$. Scopolamine decreases all FC compared to baseline, and milameline recovers scopolamine-induced FC impairments completely or partially.

scopolamine could be completely recovered by administering a mAChR agonist milameline, while other FC deficits were not completely recovered. This result was consistent with the merely partial recovery of scopolamine-induced contextual memory deficits by milameline. This study showed how phMRI and rsfMRI can possibly be used as a non-invasive indicator of alterations in neurotransmitter systems induced by pathology or treatment.

Finally, the pharmacologically induced model that has been studied most extensively by fMRI, phMRI, and rsfMRI is **addiction**. The following exemplary addiction studies will illustrate the power and biological versatility of different fMRI techniques. First of all, fMRI can be used to pinpoint the neural substrate for addiction. For example, acute nicotine administration potentiates the brain reward function and enhances motor and cognitive function. This coincides with an increased BOLD signal in brain areas implicated in reward signaling (Johnson et al., 2013) (i.e., the striato-thalamo-orbitofrontal circuit, which plays a role in compulsive drug intake, and in the insular cortex, which contributes to craving and relapse) (Bruijnzeel et al., 2014). Second, including transgenic mouse models in fMRI experiments could be useful in explaining the contribution of certain receptor types in altered behavior induced by a drug. For example, acute nicotine injection results in increased brain activation in all cortical and subcortical regions of nicotine-naïve mice, which is not observed in knockout mice for the β2-containing nicotinic receptor. This nicotine injection triggered change in activation pattern can explain observed behavioral effects such as altered spatial learning, conflict solving etc., (Suarez et al., 2009).

Third, fMRI allows for the investigation of factors that modulate addictive behaviors and their neural substrates. For example, a differential sensitivity to cocaine is seen in female rats not only as a result of hormonal changes during/throughout the estrous cycle, but also in association with changes in sexual receptivity and presence of pups (Febo et al., 2011; Caffrey and Febo, 2014). FC analyses show connectivity effects in the brain which depend on the amount of time that has passed since the previous dosage of the drug, which implies that the same dose of nicotine might have a different impact on the brain depending on the time elapsed from the previous exposure (Huang et al., 2015). Finally, long term effects of addiction are extensively studied. FC analysis provided evidence of plasticity in addicted animals learned to self-administer cocaine, consistent with results in human drug addicts (Lu et al., 2014).

(rs)fMRI Studies in Lesion Models and Transgenic Models

Both **stroke** and **neurological trauma (brain trauma and peripheral nerve injury)** are clear examples of pathologies where severe neurological damage occurs. St-fMRI and rsfMRI can detect the resulting loss of functionality (Pawela et al., 2010; Yao et al., 2012; Niskanen et al., 2013; Stephenson et al., 2013; Li et al., 2014; Shih et al., 2014) and connectivity on a functional level (van Meer et al., 2010a; Baliki et al., 2014; Mishra et al., 2014). Interestingly, in most cases this loss of functionality is partially recovered depending on the lesion severity (Niskanen et al., 2013; Shih et al., 2014). The process of recovery which relates to neuroplasticity and network reorganization, can be monitored using the same techniques (van Meer et al., 2010b, 2012; Li et al., 2014). Finally, rsfMRI can be used as a read-out for treatment efficacy resulting in different strategies to ameliorate recovery (Wang et al., 2012; Suzuki et al., 2013).

A lot of preclinical neuroscience work is performed on transgenic rodent models for **neurodegenerative diseases** such as: AD, PD, and HD, which are characterized by deposition of misfolded proteins (proteinopathies) in the brain. In AD and HD, the presence of amyloid plaques and huntingtin, respectively, are hypothesized to affect cortical functioning as shown by diminished fMRI responses to sensory stimuli (Lewandowski et al., 2013; Sanganahalli et al., 2013; see **Figure** for an example). Moreover, entire neuronal networks seem affected (Liu et al., 2014), as shown by altered functional connectivity during rsfMRI (Shah et al., 2013; Ferris et al., 2014; **Figure**) even in early disease stages before the proteinopathy establishes (Grandjean et al., 2014b). Compared with wild-type mice, FC deficits are also reported in both adult and old apoE4 and apoE-KO mice. This finding could be related to the fact that the risk of developing neurodegeneration is dependent on the present cholesterol-transporter apolipoprotein ε (APOE) genotype (Zerbi et al., 2014).

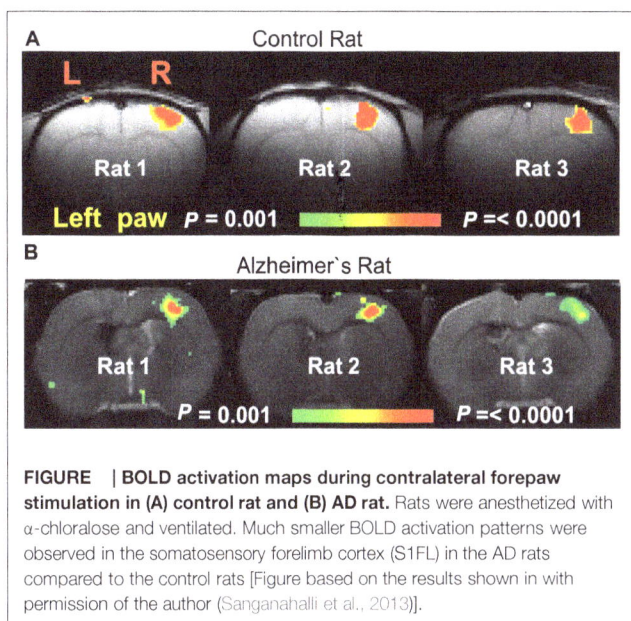

FIGURE | BOLD activation maps during contralateral forepaw stimulation in (A) control rat and (B) AD rat. Rats were anesthetized with α-chloralose and ventilated. Much smaller BOLD activation patterns were observed in the somatosensory forelimb cortex (S1FL) in the AD rats compared to the control rats [Figure based on the results shown in with permission of the author (Sanganahalli et al., 2013)].

Functional magnetic resonance imaging tools are equally suited to study which factors, for example environmental enrichment, stressors, etc., could interfere with neuronal network modulation over time (Little et al., 2012). Similarly, the effects of exercise on ameliorating the affected FC network in Parkinsonian rats was studied (Wang et al., 2015). Clearly both st-fMRI and rsfMRI could be used as read-outs for the efficacy of new therapies in neurodegenerative diseases.

Translation of Application of fMRI Techniques in Pharmacological Research from Rodents to Humans

The non-invasive nature of fMRI renders the technique valuable in terms of translation to the clinic. Though the results in animal models can be translated to the pathology in humans, daily application into the clinic is still hampered by the required sophisticated data analysis. Nevertheless, in clinical research, both st-fMRI and rsfMRI protocols are well established, but phMRI following an acute pharmacological compound injection in the magnet, to characterize the target regions of this compound, is used to a lesser extent. For st-fMRI, an important difference is the type of stimulus used since in rodents typically sensory stimulation is used while in humans also other (complex cognitive) tasks could be used as stimulus.

On the other hand, the fact that rsfMRI requires no action or cooperation of the patient – which is sometimes not feasible under pathological conditions –encouraged clinical research in measuring the brain's resting state clearly before it was even applied on a preclinical level.

It is important to notice that most of the clinical FC research is focusing on the default mode network. A DMN-like network, covering to a certain extent the same anatomical regions, was also observed in rodent models making the technique even more translational. However, the majority of preclinical studies apply a

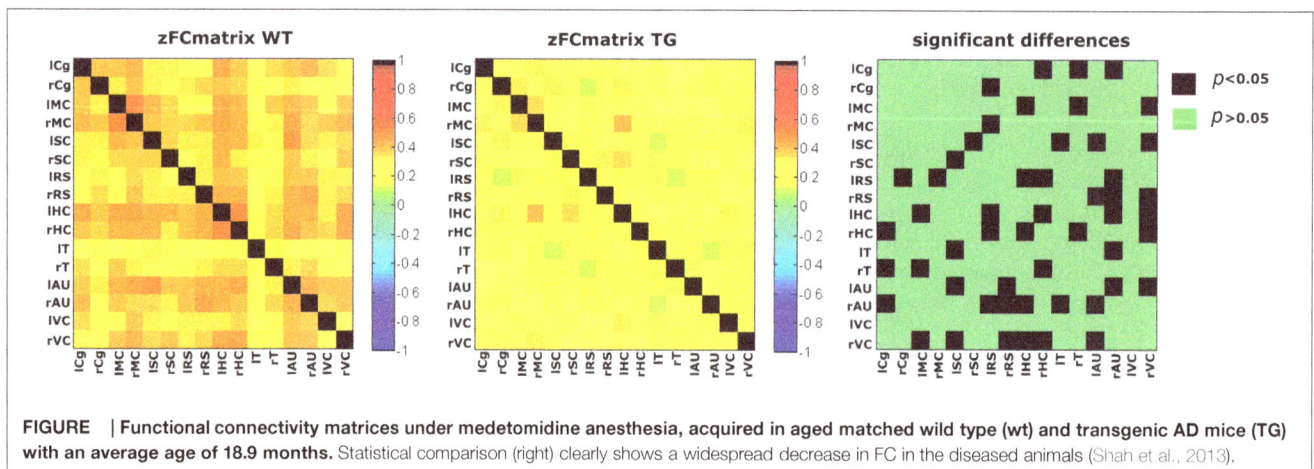

FIGURE | Functional connectivity matrices under medetomidine anesthesia, acquired in aged matched wild type (wt) and transgenic AD mice (TG) **with an average age of 18.9 months.** Statistical comparison (right) clearly shows a widespread decrease in FC in the diseased animals (Shah et al., 2013).

whole brain approach making use of the advantage of rsfMRI to have information on all brain networks obtained within a single short MRI scan.

Some important differences have to be taken into account when comparing acquisition of rodent fMRI with human fMRI. Most small animal MRI systems operate at 4.7–9.4 Tesla and even 11.4T field strengths. Although very recently high field human MRI systems are installed in clinical research centers, typically lower field strengths are used (1.5–3T) in the clinic. The higher field strength clearly results in a higher signal-to-noise ratio, which enables a higher spatial resolution as needed for rodents. On the other hand, artifacts are typically more prominent. For example in the head, which is comprised of multiple compartments with different physico-chemical properties, artifacts can be generated due to susceptibility and different relaxation properties at the higher field strength resulting in image distortions at the level of the ear cavities (Bernstein et al., 2006). As discussed in detail most animal experiments are performed under anesthesia, enabling complete immobilization of the subject, minimizing motion artifacts which can even be improved by mechanical ventilation of the animal.

For most of the applications reviewed above, convergent studies are available in humans demonstrating the clear translational quality of fMRI research. As clinical research is beyond the scope of this review, we only provide some representative illustrations and related references of key reviews in clinical research.

As outlined above, fMRI is capable of unraveling the neuronal substrate of **schizophrenia.** Similarly in humans, functional neuroimaging helped to unravel the neuronal basis of the positive, negative and cognitive symptoms of the disease. Moreover, fMRI studies assisted in developing therapeutic strategies and defining promising targets. For example, both the reported animal work and human studies pinpointed the importance of NMDA receptors in schizophrenia (Gruber et al., 2014).

fMRI can also be used to localize and monitor **epileptic** seizures, similarly as pharmacologically induced seizures in rodents. Additionally, on a clinical level, both st-fMRI and

rsfMRI can be used to explore how seizures modulate the brain and its organization (Chaudhary and Duncan, 2014).

In MDD, changed brain activation (st-fMRI) and FC anomalies were reported both in humans and animal models (Dutta et al., 2014; Kerestes et al., 2014). Moreover clinical trials have also examined the immediate or delayed effects of antidepressants on resting state networks (Dichter et al., 2014).

In the past two decades, imaging studies of drug **addiction** have demonstrated functional brain abnormalities by studying drug-addicted human populations (Parvaz et al., 2011) and rodents. Moreover, acute brain response to addictive substances are studied in humans (Hommer et al., 2011).

For **stroke** imaging there is, both in preclinical and clinical research, a clear research-focus on network reorganization after the insult and during recovery. Moreover fMRI can contribute to improve prognostic ability and the development of therapeutic interventions (Carter et al., 2012). Although in animals both rsfMRI and st-fMRI has been performed, most studies in stroke patients report rsfMRI data (Veldsman et al., 2015). Evidently, acute modulations of the brain immediately after the insult are more convenient to study in rodents than in humans.

For **neurodegenerative** diseases, st-fMRI upon a conscious task can be highly compromised by the mental status of the patients. Studies in cognitively healthy individuals with brain amyloidosis or genetic risk factors for AD have shown functional connectivity abnormalities in preclinical disease stages (Pievani et al., 2014) in convergence with the findings of Grandjean et al. (2014b) in mice. An important difference between animal models and humans is that human neurodegenerative diseases (e.g., AD) are complex diseases manifesting different features. Using animal models, one can differentiate pathological features in separate models which show one key aspect of the disease (e.g., tau and amyloid pathology in AD). In this way, the observed differences in humans may be linked to a certain hallmark of the disease.

FUTURE PERSPECTIVES

Since its first implementation, the field of fMRI has grown exponentially. st-fMRI, rsfMRI, and phMRI have been used intensively to not only characterize the functional properties and organization of healthy brains but also to evaluate pathogenesis and inspect treatment efficacy both in humans and animal models. In addition, many fascinating advanced processing techniques have become available that allow researchers to comprehend complex network topology and infer effective connectivity.

Modern brain mapping techniques, such as rsfMRI, produce increasingly large datasets of functional connection patterns underlying the large-scale functional organization of the brain[5].

Concurrent technological advances are generating similarly large connection datasets in biological, technological, social, and other scientific fields. Attempts to characterize these datasets have, over the last decade, led to the emergence of a new, multidisciplinary approach to the study of complex systems. This approach, known as **complex network analysis**, describes important properties of complex systems by quantifying topologies of their respective network representations (Rubinov and Sporns, 2010).

Secondly, new developments in **brain circuit modulations** such as deep brain stimulation (Younce et al., 2014; Lai et al., 2015) and the more targeted optogenetic modulations of neuronal populations (ofMRI) can be used to study brain networks. Brain circuit elements can be selectively triggered with temporal precision while the resulting network response is monitored non-invasively with high spatial and temporal accuracy (Lee, 2011).

Most resting-state fMRI investigations were based upon static descriptions of FC. However, since the brain must dynamically integrate, coordinate, and respond to internal and external stimuli across multiple time scales, recent studies have begun to study the dynamics of FC over time. Emerging evidence suggests that using **dynamic rsfMRI,** FC changes in macroscopic neural activity patterns can be discovered which may underlie critical aspects of cognition and behavior. Nevertheless limitations with regard to analysis and interpretation should be taken into account (Hutchison et al., 2013).

Though the focus of this review lies on BOLD-based neuronal activity measurements, we want to emphasize that **ASL,** which was briefly introduced earlier in this review, provides a non-invasive, absolute quantification of CBF both at rest and during task/drug activation. These CBF measurement are very stable over time, and as such ASL allows a relatively straightforward physiological interpretation of drug-induced changes in neuronal activation. ASL studies which follow CBF changes in response to a specific stimulus/task or pharmacological modulation are available for human research [see review, (Wang et al., 2011)]. These techniques can be translated from clinical to rodent research to detect either the central effects of a drug or the change in neuronal response following drug administration. One recently published study, presents data from 1400 rats following a standardized ASL-phMRI protocol using different known compounds (Bruns et al., 2015). Based on these data, a new method was proposed to quantitatively characterize new psychotropics in which typical and differential activation

profiles after antipsychotic, antidepressant, and anxiolytic drug injection could be defined. Similar approaches could be used for BOLD fMRI as well with interesting opportunities for future pharmacological research. The acquired 'typical activation patterns' can be used to classify drug induced brain activations of unknown psychotropics which further facilitates biological understanding and decision making in drugdiscovery (Bruns et al., 2015).

The current developments in measuring CBF by pseudo-continuous ASL on clinical scanners (Alsop et al., 2014) have dramatically improved the sensitivity and essential high temporal resolution of perfusion imaging to allow the detection of CBF based functional connectivity changes (Chuang et al., 2008; Fernandez-Seara et al., 2011). However, similar ASL acquisition protocols on preclinical scanners still need to be optimized to provide stable CBF measurements with a high spatial and temporal resolution to allow similar FC-analysis. This would create new avenues in pharmacological rodent research coming from the combination of BOLD and ASL-based MRI. Combining both BOLD and ASL-based rsfMRI in rodents would allow to perform joint FC-analysis (Jann et al., 2015) to characterize the spatiotemporal brain networks within phMRI studies. On the other hand, from the BOLD and ASL-data, it is possible to extract a third read-out of neuronal activity, being the cerebral metabolic rate of oxygen (CMRO2), which is less sensitive to vascular dynamics. Similar to BOLD and ASL experiments, one can follow drug induced changes of CMRO2 within a rsfMRI, st-fMRI, or phMRI design.

In conclusion, fMRI based on the BOLD response can be used in a wide range of different applications. Recently, sensory and pharmacologically induced fMRI were extended with fMRI measured during rest. The interest in rsfMRI is growing, resulting in an increasing number of methods to analyze and interpret the data. This review clearly shows the potential of MRI to study neuro-modulation, particularly induced by pharmacological agents. Functional MRI techniques enable researchers to obtain a vast amount of information in a relatively short amount of time compared to other imaging techniques. Moreover, we are at the beginning of fMRI's application to preclinical treatment testing, especially rsfMRI.

Another important feature which makes fMRI a unique and highly exceptional method compared to other 'brain targeting tools' such as electrophysiology, is its translational character. Indeed, many similarities have been reported between human and small animal findings. However, in general, animal studies are lagging behind studies in humans when it comes down to assessing the effects of specific pathologies on functional characteristics of the brain. With this review, we hope to have convinced and maybe even inspired neuroscientists to further exploit fMRI and its many applications in (pre)clinical setting.

ACKNOWLEDGMENTS

The authors acknowledge the Institute for the Promotion of Innovation by Science and Technology (IWT) in Flanders grant agreement 131060, Molecular Imaging of Brain Pathophysiology

---

[5]https://www.humanbrainproject.eu/

(BRAINPATH) under grant agreement number 612360 within the Marie Curie Actions-Industry-Academia Partnerships and Pathways (IAPP) program; DS is holder of an IWT PhD grant, the European Union's Seventh Framework Programme

under grant agreement number 278850 (INMiND), the Research Foundation-Flanders (FWO) (project Nr G030213N and G044311N), the Hercules Foundation (Grant Nr AUHA0012)

REFERENCES

Adamczak, J. M., Farr, T. D., Seehafer, J. U., Kalthoff, D., and Hoehn, M. (2010). High field BOLD response to forepaw stimulation in the mouse. *Neuroimage* 51, 704–712. doi: 10.1016/j.neuroimage.2010.02.083

Airaksinen, A. M., Hekmatyar, S. K., Jerome, N., Niskanen, J. P., Huttunen, J. K., Pitkanen, A., et al. (2012). Simultaneous BOLD fMRI and local field potential measurements during kainic acid-induced seizures. *Epilepsia* 53, 1245–1253. doi: 10.1111/j.1528-1167.2012.03539.x

Airaksinen, A. M., Niskanen, J. P., Chamberlain, R., Huttunen, J. K., Nissinen, J., Garwood, M., et al. (2010). Simultaneous fMRI and local field potential measurements during epileptic seizures in medetomidine-sedated rats using raser pulse sequence. *Magn. Reson. Med.* 64, 1191–1199. doi: 10.1002/mrm.22508

Alonso Bde, C., Makarova, T., and Hess, A. (2011). On the use of alpha-chloralose for repeated BOLD fMRI measurements in rats. *J. Neurosci. Methods* 195, 236–240. doi: 10.1016/j.jneumeth.2010.12.010

Alsop, D. C., Detre, J. A., Golay, X., Gunther, M., Hendrikse, J., Hernandez-Garcia, L., et al. (2014). Recommended implementation of arterial spin-labeled perfusion MRI for clinical applications: a consensus of the ISMRM perfusion study group and the European consortium for ASL in dementia. *Magn. Reson. Med.* 73, 102–116. doi: 10.1002/mrm.25197

Amaro, E. Jr., and Barker, G. J. (2006). Study design in fMRI: basic principles. *Brain Cogn.* 60, 220–232. doi: 10.1016/j.bandc.2005.11.009

Austin, V. C., Blamire, A. M., Allers, K. A., Sharp, T., Styles, P., Matthews, P. M., et al. (2005). Confounding effects of anesthesia on functional activation in rodent brain: a study of halothane and alpha-chloralose anesthesia. *Neuroimage* 24, 92–100. doi: 10.1016/j.neuroimage.2004.08.011

Baker, H. J., Lindsey, J. R., and Weisbroth, S. H. (1979). "Housing to control research variables," in *The Laboratory Rat*, Vol. I, *Biology and Diseases*, eds H. J. Baker, J. R. Lindsey, and S. H. Weisbroth (New York, NY: Academic Press).

Baliki, M. N., Chang, P. C., Baria, A. T., Centeno, M. V., and Apkarian, A. V. (2014). Resting-sate functional reorganization of the rat limbic system following neuropathic injury. *Sci. Rep.* 4:6186. doi: 10.1038/srep06186

Bandettini, P. A. (2012). Twenty years of functional MRI: the science and the stories. *Neuroimage* 62, 575–588. doi: 10.1016/j.neuroimage.2012.04.026

Becerra, L., Pendse, G., Chang, P. C., Bishop, J., and Borsook, D. (2011). Robust reproducible resting state networks in the awake rodent brain. *PLoS ONE* 6:e25701. doi: 10.1371/journal.pone.0025701

Beckmann, C. F., and Smith, S. M. (2004). Probabilistic independent component analysis for functional magnetic resonance imaging. *IEEE Trans. Med. Imaging* 23, 137–152. doi: 10.1109/TMI.2003.822821

Ben-Ari, Y., Tremblay, E., Riche, D., Ghilini, G., and Naquet, R. (1981). Electrographic, clinical and pathological alterations following systemic administration of kainic acid, bicuculline or pentetrazole: metabolic mapping using the deoxyglucose method with special reference to the pathology of epilepsy. *Neuroscience* 6, 1361–1391. doi: 10.1016/0306-4522(81)90193-7

Bernstein, M. A., Huston, J. 3rd., and Ward, H. A. (2006). Imaging artifacts at 3.0T. *J. Magn. Reson. Imaging* 24, 735–746. doi: 10.1002/jmri.20698

Bernstein, S. E. (1966). "Physiological characteristics," *Biology of the Laboratory Mouse*, ed. E. L. Green (New York, NY: Dover Publications, Inc.).

Bettinardi, R. G., Tort-Colet, N., Ruiz-Mejias, M., Sanchez-Vives, M. V., and Deco, G. (2015). Gradual emergence of spontaneous correlated brain activity during fading of general anesthesia in rats: evidences from fMRI and local field potentials. *Neuroimage* 114, 185–198. doi: 10.1016/j.neuroimage.2015.03.037

Bifone, A., and Gozzi, A. (2012). Neuromapping techniques in drug discovery: pharmacological MRI for the assessment of novel antipsychotics. *Expert Opin. Drug Discov.* 7, 1071–1082. doi: 10.1517/17460441.2012.724057

Biswal, B., Yetkin, F. Z., Haughton, V. M., and Hyde, J. S. (1995). Functional connectivity in the motor cortex of resting human brain using echo-planar MRI. *Magn. Reson. Med.* 34, 537–541. doi: 10.1002/mrm.1910340409

Borsook, D., and Becerra, L. (2011). CNS animal fMRI in pain and analgesia. *Neurosci. Biobehav. Rev.* 35, 1125–1143. doi: 10.1016/j.neubiorev.2010.11.005

Boubela, R. N., Kalcher, K., Huf, W., Kronnerwetter, C., Filzmoser, P., and Moser E. (2013). Beyond noise: using temporal ICA to extract meaningful information from high-frequency fMRI signal fluctuations during rest. *Front. Hum. Neurosci.* 7:168. doi: 10.3389/fnhum.2013.00168

Bruhn, H., Kleinschmidt, A., Boecker, H., Merboldt, K. D., Hanicke, W., and Frahm, J. (1994). The effect of acetazolamide on regional cerebral blood oxygenation at rest and under stimulation as assessed by MRI. *J. Cereb. Blood Flow Metab.* 14, 742–748. doi: 10.1038/jcbfm.1994.95

Bruijnzeel, A. W., Alexander, J. C., Perez, P. D., Bauzo-Rodriguez, R., Hall, G., Klausner, R., et al. (2014). Acute nicotine administration increases BOLD fMRI signal in brain regions involved in reward signaling and compulsive drug intake in rats. *Int. J. Neuropsychopharmacol.* 18, 1–13. doi: 10.1093/ijnp/pyu011

Bruns, A., Mueggler, T., Kunnecke, B., Risterucci, C., Prinssen, E. P., Wettstein, J. G., et al. (2015). Domain gauges: a reference system for multivariate profiling of brain fMRI activation patterns induced by psychoactive drugs in rats. *Neuroimage* 112, 70–85. doi: 10.1016/j.neuroimage.2015.02.032

Buxton, R. B., and Frank, L. R. (1997). A model for the coupling between cerebral blood flow and oxygen metabolism during neural stimulation. *J. Cereb. Blood Flow Metab.* 17, 64–72. doi: 10.1097/00004647-199701000-00009

Caffrey, M. K., and Febo, M. (2014). Cocaine-associated odor cue re-exposure increases blood oxygenation level dependent signal in memory and reward regions of the maternal rat brain. *Drug Alcohol Depend.* 134, 167–177. doi: 10.1016/j.drugalcdep.2013.09.032

Calhoun, V. D., Adali, T., Pearlson, G. D., and Pekar, J. J. (2001). A method for making group inferences from functional MRI data using independent component analysis. *Hum. Brain Mapp.* 14, 140–151. doi: 10.1002/hbm.1048

Canese, R., Marco, E. M., De Pasquale, F., Podo, F., Laviola, G., and Adriani, W. (2011). Differential response to specific 5-Ht(7) versus whole-serotonergic drugs in rat forebrains: a phMRI study. *Neuroimage* 58, 885–894. doi: 10.1016/j.neuroimage.2011.06.089

Carter, A. R., Shulman, G. L., and Corbetta, M. (2012). Why use a connectivity-based approach to study stroke and recovery of function? *Neuroimage* 62, 2271–2280. doi: 10.1016/j.neuroimage.2012.02.070

Cassidy, P. J., Schneider, J. E., Grieve, S. M., Lygate, C., Neubauer, S., and Clarke, K. (2004). Assessment of motion gating strategies for mouse magnetic resonance at high magnetic fields. *J. Magn. Reson. Imaging* 19, 229–237. doi: 10.1002/jmri.10454

Chaudhary, U. J., and Duncan, J. S. (2014). Applications of blood-oxygen-level-dependent functional magnetic resonance imaging and diffusion tensor imaging in epilepsy. *Neuroimaging Clin. N. Am.* 24, 671–694. doi: 10.1016/j.nic.2014.07.001

Chavarrias, C., Garcia-Vazquez, V., Aleman-Gomez, Y., Montesinos, P., Pascau, J., and Desco, M. (2015). fMRat: an extension of SPM for a fully automatic analysis of rodent brain functional magnetic resonance series. *Med. Biol. Eng. Comput.* doi: 10.1007/s11517-015-1365-9 [Epub ahead of print].

Chuang, K. H., van Gelderen, P., Merkle, H., Bodurka, J., Ikonomidou, V. N., Koretsky, A. P., et al. (2008). Mapping resting-state functional connectivity using perfusion MRI. *Neuroimage* 40, 1595–1605. doi: 10.1016/j.neuroimage.2008.01.006

Ciris, P. A., Qiu, M., and Constable, R. T. (2014). Non-invasive quantification of absolute cerebral blood volume during functional activation applicable to the whole human brain. *Magn. Reson. Med.* 71, 580–590. doi: 10.1002/mrm.24694

Damoiseaux, J. S., Rombouts, S. A., Barkhof, F., Scheltens, P., Stam, C. J., Smith, S. M., et al. (2006). Consistent resting-state networks across healthy subjects. *Proc. Natl. Acad. Sci. U.S.A.* 103, 13848–13853. doi: 10.1073/pnas.0601417103

Denic, A., Macura, S. I., Mishra, P., Gamez, J. D., Rodriguez, M., and Pirko, I. (2011). MRI in rodent models of brain disorders. *Neurotherapeutics* 8, 3–18. doi: 10.1007/s13311-010-0002-4

DeSalvo, M. N., Schridde, U., Mishra, A. M., Motelow, J. E., Purcaro, M. J., Danielson, N., et al. (2010). Focal BOLD fMRI changes in bicuculline-induced tonic-clonic seizures in the rat. *Neuroimage* 50, 902–909. doi: 10.1016/j.neuroimage.2010.01.006

Detre, J. A., and Wang, J. (2002). Technical aspects and utility of fMRI using BOLD and ASL. *Clin. Neurophysiol.* 113, 621–634. doi: 10.1016/S1388-2457(02)00038-X

Dichter, G. S., Gibbs, D., and Smoski, M. J. (2014). A systematic review of relations between resting-state functional-MRI and treatment response in major depressive disorder. *J. Affect. Disord.* 172C, 8–17.

Di Salle, F., Formisano, E., Linden, D. E., Goebel, R., Bonavita, S., Pepino, A., et al. (1999). Exploring brain function with magnetic resonance imaging. *Eur. J. Radiol.* 30, 84–94. doi: 10.1016/S0720-048X(99)00047-9

Dodds, C. M., Clark, L., Dove, A., Regenthal, R., Baumann, F., Bullmore, E., et al. (2009). The dopamine D2 receptor antagonist sulpiride modulates striatal BOLD signal during the manipulation of information in working memory. *Psychopharmacology (Berl.)* 207, 35–45. doi: 10.1007/s00213-009-1634-0

Dutta, A., McKie, S., and Deakin, J. F. (2014). Resting state networks in major depressive disorder. *Psychiatry Res.* 224, 139–151. doi: 10.1016/j.pscychresns.2014.10.003

Evans, A. C., Marrett, S., Neelin, P., Collins, L., Worsley, K., Dai, W., et al. (1992). Anatomical mapping of functional activation in stereotactic coordinate space. *Neuroimage* 1, 43–53. doi: 10.1016/1053-8119(92)90006-9

Febo, M. (2011). Technical and conceptual considerations for performing and interpreting functional MRI studies in awake rats. *Front. Psychiatry* 2:43. doi: 10.3389/fpsyt.2011.00043

Febo, M., Segarra, A. C., Stolberg, T. L., and Ferris, C. F. (2011). BOLD signal response to cocaine varies with sexual receptivity in female rats. *Neuroreport* 22, 19–22. doi: 10.1097/WNR.0b013e3283416f81

Feinberg, D. A., and Yacoub, E. (2012). The rapid development of high speed, resolution and precision in fMRI. *Neuroimage* 62, 720–725. doi: 10.1016/j.neuroimage.2012.01.049

Fernandez-Seara, M. A., Aznarez-Sanado, M., Mengual, E., Irigoyen, J., Heukamp, F., and Pastor, M. A. (2011). Effects on resting cerebral blood flow and functional connectivity induced by metoclopramide: a perfusion MRI study in healthy volunteers. *Br. J. Pharmacol.* 163, 1639–1652. doi: 10.1111/j.1476-5381.2010.01161.x

Ferris, C. F., Kulkarni, P., Toddes, S., Yee, J., Kenkel, W., and Nedelman, M. (2014). Studies on the Q175 knock-in model of huntington's disease using functional imaging in awake mice: evidence of olfactory dysfunction. *Front Neurol* 5:94. doi: 10.3389/fneur.2014.00094

Ferris, C. F., Smerkers, B., Kulkarni, P., Caffrey, M., Afacan, O., Toddes, S., et al. (2011). Functional magnetic resonance imaging in awake animals. *Rev. Neurosci.* 22, 665–674. doi: 10.1515/rns.2011.050

Fox, M. D., Zhang, D., Snyder, A. Z., and Raichle, M. E. (2009). The global signal and observed anticorrelated resting state brain networks. *J. Neurophysiol.* 101, 3270–3283. doi: 10.1152/jn.90777.2008

Fransson P. (2005). Spontaneous low-frequency BOLD signal fluctuations: an fMRI investigation of the resting-state default mode of brain function hypothesis. *Hum. Brain Mapp.* 26, 15–29. doi: 10.1002/hbm.20113

Friston, K. J., Harrison, L., and Penny, W. (2003). Dynamic causal modelling. *Neuroimage* 19, 1273–1302. doi: 10.1016/S1053-8119(03)00202-7

Fritsch, B., Reis, J., Gasior, M., Kaminski, R. M., and Rogawski, M. A. (2014). Role of GluK1 kainate receptors in seizures, epileptic discharges, and epileptogenesis. *J. Neurosci.* 34, 5765–5775. doi: 10.1523/JNEUROSCI.5307-13.2014

Fukuda, M., Vazquez, A. L., Zong, X., and Kim, S. G. (2013). Effects of the alpha(2)-adrenergic receptor agonist dexmedetomidine on neural, vascular and BOLD fMRI responses in the somatosensory cortex. *Eur. J. Neurosci.* 37, 80–95. doi: 10.1111/ejn.12024

Garrett, K. M., and Gan, J. (1998). Enhancement of gamma-aminobutyric acidA receptor activity by alpha-chloralose. *J. Pharmacol. Exp. Ther.* 285, 680–686.

Grandjean, J., Schroeter, A., Batata, I., and Rudin, M. (2014a). Optimization of anesthesia protocol for resting-state fMRI in mice based on differential effects of anesthetics on functional connectivity patterns. *Neuroimage* 102(Pt. 2), 838–847. doi: 10.1016/j.neuroimage.2014.08.043

Grandjean, J., Schroeter, A., He, P., Tanadini, M., Keist, R., Krstic, D., et al. (2014b). Early alterations in functional connectivity and white matter structure in a transgenic mouse model of cerebral amyloidosis. *J. Neurosci.* 34, 13780–13789. doi: 10.1523/JNEUROSCI.4762-13.2014

Gruber, O., Santuccione, A. C., and Aach, H. (2014). Magnetic resonance imaging in studying schizophrenia, negative symptoms, and the glutamate system. *Front. Psychiatry* 5:32. doi: 10.3389/fpsyt.2014.00032

Hodkinson, D. J., de Groote, C., McKie, S., Deakin, J. F., and Williams, S. R. (2012). Differential effects of anaesthesia on the phMRI response to acute ketamine challenge. *Br. J. Med. Med. Res.* 2, 373–385. doi: 10.9734/BJMMR/2012/1412

Hommer, D. W., Bjork, J. M., and Gilman, J. M. (2011). Imaging brain response to reward in addictive disorders. *Ann. N. Y. Acad. Sci.* 1216, 50–61. doi: 10.1111/j.1749-6632.2010.05898.x

Huang, W., Heffernan, M. E., Li, Z., Zhang, N., Overstreet, D. H., and King, J. A. (2011). Fear induced neuronal alterations in a genetic model of depression: an fMRI study on awake animals. *Neurosci. Lett.* 489, 74–78. doi: 10.1016/j.neulet.2010.11.069

Huang, W., Tam, K., Fernando, J., Heffernan, M., King, J., and DiFranza, J. R. (2015). Nicotine and resting-state functional connectivity: effects of intermittent doses. *Nicotine Tob. Res.* doi: 10.1093/ntr/ntv009 [Epub ahead of print].

Hutchison, R. M., Mirsattari, S. M., Jones, C. K., Gati, J. S., and Leung, L. S. (2010). Functional networks in the anesthetized rat brain revealed by independent component analysis of resting-state FMRI. *J. Neurophysiol.* 103, 3398–3406. doi: 10.1152/jn.00141.2010

Hutchison, R. M., Womelsdorf, T., Allen, E. A., Bandettini, P. A., Calhoun, V. D., Corbetta, M., et al. (2013). Dynamic functional connectivity: promise, issues, and interpretations. *Neuroimage* 80, 360–378. doi: 10.1016/j.neuroimage.2013.05.079

Huttunen, J. K., Grohn, O., and Penttonen, M. (2008). Coupling between simultaneously recorded BOLD response and neuronal activity in the rat somatosensory cortex. *Neuroimage* 39, 775–785. doi: 10.1016/j.neuroimage.2007.06.042

Huttunen, J. K., Niskanen, J. P., Lehto, L. J., Airaksinen, A. M., Niskanen, E. I., Penttonen, M., et al. (2011). Evoked local field potentials can explain temporal variation in blood oxygenation level-dependent responses in rat somatosensory cortex. *NMR Biomed.* 24, 209–215. doi: 10.1002/nbm.1575

Hyder, F., Behar, K. L., Martin, M. A., Blamire, A. M., and Shulman, R. G. (1994). Dynamic magnetic resonance imaging of the rat brain during forepaw stimulation. *J. Cereb. Blood Flow Metab.* 14, 649–655. doi: 10.1038/jcbfm.1994.81

Iannetti, G. D., and Wise, R. G. (2007). BOLD functional MRI in disease and pharmacological studies: room for improvement? *Magn. Reson. Imaging* 25, 978–988. doi: 10.1016/j.mri.2007.03.018

James, J. S., Rajesh, P., Chandran, A. V., and Kesavadas, C. (2014). fMRI paradigm designing and post-processing tools. *Indian J. Radiol. Imaging* 24, 13–21. doi: 10.4103/0971-3026.130686

Jann, K., Gee, D. G., Kilroy, E., Schwab, S., Smith, R. X., Cannon, T. D., et al. (2015). Functional connectivity in BOLD and CBF data: similarity and reliability of resting brain networks. *Neuroimage* 106, 111–122. doi: 10.1016/j.neuroimage.2014.11.028

Jenkins, B. G. (2012). Pharmacologic magnetic resonance imaging (phMRI): imaging drug action in the brain. *Neuroimage* 62, 1072–1085. doi: 10.1016/j.neuroimage.2012.03.075

Johnson, T. R., Smerkers, B., Moulder, J. K., Stellar, J. R., and Febo, M. (2013). Neural processing of a cocaine-associated odor cue revealed by functional MRI in awake rats. *Neurosci. Lett.* 534, 160–165. doi: 10.1016/j.neulet.2012.11.054

Jonckers, E., Delgado, Y. P. R., Shah, D., Guglielmetti, C., Verhoye, M., and Van der Linden, A. (2013a). Different anesthesia regimes modulate the functional connectivity outcome in mice. *Magn. Reson. Med.* 72, 1103–11012. doi: 10.1002/mrm.24990

Jonckers, E., Van der Linden, A., and Verhoye, M. (2013b). Functional magnetic resonance imaging in rodents: an unique tool to study in vivo pharmacologic neuromodulation. *Curr. Opin. Pharmacol.* 13, 813–820. doi: 10.1016/j.coph.2013.06.008

Jonckers, E., Van Audekerke, J., De Visscher, G., Van der Linden, A., and Verhoye, M. (2011). Functional connectivity FMRI of the rodent brain: comparison of functional connectivity networks in rat and mouse. *PLoS ONE* 6:e18876. doi: 10.1371/journal.pone.0018876

Kalthoff, D., Po, C., Wiedermann, D., and Hoehn, M. (2013). Reliability and spatial specificity of rat brain sensorimotor functional connectivity networks are superior under sedation compared with general anesthesia. *NMR Biomed.* 26, 638–650. doi: 10.1002/nbm.2908

Kerestes, R., Davey, C. G., Stephanou, K., Whittle, S., and Harrison, B. J. (2014). Functional brain imaging studies of youth depression: a systematic review. *Neuroimage Clin.* 4, 209–231. doi: 10.1016/j.nicl.2013.11.009

Kim, T., Masamoto, K., Fukuda, M., Vazquez, A., and Kim, S. G. (2010). Frequency-dependent neural activity, CBF, and BOLD fMRI to somatosensory stimuli in isoflurane-anesthetized rats. *Neuroimage* 52, 224–233. doi: 10.1016/j.neuroimage.2010.03.064

King, J. A., Garelick, T. S., Brevard, M. E., Chen, W., Messenger, T. L., Duong, T. Q., et al. (2005). Procedure for minimizing stress for fMRI studies in conscious rats. *J. Neurosci. Methods* 148, 154–160. doi: 10.1016/j.jneumeth.2005.04.011

Klinkenberg, I., and Blokland, A. (2010). The validity of scopolamine as a pharmacological model for cognitive impairment: a review of animal behavioral studies. *Neurosci. Biobehav. Rev.* 34, 1307–1350. doi: 10.1016/j.neubiorev.2010.04.001

Klomp, A., Tremoleda, J. L., Schrantee, A., Gsell, W., and Reneman, L. (2012a). The use of pharmacological-challenge fMRI in pre-clinical research: application to the 5-HT system. *J. Vis. Exp.* 62:3956. doi: 10.3791/3956

Klomp, A., Tremoleda, J. L., Wylezinska, M., Nederveen, A. J., Feenstra, M., Gsell, W., et al. (2012b). Lasting effects of chronic fluoxetine treatment on the late developing rat brain: age-dependent changes in the serotonergic neurotransmitter system assessed by pharmacological MRI. *Neuroimage* 59, 218–226. doi: 10.1016/j.neuroimage.2011.07.082

Kwong, K. K., Belliveau, J. W., Chesler, D. A., Goldberg, I. E., Weisskoff, R. M., Poncelet, B. P., et al. (1992). Dynamic magnetic resonance imaging of human brain activity during primary sensory stimulation. *Proc. Natl. Acad. Sci. U.S.A.* 89, 5675–5679. doi: 10.1073/pnas.89.12.5675

Lahti, K. M., Ferris, C. F., Li, F., Sotak, C. H., and King, J. A. (1999). Comparison of evoked cortical activity in conscious and propofol-anesthetized rats using functional MRI. *Magn. Reson. Med.* 41, 412–416. doi: 10.1002/(SICI)1522-2594(199902)41:2<412::AID-MRM28>3.0.CO;2-3

Lai, H. Y., Albaugh, D. L., Kao, Y. C., Younce, J. R., and Shih, Y. Y. (2015). Robust deep brain stimulation functional MRI procedures in rats and mice using an MR-compatible tungsten microwire electrode. *Magn. Reson. Med.* 73, 1246–1251. doi: 10.1002/mrm.25239

Larsen, M., and Langmoen, I. A. (1998). The effect of volatile anaesthetics on synaptic release and uptake of glutamate. *Toxicol. Lett.* 100–101, 59–64. doi: 10.1016/S0378-4274(98)00165-9

Lee, J. H. (2011). Tracing activity across the whole brain neural network with optogenetic functional magnetic resonance imaging. *Front. Neuroinform.* 5:21. doi: 10.3389/fninf.2011.00021

Lewandowski, N. M., Bordelon, Y., Brickman, A. M., Angulo, S., Khan, U., Muraskin, J., et al. (2013). Regional vulnerability in Huntington's disease: fMRI-guided molecular analysis in patients and a mouse model of disease. *Neurobiol. Dis.* 52, 84–93. doi: 10.1016/j.nbd.2012.11.014

Li, B., Zhou, F., Luo, Q., and Li, P. (2012). Altered resting-state functional connectivity after cortical spreading depression in mice. *Neuroimage* 63, 1171–1177. doi: 10.1016/j.neuroimage.2012.08.024

Li, R., Hettinger, P. C., Liu, X., Machol, J. T., Yan, J. G., Matloub, H. S., et al. (2014). Early evaluation of nerve regeneration after nerve injury and repair using functional connectivity MRI. *Neurorehabil. Neural Repair* 28, 707–715. doi: 10.1177/1545968314521002

Liang, Z., King, J., and Zhang, N. (2012). Anticorrelated resting-state functional connectivity in awake rat brain. *Neuroimage* 59, 1190–1199. doi: 10.1016/j.neuroimage.2011.08.009

Lindquist, M. A., Meng Loh, J., Atlas, L. Y., and Wager, T. D. (2009). Modeling the hemodynamic response function in fMRI: efficiency, bias and mis-modeling. *Neuroimage* 45, S187–S198. doi: 10.1016/j.neuroimage.2008.10.065

Liska, A., Galbusera, A., Schwarz, A. J., and Gozzi, A. (2015). Functional connectivity hubs of the mouse brain. *Neuroimage* 115, 281–291. doi: 10.1016/j.neuroimage.2015.04.033

Little, D. M., Foxely, S., and Lazarov, O. (2012). A preliminary study targeting neuronal pathways activated following environmental enrichment by resting state functional magnetic resonance imaging. *J. Alzheimer's Dis.* 32, 101–107.

Liu, T., Bai, W., Yi, H., Tan, T., Wei, J., Wang, J., and Tian, X. (2014). Functional connectivity in a rat model of Alzheimer's disease during a working memory task. *Curr. Alzheimer Res.* 11, 981–991. doi: 10.2174/1567205011666141107125912

Liu, X., Pillay, S., Li, R., Vizuete, J. A., Pechman, K. R., Schmainda, K. M., et al. (2013). Multiphasic modification of intrinsic functional connectivity of the rat brain during increasing levels of propofol. *Neuroimage* 83, 581–592. doi: 10.1016/j.neuroimage.2013.07.003

Logothetis, N. K. (2002). The neural basis of the blood-oxygen-level-dependent functional magnetic resonance imaging signal. *Philos. Trans. R. Soc. Lond B Biol. Sci.* 357, 1003–1037. doi: 10.1098/rstb.2002.1114

Logothetis, N. K. (2008). What we can do and what we cannot do with fMRI. *Nature* 453, 869–878. doi: 10.1038/nature06976

Logothetis, N. K., Pauls, J., Augath, M., Trinath, T., and Oeltermann, A. (2001). Neurophysiological investigation of the basis of the fMRI signal. *Nature* 412, 150–157. doi: 10.1038/35084005

Logothetis, N. K., and Wandell, B. A. (2004). Interpreting the BOLD signal. *Annu. Rev. Physiol.* 66, 735–769. doi: 10.1146/annurev.physiol.66.082602.092845

Lowe, M. J., Dzemidzic, M., Lurito, J. T., Mathews, V. P., and Phillips, M. D. (2000). Correlations in low-frequency BOLD fluctuations reflect cortico-cortical connections. *Neuroimage* 12, 582–587. doi: 10.1006/nimg.2000.0654

Lu, H., Zou, Q., Chefer, S., Ross, T. J., Vaupel, D. B., Guillem, K., et al. (2014). Abstinence from cocaine and sucrose self-administration reveals altered mesocorticolimbic circuit connectivity by resting state MRI. *Brain Connect.* 4, 499–510. doi: 10.1089/brain.2014.0264

Lu, H., Zou, Q., Gu, H., Raichle, M. E., Stein, E. A., and Yang, Y. (2012). Rat brains also have a default mode network. *Proc. Natl. Acad. Sci. U.S.A.* 109, 3979–3984. doi: 10.1073/pnas.1200506109

Magnuson, M. E., Thompson, G. J., Pan, W. J., and Keilholz, S. D. (2014). Time-dependent effects of isoflurane and dexmedetomidine on functional connectivity, spectral characteristics, and spatial distribution of spontaneous BOLD fluctuations. *NMR Biomed.* 27, 291–303. doi: 10.1002/nbm.3062

Mandeville, J. B. (2012). IRON fMRI measurements of CBV and implications for BOLD signal. *Neuroimage* 62, 1000–1008. doi: 10.1016/j.neuroimage.2012.01.070

Mandeville, J. B., Marota, J. J., Kosofsky, B. E., Keltner, J. R., Weissleder, R., Rosen, B. R., et al. (1998). Dynamic functional imaging of relative cerebral blood volume during rat forepaw stimulation. *Magn. Reson. Med.* 39, 615–624. doi: 10.1002/mrm.1910390415

Margulies, D. S., Bottger, J., Long, X., Lv, Y., Kelly, C., Schafer, A., et al. (2010). Resting developments: a review of fMRI post-processing methodologies for spontaneous brain activity. *MAGMA* 23, 289–307. doi: 10.1007/s10334-010-0228-5

Mishra, A. M., Bai, X., Motelow, J. E., Desalvo, M. N., Danielson, N., Sanganahalli, B. G., et al. (2013). Increased resting functional connectivity in spike-wave epilepsy in WAG/Rij rats. *Epilepsia* 54, 1214–1222. doi: 10.1111/epi.12227

Mishra, A. M., Bai, X., Sanganahalli, B. G., Waxman, S. G., Shatillo, O., Grohn, O., et al. (2014). Decreased resting functional connectivity after traumatic brain injury in the rat. *PLoS ONE* 9:e95280. doi: 10.1371/journal.pone.0095280

Mueggler, T., Baumann, D., Rausch, M., and Rudin, M. (2001). Bicuculline-induced brain activation in mice detected by functional magnetic resonance imaging. *Magn. Reson. Med.* 46, 292–298. doi: 10.1002/mrm.1190

Muller, K., Lohmann, G., Bosch, V., and von Cramon, D. Y. (2001). On multivariate spectral analysis of fMRI time series. *Neuroimage* 14, 347–356. doi: 10.1006/nimg.2001.0804

Nakai, M., Yamamoto, J., and Matsui, Y. (1986). Acute systemic and regional hemodynamic effects of alpha 1-adrenoceptor blockade in conscious spontaneously hypertensive rats. *Clin. Exp. Hypertens. A* 8, 981–996. doi: 10.3109/10641968609044081

Nasrallah, F. A., Lew, S. K., Low, A. S., and Chuang, K. H. (2014). Neural correlate of resting-state functional connectivity under alpha2 adrenergic receptor agonist, medetomidine. *Neuroimage* 84, 27–34. doi: 10.1016/j.neuroimage.2013.08.004

Niskanen, J. P., Airaksinen, A. M., Sierra, A., Huttunen, J. K., Nissinen, J., Karjalainen, P. A., et al. (2013). Monitoring functional impairment and recovery after traumatic brain injury in rats by FMRI. *J. Neurotrauma* 30, 546–556. doi: 10.1089/neu.2012.2416

Ogawa, S., Lee, T. M., Kay, A. R., and Tank, D. W. (1990). Brain magnetic resonance imaging with contrast dependent on blood oxygenation. *Proc. Natl. Acad. Sci. U.S.A.* 87, 9868–9872. doi: 10.1073/pnas.87.24.9868

Pan, W. J., Thompson, G. J., Magnuson, M. E., Jaeger, D., and Keilholz, S. (2013). Infraslow LFP correlates to resting-state fMRI BOLD signals. *Neuroimage* 74, 288–297. doi: 10.1016/j.neuroimage.2013.02.035

Pan, W. J., Thompson, G., Magnuson, M., Majeed, W., Jaeger, D., and Keilholz S. (2010). Simultaneous FMRI and electrophysiology in the rodent brain. *J. Vis. Exp.* 42:1901. doi: 10.3791/1901

Parvaz, M. A., Alia-Klein, N., Woicik, P. A., Volkow, N. D., and Goldstein, R. Z. (2011). Neuroimaging for drug addiction and related behaviors. *Rev. Neurosci.* 22, 609–624. doi: 10.1515/rns.2011.055

Pawela, C. P., Biswal, B. B., Hudetz, A. G., Li, R., Jones, S. R., Cho, Y. R., et al. (2010). Interhemispheric neuroplasticity following limb deafferentation detected by resting-state functional connectivity magnetic resonance imaging (fcMRI) and functional magnetic resonance imaging (fMRI). *Neuroimage* 49, 2467–2478. doi: 10.1016/j.neuroimage.2009.09.054

Peper, J. S., van den Heuvel, M. P., Mandl, R. C., Hulshoff Pol, H. E., and van Honk, J. (2011). Sex steroids and connectivity in the human brain: a review of neuroimaging studies. *Psychoneuroendocrinology* 36, 1101–1113. doi: 10.1016/j.psyneuen.2011.05.004

Pievani, M., Filippini, N., van den Heuvel, M. P., Cappa, S. F., and Frisoni, G. B. (2014). Brain connectivity in neurodegenerative diseases–from phenotype to proteinopathy. *Nat. Rev. Neurol.* 10, 620–633. doi: 10.1038/nrneurol.2014.178

Ratering, D., Baltes, C., Nordmeyer-Massner, J., Marek, D., and Rudin, M. (2008). Performance of a 200-MHz cryogenic RF probe designed for MRI and MRS of the murine brain. *Magn. Reson. Med.* 59, 1440–1447. doi: 10.1002/mrm.21629

Razoux, F., Baltes, C., Mueggler, T., Seuwen, A., Russig, H., Mansuy, I., et al. (2013). Functional MRI to assess alterations of functional networks in response to pharmacological or genetic manipulations of the serotonergic system in mice. *Neuroimage* 74, 326–336. doi: 10.1016/j.neuroimage.2013.02.031

Roebroeck, A., Formisano, E., and Goebel, R. (2005). Mapping directed influence over the brain using Granger causality and fMRI. *Neuroimage* 25, 230–242. doi: 10.1016/j.neuroimage.2004.11.017

Rubinov, M., and Sporns, O. (2010). Complex network measures of brain connectivity: uses and interpretations. *Neuroimage* 52, 1059–1069. doi: 10.1016/j.neuroimage.2009.10.003

Salimi-Khorshidi, G., Douaud, G., Beckmann, C. F., Glasser, M. F., Griffanti, L., and Smith, S. M. (2014). Automatic denoising of functional MRI data: combining independent component analysis and hierarchical fusion of classifiers. *Neuroimage* 90, 449–468. doi: 10.1016/j.neuroimage.2013.11.046

Sanganahalli, B. G., Herman, P., Behar, K. L., Blumenfeld, H., Rothman, D. L., and Hyder, F. (2013). Functional MRI and neural responses in a rat model of Alzheimer's disease. *Neuroimage* 79, 404–411. doi: 10.1016/j.neuroimage.2013.04.099

Sawiak, S. J., Wood, N. I., Williams, G. B., Morton, A. J., and Carpenter, T. A. (2009). Voxel-based morphometry in the R6/2 transgenic mouse reveals differences between genotypes not seen with manual 2D morphometry. *Neurobiol. Dis.* 33, 20–27. doi: 10.1016/j.nbd.2008.09.016

Scheinin, M., Kallio, A., Koulu, M., Viikari, J., and Scheinin, H. (1987). Sedative and cardiovascular effects of medetomidine, a novel selective alpha 2-adrenoceptor agonist, in healthy volunteers. *Br. J. Clin. Pharmacol.* 24, 443–451. doi: 10.1111/j.1365-2125.1987.tb03196.x

Schlegel, F., Schroeter, A., and Rudin, M. (2015). The hemodynamic response to somatosensory stimulation in mice depends on the anesthetic used: implications on analysis of mouse fMRI data. *Neuroimage* 116, 40–49. doi: 10.1016/j.neuroimage.2015.05.013

Schneider, L. S., Mangialasche, F., Andreasen, N., Feldman, H., Giacobini, E., Jones, R., et al. (2014). Clinical trials and late-stage drug development for Alzheimer's disease: an appraisal from 1984 to 2014. *J. Intern. Med.* 275, 251–283. doi: 10.1111/joim.12191

Schroeter, A., Schlegel, F., Seuwen, A., Grandjean, J., and Rudin, M. (2014). Specificity of stimulus-evoked fMRI responses in the mouse: the influence of systemic physiological changes associated with innocuous stimulation under four different anesthetics. *Neuroimage* 94, 372–384. doi: 10.1016/j.neuroimage.2014.01.046

Schwarz, A. J., Gozzi, A., Reese, T., and Bifone, A. (2007a). Functional connectivity in the pharmacologically activated brain: resolving networks of correlated responses to d-amphetamine. *Magn. Reson. Med.* 57, 704–713. doi: 10.1002/mrm.21179

Schwarz, A. J., Gozzi, A., Reese, T., and Bifone, A. (2007b) In vivo mapping of functional connectivity in neurotransmitter systems using pharmacological MRI. *Neuroimage* 34, 1627–1636. doi: 10.1016/j.neuroimage.2006.11.010

Schwarz, A. J., Gozzi, A., Reese, T., Heidbreder, C. A., and Bifone, A. (2007c). Pharmacological modulation of functional connectivity: the correlation structure underlying the phMRI response to d-amphetamine modified by selective dopamine D3 receptor antagonist SB277011A. *Magn. Reson. Imaging* 25, 811–820. doi: 10.1016/j.mri.2007.02.017

Sekar, S., Van Audekerke, J., Vanhoutte, G., Lowe, A. S., Blamire, A. M., Van der Linden, A., et al. (2011a). Neuroanatomical targets of reboxetine and bupropion as revealed by pharmacological magnetic resonance imaging. *Psychopharmacology (Berl.)* 217, 549–557. doi: 10.1007/s00213-011-2311-7

Sekar, S., Verhoye, M., Van Audekerke, J., Vanhoutte, G., Lowe, A. S., Blamire, A. M., et al. (2011b). Neuroadaptive responses to citalopram in rats using pharmacological magnetic resonance imaging. *Psychopharmacology (Berl.)* 213, 521–531. doi: 10.1007/s00213-010-2084-4

Sekar, S., Verhoye, M., Van Audekerke, J., Tahon, K., Wuyts, K., Mackie, M., et al. (2010). Acute and sub-chronic neuronal effects of NMDA receptor antagonist, memantine using pharmacological magnetic resonance imaging. *Proc. Intl. Soc. Mag. Reson. Med.* 18, 2355.

Sforazzini, F., Schwarz, A. J., Galbusera, A., Bifone, A., and Gozzi, A. (2014). Distributed BOLD and CBV-weighted resting-state networks in the mouse brain. *Neuroimage* 87, 403–415. doi: 10.1016/j.neuroimage.2013.09.050

Shah, D., Blockx, I., Guns, P. J., De Deyn, P. P., Van Dam, D., Jonckers, E., et al. (2015a). Acute modulation of the cholinergic system in the mouse brain detected by pharmacological resting-state functional MRI. *Neuroimage* 109, 151–159. doi: 10.1016/j.neuroimage.2015.01.009

Shah, D., Blockx, I., Keliris, G. A., Kara, F., Jonckers, E., Verhoye, M., et al. (2015b). Cholinergic and serotonergic modulations differentially affect large-scale functional networks in the mouse brain. *Brain Struct. Funct.* doi: 10.1007/s00429-015-1087-7 [Epub ahead of print].

Shah, D., Jonckers, E., Praet, J., Vanhoutte, G., Delgado, Y. P. R., Bigot, C., et al. (2013). Resting state FMRI reveals diminished functional connectivity in a mouse model of amyloidosis. *PLoS ONE* 8:e84241. doi: 10.1371/journal.pone.0084241

Shih, Y. Y., Huang, S., Chen, Y. Y., Lai, H. Y., Kao, Y. C., Du, F., et al. (2014). Imaging neurovascular function and functional recovery after stroke in the rat striatum using forepaw stimulation. *J. Cereb. Blood Flow Metab.* 34, 1483–1492. doi: 10.1038/jcbfm.2014.103

Sierakowiak, A., Monnot, C., Aski, S. N., Uppman, M., Li, T. Q., Damberg, P., et al. (2015). Default mode network, motor network, dorsal and ventral basal ganglia networks in the rat brain: comparison to human networks using resting state-fMRI. *PLoS ONE* 10:e0120345. doi: 10.1371/journal.pone.0120345

Silverman, J., and Muir, W. W. III. (1993). A review of laboratory animal anesthesia with chloral hydrate and chloralose. *Lab. Anim. Sci.* 43, 210–216.

Sloan, H. L., Austin, V. C., Blamire, A. M., Schnupp, J. W., Lowe, A. S., Allers, K. A., et al. (2010). Regional differences in neurovascular coupling in rat brain as determined by fMRI and electrophysiology. *Neuroimage* 53, 399–411. doi: 10.1016/j.neuroimage.2010.07.014

Smirnakis, S. M., Schmid, M. C., Weber, B., Tolias, A. S., Augath, M., and Logothetis, N. K. (2007). Spatial specificity of BOLD versus cerebral blood volume fMRI for mapping cortical organization. *J. Cereb. Blood Flow Metab.* 27, 1248–1261. doi: 10.1038/sj.jcbfm.9600434

Song, T., Nie, B., Ma, E., Che, J., Sun, S., Wang, Y., et al. (2015). Functional magnetic resonance imaging reveals abnormal brain connectivity in EGR3 gene transfected rat model of schizophrenia. *Biochem. Biophys. Res. Commun.* 460, 678–683. doi: 10.1016/j.bbrc.2015.03.089

Squillace, M., Dodero, L., Federici, M., Migliarini, S., Errico, F., Napolitano, F., et al. (2014). Dysfunctional dopaminergic neurotransmission in asocial BTBR mice. *Transl. Psychiatry* 4:e427. doi: 10.1038/tp.2014.69

Stephenson, J. B. T., Li, R., Yan, J. G., Hyde, J., and Matloub, H. (2013). Transhemispheric cortical plasticity following contralateral C7 nerve transfer:

a rat functional magnetic resonance imaging survival study. *J. Hand. Surg. Am.* 38, 478–487. doi: 10.1016/j.jhsa.2012.12.018

Suarez, S. V., Amadon, A., Giacomini, E., Wiklund, A., Changeux, J. P., Le Bihan, D., et al. (2009). Brain activation by short-term nicotine exposure in anesthetized wild-type and beta2-nicotinic receptors knockout mice: a BOLD fMRI study. *Psychopharmacology (Berl.)* 202, 599–610. doi: 10.1007/s00213-008-1338-x

Sumiyoshi, A., Suzuki, H., Shimokawa, H., and Kawashima, R. (2012). Neurovascular uncoupling under mild hypoxic hypoxia: an EEG-fMRI study in rats. *J. Cereb. Blood Flow Metab.* 32, 1853–1858. doi: 10.1038/jcbfm.2012.111

Suzuki, J., Sasaki, M., Harada, K., Bando, M., Kataoka, Y., Onodera, R., et al. (2013). Bilateral cortical hyperactivity detected by fMRI associates with improved motor function following intravenous infusion of mesenchymal stem cells in a rat stroke model. *Brain Res.* 1497, 15–22. doi: 10.1016/j.brainres.2012.12.028

Tamminga, C. A. (2006). The neurobiology of cognition in schizophrenia. *J. Clin. Psychiatry* 67(Suppl. 9), 9–13; discussion 36–42. doi: 10.4088/jcp.0906e11

Tu, Y., Yu, T., Fu, X. Y., Xie, P., Lu, S., Huang, X. Q., et al. (2011). Altered thalamocortical functional connectivity by propofol anesthesia in rats. *Pharmacology* 88, 322–326. doi: 10.1159/000334168

Upadhyay, J., Baker, S. J., Chandran, P., Miller, L., Lee, Y., Marek, G. J., et al. (2011). Default-mode-like network activation in awake rodents. *PLoS ONE* 6:e27839. doi: 10.1371/journal.pone.0027839

Van Camp, N., Peeters, R. R., and Van der Linden, A. (2005). A comparison between blood oxygenation level-dependent and cerebral blood volume contrast in the rat cerebral and cerebellar somatosensoric cortex during electrical paw stimulation. *J. Magn. Reson. Imaging* 22, 483–491. doi: 10.1002/jmri.20417

Van Der Linden, A., van Camp, N., Ramos-Cabrer, P., and Hoehn, M. (2007). Current status of functional MRI on small animals: application to physiology, pathophysiology, and cognition. *NMR Biomed.* 20, 522–545. doi: 10.1002/nbm.1131

Vanhoutte, G., Verhoye, M., and Van der Linden, A. (2006). Changing body temperature affects the T2* signal in the rat brain and reveals hypothalamic activity. *Magn. Reson. Med.* 55, 1006–1012. doi: 10.1002/mrm.20861

van Meer, M. P., Otte, W. M., van der Marel, K., Nijboer, C. H., Kavelaars, A., van der Sprenkel, J. W., et al. (2012). Extent of bilateral neuronal network reorganization and functional recovery in relation to stroke severity. *J. Neurosci.* 32, 4495–4507. doi: 10.1523/JNEUROSCI.3662-11.2012

van Meer, M. P. M., van der Marel, K. M., Otte, W. M., van der Sprenkel, J. W. B., and Dijkhuizen, R. M. (2010a). Correspondence between altered functional and structural connectivity in the contralesional sensorimotor cortex after unilateral stroke in rats: a combined resting-state functional MRI and manganese-enhanced MRI study. *J. Cereb. Blood Flow Metab.* 30, 1707–1711. doi: 10.1038/jcbfm.2010.124

van Meer, M. P., van der Marel, K., Wang, K., Otte, W. M., El Bouazati, S., Roeling, T. A., et al. (2010b). Recovery of sensorimotor function after experimental stroke correlates with restoration of resting-state interhemispheric functional connectivity. *J. Neurosci.* 30, 3964–3972. doi: 10.1523/JNEUROSCI.5709-09.2010

Veldsman, M., Cumming, T., and Brodtmann, A. (2015). Beyond BOLD: optimizing functional imaging in stroke populations. *Hum. Brain Mapp.* 36, 1620–1636. doi: 10.1002/hbm.22711

Vuong, J., Henderson, A. K., Tuor, U. I., Dunn, J. F., and Teskey, G. C. (2011). Persistent enhancement of functional MRI responsiveness to sensory stimulation following repeated seizures. *Epilepsia* 52, 2285–2292. doi: 10.1111/j.1528-1167.2011.03317.x

Wang, D. J., Chen, Y., Fernandez-Seara, M. A., and Detre, J. A. (2011). Potentials and challenges for arterial spin labeling in pharmacological magnetic resonance imaging. *J. Pharmacol. Exp. Ther.* 337, 359–366. doi: 10.1124/jpet.110.172577

Wang, Z., Guo, Y., Myers, K. G., Heintz, R., Peng, Y. H., Maarek, J. M., et al. (2015). Exercise alters resting-state functional connectivity of motor circuits in parkinsonian rats. *Neurobiol. Aging* 36, 536–544. doi: 10.1016/j.neurobiolaging.2014.08.016

Wang, Z., Tsai, L. K., Munasinghe, J., Leng, Y., Fessler, E. B., Chibane, F., et al. (2012). Chronic valproate treatment enhances postischemic angiogenesis and promotes functional recovery in a rat model of ischemic stroke. *Stroke* 43, 2430–2436. doi: 10.1161/STROKEAHA.112.652545

Wehrl, H. F., Hossain, M., Lankes, K., Liu, C. C., Bezrukov, I., Martirosian, P., et al. (2013). Simultaneous PET-MRI reveals brain function in activated and resting state on metabolic, hemodynamic and multiple temporal scales. *Nat. Med.* 19, 1184–1189. doi: 10.1038/nm.3290

Wehrl, H. F., Martirosian, P., Schick, F., Reischl, G., and Pichler, B. J. (2014). Assessment of rodent brain activity using combined [(15)O]H2O-PET and BOLD-fMRI. *Neuroimage* 89, 271–279. doi: 10.1016/j.neuroimage.2013.11.044

Weis, S., Hausmann, M., Stoffers, B., and Sturm, W. (2011). Dynamic changes in functional cerebral connectivity of spatial cognition during the menstrual cycle. *Hum. Brain Mapp.* 32, 1544–1556. doi: 10.1002/hbm.21126

Williams, D. S., Detre, J. A., Leigh, J. S., and Koretsky, A. P. (1992). Magnetic resonance imaging of perfusion using spin inversion of arterial water. *Proc. Natl. Acad. Sci. U.S.A.* 89, 212–216. doi: 10.1073/pnas.89.1.212

Williams, K. A., Magnuson, M., Majeed, W., Laconte, S. M., Peltier, S. J., Hu, X., et al. (2010). Comparison of alpha-chloralose, medetomidine and isoflurane anesthesia for functional connectivity mapping in the rat. *Magn. Reson. Imaging* 28, 995–1003. doi: 10.1016/j.mri.2010.03.007

Williams, K. A., Mehta, N. S., Redei, E. E., Wang, L., and Procissi, D. (2014). Aberrant resting-state functional connectivity in a genetic rat model of depression. *Psychiatry Res.* 222, 111–113. doi: 10.1016/j.pscychresns.2014.02.001

Wu, C. W., Gu, H., Lu, H., Stein, E. A., Chen, J. H., and Yang, Y. (2008). Frequency specificity of functional connectivity in brain networks. *Neuroimage* 42, 1047–1055. doi: 10.1016/j.neuroimage.2008.05.035

Yao, Q. L., Zhang, H. Y., Nie, B. B., Fang, F., Jiao, Y., and Teng, G. J. (2012). MRI assessment of amplitude of low-frequency fluctuation in rat brains with acute cerebral ischemic stroke. *Neurosci. Lett.* 509, 22–26. doi: 10.1016/j.neulet.2011.12.036

Younce, J. R., Albaugh, D. L., and Shih, Y. Y. (2014). Deep brain stimulation with simultaneous FMRI in rodents. *J. Vis. Exp.* 84:e51271. doi: 10.3791/51271

Zerbi, V., Wiesmann, M., Emmerzaal, T. L., Jansen, D., Van Beek, M., Mutsaers, M. P., et al. (2014). Resting-state functional connectivity changes in aging apoE4 and apoE-KO mice. *J. Neurosci.* 34, 13963–13975. doi: 10.1523/JNEUROSCI.0684-14.2014

Zhang, F., Eckman, C., Younkin, S., Hsiao, K. K., and Iadecola, C. (1997). Increased susceptibility to ischemic brain damage in transgenic mice overexpressing the amyloid precursor protein. *J. Neurosci.* 17, 7655–7661.

Zhang, N., Rane, P., Huang, W., Liang, Z., Kennedy, D., Frazier, J. A., et al. (2010). Mapping resting-state brain networks in conscious animals. *J. Neurosci. Methods* 189, 186–196. doi: 10.1016/j.jneumeth.2010.04.001

Conflict of Interest Statement: The authors declare that the research was conducted in the absence of any commercial or financial relationships that could be construed as a potential conflict of interest.

11

In vivo Small Animal Micro-CT using Nanoparticle Contrast Agents

Jeffrey R. Ashton[1,2], Jennifer L. West[1] and Cristian T. Badea[2]*

[1] *Department of Biomedical Engineering, Duke University, Durham, NC, USA,* [2] *Department of Radiology, Center for In Vivo Microscopy, Duke University Medical Center, Durham, NC, USA*

Computed tomography (CT) is one of the most valuable modalities for *in vivo* imaging because it is fast, high-resolution, cost-effective, and non-invasive. Moreover, CT is heavily used not only in the clinic (for both diagnostics and treatment planning) but also in preclinical research as micro-CT. Although CT is inherently effective for lung and bone imaging, soft tissue imaging requires the use of contrast agents. For small animal micro-CT, nanoparticle contrast agents are used in order to avoid rapid renal clearance. A variety of nanoparticles have been used for micro-CT imaging, but the majority of research has focused on the use of iodine-containing nanoparticles and gold nanoparticles. Both nanoparticle types can act as highly effective blood pool contrast agents or can be targeted using a wide variety of targeting mechanisms. CT imaging can be further enhanced by adding spectral capabilities to separate multiple co-injected nanoparticles *in vivo*. Spectral CT, using both energy-integrating and energy-resolving detectors, has been used with multiple contrast agents to enable functional and molecular imaging. This review focuses on new developments for *in vivo* small animal micro-CT using novel nanoparticle probes applied in preclinical research.

Keywords: micro-CT, small animal imaging, nanoparticles, contrast agents, spectral imaging

Edited by:
*Nicolau Beckmann,
Novartis Institutes for BioMedical
Research, Switzerland*

Reviewed by:
*David Cormode,
University of Pennsylvania, USA
Detlef Stiller,
Boehringer Ingelheim
Pharmaceuticals, Germany*

***Correspondence:**
*Cristian T. Badea
cristian.badea@duke.edu*

INTRODUCTION

X-ray computed tomography (CT) is one of the most powerful and widely used imaging modalities in modern clinical practice. CT provides non-invasive three-dimensional imaging capabilities at lower cost and higher spatial and temporal resolution than other imaging modalities such as MRI and PET (Kircher and Willmann, 2012). CT imaging can reveal a patient's anatomy in exquisite detail and is extremely useful in the diagnosis of a wide variety of diseases. CT systems with high resolution (also known as micro-CT systems) have been developed over the last few decades and have been used with great success in small animal studies. With micro-CT, animals can be non-invasively imaged *in vivo* multiple times over the course of a preclinical study, which significantly decreases the number of animals required compared to methods requiring *ex vivo* analysis. Additionally, the continued development of micro-CT can help to test and optimize imaging advances for translation to clinical CT. This review provides an overview of micro-CT imaging principles and applications of micro-CT in preclinical small animal studies, with a special emphasis on the use of nanoparticle contrast agents and spectral imaging methods that could serve well in drug discovery and pharmacological research.

MICRO-CT IMAGING PRINCIPLES

Imaging System

A CT system consists of an x-ray source and x-ray detectors, between which the subject is placed. In clinical CT, the x-ray source and detectors rotate around the subject to produce projections of x-ray attenuation through the body at many different angles. For micro-CT, the x-ray source and detectors may also be static, while the small animal is rotated between them. The x-ray projections acquired at each angle of rotation are then used to reconstruct tomographic images, which are visualized as 2D slices or 3D volumes of the specimen. The most common reconstruction method for micro-CT is a cone-beam implementation of filtered back projection (Feldkamp et al., 1984). A schematic of a micro-CT system and reconstruction process is shown in **Figure** .

X-ray Generation

X-rays are generated by accelerating electrons across a high voltage to collide with an anode composed of a high atomic number, high melting point material (commonly tungsten). Interactions between the electrons and the tungsten anode lead to the production of x-rays with a broad energy spectrum. The maximum energy of the x-ray spectrum is determined by the voltage applied in the x-ray tube. As tube voltage increases, the mean x-ray energy and number of photons produced both increase. This is demonstrated in **Figure** for a tungsten anode operating at two different voltages: 80 and 140 kV. The energy of the produced x-rays is an important determinant of their absorption by a given material. This energy spectrum can be modified by filtration through metal filters. Filtration is primarily used to increase the mean energy of the x-ray spectrum by removing low energy photons. Filtration can be used to both reduce radiation dose and improve image quality, and filtration can be optimized depending on the imaging task (Hupfer et al., 2012). Micro-CT x-ray tubes differ from clinical x-ray tubes in that they usually have a much smaller focal spot (area where the electron beam interacts with the anode), which reduces the source function blur (i.e., penumbra blurring) and thereby greatly improves the maximum image resolution. This increased resolution is necessary for imaging small animals which have much smaller features than humans.

X-ray Attenuation

X-rays travel from the focal point of the x-ray tube, through the subject, and on to the x-ray detector. The x-ray detector measures the relative amount of x-rays absorbed by the subject at any given position. X-ray attenuation is given by

$$I = I_0\, e^{-\mu x}$$

where I is the intensity of the x-rays transmitted through the subject, I_0 is the original intensity of the x-rays incident on the object, μ is the linear attenuation coefficient of the object, and x is the thickness of the object. Therefore, absorption of x-rays by a material is dependent on the thickness of the material and on the material-dependent attenuation coefficient. Diagnostic x-rays can be absorbed by a material via two primary mechanisms: compton scattering and the photoelectric effect.

Compton scattering occurs when an x-ray photon collides with an outer shell electron within the subject. Upon collision, the electron absorbs a portion of the x-ray energy and is ejected from the atom. The x-ray photon is deflected from its original direction and loses some energy. This scattering can occur in all directions and can lead to noise at the detector. The amount of Compton scattering that occurs within an object depends primarily on the energy of the incident x-ray photon and the density of the object. Compton scattering decreases slightly with increasing photon energy, so higher energy x-rays are better able to pass through a patient without attenuation. The density of outer shell electrons increases with the mass density of a material, so denser materials tend to have more Compton scattering and therefore more x-ray attenuation.

The photoelectric effect occurs when an x-ray photon transfers all of its energy to an inner shell electron within the subject. This electron is ejected from the atom and its vacancy is subsequently filled by an outer-shell electron, which leads to the release of a secondary photon. The photoelectric effect is highly dependent on both the energy of the incident x-ray and the atomic weight of the object. The photoelectric effect is strongest when the x-ray energy matches the binding energy of the inner-shell electrons. As x-ray energy increases, the likelihood of the photoelectric effect drops rapidly, proportional to the inverse cube of the x-ray energy ($1/E^3$). If the x-ray energy is below the energy of a particular electron shell, then none of those electrons can participate in the photoelectric effect because the x-ray does not have enough energy to overcome the electron binding energy. This leads to the K-edge effect, where the probability of absorption due to the photoelectric effect jumps abruptly as the x-ray energy increases above the K-shell electron binding energy. The photoelectric effect is also proportional to the cube of a material's atomic number (Z^3), so high atomic weight materials exhibit a much stronger photoelectric effect than low atomic weight materials. This is why contrast agents for CT traditionally include high atomic weight elements (e.g., iodine, barium). The K-edge effect is shown in **Figure** , which demonstrates the relative probability of x-ray photon attenuation at different x-ray energies for several high Z materials such as iodine, gold, barium, gadolinium, bismuth.

APPLICATIONS OF NON-CONTRAST-ENHANCED MICRO-CT

Micro-CT images only demonstrate high contrast when there are large differences between material densities (Compton scattering) or atomic weights (photoelectric effect) within the patient. In the case of soft tissue imaging, there is very little natural contrast so an exogenous high atomic weight contrast agent must be administered for effective imaging (Yu and Watson, 1999). However, non-contrast-enhanced micro-CT performs well for bone and lung imaging, both of which have high inherent contrast in the absence of exogenous contrast agents.

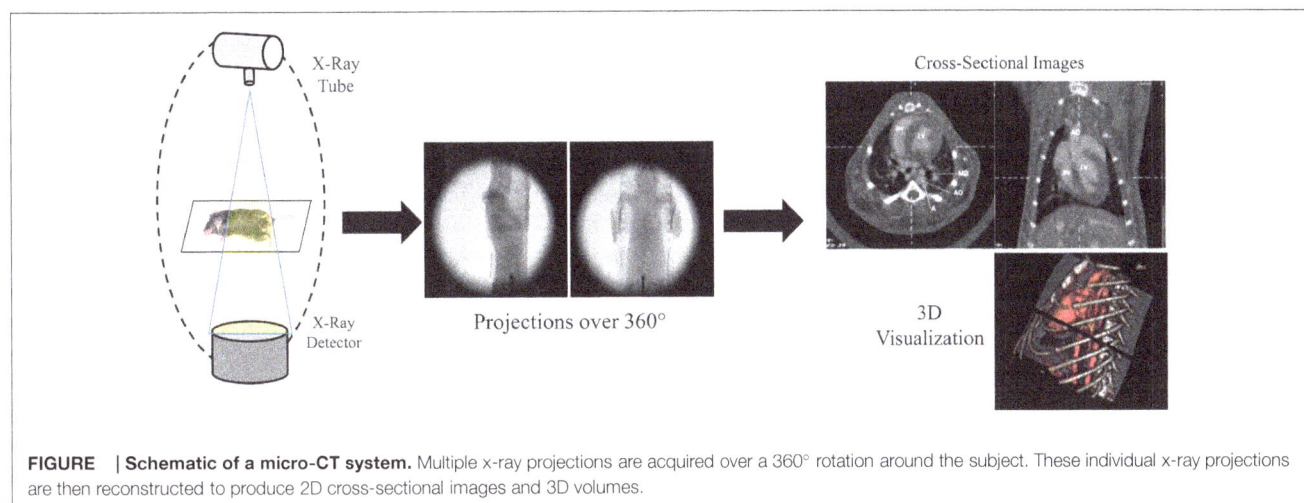

FIGURE | **Schematic of a micro-CT system.** Multiple x-ray projections are acquired over a 360° rotation around the subject. These individual x-ray projections are then reconstructed to produce 2D cross-sectional images and 3D volumes.

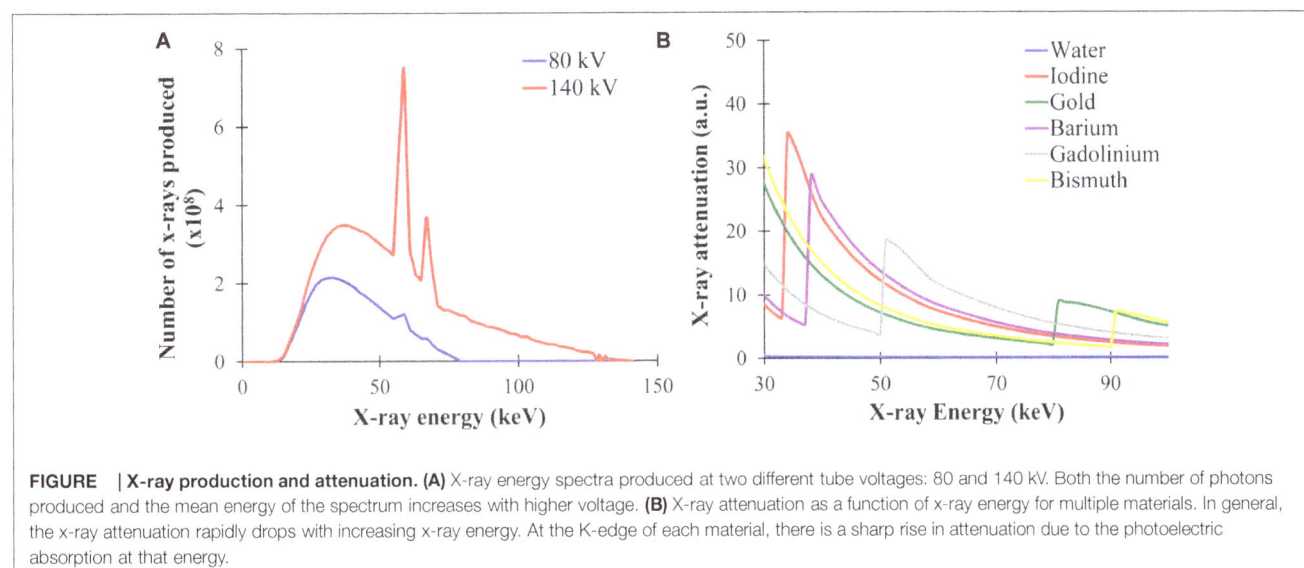

FIGURE | **X-ray production and attenuation. (A)** X-ray energy spectra produced at two different tube voltages: 80 and 140 kV. Both the number of photons produced and the mean energy of the spectrum increases with higher voltage. **(B)** X-ray attenuation as a function of x-ray energy for multiple materials. In general, the x-ray attenuation rapidly drops with increasing x-ray energy. At the K-edge of each material, there is a sharp rise in attenuation due to the photoelectric absorption at that energy.

Bone Imaging

Micro-CT is well-suited for bone imaging because of the natural contrast between bone and soft tissues, which is due to the high effective atomic weight of bone. This makes micro-CT extremely valuable for non-invasive, high-resolution bone imaging without the need of an exogenous contrast agent. Bone imaging was one of the very first common applications of micro-CT for small animal imaging (Feldkamp et al., 1989; Kinney et al., 1995). Micro-CT can accurately quantify a variety of bone parameters, including cross-sectional area, cortical thickness, bone mineral density, bone volume, bone surface ratio, and trabecular thickness (Bouxsein et al., 2010). Structural micro-CT studies have examined bone architecture (Waarsing et al., 2005; Hsu et al., 2014), bone remodeling (David et al., 2003; Cowan et al., 2007), and osteoarthritis (Appleton et al., 2007; McErlain et al., 2008). Micro-CT has also been used to monitor bone healing after treatment with basic fibroblast growth factor (Yao et al., 2005), vascular endothelial growth factor gene therapy (Li et al., 2009), or stem cell therapy (Lee et al., 2009). Micro-CT can also

be used to longitudinally track bone loss and structural changes following radiation therapy and bone marrow transplantation (Dumas et al., 2009) or after spinal cord injury (Jiang et al., 2006). In the case of osteoporosis, micro-CT measurements have been used to study disease progression after ovariectomy (Laib et al., 2001) or immobilization (Laib et al., 2000). Micro-CT has also been used to study early bone development and growth (Guldberg et al., 2004). Additionally, micro-CT has been used extensively in studies of bone regeneration (Umoh et al., 2009) and bone tissue engineering (Lin et al., 2005; Ho and Hutmacher, 2006). In these cases, micro-CT can quantify mineral content, porosity, and connectivity, as well as accurately determine three-dimensional structures. **Figure** illustrates the use of micro-CT to evaluate healing of a tibial bone defect after treatment with an osteoinductive gel scaffold (Sagar et al., 2013). This study shows the ability of micro-CT to produce both 2D cross-sectional bone images as well 3D reconstructions of entire bones. Within the 3D reconstructions, bone microarchitecture is clearly visualized.

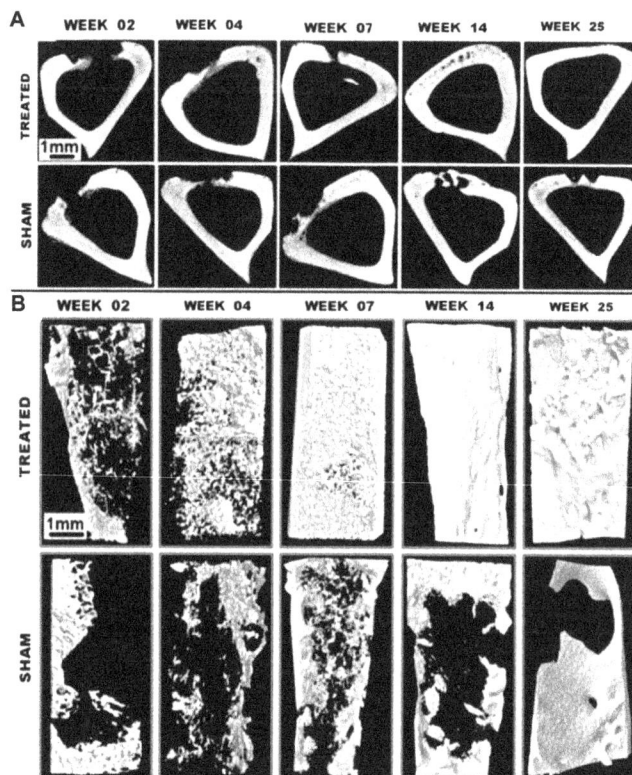

FIGURE | Tibial bone defect micro-CT imaging. (A) Axial micro-CT cross-sections and **(B)** 3D reconstructions of tibial bone defects after treatment with an osteoinductive gel scaffold. Longitudinal imaging was performed up to 25 weeks. Addition of the treatment gel significantly improves healing of the bone defect.

Lung Imaging

The large difference in density between air-filled lungs and soft tissues creates high contrast for lung imaging, which makes CT an extremely useful modality for studying the lung. The primary difficulty in imaging the lungs is respiratory motion. Small animal respiratory rates are 3–4 times the average human respiratory rate, so completing an entire scan between breaths is not practical. Instead, various gating strategies are used which allow researchers to acquire each projection at the same stage in the respiratory cycle, so that there is only minimal motion from one projection to the next. One of the most effective methods of respiratory gating is to intubate the animal and control the respiration by mechanical ventilation (Hedlund and Johnson, 2002; Namati et al., 2006). This allows projections to be acquired at exactly the same point in each respiratory cycle. For a less invasive approach, the respirations of a freely breathing animal can be monitored using a pressure transducer. The x-ray projections can then be acquired automatically at the same point in the measured respiratory cycle (Badea et al., 2004). This method does not perfectly eliminate respiratory motion, but it is much less invasive than mechanical ventilation and can still resolve features down to ~150 microns (Namati et al., 2006). Retrospective gating is also possible, in which many projections are acquired rapidly and sorted post-acquisition according to phase of the respiratory cycle. Subsequently, these sorted projections are used for the reconstruction of tomographic images corresponding to each phase of the respiratory cycle (Ford et al., 2007).

Micro-CT with respiratory gating has been used to study a wide variety of lung diseases. Micro-CT can be used to longitudinally monitor mice for the presence of lung metastases (Li et al., 2006) as well as follow the growth of lung tumors (Hori et al., 2008; Namati et al., 2010; Li et al., 2013a; Rudyanto et al., 2013). The treatment efficacy of chemotherapy (Ueno et al., 2012) or radiation therapy (Perez et al., 2009, 2013; Kirsch et al., 2010) on lung tumors can be measured using micro-CT, and lung injury resulting from radiation therapy can also be assessed (Saito and Murase, 2012). In addition to tumor characterization, micro-CT is also useful for imaging diseases of the lung parenchyma. Mouse models of emphysema created by intra-tracheal instillation of elastase (Postnov et al., 2005; Artaechevarria et al., 2011; De Langhe et al., 2012; Munoz-Barrutia et al., 2012) or exposure to cigar smoke (Sasaki et al., 2015) have been developed and characterized by micro-CT. In emphysema, CT values decrease compared to normal lung due to the loss of soft tissue parenchyma and increased air-trapping. A mouse model of bleomycin-induced lung fibrosis has also been studied extensively by micro-CT (Shofer et al., 2007, 2008; De Langhe et al., 2012) and this model has been used with micro-CT for the preclinical evaluation of drug efficacy (Scotton et al., 2013; Choi et al., 2014; Zhou et al., 2015). In fibrosis, CT values increase due to an expansion of the parenchyma tissue. Lung compliance and lung volume, which are important factors in both emphysema and fibrosis, can also be measured by micro-CT. Animals are mechanically ventilated at multiple pressures and the lung volume at each pressure is measured. The resulting lung pressure-volume curve can be used to calculate lung compliance (Guerrero et al., 2006; Shofer et al., 2007). **Figure** shows an example of automatic quantification of lung air volumes using micro-CT in normal mice and in mice with bleomycin-induced fibrosis (De Langhe et al., 2012). Micro-CT has also been used to detect chronic silicosis (Artaechevarria et al., 2010) and acute respiratory distress syndrome (Voelker et al., 2014).

MICRO-CT CONTRAST AGENTS

Because of the lack of inherent contrast for soft tissue imaging, the majority of CT scans make use of high atomic weight contrast agents. In current clinical practice, iodine is the most commonly used element for intravascular CT contrast. Iodine contrast agents are made up of water-soluble aromatic iodinated compounds. These compounds provide effective contrast due to their high atomic number, which produces a strong photoelectric effect. Because CT is relatively insensitive to contrast, high concentrations of contrast agent (up to 400 mg iodine/mL) must be injected in order to produce adequate image enhancement. Clinical CT contrast agents are generally safe, but severe adverse reactions sometimes occur. These adverse reactions are generally divided into two types: allergic reactions and contrast-induced nephropathy (CIN). CIN occurs due to the high osmolality and viscosity of clinical contrast agents and is more common in patients with chronic renal disease (Namasivayam et al., 2006; Tepel et al., 2006; Wang et al., 2007). Iodinated contrast agents are rapidly cleared from the bloodstream by the kidneys (Bourin et al., 1997), so there is only a very short window for imaging after injection. Additionally, these agents quickly distribute from

the intravascular to the extravascular space throughout the body. Initially, this provides useful contrast, but after a short time this nonspecific uptake leads to uniform enhancement throughout most of the body. Development and optimization of these small molecule contrast agents continues in order to address some of these limitations, but no breakthroughs have occurred in clinical contrast agents for many years (Lusic and Grinstaff, 2013). This lack of progress is primarily due to the significant hurdle of developing high atomic weight agents that simultaneously demonstrate low toxicity, high efficacy, and low cost.

For small animal imaging, the use of clinical contrast agents is particularly difficult. Small animals have much higher renal clearance rates than humans, so injected contrast agents are rapidly excreted. This can be illustrated for the case of a mouse. In the average adult mouse, blood volume is approximately 1.5–2.0 mL (Diehl et al., 2001), and the glomerular filtration rate (the volume of plasma filtered by the kidneys per time) is approximately 0.4 mL/s (Cervenka et al., 1999). Therefore, the whole mouse blood volume is filtered by the kidneys in less than 5 s. Consistent with this filtration rate, it has been shown that clinical iodine contrast agents drop to undetectable levels in the bloodstream within 4 s of injection in a mouse (Lin et al., 2009). This rapid clearance of contrast agent severely limits the useful application of clinical contrast agents in small animals.

To overcome the rapid clearance of traditional contrast agents, blood pool contrast agents have been developed which exhibit prolonged blood residence time and stable enhancement for minutes to hours. Blood pool agents are made up of a wide variety of high molecular weight compounds or nanoparticles that avoid renal clearance due to their large size. Iodine-based blood pool agents include iodine-containing polymers (Galperin et al., 2007; Aviv et al., 2009), micelles (Trubetskoy et al., 1997; Torchilin et al., 1999), emulsions (de Vries et al., 2010; Hallouard et al., 2013; Li et al., 2013b), and liposomes (Krause et al., 1993; Petersein et al., 1999; Mukundan et al., 2006; Ghaghada et al.,

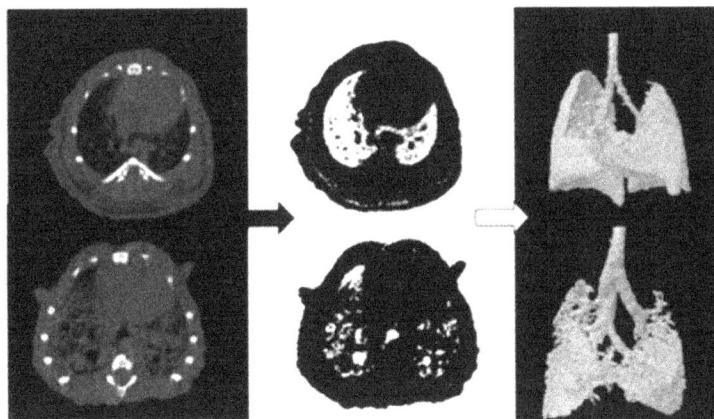

FIGURE | **Automated analysis of lung air volumes for a normal mouse and a mouse with lung fibrosis.** CT cross-sections of the lungs are thresholded to include only those voxels which primarily contain air. These binary images are then converted to 3D volumes to visualize and quantify the aerated lung volumes. The fibrotic lung has significantly reduced air volume compared to the normal lung.

2011). A schematic demonstrating the configuration of several iodine-containing nanoparticle agents is shown in **Figure** . Historically, these iodine nanoparticles have been the most used contrast agents for micro-CT imaging. The development and use of these iodine-containing blood pool contrast agents have been reviewed elsewhere (Hallouard et al., 2010; Annapragada et al., 2012; Cormode et al., 2014; Li et al., 2014). Some iodine-containing blood pool agents are commercially available for small animal research, including *Fenestra®* (MediLumine, Montreal, QC, Canada) and *Exia*^{TM} (Binitio Biomedical, Inc., Ottawa, ON, Canada), and *Exitron*^{TM} *P* (Miltenyi Biotec, San Diego, CA, USA).

Over the past several years, metal nanoparticle contrast agents have been developed incorporating a wide variety of elements. The most commonly used metal nanoparticles for micro-CT consist of gold. Gold nanoparticles produce greater CT enhancement than iodinated contrast agents because of the high atomic number of gold ($Z = 79$) compared to iodine ($Z = 53$). Gold nanoparticles are particularly promising for *in vivo* imaging applications because gold is extremely inert and gold nanoparticles can be readily modified with surface-linked molecules to render them biocompatible (Li et al., 2012). Bismuth is another promising element for use as contrast agent because it is plentiful, inexpensive, and has a high atomic number ($Z = 83$). Multiple formulations of bismuth nanoparticles have been proposed for use as CT contrast agents (Rabin et al., 2006; Ai et al., 2011; Perera et al., 2011; Swy et al., 2014). Nanoparticles for micro-CT have also been developed using other metals, including bismuth, barium, tantalum, silver, gadolinium, ytterbium, and thorium (Jakhmola et al., 2012). Some metal nanoparticle contrast agents are commercially available, including the gold nanoparticle agent AuroVist^{TM} (Nanoprobes, Inc., Yaphank, NY, USA)

and the barium nanoparticle agent *Exitron*^{TM} *Nano* (Miltenyi Biotec).

Surface conjugation is important for nanoparticle contrast agents, because bare nanoparticles adsorb serum proteins and are readily recognized and cleared by the immune system. A variety of molecules can be added to the nanoparticle surface to decrease nanoparticle clearance, but the most common modification strategy is the addition of polyethylene glycol (PEG; Jokerst et al., 2011). Surface PEGylation significantly increases nanoparticles' blood residence time, which allows them to be used as blood pool contrast agents. Nanoparticles' blood residence time and biodistribution are also heavily influenced by their size and shape, with smaller nanoparticles tending to have longer blood residence times.

APPLICATIONS OF CONTRAST-ENHANCED MICRO-CT

The development of nanoparticle contrast agents has opened the door for many exciting applications in small animal imaging. While imaging applications using low molecular weight contrast agents have been limited, blood pool contrast agents have now been used for a wide range of imaging applications. Important modern applications for contrast-enhanced micro-CT in small animals include imaging of the vasculature, heart, abdomen and tumors. Current micro-CT contrast agent research is now focused on developing agents with active targeting, multi-modal, or theranostic capabilities.

Vascular Imaging

Vascular imaging for micro-CT is done primarily using blood pool contrast agents. Micro-CT scan times must be longer

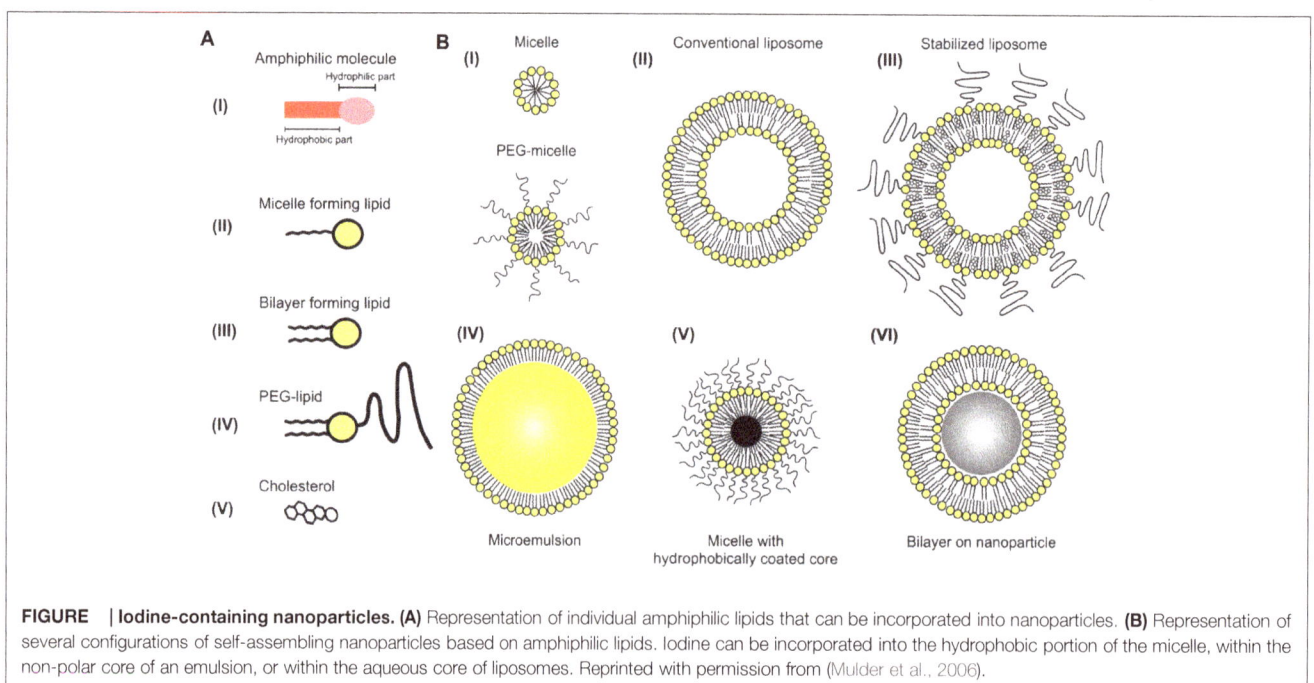

FIGURE | **Iodine-containing nanoparticles. (A)** Representation of individual amphiphilic lipids that can be incorporated into nanoparticles. **(B)** Representation of several configurations of self-assembling nanoparticles based on amphiphilic lipids. Iodine can be incorporated into the hydrophobic portion of the micelle, within the non-polar core of an emulsion, or within the aqueous core of liposomes. Reprinted with permission from (Mulder et al., 2006).

than clinical CT scan times due to the requirement for much higher resolution. Higher resolution implies a need for more x-ray flux, which is achieved with a longer integration time per projection. Early micro-CT scanners required up to an hour to complete a scan. In these cases, low molecular weight contrast agents could not be used for vascular imaging, as they would be cleared from the bloodstream long before the image acquisition was completed. For current micro-CT scanners, scan times of under a minute are now possible. Using these fast protocols, low molecular weight contrast agents have been successfully used for vascular imaging (Kiessling et al., 2004; Badea et al., 2006; Schambach et al., 2010). However, these contrast agents must be either repeatedly or continuously administered over the course of a scan to achieve a constant level of vascular enhancement. This increases the difficulty of imaging and may significantly increase the injected dose of contrast agent. As an alternative to low molecular weight contrast agents, blood pool contrast agents have been successfully used for a variety of vascular applications, including measurements of vascular morphology, diameter, and branching (Vandeghinste et al., 2011), imaging pulmonary vasculature (Johnson, 2007), imaging hepatic vasculature (Chouker et al., 2008), imaging tumor vasculature (Badea et al., 2006; Graham et al., 2008), and measuring vascular permeability (Langheinrich and Ritman, 2006). By providing a constant level of enhancement within the vasculature over a prolonged period of time (minutes to hours), these contrast agents simplify the acquisition of vascular images using micro-CT and allow for a wider range of imaging protocols to be used. **Figure** shows an example of vascular imaging. In this study, micro-CT was used with a liposomal iodine contrast agent in order to study the vasculature associated with primary soft tissue sarcomas of the hindlimb (Moding et al., 2013).

Cardiac Imaging

Cardiac imaging is challenging in small animals due to their rapid heart rate ($\sim$600 bpm for mice). Like respiratory gating (see Lung Imaging), cardiac gating can be used to minimize artifacts due to cardiac motion in the resulting CT images. Cardiac gating can be performed either prospectively (Badea et al., 2005, 2008a, 2011b; Ford et al., 2005; Guo et al., 2011) or retrospectively (Bartling et al., 2007; Song et al., 2007; Badea et al., 2008a, 2011c; Ashton et al., 2014a). In both cases, the ECG of the animal is continuously monitored. In prospective gating, each projection is triggered at a pre-defined point of the cardiac cycle, so that the heart is in the same position in each of the projections. In retrospective gating, projections are acquired rapidly over several rotations and then the timing of the images is compared to the ECG tracing. Each of the images is sorted into projections belonging to different points in the cardiac cycle. Each set of projections can then be compiled together for tomographic reconstruction. Retrospective gating is much more rapid, but produces an irregular angular distribution of projections, which can cause artifacts during the reconstruction process. Because prospectively gated images are acquired over many cardiac cycles, they require several minutes to perform. Many cardiac imaging protocols incorporate both respiratory and cardiac gating to minimize overall thoracic

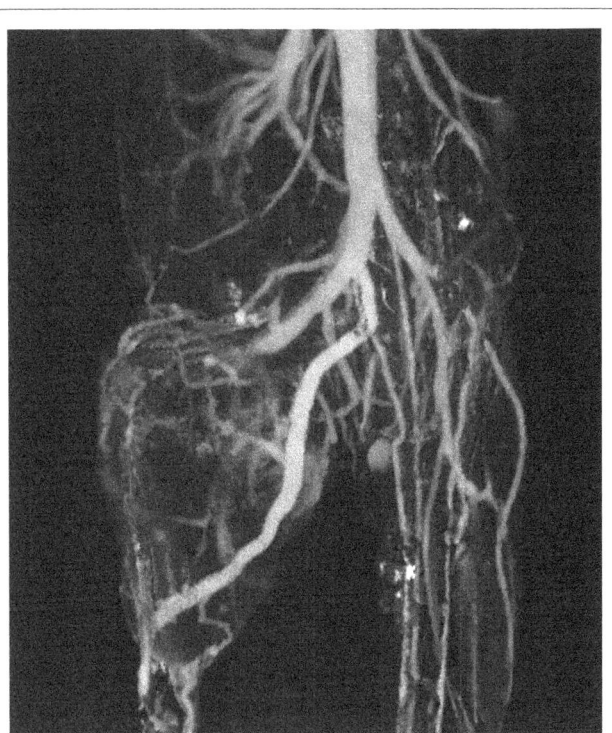

FIGURE | **Coronal maximum intensity projection of intravascular iodine in a mouse with a soft-tissue sarcoma in the right hindlimb.** Micro-CT imaging (88 μm voxel size) was performed immediately after injection of a liposomal iodine contrast agent.

motion during the scan (Badea et al., 2004). We note that intrinsic retrospective gating can also be implemented with cardiac and respiratory motion signals derived from information within each of the acquired projections, thus avoiding the complications of having ECG or respiratory sensors attached to the mouse (Bartling et al., 2008; Johnston et al., 2010; Kuntz et al., 2010).

For all cardiac imaging, contrast agents are necessary to differentiate the myocardium from the heart lumen. Because cardiac-gated scans can require several minutes to perform, enhancement of the blood within the heart must remain constant for a prolonged period of time to produce high quality scans. Such imaging is possible with low molecular weight contrast agents by using continuous administration or repeated injections (Sawall et al., 2012), but the vast majority of studies have made use of blood pool contrast agents, which make cardiac-gated CT protocols practical. Because images can be acquired over multiple phases of the cardiac cycle, cardiac micro-CT can produce 4D images of the beating heart. These datasets can be used to measure cardiac function, including ventricular volumes, stroke volume, ejection fraction, wall motion, and cardiac output (Badea et al., 2005, 2007, 2008b, 2011b; Wetzel et al., 2007). Measurements of cardiac function by micro-CT can be used to evaluate the effect of drugs in preclinical studies. Cardiac micro-CT has been used to measure changes in cardiac function as a result of dobutamine-induced cardiac stress (Badea et al., 2011c), as shown in **Figure** . Cardiac micro-CT can also be used to longitudinally measure changes in cardiac function over time. For example, left ventricular remodeling following a coronary ligation-induced myocardial infarction has been tracked by micro-CT (Sheikh et al., 2010). Measurements of cardiac function and infarct size have also been performed in coronary ligation mouse models using either a combination of blood pool agent (Fenestra VC) and a low molecular contrast agent (Nahrendorf et al., 2007) or a blood pool contrast agent (Exia 160) which shows specific uptake in myocardium (Ashton et al., 2014a). An example of micro-CT imaging of myocardial infarction using a delayed hyperenhancement protocol (Nahrendorf et al., 2007) is shown in **Figure** .

Liver and Spleen Imaging

Blood-pool contrast agents, which avoid renal clearance due to their large size (>6 nm), are eventually cleared from the bloodstream by phagocytic cells in the reticuloendothelial system (Moghimi et al., 2001). This clearance occurs primarily in the liver and spleen, which leads to accumulation of contrast in those organs over time. This leads to high enhancement of these organs for liver and spleen-specific imaging. One of the most commonly used micro-CT contrast agents, Fenestra LC, is composed of iodinated phospholipids which are recognized by the ApoE receptor on hepatocytes and internalized in the liver, which provides additional specificity for liver imaging. Because these blood pool contrast agents get taken up by normal-functioning liver and spleen, they can be used to identify necrotic regions (Chouker et al., 2008), liver tumors (Almajdub et al., 2007; Montet et al., 2007; Desnoyers et al., 2008; Graham et al., 2008; Kim et al., 2008; Boll et al., 2011), and spleen tumors (Almajdub et al., 2007), as well as to measure organ volume, quantify hepatic necrosis (Varenika et al., 2013), and determine liver anatomy (Fiebig et al., 2012). **Figure** shows longitudinal imaging of liver metastases as they increase in size over time following a single injection of nanoparticle contrast agent (Boll et al., 2011).

Cancer Imaging

Because tumors generally have the same density as their surrounding tissues, contrast agents are necessary for tumor identification and characterization by micro-CT. The vast majority of cancer imaging studies have been performed using blood pool nanoparticle contrast agents. Nanoparticles tend to accumulate in tumors due to the enhanced permeability and retention (EPR) effect (Maeda et al., 2000; Maeda, 2001). Rapid angiogenesis within a tumor leads to the development of immature, poorly organized, leaky vasculature. Gaps in this leaky vasculature are large enough that nanoparticles (up to 200–300 nm) can readily extravasate into the tumor tissue. Tumors also tend to have very poorly developed lymphatic drainage, so the nanoparticles are not cleared from the tumor once they extravasate. This effect leads to the gradual passive accumulation of nanoparticles in the tumor perivascular space over the course of hours to days. EPR has been widely exploited for both tumor imaging and therapy using nanoparticle agents.

Using micro-CT, dynamic biodistribution of contrast agent within small animal tumor models can be tracked. A liposomal iodine contrast agent was used in a rabbit tumor model for contrast agent tracking and biodistribution analysis (Zheng et al., 2009). Quantitative analysis was performed to determine the percent contrast agent uptake within each organ, including the tumor. Liposomal iodine was also used in two mouse models of breast cancer to demonstrate dynamic changes in enhancement within tumor vasculature and tumor parenchyma (Samei et al., 2009; Ghaghada et al., 2011). Immediately after injection, the contrast agent is entirely intravascular, with no significant enhancement within the tumor tissue. This early phase allows for the analysis of tumor vascular morphology, location, and density. After the contrast agent was cleared from the bloodstream, late phase imaging was performed to demonstrate passive accumulation of the contrast agent in the tumors due to EPR. The tumors showed heterogeneous enhancement throughout their volumes, demonstrating spatial heterogeneity in tumor perfusion and vascular permeability. **Figure** shows an example of

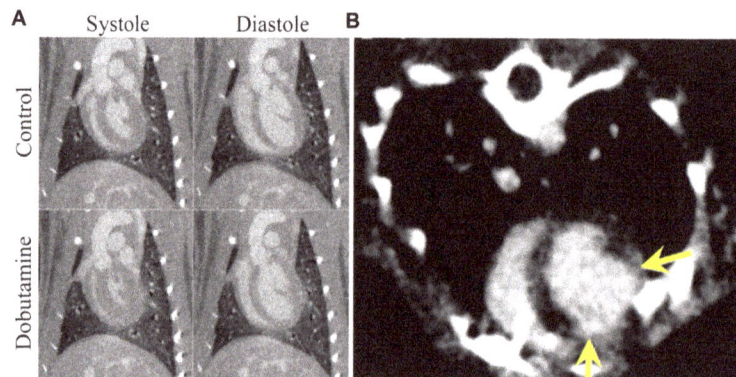

FIGURE | **Cardiac micro-CT imaging. (A)** Coronal micro-CT images through the left ventricle of a rat showing the heart in systole (left) and diastole (right) with and without the administration of dobutamine (10 µg/kg/min). End systolic volume is significantly decreased and stroke volume and cardiac output are both significantly increased. End diastolic volume is relatively unchanged after administration of dobutamine. **(B)** An axial image showing myocardial infarction in a rat using delayed hyper enhancement. The yellow arrows show the boundaries of the region of myocardial infarction.

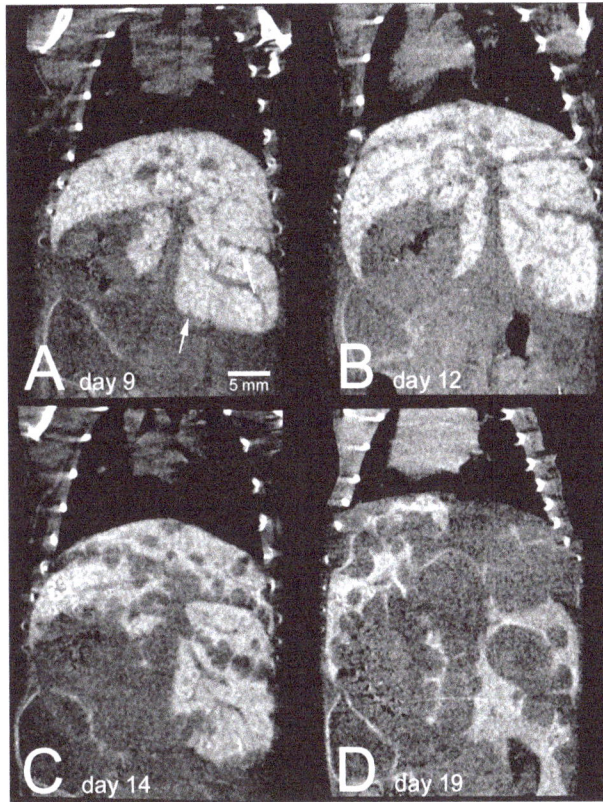

FIGURE | **Longitudinal micro-CT imaging of liver metastases in a mouse following injection of a nanoparticle contrast agent.** A single mouse is shown at 9 days **(A)**, 12 day s **(B)**, 14 day s **(C)**, and 19 days **(D)** after intrasplenic injection of tumor cells. Normal liver tissue is highly enhancing due to nanoparticle uptake, while the tumor regions show no enhancement. The enhancement remains high within the normal liver over the entire course of the experiment. By day 19, metastatic tumors take up the majority of the liver volume.

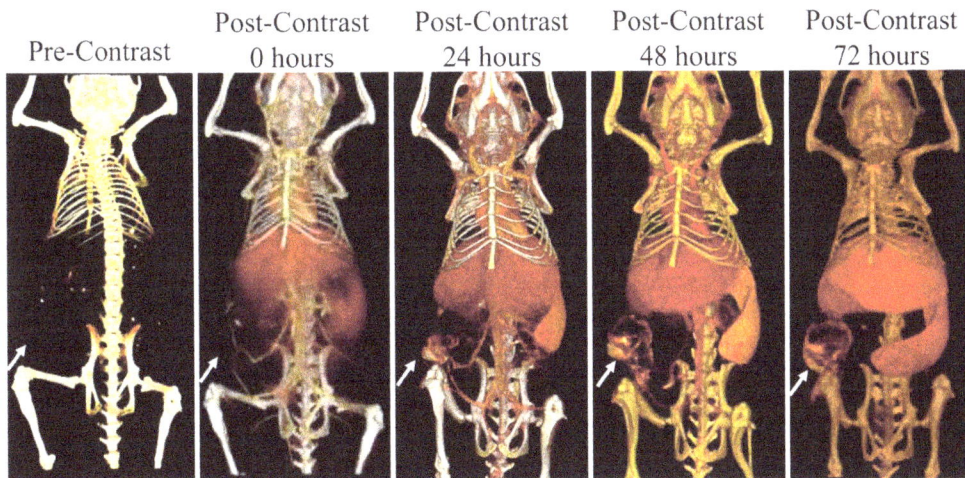

FIGURE | **Longitudinal micro-CT imaging of liposomal iodine biodistribution.** Liposomes slowly accumulate in the subcutaneous tumor, liver, and spleen over the course of 72 h. The white arrow points to the location of the tumor in each image.

nanoparticle dynamic biodistribution and tumor accumulation for a mouse injected with liposomal iodine (Ghaghada et al., 2011). Immediately after liposome injection, blood vessels are clearly outlined. At later time points, the liposomes accumulate both in the flank tumor and in the liver and spleen. Further studies have been done in mouse xenograft tumor models to carefully map the spatial and temporal distribution of liposome uptake by micro-CT (Ekdawi et al., 2015), which has important implications for nanoparticle-based drug delivery. Measurements of tumor vascular density in early phase imaging and total contrast accumulation in late phase imaging have also been used in two mouse models of lung cancer to differentiate between benign and malignant cancer types (Badea et al., 2012). Iodine-containing nanoparticle contrast agents have also been used for tumor imaging in two other models of lung cancer (Kindlmann et al., 2005; Anayama et al., 2013) and a mouse model of liver cancer (Rothe et al., 2015). Gold nanoparticles have also been used for passive tumor targeting in mouse models of breast and brain cancer (Hainfeld et al., 2006, 2013).

Active Targeting

In addition to the passive accumulation of nanoparticles in the reticuloendothelial system or tumors, active targeting of nanoparticles can be accomplished by conjugating specific ligands to the nanoparticle surface which can then link to their binding partners *in vivo* (Erathodiyil and Ying, 2011). Typically, these binding partners are cellular receptors or extracellular matrix proteins that are overexpressed in a pathological condition, so binding is specific to the region of pathology. Potential ligands for conjugation to the nanoparticle surface include antibodies, antibody fragments, other proteins, peptides, aptamers, lipids, carbohydrates, and other small molecules. The use of targeted contrast agents for micro-CT has recently been reviewed (Li et al., 2014). Gold nanoparticles have been used extensively for active targeting due to the ease of gold surface modification via gold-thiol bond formation. Gold nanoparticles have been used as a micro-CT contrast agent for the targeting of multiple tumor markers, including Her2 (Hainfeld et al., 2011), the gastrin-releasing peptide (GRP) receptor (Chanda et al., 2010), the epidermal growth factor receptor (EGFR) (Reuveni et al., 2011b), the folic acid receptor (FAR) (Wang et al., 2013), and tumor microcalcifications (Cole et al., 2014). **Figure** demonstrates the use of EGFR-antibody conjugated gold nanoparticles to target an EGFR-expressing subcutaneous tumor. Tumor enhancement was significantly increased with targeted gold nanoparticles compared to non-targeted gold nanoparticles (190 HU vs. 78 HU). Gold nanoparticles have also been used for CT imaging of lymph nodes by targeting CD4 (Eck et al., 2010), imaging of inflammation by targeting intravascular E-selectin (Wyss et al., 2009), imaging of atherosclerosis by targeting fibrin (Winter et al., 2005), imaging of myocardial scars by targeting collagen (Danila et al., 2013), and imaging of other cardiovascular disease (Ghann et al., 2012). In addition to targeting by the surface conjugation of a ligand, some nanoparticles have inherent targeting abilities due to their nanoparticle chemistry. Gold nanoparticle encapsulated within HDL particles are naturally recognized by HDL receptors and taken up in atherosclerotic plaques (Cormode et al., 2010). Exia-160 consists of iodinated molecules which can be fully metabolized by the body, and therefore the contrast agent accumulates in metabolically active tissues, including the myocardium and brown adipose tissue. This effect has been used to discriminate between healthy and infarcted myocardium (Ashton et al., 2014a).

Targeted CT imaging can also be accomplished by labeling cells with nanoparticle contrast agents. Cell labeling with nanoparticles has been successfully used for MRI and other imaging modalities, but has only recently been demonstrated for CT (Betzer et al., 2014). In this study mesenchymal stem cells were labeled with gold nanoparticles prior to injection into a rat model of depression. Cell migration into depression-related bring regions was successfully tracked up to 1 month post-transplantation using micro-CT. The continued development of CT contrast agents for targeted imaging and cell tracking will improve the specificity of CT imaging for a wide range of pathologies and cell therapies and will make molecular imaging with CT a reality.

Multi-modality Imaging

Micro-CT can also be combined with other imaging modalities in order to better study molecular and anatomical information simultaneously. A micro-CT system can be combined with single photon emission computed tomography (SPECT), positron emission tomography (PET), or fluorescence molecular tomography (FMT) into a single unit (Goertzen et al., 2002; Liang et al., 2007). SPECT, PET, and FMT are all highly sensitive, so targeted molecular imaging with radio-labeled or fluorescently labeled small molecules or biomolecules is readily accomplished. However, these modalities are all limited by poor spatial resolution and poor anatomical imaging. By combining these systems with micro-CT, high resolution anatomical images can be co-registered with molecular images to produce highly useful datasets. Combining micro-SPECT and micro-PET with micro-CT can also improve the image quality of the resultant SPECT and PET images by allowing for attenuation correction (Chow et al., 2005; Hwang and Hasegawa, 2005). **Figure** shows a combined micro-CT/micro-PET image for a tumor-bearing mouse soon after injection of both liposomal iodine and ^{18}F-fluorodeoxyglucose (FDG) (Badea et al., 2011a). The micro-CT image provides high resolution anatomical detail to give context to the tumor signal seen in the micro-PET image.

A second application of multi-modal imaging which has gained much attention recently is the use of agents that produce contrast for multiple imaging modalities simultaneously. Thus, multiple imaging modalities can be used after injection of a single contrast agent. This helps to improve registration between the different modalities, and increase the amount of information gained from hybrid imaging systems. Many different formulations of multi-modal contrast agents have been developed, and the development of these agents has been reviewed previously (Key and Leary, 2014). Combined CT/MR contrast agents have been developed using gadolinium chelates conjugated to gold nanoparticles (Alric et al., 2008) or gold nanoshells (Coughlin et al., 2014), liposomes containing both gadolinium and iodine-based contrast agents (Zheng et al., 2006), and iron oxide core nanoparticles surrounded by either a gold shell (Carril et al., 2014) or a mesoporous silica shell filled with iodinated oil (Xue et al., 2014). A combined CT/SPECT agent has been developed using a dendrimer linked to both iodinated organic molecules and SPECT agent chelators (Criscione et al., 2011). A combined PET/CT agent has been demonstrated using

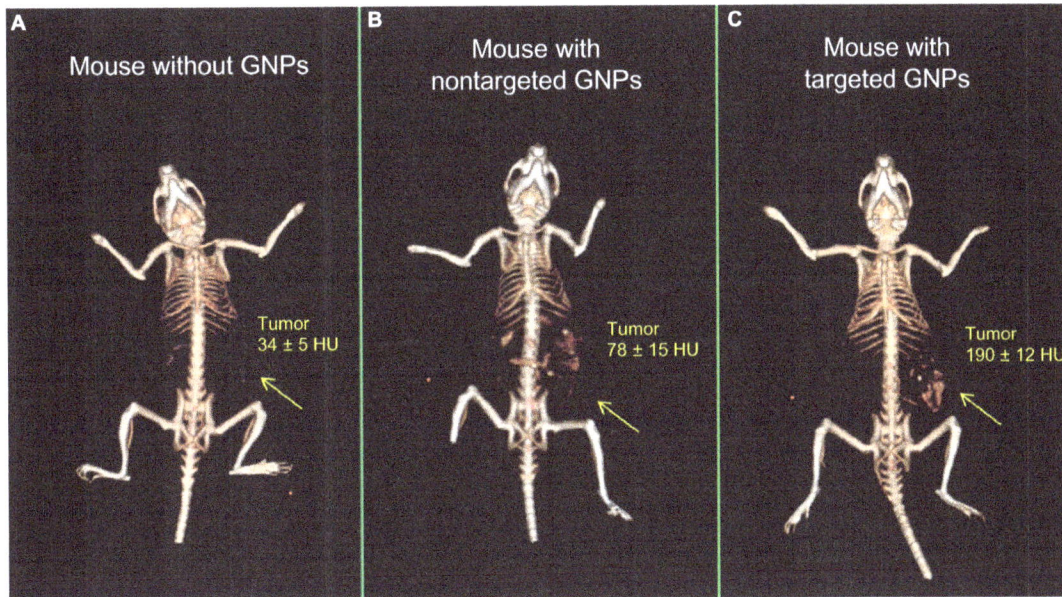

FIGURE | **3D micro-CT reconstructions of mice with EGFR-expressing tumors.** Mice were injected with **(A)** saline, **(B)** non-targeted gold nanoparticles, or **(C)** EGFR-antibody targeted gold nanoparticles. Increased CT enhancement was seen for both types of nanoparticles, but targeted nanoparticles showed significantly higher enhancement than non-targeted controls. Reprinted from with permission from (Reuveni et al., 2011a)

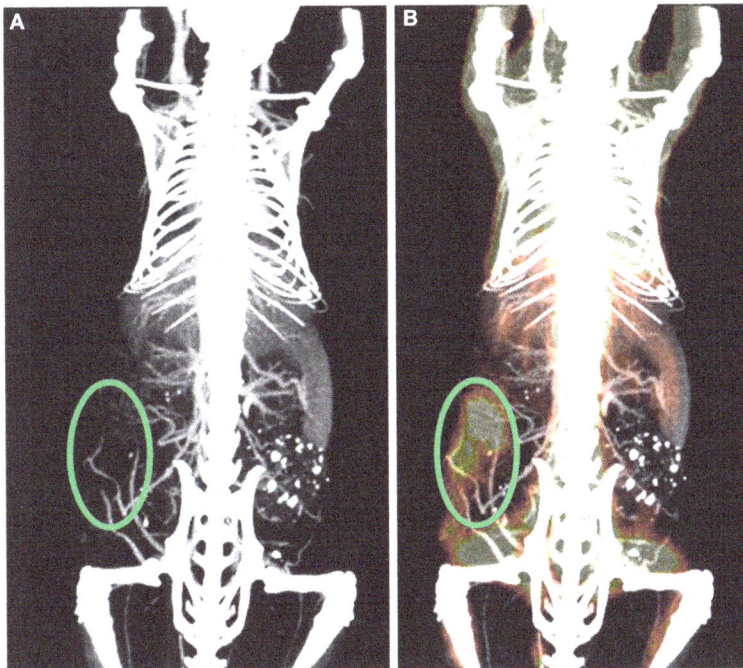

FIGURE | **Multi-modal micro-CT/micro-PET imaging. (A)** Maximum intensity projection rendered micro-CT image acquired 1 h post-administration of PEGylated liposomal-iodixanol. **(B)** The overlaid PET/CT image shows the metabolically active tumor (green ellipse).

gold nanoparticles conjugated to both glucose and ^{18}F-FDG for targeting of metabolically active tumors (Roa et al., 2012; Feng et al., 2014). All of these formulations have been successfully tested *in vivo* with multi-modal small animal imaging.

Theranostics

Another exciting topic of current research is the development of theranostic nanoparticles – nanoparticles that can be used for both therapy and diagnostic imaging. Many nanoparticles used as micro-CT contrast agents can easily be adapted to incorporate therapeutics or act directly as a therapeutic agent themselves. Gold nanoparticles, for example, have the inherent ability to increase the effectiveness of radiation therapy, because they absorb therapeutic x-rays efficiently and then release that energy to the surrounding tissues. This can significantly increase the locally delivered dose in regions of high nanoparticle concentration. This has been used by several groups to effectively treat cancer in multiple animal models (Hainfeld et al., 2004, 2008, 2010, 2013, 2014; Jeremic et al., 2013; Park et al., 2015; Wolfe et al., 2015). Gold nanoparticles also exhibit high absorbance of light at their surface plasmon resonance wavelength, which can be tuned by altering the shape and size of the nanoparticle. For many gold nanoparticle shapes (i.e., nanorods, nanoshells, nanostars), this plasmon resonance occurs in the near infrared region, which is optimal for use with photothermal heating. In photothermal heating, nanoparticles convert laser light into heat, which leads to local hyperthermia. This can be used for tumor ablation when nanoparticles are accumulated within a tumor. The use of nanoparticle for combined CT imaging and photothermal therapy has been recently reviewed (Curry et al., 2014). Gold nanorods (Huang et al., 2011) and hollow gold nanoshells (Park et al., 2015) have both been used for combined CT imaging, radiation therapy, and photothermal therapy. **Figure** shows a gold nanostar theranostic probe which was used for CT imaging and photothermal therapy in a mouse model of primary soft tissue sarcoma (Liu et al., 2015). This probe showed high tumor accumulation and CT enhancement as well as effective tumor ablation following photothermal therapy. Therapeutics can also be incorporated into nanoparticles by direct conjugation to the nanoparticle surface or by co-encapsulation of the therapeutic with the imaging agent (e.g., within the aqueous core of a liposome). Both methods have been used for the addition of therapeutic radioisotopes or chemotherapy drugs to nanoparticle contrast agents (Chen et al., 2014; Lu, 2014; Ryu et al., 2014; Zhu et al., 2014).

FUTURE DIRECTIONS – SPECTRAL CT

Much effort has been made to overcome the low contrast sensitivity inherent in CT imaging. The primary method, as discussed above, is to add large amounts of an exogenous contrast agent. However, significant developments have also been made in imaging system design which can potentially improve CT image contrast. One of the most promising recent developments in CT has been the use of spectral information to improve contrast discrimination. In traditional CT imaging, the overall attenuation of x-ray intensity is measured by the detector, but the detected x-rays are not spectrally resolved. The spectrum of transmitted x-rays is important because the absorption of x-rays by different materials is highly dependent on x-ray energy, so the transmitted x-ray spectrum depends on what materials are present along the x-ray path. Therefore, there is a significant amount of information that can be gained by including spectral data in the CT reconstruction process. Based on differences in

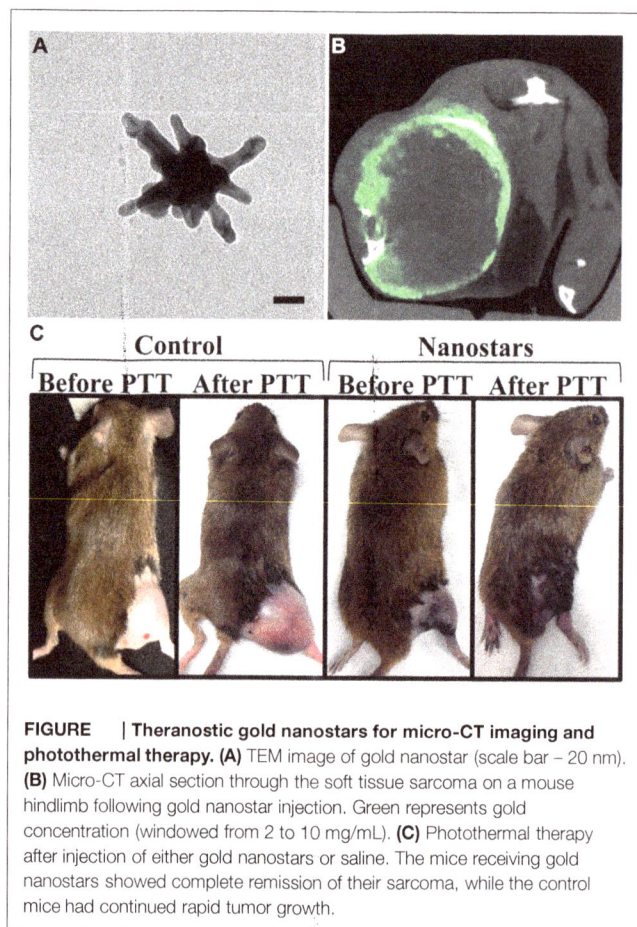

FIGURE | **Theranostic gold nanostars for micro-CT imaging and photothermal therapy. (A)** TEM image of gold nanostar (scale bar – 20 nm). **(B)** Micro-CT axial section through the soft tissue sarcoma on a mouse hindlimb following gold nanostar injection. Green represents gold concentration (windowed from 2 to 10 mg/mL). **(C)** Photothermal therapy after injection of either gold nanostars or saline. The mice receiving gold nanostars showed complete remission of their sarcoma, while the control mice had continued rapid tumor growth.

x-ray absorption, multiple materials can be differentiated and quantified within a single scan using spectral CT.

There are two primary methods used to obtain spectral CT data. The first method, dual-energy (DE) CT, uses x-ray sources with two different energy spectra and traditional energy integrating x-ray detectors. The second method uses a single x-ray source but has energy-resolving detectors (photon counting detectors) that can measure the energy of each detected photons. DE CT is currently used clinically and has been successful in improving imaging for a variety of applications (Jepperson et al., 2013; Aran et al., 2014; Marin et al., 2014; Mileto et al., 2014; Ohana et al., 2014; Paul et al., 2014; Bongartz et al., 2015)

Dual-energy CT

DE CT can use either a single x-ray source which rapidly switches between two tube voltages or two separate sources (offset from one another by 90°) that each operate at a unique voltage. In either case, x-ray projections are acquired at each rotation angle using both x-ray sources. Additionally, a double-layer or "sandwich" detector is sometimes used to separate low and high energy x-rays. In DE CT, a complete CT dataset is acquired for two different x-ray energy spectra. Most of a patient's body appears the same on both images, because absorption of x-rays by low atomic weight materials, which is primarily due to Compton scattering, is very weakly dependent on x-ray energy. However, the photoelectric effect in high atomic weight materials is highly dependent on x-ray energy. Therefore, the attenuation coefficient of high atomic weight materials (calcium in bone, iodine, gold) will depend on the energy spectrum of the incident x-rays. This effect is particularly pronounced if the two energy spectra fall on either side of the K-edge for one of the materials. Because there is a large increase in attenuation at energies above the K-edge (see **Figure**   ), this leads to a large difference in signal between the two scans. By combining data from the two energy sets, these high Z materials can be differentiated from one another and quantified. This process is demonstrated in **Figure**   , which shows scans of an *in vitro* phantom containing vials of water, gold, iodine, or a mixture of gold and iodine. Scans at two different energies were simultaneously acquired. These two scans were then mathematically decomposed into a map of iodine concentration and a map of gold concentration (Clark et al., 2013). We note that although the K-edges have helped with the separation between iodine and gold, we are not able to deliver true K-edge imaging as is possible with synchrotron mono-energetic beams.

Spectral separation using DE CT is somewhat limited by our ability to minimize the overlap of x-ray spectra using polychromatic sources. Although the peak tube voltage can be changed over a wide range, the average energy of the resulting spectrum does not change significantly, as was shown for the two energy spectra in **Figure**   . The separation between the two energy spectra can be improved by applying additional filtration to the x-ray tubes, which can preferentially remove low energy photons and further increase the average energy of the x-ray spectrum. The other limitation for DE CT is its ability to discriminate between closely related elements. Discrimination of two elements using DE CT is best when there is a large difference in their attenuations at the two x-ray energies. This works very well for elements with widely different k-edges (gold and iodine), but does not work for elements with very similar k-edges (barium

and iodine). By careful selection and design of contrast agents, this limitation can be avoided.

Although DE CT is commonly used in the clinic, its use has been limited to date in preclinical micro-CT imaging. The primary challenge with translating CT to micro-CT is the significant increase in resolution. Because voxel size is much smaller, the noise is much higher for micro-CT than for clinical CT. This could be improved by significantly increasing the number of x-ray photons delivered in order to get the same photon flux through each voxel. However, the radiation dose must be limited for *in vivo* studies, so noise cannot be decreased to the levels seen in clinical scans. This presents a problem for DE reconstruction, because the mathematical decomposition of multiple materials depends on having high quality (low noise) measurements of attenuation at each voxel. High levels of noise make material decomposition inaccurate. By minimizing scatter during acquisition and applying post-acquisition image processing strategies, beam hardening and noise can be reduced to allow for successful DE decomposition. It has been shown that applying joint domain bilateral filtration (an edge-preserving, smoothing filter that incorporates data from both energy sets) prior to DE decomposition significantly improves the DE decomposition accuracy, precision, and limits of detectability (Clark et al., 2013). The mean limits of detectability for each element were determined to be 2.3 mg/mL (18 mM) for iodine and 1.0 mg/mL (5.1 mM) for gold, well within the observed *in vivo* concentrations of each element (I: 0–24 mg/mL, Au: 0–9 mg/mL) and a factor of 10 improvement over the limits without post-reconstruction joint bilateral filtration. *In vitro* testing of this method using imaging phantoms containing both gold and iodine is shown in **Figure**   (Clark et al., 2013). Using this method, DE micro-CT has been used successfully for a variety of applications in mice. DE CT was used for atherosclerosis imaging to differentiate liposomal iodine accumulated in plaque macrophages from calcium within the plaque (Bhavane et al., 2013). Iodine accumulated within the myocardium has been separated from other soft tissues and from calcium in the bone for imaging of myocardial infarction (Ashton et al., 2014a). DE CT has been used to separate gold nanoparticles accumulated within soft-tissue sarcomas (Clark et al., 2013) or primary lung tumors (Ashton et al., 2014b) from liposomal iodine within the vasculature. Images of the decomposed gold and iodine maps for a soft-tissue sarcoma are shown in **Figure**   . In these studies, the simultaneous measurement of two different nanoparticle concentrations was used to calculate tumor vascular density and vascular permeability. Validation of the calculated results was performed using histology and *ex vivo* measurements of tissue gold and iodine concentrations (Ashton et al., 2014b). In two additional studies, DE CT was used to assess vascular changes following radiation therapy. In the first, the increase in vascular permeability in a soft-tissue sarcoma was determined by measuring accumulation of liposomal iodine (Moding et al., 2013). In the second study, cardiac injury following radiation therapy was assessed using gold nanoparticles and liposomal iodine (Lee et al., 2014). Cardiac-gated CT imaging was performed to obtain a DE decomposition of the myocardium at each phase of the cardiac cycle. This data

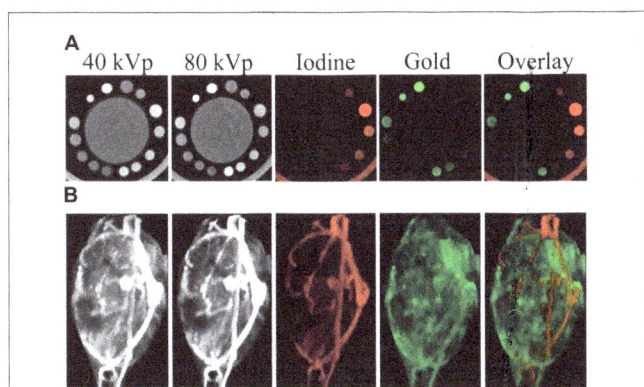

FIGURE | **Dual energy micro-CT material decomposition. (A)**, *In vitro* phantom consisting of a large tube of water surrounded by vials containing gold, iodine, or a mixture of the two. **(B)**, *In vivo* imaging of gold nanoparticles and iodine-containing liposomes within a mouse soft tissue sarcoma. The iodine (shown in red) and gold (shown in green) maps are the result of dual energy decomposition. In both cases, the decomposition was able to successfully differentiate the signals from the gold and iodine contrast agents.

was used to assess both extent of cardiac injury and change in cardiac function.

Our group has recently also demonstrated triple-energy micro-CT for the differentiation of three materials: gold, iodine, and gadolinium. Using a novel algorithm called spectral diffusion (Clark and Badea, 2014), these three materials were successfully separated and quantified both in an *in vitro* phantom and *in vivo*. **Figure** shows *in vivo* images with decomposed concentration maps depicting liposomal iodine accumulated within the liver and spleen, gold nanoparticles within the vasculature, and a low molecular weight gadolinium contrast agent in the kidneys. Dual and triple-energy CT have the potential to be particularly useful with targeted contrast agents, so that contrast agents with multiple different targets can be co-injected and individually quantified using a single scan.

Photon Counting X-ray Detectors

The alternative to DE CT is the use of energy-resolving photon-counting x-ray detectors (PCXDs) for spectral CT imaging. The PCXDs acquire data for each projection using multiple energy bins. These detectors directly convert photons to a digital signal, which decreases the noise that is inherent in traditional energy-integrating detectors (Schirra et al., 2014). Each photon that is counted by the detector is assigned into one of the energy bins, which provides an approximation of the energy spectrum of the transmitted x-rays. Energy bins can be chosen to include regions of the spectrum above and below the K-edge of the elements of interest. The measured attenuations from each energy bin can then be used to simultaneously solve for the concentration of one or more high atomic weight materials within a single voxel. This method can also be used quantify the contribution of either Compton scattering or the photoelectric effect within any given voxel, which allows accurate separation between signal from soft tissues and signal from high Z materials.

Photon-counting x-ray detectors are not yet used in standard clinical CT imaging, but prototype photon counting CT scanners have been deployed in some research hospitals. It is expected that PCXDs will likely be generally adopted in the clinical realm once the technology has further advanced (Taguchi and Iwanczyk, 2013). The primary drawback of current PCXDs is the relatively low photon count rate for each individual detector. Because it takes a finite amount of time to count a single photon, the hardware can fall behind when photon flux is high. This leads to pulse pileup, which can cause saturation of the detectors and loss of spectral sensitivity and accuracy (Schirra et al., 2014). Clinical CT operates at very high photon flux, so this problem must be resolved before PCXDs can be effectively used clinically. The most obvious solution is to decrease the detector size, which will decrease the flux incident on each detector. However, as detectors become smaller, the charge sharing between detectors increases, which can lead to multiple counts for single x-rays and counts at the wrong energies. This leads to spectral distortions and high noise. Therefore, many researchers are focused on improving both the hardware and reconstruction algorithms necessary for optimal spectral imaging with PCXDs.

Although PCXDs are still experimental for clinical CT, their use in preclinical small animal studies has been successfully demonstrated. Spectral CT has been used with targeted nanoparticles to image atherosclerotic plaques (Cormode et al., 2010). Gold nanoparticles were encapsulated within high-density lipoprotein (HDL) particles to target plaque macrophages. A preclinical spectral CT system (Phillips Research, Hamburg) was used to differentiate the gold from iodine, calcium, and soft tissues. This analysis was first performed in an *in vitro*

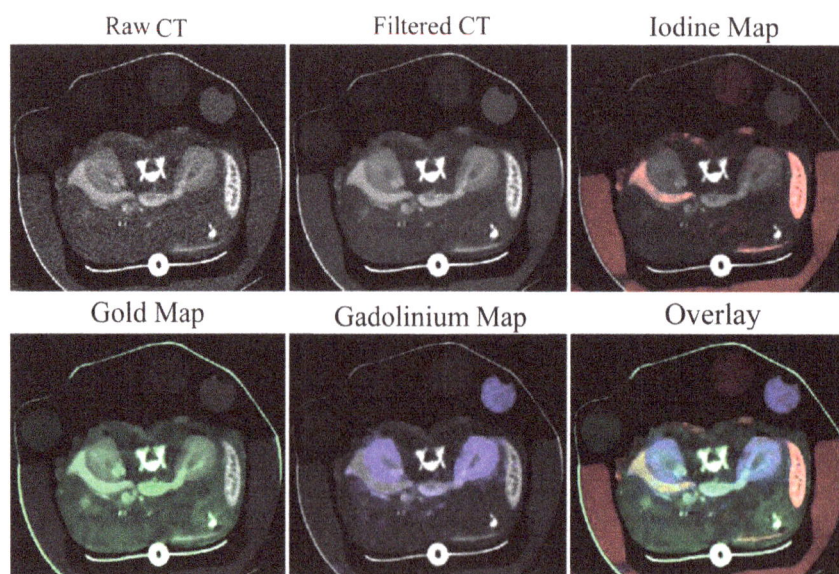

FIGURE | Three-energy micro-CT imaging in a mouse. Liposomal iodine was injected 72 h before imaging. Gold nanoparticles and low molecular weight gadolinium were injected immediately before imaging. Images were acquired at three energies, filtered, then separated into maps of iodine (red), gold (green), and gadolinium (blue) concentration.

aorta phantom, as shown in **Figure**   . Spectral CT was used to resolve the signals from gold, iodine and calcium within the tissue phantom matrix. The spectral CT system successfully differentiated the phantom regions containing gold, iodine, and calcium, with very little overlap between the signals. They also tested the targeting of their gold-HDL particles in a mouse model of atherosclerosis. Spectral CT (and subsequent histology) demonstrated that the gold successfully accumulated within the plaques and that gold could be discriminated from iodine, calcium, and soft-tissue *in vivo*, as seen in **Figure**   . The same HDL-encapsulated gold nanoparticles have been used along with a blood pool iodine contrast agent to simultaneously image the signals from gold accumulated within lymph nodes, iodine within the blood, bone, and soft tissue (Roessl et al., 2011).

Low density-lipoproteins (LDLs) labeled with gold nanoparticles have also been used to image tumors using spectral CT (Allijn et al., 2013). Gold nanoparticles accumulating in lymph nodes after subcutaneous injection have been differentiated from soft tissue and bone (Schirra et al., 2012). Iodine within the vasculature and barium within the gastrointestinal tract have been imaged and differentiated from bone and soft tissue (Anderson et al., 2010). Spectral imaging has also been used to detect novel ytterbium nanoparticles within the vasculature (Pan et al., 2012) and organic bismuth nanocolloids targeted to fibrin-rich clots (Pan et al., 2010). In both cases, spectral CT was used to differentiate contrast agent signal from soft tissue and bone. The primary limitation in all of these studies was that the low photon-count rate limitations of the PCXD

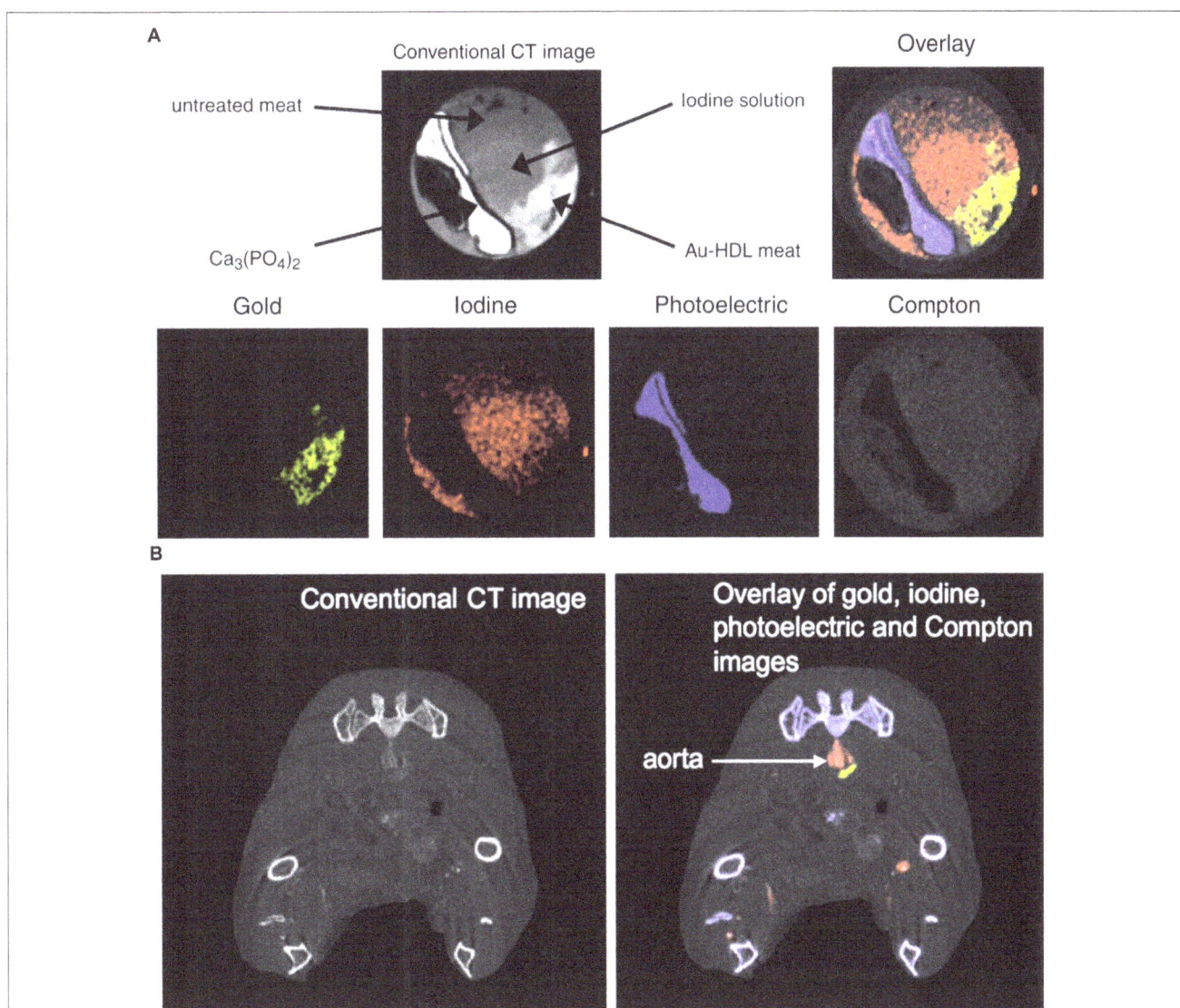

FIGURE | Spectral micro-CT imaging using photon counting x-ray detectors and HDL-encapsulated gold nanoparticles. (A) In vitro aorta phantom study demonstrating the conventional CT image along with the decomposition of the CT image into gold, iodine, photoelectric, and Compton components. **(B)** *In vivo* imaging of targeted gold nanoparticles and blood pool iodine in a mouse model of atherosclerosis. The iodine (red) can be clearly visualized within the aorta, while the gold signal (yellow) is immediately adjacent to the aorta lumen in the atherosclerotic plaque. Reprinted with permission from (Cormode et al., 2010).

system resulted in a long scan time. Because the scan time was so long, the imaging was done after sacrificing the animals in order to prevent motion over the course of the long acquisition. Despite the limitations, these studies demonstrate that spectral CT using a PCXD system has the potential for high quality *in vivo* imaging and material discrimination. Some technical problems remain to be solved, but PCXD systems have great promise for use in both preclinical and clinical CT imaging.

RADIATION DOSE CONSIDERATIONS

One of the primary drawbacks of x-ray CT imaging is exposure to radiation. X-ray radiation exposure can lead to biological damage and long-term health effects (Boone et al., 2004). Radiation exposure is particularly important to consider for micro-CT applications, because higher radiation doses are required for high resolution CT scans. Signal-to-noise ratio in CT is inversely proportional to the square root of the number of x-rays passing through each voxel. As voxel size decreases, the number of x-rays necessary to maintain a constant signal-to-noise ratio increases significantly. In planning micro-CT studies, a balance must be made between desired image quality and radiation exposure.

The $LD_{50/30}$ radiation dose in mice (the dose required to kill 50% of mice within 30 days) depends on many factors, but tends to be between 5 and 8 Gy (Ritman, 2004; Carlson et al., 2007). The typical radiation dose for a single micro-CT scan can vary widely and reported values in the literature range from 0.017 Gy to 0.78 Gy (Carlson et al., 2007). Rodents have the ability to repair damage from low doses of radiation (~0.3 Gy) over the course of several hours (Parkins et al., 1985), so most low dose micro-CT scans should have limited biological impact, even when the same animals are longitudinally scanned over the course of a study. But for higher dose scans, longitudinal imaging can potentially lead to a cumulative dose that could affect biological function (particularly immune function and tumor response) and long-term health (Boone et al., 2004). Therefore, careful consideration must be made to determine the optimal imaging protocol for each individual application to minimize the effects of radiation dose on the experiment. With additional advances in micro-CT technology and reconstruction algorithms, radiation doses should further decrease, which will help to overcome radiation as a limitation of micro-CT imaging.

NANOPARTICLE CONTRAST AGENT SAFETY

Understanding the potential toxicity of nanoparticles is essential in order to apply nanoparticle contrast agents *in vivo* and eventually translate these contrast agents to the clinic. Because blood pool contrast agents are not rapidly cleared from the body by the kidneys, they have much more opportunity to interact with the body and accumulate in various organs.

Since each nanoparticle formulation is unique, rigorous toxicity testing must be performed for any proposed contrast agent in order to fully understand its usefulness for both preclinical research and potential clinical translation. For example, there is strong evidence regarding bio-compatibility of gold (Cervenka et al., 1999; Hainfeld et al., 2006; Lin et al., 2009). Gold-based nano-products are now undergoing clinical trials, e.g., colloidal Au-based tumor necrosis factor (CYT-6091, CytImmune, Inc., Rockville, MD, USA) and gold nanoshells (Nanospectra, Inc., Houston, TX, USA). However, there is still uncertainty regarding the toxicity of many of the recently proposed nanoparticle contrast agents; although most of the studies reviewed here have stated that no toxicity has been observed, comprehensive prospective toxicity studies are still required to be performed. Because many nanoparticles can accumulate in the body for up to several months, in depth studies of long term toxicity are particularly important. A better understanding of nanoparticle toxicity is necessary for the further advancement of the field of nanoparticle CT contrast agents.

CONCLUSION

Micro-CT has become an extremely important tool in small animal research. Micro-CT produces non-invasive, three-dimensional, high resolution anatomical images, which can provide a wealth of information about normal animal function and pathology. Although x-ray CT is limited by low tissue contrast, developments in contrast agent design show great promise for use in imaging a wide range of organ systems and pathologies. Additional new developments in spectral imaging will further improve the usefulness of micro-CT in acquiring functional and molecular information. This will greatly expand the potential applications for micro-CT in small animal research. The increasing availability and low cost of micro-CT scanners promises to greatly increase the use and impact of micro-CT imaging on small animal studies. Given the common use of mouse models of disease to validate potential drug targets, to assess therapeutic efficacy, and to identify and validate biomarkers of drug efficacy and/or safety, micro-CT with nanoparticle based contrast agents can have far-reaching applications in drug discovery and pharmacology. Continuous development of novel CT/micro-CT imaging technology and contrast agents will serve well drug discovery and result in better medicines. Contrast agents and technology developed for preclinical micro-CT also have the potential to translate to significant improvements in clinical CT imaging.

FUNDING

This work was supported by the Duke Center for In Vivo Microscopy, an NIH/NIBIB National Biomedical Technology Resource Center (P41 EB015897) and by NCI R01 CA196667. JA was supported by an American Heart Association Predoctoral Fellowship (14PRE20110008).

REFERENCES

Ai, K., Liu, Y., Liu, J., Yuan, Q., He, Y., and Lu, L. (2011). Large-scale synthesis of Bi(2)S(3) nanodots as a contrast agent for in vivo X-ray computed tomography imaging. *Adv. Mater.* 23, 4886–4891. doi: 10.1002/adma.201103289

Allijn, I. E., Leong, W., Tang, J., Gianella, A., Mieszawska, A. J., Fay, F., et al. (2013). Gold nanocrystal labeling allows low-density lipoprotein imaging from the subcellular to macroscopic level. *ACS Nano* 7, 9761–9770. doi: 10.1021/nn403258w

Almajdub, M., Nejjari, M., Poncet, G., Magnier, L., Chereul, E., Roche, C., et al. (2007). In-vivo high-resolution X-ray microtomography for liver and spleen tumor assessment in mice. *Contrast Media Mol. Imaging* 2, 88–93. doi: 10.1002/cmmi.130

Alric, C., Taleb, J., Le Duc, G., Mandon, C., Billotey, C., Le Meur-Herland, A., et al. (2008). Gadolinium chelate coated gold nanoparticles as contrast agents for both X-ray computed tomography and magnetic resonance imaging. *J. Am. Chem. Soc.* 130, 5908–5915. doi: 10.1021/ja078176p

Anayama, T., Nakajima, T., Dunne, M., Zheng, J., Allen, C., Driscoll, B., et al. (2013). A novel minimally invasive technique to create a rabbit VX2 lung tumor model for nano-sized image contrast and interventional studies. *PLoS ONE* 8:e67355. doi: 10.1371/journal.pone.0067355

Anderson, N. G., Butler, A. P., Scott, N. J. A., Cook, N. J., Butzer, J. S., Schleich, N., et al. (2010). Spectroscopic (multi-energy) CT distinguishes iodine and barium contrast material in MICE. *Eur. Radiol.* 20, 2126–2134. doi: 10.1007/s00330-010-1768-9

Annapragada, A. V., Hoffman, E., Divekar, A., Karathanasis, E., and Ghaghada, K. B. (2012). High-resolution CT vascular imaging using blood pool contrast agents. *Methodist Debakey Cardiovasc. J.* 8, 18–22. doi: 10.14797/mdcj-8-1-18

Appleton, C. T., Mcerlain, D. D., Pitelka, V., Schwartz, N., Bernier, S. M., Henry, J. L., et al. (2007). Forced mobilization accelerates pathogenesis: characterization of a preclinical surgical model of osteoarthritis. *Arthritis Res. Ther.* 9:R13. doi: 10.1186/ar2120

Aran, S., Daftari Besheli, L., Karcaaltincaba, M., Gupta, R., Flores, E. J., and Abujudeh, H. H. (2014). Applications of dual-energy CT in emergency radiology. *AJR Am. J. Roentgenol.* 202, W314–W324. doi: 10.2214/AJR.13.11682

Artaechevarria, X., Blanco, D., De Biurrun, G., Ceresa, M., Perez-Martin, D., Bastarrika, G., et al. (2011). Evaluation of micro-CT for emphysema assessment in mice: comparison with non-radiological techniques. *Eur. Radiol.* 21, 954–962. doi: 10.1007/s00330-010-1982-5

Artaechevarria, X., Blanco, D., Perez-Martin, D., De Biurrun, G., Montuenga, L. M., De Torres, J. P., et al. (2010). Longitudinal study of a mouse model of chronic pulmonary inflammation using breath hold gated micro-CT. *Eur. Radiol.* 20, 2600–2608. doi: 10.1007/s00330-010-1853-0

Ashton, J. R., Befera, N., Clark, D., Qi, Y., Mao, L., Rockman, H. A., et al. (2014a). Anatomical and functional imaging of myocardial infarction in mice using micro-CT and eXIA 160 contrast agent. *Contrast Media Mol. Imaging* 9, 161–168. doi: 10.1002/cmmi.1557

Ashton, J. R., Clark, D. P., Moding, E. J., Ghaghada, K., Kirsch, D. G., West, J. L., et al. (2014b). Dual-energy micro-CT functional imaging of primary lung cancer in mice using gold and iodine nanoparticle contrast agents: a validation study. *PLoS ONE* 9:e88129. doi: 10.1371/journal.pone.0088129

Aviv, H., Bartling, S., Kiessling, F., and Margel, S. (2009). Radiopaque iodinated copolymeric nanoparticles for X-ray imaging applications. *Biomaterials* 30, 5610–5616. doi: 10.1016/j.biomaterials.2009.06.038

Badea, C. T., Athreya, K. K., Espinosa, G., Clark, D., Ghafoori, A. P., Li, Y., et al. (2012). Computed tomography imaging of primary lung cancer in mice using a liposomal-iodinated contrast agent. *PLoS ONE* 7:e34496. doi: 10.1371/journal.pone.0034496

Badea, C., Fubara, B., Hedlund, L., and Johnson, G. (2005). 4D micro-CT of the mouse heart. *Mol. Imaging* 4, 110–116.

Badea, C., Hedlund, L. W., and Johnson, G. A. (2004). Micro-CT with respiratory and cardiac gating. *Med. Phys.* 31, 3324–3329. doi: 10.1118/1.1812604

Badea, C., Schreibmann, E., and Fox, T. (2008a). A registration based approach for 4D cardiac micro-CT using combined prospective and retrospective gating. *Med. Phys.* 35, 1170–1179. doi: 10.1118/1.2868778

Badea, C. T., Wetzel, A. W., Mistry, N., Pomerantz, S., Nave, D., and Johnson, G. A. (2008b). Left ventricle volume measurements in cardiac micro-CT: the

impact of radiation dose and contrast agent. *Comput. Med. Imaging Graph.* 32, 239–250. doi: 10.1016/j.compmedimag.2007.12.004

Badea, C. T., Ghaghada, K., Espinosa, G., Strong, L., and Annapragada, A. (2011a). "Multi-modality PET-CT imaging of breast cancer in an animal model using nanoparticle x-ray contrast agent and 18F-FDG," in *Proceedings of the SPIE 7965, Medical Imaging 2011: Biomedical Applications in Molecular, Structural, and Functional Imaging*, Vol. 796511 (Lake Buena Vista, FL: SPIE Digital Library).

Badea, C. T., Hedlund, L. W., Cook, J., Berridge, B. R., and Johnson, G. A. (2011b). Micro-CT imaging assessment of dobutamine-induced cardiac stress in rats. *J. Pharmacol. Toxicol. Methods* 63, 24–29. doi: 10.1016/j.vascn.2010.04.002

Badea, C. T., Johnston, S. M., Qi, Y., and Johnson, G. A. (2011c). 4D micro-CT for cardiac and perfusion applications with view under sampling. *Phys. Med. Biol.* 56, 3351–3369. doi: 10.1088/0031-9155/56/11/011

Badea, C. T., Hedlund, L. W., De Lin, M., Boslego Mackel, J. F., and Johnson, G. A. (2006). Tumor imaging in small animals with a combined micro-CT/micro-DSA system using iodinated conventional and blood pool contrast agents. *Contrast Media Mol. Imaging* 1, 153–164. doi: 10.1002/cmmi.103

Badea, C. T., Hedlund, L. W., Mackel, J. F., Mao, L., Rockman, H. A., and Johnson, G. A. (2007). Cardiac micro-computed tomography for morphological and functional phenotyping of muscle LIM protein null mice. *Mol. Imaging* 6, 261–268.

Bartling, S. H., Dinkel, J., Stiller, W., Grasruck, M., Madisch, I., Kauczor, H. U., et al. (2008). Intrinsic respiratory gating in small-animal CT. *Eur. Radiol.* 18, 1375–1384. doi: 10.1007/s00330-008-0903-3

Bartling, S. H., Stiller, W., Grasruck, M., Schmidt, B., Peschke, P., Semmler, W., et al. (2007). Retrospective motion gating in small animal CT of mice and rats. *Invest. Radiol.* 42, 704–714. doi: 10.1097/RLI.0b013e318070dcad

Betzer, O., Shwartz, A., Motiei, M., Kazimirsky, G., Gispan, I., Damti, E., et al. (2014). Nanoparticle-based CT imaging technique for longitudinal and quantitative stem cell tracking within the brain: application in neuropsychiatric disorders. *ACS Nano* 8, 9274–9285. doi: 10.1021/nn503131h

Bhavane, R., Badea, C., Ghaghada, K. B., Clark, D., Vela, D., Moturu, A., et al. (2013). Dual-energy computed tomography imaging of atherosclerotic plaques in a mouse model using a liposomal-iodine nanoparticle contrast agent. *Circ. Cardiovasc. Imaging* 6, 285–294. doi: 10.1161/CIRCIMAGING.112.000119

Boll, H., Nittka, S., Doyon, F., Neumaier, M., Marx, A., Kramer, M., et al. (2011). Micro-CT based experimental liver imaging using a nanoparticulate contrast agent: a longitudinal study in mice. *PLoS ONE* 6:e25692. doi: 10.1371/journal.pone.0025692

Bongartz, T., Glazebrook, K. N., Kavros, S. J., Murthy, N. S., Merry, S. P., Franz, W. B., et al. (2015). Dual-energy CT for the diagnosis of gout: an accuracy and diagnostic yield study. *Ann. Rheum. Dis.* 74, 1072–1077. doi: 10.1136/annrheumdis-2013-205095

Boone, J. M., Velazquez, O., and Cherry, S. R. (2004). Small-animal X-ray dose from micro-CT. *Mol. Imaging* 3, 149–158. doi: 10.1162/1535350042380326

Bourin, M., Jolliet, P., and Ballereau, F. (1997). An overview of the clinical pharmacokinetics of x-ray contrast media. *Clin. Pharmacokinet.* 32, 180–193. doi: 10.2165/00003088-199732030-00002

Bouxsein, M. L., Boyd, S. K., Christiansen, B. A., Guldberg, R. E., Jepsen, K. J., and Muller, R. (2010). Guidelines for assessment of bone microstructure in rodents using micro-computed tomography. *J. Bone Miner. Res.* 25, 1468–1486. doi: 10.1002/jbmr.141

Carlson, S. K., Classic, K. L., Bender, C. E., and Russell, S. J. (2007). Small animal absorbed radiation dose from serial micro-computed tomography imaging. *Mol. Imaging Biol.* 9, 78–82. doi: 10.1007/s11307-007-0080-9

Carril, M., Fernandez, I., Rodriguez, J., Garcia, I., and Penades, S. (2014). Gold-coated iron oxide glyconanoparticles for MRI, CT, and US Multimodal Imaging. *Parti. Part. Syst. Charact.* 31, 81–87. doi: 10.1002/ppsc.201300239

Cervenka, L., Mitchell, K. D., and Navar, L. G. (1999). Renal function in mice: effects of volume expansion and angiotensin II. *J. Am. Soc. Nephrol.* 10, 2631–2636.

Chanda, N., Kattumuri, V., Shukla, R., Zambre, A., Katti, K., Upendran, A., et al. (2010). Bombesin functionalized gold nanoparticles show in vitro and in vivo cancer receptor specificity. *Proc. Natl. Acad. Sci. U.S.A.* 107, 8760–8765. doi: 10.1073/pnas.1002143107

Chen, F., Ehlerding, E. B., and Cai, W. (2014). Theranostic nanoparticles. *J. Nucl. Med.* 55, 1919–1922. doi: 10.2967/jnumed.114.146019

Choi, E. J., Jin, G. Y., Bok, S. M., Han, Y. M., Lee, Y. S., Jung, M. J., et al. (2014). Serial micro-CT assessment of the therapeutic effects of rosiglitazone in a bleomycin-induced lung fibrosis mouse model. *Korean J. Radiol.* 15, 448–455. doi: 10.3348/kjr.2014.15.4.448

Chouker, A., Lizak, M., Schimel, D., Helmberger, T., Ward, J. M., Despres, D., et al. (2008). Comparison of Fenestra VC Contrast-enhanced computed tomography imaging with gadopentetate dimeglumine and ferucarbotran magnetic resonance imaging for the in vivo evaluation of murine liver damage after ischemia and reperfusion. *Invest. Radiol.* 43, 77–91. doi: 10.1097/RLI.0b013e318155aa2e

Chow, P. L., Rannou, F. R., and Chatziioannou, A. F. (2005). Attenuation correction for small animal PET tomographs. *Phys. Med. Biol.* 50, 1837–1850. doi: 10.1088/0031-9155/50/8/014

Clark, D. P., and Badea, C. T. (2014). Spectral diffusion: an algorithm for robust material decomposition of spectral CT data. *Phys. Med. Biol.* 59, 6445–6466. doi: 10.1088/0031-9155/59/21/6445

Clark, D., Ghaghada, K., Moding, E., Kirsch, D., and Badea, C. (2013). In vivo characterization of tumor vasculature using iodine and gold nanoparticles and dual energy micro-CT. *Phys. Med. Biol.* 58, 1683–1704. doi: 10.1088/0031-9155/58/6/1683

Cole, L. E., Vargo-Gogola, T., and Roeder, R. K. (2014). Bisphosphonate-functionalized gold nanoparticles for contrast-enhanced X-ray detection of breast microcalcifications. *Biomaterials* 35, 2312–2321. doi: 10.1016/j.biomaterials.2013.11.077

Cormode, D. P., Naha, P. C., and Fayad, Z. A. (2014). Nanoparticle contrast agents for computed tomography: a focus on micelles. *Contrast Media Mol. Imaging* 9, 37–52. doi: 10.1002/cmmi.1551

Cormode, D. P., Roessl, E., Thran, A., Skajaa, T., Gordon, R. E., Schlomka, J. P., et al. (2010). Atherosclerotic plaque composition: analysis with multicolor CT and targeted gold nanoparticles. *Radiology* 256, 774–782. doi: 10.1148/radiol.10092473

Coughlin, A. J., Ananta, J. S., Deng, N., Larina, I. V., Decuzzi, P., and West, J. L. (2014). Gadolinium-conjugated gold nanoshells for multimodal diagnostic imaging and photothermal cancer therapy. *Small* 10, 556–565. doi: 10.1002/smll.201302217

Cowan, C. M., Aghaloo, T., Chou, Y. F., Walder, B., Zhang, X., Soo, C., et al. (2007). MicroCT evaluation of three-dimensional mineralization in response to BMP-2 doses in vitro and in critical sized rat calvarial defects. *Tissue Eng.* 13, 501–512. doi: 10.1089/ten.2006.0141

Criscione, J. M., Dobrucki, L. W., Zhuang, Z. W., Papademetris, X., Simons, M., Sinusas, A. J., et al. (2011). Development and application of a multimodal contrast agent for SPECT/CT hybrid imaging. *Bioconjug. Chem.* 22, 1784–1792. doi: 10.1021/bc200162r

Curry, T., Kopelman, R., Shilo, M., and Popovtzer, R. (2014). Multifunctional theranostic gold nanoparticles for targeted CT imaging and photothermal therapy. *Contrast Media Mol. Imaging* 9, 53–61. doi: 10.1002/cmmi.1563

Danila, D., Johnson, E., and Kee, P. (2013). CT imaging of myocardial scars with collagen-targeting gold nanoparticles. *Nanomedicine* 9, 1067–1076. doi: 10.1016/j.nano.2013.03.009

David, V., Laroche, N., Boudignon, B., Lafage-Proust, M. H., Alexandre, C., Ruegsegger, P., et al. (2003). Noninvasive in vivo monitoring of bone architecture alterations in hindlimb-unloaded female rats using novel three-dimensional microcomputed tomography. *J. Bone Miner. Res.* 18, 1622–1631. doi: 10.1359/jbmr.2003.18.9.1622

De Langhe, E., Vande Velde, G., Hostens, J., Himmelreich, U., Nemery, B., Luyten, F. P., et al. (2012). Quantification of lung fibrosis and emphysema in mice using automated micro-computed tomography. *PLoS ONE* 7:e43123. doi: 10.1371/journal.pone.0043123

Desnoyers, L. R., Pai, R., Ferrando, R. E., Hotzel, K., Le, T., Ross, J., et al. (2008). Targeting FGF19 inhibits tumor growth in colon cancer xenograft and FGF19 transgenic hepatocellular carcinoma models. *Oncogene* 27, 85–97. doi: 10.1038/sj.onc.1210623

de Vries, A., Custers, E., Lub, J., Van Den Bosch, S., Nicolay, K., and Grull, H. (2010). Block-copolymer-stabilized iodinated emulsions for use as CT contrast agents. *Biomaterials* 31, 6537–6544. doi: 10.1016/j.biomaterials.2010.04.056

Diehl, K. H., Hull, R., Morton, D., Pfister, R., Rabemampianina, Y., Smith, D., et al. (2001). A good practice guide to the administration of substances and removal of blood, including routes and volumes. *J. Appl. Toxicol.* 21, 15–23. doi: 10.1002/jat.727

Dumas, A., Brigitte, M., Moreau, M. F., Chretien, F., Basle, M. F., and Chappard, D. (2009). Bone mass and microarchitecture of irradiated and bone marrow-transplanted mice: influences of the donor strain. *Osteoporos. Int.* 20, 435–443. doi: 10.1007/s00198-008-0658-3

Eck, W., Nicholson, A. I., Zentgraf, H., Semmler, W., and Bartling, S. (2010). Anti-CD4-targeted gold nanoparticles induce specific contrast enhancement of peripheral lymph nodes in X-ray computed tomography of live mice. *Nano Lett.* 10, 2318–2322. doi: 10.1021/nl101019s

Ekdawi, S. N., Stewart, J. M., Dunne, M., Stapleton, S., Mitsakakis, N., Dou, Y. N., et al. (2015). Spatial and temporal mapping of heterogeneity in liposome uptake and microvascular distribution in an orthotopic tumor xenograft model. *J. Control. Release* 207, 101–111. doi: 10.1016/j.jconrel.2015.04.006

Erathodiyil, N., and Ying, J. Y. (2011). Functionalization of inorganic nanoparticles for bioimaging applications. *Acc. Chem. Res.* 44, 925–935. doi: 10.1021/ar2000327

Feldkamp, L. A., Davis, L. C., and Kress, J. W. (1984). Practical cone-beam algorithm. *J. Opt. Soc. Am.* 1, 612–619. doi: 10.1364/JOSAA.1.000612

Feldkamp, L. A., Goldstein, S. A., Parfitt, A. M., Jesion, G., and Kleerekoper, M. (1989). The direct examination of three-dimensional bone architecture in vitro by computed tomography. *J. Bone Miner. Res.* 4, 3–11. doi: 10.1002/jbmr.5650040103

Feng, G., Kong, B., Xing, J., and Chen, J. (2014). Enhancing multimodality functional and molecular imaging using glucose-coated gold nanoparticles. *Clin. Radiol.* 69, 1105–1111. doi: 10.1016/j.crad.2014.05.112

Fiebig, T., Boll, H., Figueiredo, G., Kerl, H. U., Nittka, S., Groden, C., et al. (2012). Three-dimensional in vivo imaging of the murine liver: a micro-computed tomography-based anatomical study. *PLoS ONE* 7:e31179. doi: 10.1371/journal.pone.0031179

Ford, N. L., Nikolov, H. N., Norley, C. J., Thornton, M. M., Foster, P. J., Drangova, M., et al. (2005). Prospective respiratory-gated micro-CT of free breathing rodents. *Med. Phys.* 32, 2888–2898. doi: 10.1118/1.2013007

Ford, N. L., Wheatley, A. R., Holdsworth, D. W., and Drangova, M. (2007). Optimization of a retrospective technique for respiratory-gated high speed micro-CT of free-breathing rodents. *Phys. Med. Biol.* 52, 5749–5769. doi: 10.1088/0031-9155/52/19/002

Galperin, A., Margel, D., Baniel, J., Dank, G., Biton, H., and Margel, S. (2007). Radiopaque iodinated polymeric nanoparticles for X-ray imaging applications. *Biomaterials* 28, 4461–4468. doi: 10.1016/j.biomaterials.2007.06.032

Ghaghada, K. B., Badea, C. T., Karumbaiah, L., Fettig, N., Bellamkonda, R. V., Johnson, G., et al. (2011). Evaluation of tumor microenvironment in an animal model using a nanoparticle contrast agent in computed tomography imaging. *Acad. Radiol.* 18, 20–30. doi: 10.1016/j.acra.2010.09.003

Ghann, W. E., Aras, O., Fleiter, T., and Daniel, M. C. (2012). Syntheses and characterization of lisinopril-coated gold nanoparticles as highly stable targeted CT contrast agents in cardiovascular diseases. *Langmuir* 28, 10398–10408. doi: 10.1021/la301694q

Goertzen, A. L., Meadors, A. K., Silverman, R. W., and Cherry, S. R. (2002). Simultaneous molecular and anatomical imaging of the mouse in vivo. *Phys. Med. Biol.* 47, 4315–4328. doi: 10.1088/0031-9155/47/24/301

Graham, K. C., Ford, N. L., Mackenzie, L. T., Postenka, C. O., Groom, A. C., Macdonald, I. C., et al. (2008). Noninvasive quantification of tumor volume in preclinical liver metastasis models using contrast-enhanced x-ray computed tomography. *Invest. Radiol.* 43, 92–99. doi: 10.1097/RLI.0b013e31815603d7

Guerrero, T., Castillo, R., Sanders, K., Price, R., Komaki, R., and Cody, D. (2006). Novel method to calculate pulmonary compliance images in rodents from computed tomography acquired at constant pressures. *Phys. Med. Biol.* 51, 1101–1112. doi: 10.1088/0031-9155/51/5/003

Guldberg, R. E., Lin, A. S., Coleman, R., Robertson, G., and Duvall, C. (2004). Microcomputed tomography imaging of skeletal development and growth. *Birth Defects Res. C Embryo Today* 72, 250–259. doi: 10.1002/bdrc.20016

Guo, X., Johnston, S. M., Qi, Y., Johnson, G. A., and Badea, C. T. (2011). 4D micro-CT using fast prospective gating. *Phys. Med. Biol.* 57, 257–271. doi: 10.1088/0031-9155/57/1/257

Hainfeld, J. F., Dilmanian, F. A., Slatkin, D. N., and Smilowitz, H. M. (2008). Radiotherapy enhancement with gold nanoparticles. *J. Pharm. Pharmacol.* 60, 977–985. doi: 10.1211/jpp.60.8.0005

Hainfeld, J. F., Dilmanian, F. A., Zhong, Z., Slatkin, D. N., Kalef-Ezra, J. A., and Smilowitz, H. M. (2010). Gold nanoparticles enhance the radiation therapy of a murine squamous cell carcinoma. *Phys. Med. Biol.* 55, 3045–3059. doi: 10.1088/0031-9155/55/11/004

Hainfeld, J. F., Lin, L., Slatkin, D. N., Avraham Dilmanian, F., Vadas, T. M., and Smilowitz, H. M. (2014). Gold nanoparticle hyperthermia reduces radiotherapy dose. *Nanomedicine* 10, 1609–1617. doi: 10.1016/j.nano.2014.05.006

Hainfeld, J. F., O'Connor, M. J., Dilmanian, F. A., Slatkin, D. N., Adams, D. J., and Smilowitz, H. M. (2011). Micro-CT enables microlocalisation and quantification of Her2-targeted gold nanoparticles within tumour regions. *Br. J. Radiol.* 84, 526–533. doi: 10.1259/bjr/42612922

Hainfeld, J. F., Slatkin, D. N., Focella, T. M., and Smilowitz, H. M. (2006). Gold nanoparticles: a new X-ray contrast agent. *Br. J. Radiol.* 79, 248–253. doi: 10.1259/bjr/13169882

Hainfeld, J. F., Slatkin, D. N., and Smilowitz, H. M. (2004). The use of gold nanoparticles to enhance radiotherapy in mice. *Phys. Med. Biol.* 49, N309–N315. doi: 10.1088/0031-9155/49/18/N03

Hainfeld, J. F., Smilowitz, H. M., O'Connor, M. J., Dilmanian, F. A., and Slatkin, D. N. (2013). Gold nanoparticle imaging and radiotherapy of brain tumors in mice. *Nanomedicine (Lond.)* 8, 1601–1609. doi: 10.2217/nnm.12.165

Hallouard, F., Anton, N., Choquet, P., Constantinesco, A., and Vandamme, T. (2010). Iodinated blood pool contrast media for preclinical X-ray imaging applications–a review. *Biomaterials* 31, 6249–6268. doi: 10.1016/j.biomaterials.2010.04.066

Hallouard, F., Briancon, S., Anton, N., Li, X., Vandamme, T., and Fessi, H. (2013). Iodinated nano-emulsions as contrast agents for preclinical X-ray imaging: impact of the free surfactants on the pharmacokinetics. *Eur. J. Pharm. Biopharm.* 83, 54–62. doi: 10.1016/j.ejpb.2012.09.003

Hedlund, L. W., and Johnson, G. A. (2002). Mechanical ventilation for imaging the small animal lung. *ILAR J.* 43, 159–174. doi: 10.1093/ilar.43.3.159

Ho, S. T., and Hutmacher, D. W. (2006). A comparison of micro CT with other techniques used in the characterization of scaffolds. *Biomaterials* 27, 1362–1376. doi: 10.1016/j.biomaterials.2005.08.035

Hori, Y., Takasuka, N., Mutoh, M., Kitahashi, T., Kojima, S., Imaida, K., et al. (2008). Periodic analysis of urethane-induced pulmonary tumors in living A/J mice by respiration-gated X-ray microcomputed tomography. *Cancer Sci.* 99, 1774–1777. doi: 10.1111/j.1349-7006.2008.00889.x

Hsu, J. T., Chen, Y. J., Ho, J. T., Huang, H. L., Wang, S. P., Cheng, F. C., et al. (2014). A comparison of micro-CT and dental CT in assessing cortical bone morphology and trabecular bone microarchitecture. *PLoS ONE* 9:e107545. doi: 10.1371/journal.pone.0107545

Huang, P., Bao, L., Zhang, C., Lin, J., Luo, T., Yang, D., et al. (2011). Folic acid-conjugated silica-modified gold nanorods for X-ray/CT imaging-guided dual-mode radiation and photo-thermal therapy. *Biomaterials* 32, 9796–9809. doi: 10.1016/j.biomaterials.2011.08.086

Hupfer, M., Nowak, T., Brauweiler, R., Eisa, F., and Kalender, W. A. (2012). Spectral optimization for micro-CT. *Med. Phys.* 39, 3229–3239. doi: 10.1118/1.4718575

Hwang, A. B., and Hasegawa, B. H. (2005). Attenuation correction for small animal SPECT imaging using x-ray CT data. *Med. Phys.* 32, 2799–2804. doi: 10.1118/1.1984347

Jakhmola, A., Anton, N., and Vandamme, T. F. (2012). Inorganic nanoparticles based contrast agents for X-ray computed tomography. *Adv. Healthc. Mater* 1, 413–431. doi: 10.1002/adhm.201200032

Jepperson, M. A., Cernigliaro, J. G., Sella, D., Ibrahim, E., Thiel, D. D., Leng, S., et al. (2013). Dual-energy CT for the evaluation of urinary calculi: image interpretation, pitfalls and stone mimics. *Clin. Radiol.* 68, e707–e714. doi: 10.1016/j.crad.2013.07.012

Jeremic, B., Aguerri, A. R., and Filipovic, N. (2013). Radiosensitization by gold nanoparticles. *Clin. Trans. Oncol.* 15, 593–601. doi: 10.1007/s12094-013-1003-7

Jiang, S. D., Jiang, L. S., and Dai, L. Y. (2006). Spinal cord injury causes more damage to bone mass, bone structure, biomechanical properties and bone metabolism than sciatic neurectomy in young rats. *Osteoporos. Int.* 17, 1552–1561. doi: 10.1007/s00198-006-0165-3

Johnson, K. A. (2007). Imaging techniques for small animal imaging models of pulmonary disease: Micro-CT. *Toxicol. Pathol.* 35, 59–64. doi: 10.1080/01926230601184262

Johnston, S. M., Perez, B. A., Kirsch, D. G., and Badea, C. T. (2010). Phase-selective image reconstruction of the lungs in small animals using Micro-CT. *Proc. SPIE Int. Soc. Opt. Eng.* 7622, 76223G.1–76223G.9.

Jokerst, J. V., Lobovkina, T., Zare, R. N., and Gambhir, S. S. (2011). Nanoparticle PEGylation for imaging and therapy. *Nanomedicine (Lond.)* 6, 715–728. doi: 10.2217/nnm.11.19

Key, J., and Leary, J. F. (2014). Nanoparticles for multimodal in vivo imaging in nanomedicine. *Int. J. Nanomed.* 9, 711–726. doi: 10.2147/IJN.S53717

Kiessling, F., Greschus, S., Lichy, M. P., Bock, M., Fink, C., Vosseler, S., et al. (2004). Volumetric computed tomography (VCT): a new technology for noninvasive, high-resolution monitoring of tumor angiogenesis. *Nat. Med.* 10, 1133–1138. doi: 10.1038/nm1101

Kim, H. W., Cai, Q. Y., Jun, H. Y., Chon, K. S., Park, S. H., Byun, S. J., et al. (2008). Micro-CT imaging with a hepatocyte-selective contrast agent for detecting liver metastasis in living mice. *Acad. Radiol.* 15, 1282–1290. doi: 10.1016/j.acra.2008.03.021

Kindlmann, G. L., Weinstein, D. M., Jones, G. M., Johnson, C. R., Capecchi, M. R., and Keller, C. (2005). Practical vessel imaging by computed tomography in live transgenic mouse models for human tumors. *Mol. Imaging* 4, 417–424.

Kinney, J. H., Lane, N. E., and Haupt, D. L. (1995). In vivo, three-dimensional microscopy of trabecular bone. *J. Bone Miner. Res.* 10, 264–270. doi: 10.1002/jbmr.5650100213

Kircher, M. F., and Willmann, J. K. (2012). Molecular body imaging: MR imaging, CT, and US. part I. principles. *Radiology* 263, 633–643. doi: 10.1148/radiol.12102394

Kirsch, D. G., Grimm, J., Guimaraes, A. R., Wojtkiewicz, G. R., Perez, B. A., Santiago, P. M., et al. (2010). Imaging primary lung cancers in mice to study radiation biology. *Int. J. Radiat. Oncol. Biol. Phys.* 76, 973–977. doi: 10.1016/j.ijrobp.2009.11.038

Krause, W., Leike, J., Sachse, A., and Schuhmann-Giampieri, G. (1993). Characterization of iopromide liposomes. *Invest. Radiol.* 28, 1028–1032. doi: 10.1097/00004424-199311000-00011

Kuntz, J., Dinkel, J., Zwick, S., Bauerle, T., Grasruck, M., Kiessling, F., et al. (2010). Fully automated intrinsic respiratory and cardiac gating for small animal CT. *Phys. Med. Biol.* 55, 2069–2085. doi: 10.1088/0031-9155/55/7/018

Laib, A., Barou, O., Vico, L., Lafage-Proust, M. H., Alexandre, C., and Rugsegger, P. (2000). 3D micro-computed tomography of trabecular and cortical bone architecture with application to a rat model of immobilisation osteoporosis. *Med. Biol. Eng. Comput.* 38, 326–332. doi: 10.1007/BF02347054

Laib, A., Kumer, J. L., Majumdar, S., and Lane, N. E. (2001). The temporal changes of trabecular architecture in ovariectomized rats assessed by MicroCT. *Osteoporos. Int.* 12, 936–941. doi: 10.1007/s001980170022

Langheinrich, A. C., and Ritman, E. L. (2006). Quantitative imaging of microvascular permeability in a rat model of lipopolysaccharide-induced sepsis: evaluation using cryostatic micro-computed tomography. *Invest. Radiol.* 41, 645–650. doi: 10.1097/01.rli.0000227494.17444.64

Lee, C. L., Min, H., Befera, N., Clark, D., Qi, Y., Das, S., et al. (2014). Assessing cardiac injury in mice with dual energy-microCT, 4D-microCT, and microSPECT imaging after partial heart irradiation. *Int. J. Radiat. Oncol. Biol. Phys.* 88, 686–693. doi: 10.1016/j.ijrobp.2013.11.238

Lee, S. W., Padmanabhan, P., Ray, P., Gambhir, S. S., Doyle, T., Contag, C., et al. (2009). Stem cell-mediated accelerated bone healing observed with in vivo molecular and small animal imaging technologies in a model of skeletal injury. *J. Orthop. Res.* 27, 295–302. doi: 10.1002/jor.20736

Li, M., Jirapatnakul, A., Biancardi, A., Riccio, M. L., Weiss, R. S., and Reeves, A. P. (2013a). Growth pattern analysis of murine lung neoplasms by advanced semi-automated quantification of micro-CT images. *PLoS ONE* 8:e83806. doi: 10.1371/journal.pone.0083806

Li, X., Anton, N., Zuber, G., Zhao, M., Messaddeq, N., Hallouard, F., et al. (2013b). Iodinated alpha-tocopherol nano-emulsions as non-toxic contrast agents for preclinical X-ray imaging. *Biomaterials* 34, 481–491. doi: 10.1016/j.biomaterials.2012.09.026

Li, R., Stewart, D. J., Von Schroeder, H. P., Mackinnon, E. S., and Schemitsch, E. H. (2009). Effect of cell-based VEGF gene therapy on healing of a segmental bone defect. *J. Orthop. Res.* 27, 8–14. doi: 10.1002/jor.20658

Li, X., Anton, N., Zuber, G., and Vandamme, T. (2014). Contrast agents for preclinical targeted X-ray imaging. *Adv. Drug Deliv. Rev.* 76, 116–133. doi: 10.1016/j.addr.2014.07.013

Li, X. F., Zanzonico, P., Ling, C. C., and O'Donoghue, J. (2006). Visualization of experimental lung and bone metastases in live nude mice by X-ray micro-computed tomography. *Technol. Cancer Res. Treat.* 5, 147–155.

Li, X. M., Wang, L., Fan, Y. B., Feng, Q. L., and Cui, F. Z. (2012). Biocompatibility and toxicity of nanoparticles and Nanotubes. *J. Nanomater.* 2012:548389. doi: 10.1155/2012/591278

Liang, H., Yang, Y., Yang, K., Wu, Y., Boone, J. M., and Cherry, S. R. (2007). A microPET/CT system for in vivo small animal imaging. *Phys. Med. Biol.* 52, 3881–3894. doi: 10.1088/0031-9155/52/13/015

Lin, C. Y., Schek, R. M., Mistry, A. S., Shi, X., Mikos, A. G., Krebsbach, P. H., et al. (2005). Functional bone engineering using ex vivo gene therapy and topology-optimized, biodegradable polymer composite scaffolds. *Tissue Eng.* 11, 1589–1598. doi: 10.1089/ten.2005.11.1589

Lin, M. D., Marshall, C. T., Qi, Y., Badea, C., Piantadosi, C., and Johnson, G. A. (2009). Quantitative blood flow measurements in the small animal cardiopulmonary system using x-ray digital subtraction angiography. *Med. Phys.* 36, 5347–5358. doi: 10.1118/1.3231823

Liu, Y., Ashton, J. R., Moding, E. J., Yuan, H., Register, J. K., Fales, A. M., et al. (2015). A Plasmonic gold nanostar theranostic probe for in vivo tumor imaging and photothermal therapy. *Theranostics* 5, 946–960. doi: 10.7150/thno. 11974

Lu, Z. R. (2014). Theranostics: fusion of therapeutics and diagnostics. *Pharm. Res.* 31, 1355–1357. doi: 10.1007/s11095-014-1343-1

Lusic, H., and Grinstaff, M. W. (2013). X-Ray computed tomography contrast agents. *Chem. Rev.* 113, 1641–1666. doi: 10.1021/cr200358s

Maeda, H. (2001). The enhanced permeability and retention (EPR) effect in tumor vasculature: the key role of tumor-selective macromolecular drug targeting. *Adv. Enzyme Regul.* 41, 189–207. doi: 10.1016/S0065-2571(00)00013-3

Maeda, H., Wu, J., Sawa, T., Matsumura, Y., and Hori, K. (2000). Tumor vascular permeability and the EPR effect in macromolecular therapeutics: a review. *J. Control. Release* 65, 271–284. doi: 10.1016/S0168-3659(99)00248-5

Marin, D., Boll, D. T., Mileto, A., and Nelson, R. C. (2014). State of the art: dual-energy CT of the abdomen. *Radiology* 271, 327–342. doi: 10.1148/radiol.14131480

McErlain, D. D., Appleton, C. T., Litchfield, R. B., Pitelka, V., Henry, J. L., Bernier, S. M., et al. (2008). Study of subchondral bone adaptations in a rodent surgical model of OA using in vivo micro-computed tomography. *Osteoarthritis Cartilage* 16, 458–469. doi: 10.1016/j.joca.2007.08.006

Mileto, A., Marin, D., Nelson, R. C., Ascenti, G., and Boll, D. T. (2014). Dual energy MDCT assessment of renal lesions: an overview. *Eur. Radiol.* 24, 353–362. doi: 10.1007/s00330-013-3030-8

Moding, E. J., Clark, D. P., Qi, Y., Li, Y., Ma, Y., Ghaghada, K., et al. (2013). Dual-energy micro-computed tomography imaging of radiation-induced vascular changes in primary mouse sarcomas. *Int. J. Radiat. Oncol. Biol. Phys.* 85, 1353–1359. doi: 10.1016/j.ijrobp.2012.09.027

Moghimi, S. M., Hunter, A. C., and Murray, J. C. (2001). Long-circulating and target-specific nanoparticles: theory to practice. *Pharmacol. Rev.* 53, 283–318.

Montet, X., Pastor, C. M., Vallee, J. P., Becker, C. D., Geissbuhler, A., Morel, D. R., et al. (2007). Improved visualization of vessels and hepatic tumors by micro-computed tomography (CT) using iodinated liposomes. *Invest. Radiol.* 42, 652–658. doi: 10.1097/RLI.0b013e31805f445b

Mukundan, S., Ghaghada, K., Badea, C., Hedlund, L., Johnson, G., Provenzale, J., et al. (2006). A nanoscale, liposomal contrast agent for preclincal microct imaging of the mouse. *AJR Am J Roentgenol.* 186, 300–307.

Mulder, W. J., Strijkers, G. J., Van Tilborg, G. A., Griffioen, A. W., and Nicolay, K. (2006). Lipid-based nanoparticles for contrast-enhanced MRI and molecular imaging. *NMR Biomed.* 19, 142–164. doi: 10.1002/nbm.1011

Munoz-Barrutia, A., Ceresa, M., Artaechevarria, X., Montuenga, L. M., and Ortiz-De-Solorzano, C. (2012). Quantification of lung damage in an elastase-induced mouse model of emphysema. *Int. J. Biomed. Imaging* 2012, 734734. doi: 10.1155/2012/734734

Nahrendorf, M., Badea, C., Hedlund, L. W., Figueiredo, J. L., Sosnovik, D. E., Johnson, G. A., et al. (2007). High-resolution imaging of murine myocardial infarction with delayed-enhancement cine micro-CT. *Am. J. Physiol. Heart Circ. Physiol.* 292, H3172–H3178. doi: 10.1152/ajpheart.01307.2006

Namasivayam, S., Kalra, M. K., Torres, W. E., and Small, W. C. (2006). Adverse reactions to intravenous iodinated contrast media: an update. *Curr. Probl. Diagn. Radiol.* 35, 164–169. doi: 10.1067/j.cpradiol.2006.04.001

Namati, E., Chon, D., Thiesse, J., Hoffman, E. A., De Ryk, J., Ross, A., et al. (2006). In vivo micro-CT lung imaging via a computer-controlled intermittent iso-pressure breath hold (IIBH) technique. *Phys. Med. Biol.* 51, 6061–6075. doi: 10.1088/0031-9155/51/23/008

Namati, E., Thiesse, J., Sieren, J. C., Ross, A., Hoffman, E. A., and Mclennan, G. (2010). Longitudinal assessment of lung cancer progression in the mouse using in vivo micro-CT imaging. *Med. Phys.* 37, 4793–4805. doi: 10.1118/1.3476454

Ohana, M., Jeung, M. Y., Labani, A., El Ghannudi, S., and Roy, C. (2014). Thoracic dual energy CT: acquisition protocols, current applications and future developments. *Diagn. Interv. Imaging* 95, 1017–1026. doi: 10.1016/j.diii.2014.01.001

Pan, D., Roessl, E., Schlomka, J. P., Caruthers, S. D., Senpan, A., Scott, M. J., et al. (2010). Computed tomography in color: nanok-enhanced spectral CT molecular imaging. *Angewandte Chem. Int. Ed.* 49, 9635–9639. doi: 10.1002/anie.201005657

Pan, D., Schirra, C. O., Senpan, A., Schmieder, A. H., Stacy, A. J., Roessl, E., et al. (2012). An early investigation of ytterbium nanocolloids for selective and quantitative "multicolor" spectral CT imaging. *ACS Nano* 6, 3364–3370. doi: 10.1021/nn300392x

Park, J., Park, J., Ju, E. J., Park, S. S., Choi, J., Lee, J. H., et al. (2015). Multifunctional hollow gold nanoparticles designed for triple combination therapy and CT imaging. *J. Control. Release* 207, 77–85. doi: 10.1016/j.jconrel.2015.04.007

Parkins, C. S., Fowler, J. F., Maughan, R. L., and Roper, M. J. (1985). Repair in mouse lung for up to 20 fractions of X rays or neutrons. *Br. J. Radiol.* 58, 225–241. doi: 10.1259/0007-1285-58-687-225

Paul, J., Vogl, T. J., and Mbalisike, E. C. (2014). Oncological applications of dual-energy computed tomography imaging. *J. Comput. Assist. Tomogr.* 38, 834–842. doi: 10.1097/RCT.0000000000000133

Perera, V. S., Hao, J., Gao, M., Gough, M., Zavalij, P. Y., Flask, C., et al. (2011). Nanoparticles of the novel coordination polymer KBi(H2O)2[Fe(CN)6].H2O as a potential contrast agent for computed tomography. *Inorg Chem.* 50, 7910–7912. doi: 10.1021/ic200587s

Perez, B., Ghafoori, A., Johnston, S., Jeffords, L., Kim, Y., Badea, C., et al. (2009). Dissecting the mechanism of tumor response to radiation therapy with primary lung cancers in mice. *Int. J. Radiat. Oncol. Biol. Phys.* 75, S537–S537. doi: 10.1016/j.ijrobp.2009.07.1227

Perez, B. A., Ghafoori, A. P., Lee, C. L., Johnston, S. M., Li, Y., Moroshek, J. G., et al. (2013). Assessing the radiation response of lung cancer with different gene mutations using genetically engineered mice. *Front. Oncol.* 3:72. doi: 10.3389/fonc.2013.00072

Petersein, J., Franke, B., Fouillet, X., and Hamm, B. (1999). Evaluation of liposomal contrast agents for liver CT in healthy rabbits. *Invest. Radiol.* 34, 401–409. doi: 10.1097/00004424-199906000-00003

Postnov, A. A., Meurrens, K., Weiler, H., Van Dyck, D., Xu, H., Terpstra, P., et al. (2005). In vivo assessment of emphysema in mice by high resolution X-ray microtomography. *J. Microsc.* 220, 70–75. doi: 10.1111/j.1365-2818.2005.01510.x

Rabin, O., Manuel Perez, J., Grimm, J., Wojtkiewicz, G., and Weissleder, R. (2006). An X-ray computed tomography imaging agent based on long-circulating bismuth sulphide nanoparticles. *Nat. Mater.* 5, 118–122. doi: 10.1038/nma t1571

Reuveni, T., Motiei, M., Romman, Z., Popovtzer, A., and Popovtzer, R. (2011). Targeted gold nanoparticles enable molecular CT imaging of cancer: an in vivo study. *Int. J. Nanomed.* 6, 2859–2864. doi: 10.2147/IJN.S25446

Ritman, E. L. (2004). Micro-computed tomography-current status and developments. *Annu. Rev. Biomed. Eng.* 6, 185–208. doi: 10.1146/annurev.bioeng.6.040803.140130

Roa, W., Xiong, Y. P., Chen, J., Yang, X. Y., Song, K., Yang, X. H., et al. (2012). Pharmacokinetic and toxicological evaluation of multi-functional thiol-6-fluoro-6-deoxy-D-glucose gold nanoparticles in vivo. *Nanotechnology* 23:375101. doi: 10.1088/0957-4484/23/37/375101

Roessl, E., Cormode, D., Brendel, B., Engel, K. J., Martens, G., Thran, A., et al. (2011). Preclinical spectral computed tomography of gold nano-particles. *Nucl. Instrum. Methods Phys. Res. A Accelerators Spectrometers Detectors Assoc. Equipm.* 648, S259–S264. doi: 10.1016/j.nima.2010.11.072

Rothe, J. H., Rudolph, I., Rohwer, N., Kupitz, D., Gregor-Mamoudou, B., Derlin, T., et al. (2015). Time course of contrast enhancement by micro-CT with dedicated contrast agents in normal mice and mice with hepatocellular carcinoma: comparison of one iodinated and two nanoparticle-based agents. *Acad. Radiol.* 22, 169–178. doi: 10.1016/j.acra.2014.07.022

Rudyanto, R. D., Bastarrika, G., De Biurrun, G., Agorreta, J., Montuenga, L. M., Ortiz-De-Solorzano, C., et al. (2013). Individual nodule tracking in micro-CT images of a longitudinal lung cancer mouse model. *Med. Image Anal.* 17, 1095–1105. doi: 10.1016/j.media.2013.07.002

Ryu, J. H., Lee, S., Son, S., Kim, S. H., Leary, J. F., Choi, K., et al. (2014). Theranostic nanoparticles for future personalized medicine. *J. Control. Release* 190, 477–484. doi: 10.1016/j.jconrel.2014.04.027

Sagar, N., Pandey, A. K., Gurbani, D., Khan, K., Singh, D., Chaudhari, B. P., et al. (2013). In-vivo efficacy of compliant 3D nano-composite in critical-size bone defect repair: a six month preclinical study in rabbit. *PLoS ONE* 8:e77578. doi: 10.1371/journal.pone.0077578

Saito, S., and Murase, K. (2012). Detection and early phase assessment of radiation-induced lung injury in mice using micro-CT. *PLoS ONE* 7:e45960. doi: 10.1371/journal.pone.0045960

Samei, E., Saunders, R. S., Badea, C. T., Ghaghada, K. B., Hedlund, L. W., Qi, Y., et al. (2009). Micro-CT imaging of breast tumors in rodents using a liposomal, nanoparticle contrast agent. *Int. J. Nanomed.* 4, 277–282. doi: 10.2147/IJN.S7881

Sasaki, M., Chubachi, S., Kameyama, N., Sato, M., Haraguchi, M., Miyazaki, M., et al. (2015). Evaluation of cigarette smoke-induced emphysema in mice using quantitative micro computed tomography. *Am. J. Physiol. Lung Cell Mol. Physiol.* 308, L1039–L1045. doi: 10.1152/ajplung.0036 6.2014

Sawall, S., Kuntz, J., Socher, M., Knaup, M., Hess, A., Bartling, S., et al. (2012). Imaging of cardiac perfusion of free-breathing small animals using dynamic phase-correlated micro-CT. *Med. Phys.* 39, 7499–7506. doi: 10.1118/1.4 762685

Schambach, S. J., Bag, S., Groden, C., Schilling, L., and Brockmann, M. A. (2010). Vascular imaging in small rodents using micro-CT. *Methods* 50, 26–35. doi: 10.1016/j.ymeth.2009.09.003

Schirra, C. O., Brendel, B., Anastasio, M. A., and Roessl, E. (2014). Spectral CT: a technology primer for contrast agent development. *Contrast Media Mol. Imaging* 9, 62–70. doi: 10.1002/cmmi.1573

Schirra, C. O., Pan, D. P. J., Roessl, E., Senpan, A., Schmirder, A. H., Scott, M., et al. (2012). Optimized ruptured plaque detection with ytterbium nanocolloids and spectral CT. *Circulation* 126, A13493.

Scotton, C. J., Hayes, B., Alexander, R., Datta, A., Forty, E. J., Mercer, P. F., et al. (2013). Ex vivo micro-computed tomography analysis of bleomycin-induced lung fibrosis for preclinical drug evaluation. *Eur. Respir. J.* 42, 1633–1645. doi: 10.1183/09031936.00182412

Sheikh, A. Y., Van Der Bogt, K. E. A., Doyle, T. C., Sheikh, M. K., Ransohoff, K. J., Ali, Z. A., et al. (2010). Micro-CT for Characterization of Murine CV Disease Models. *Jacc-Cardiovasc. Imaging* 3, 783–785. doi: 10.1016/j.jcmg.201 0.01.012

Shofer, S., Badea, C., Auerbach, S., Schwartz, D. A., and Johnson, G. A. (2007). A micro-computed tomography-based method for the measurement of pulmonary compliance in healthy and bleomycin-exposed mice. *Exp. Lung. Res.* 33, 169–183. doi: 10.1080/01902140701364458

Shofer, S., Badea, C., Qi, Y., Potts, E., Foster, W. M., and Johnson, G. A. (2008). A micro-CT analysis of murine lung recruitment in bleomycin-induced lung injury. *J. Appl. Physiol.* 105, 669–677. doi: 10.1152/japplphysiol.0098 0.2007

Song, J., Liu, Q. H., Johnson, G. A., and Badea, C. T. (2007). Sparseness prior based iterative image reconstruction for retrospectively gated cardiac micro-CT. *Med. Phys.* 34, 4476–4483. doi: 10.1118/1.2795830

Swy, E. R., Schwartz-Duval, A. S., Shuboni, D. D., Latourette, M. T., Mallet, C. L., Parys, M., et al. (2014). Dual-modality, fluorescent, PLGA encapsulated bismuth nanoparticles for molecular and cellular fluorescence imaging and computed tomography. *Nanoscale* 6, 13104–13112. doi: 10.1039/c4nr 01405g

Taguchi, K., and Iwanczyk, J. S. (2013). Vision 20/20: single photon counting x-ray detectors in medical imaging. *Med. Phys.* 40:100901. doi: 10.1118/1.4 820371

Tepel, M., Aspelin, P., and Lameire, N. (2006). Contrast-induced nephropathy: a clinical and evidence-based approach. *Circulation* 113, 1799–1806. doi: 10.1161/CIRCULATIONAHA.105.595090

Torchilin, V. P., Frank-Kamenetsky, M. D., and Wolf, G. L. (1999). CT visualization of blood pool in rats by using long-circulating, iodine-containing micelles. *Acad. Radiol.* 6, 61–65. doi: 10.1016/S1076-6332(99)80 063-4

Trubetskoy, V. S., Gazelle, G. S., Wolf, G. L., and Torchilin, V. P. (1997). Block-copolymer of polyethylene glycol and polylysine as a carrier of organic iodine: design of long-circulating particulate contrast medium for X-ray computed tomography. *J. Drug Target.* 4, 381–388. doi: 10.3109/1061186970901 7895

Ueno, T., Imaida, K., Yoshimoto, M., Hayakawa, T., Takahashi, M., Imai, T., et al. (2012). Non-invasive X-ray micro-computed tomographic evaluation of indomethacin on urethane-induced lung carcinogenesis in mice. *Anticancer Res.* 32, 4773–4780.

Umoh, J. U., Sampaio, A. V., Welch, I., Pitelka, V., Goldberg, H. A., Underhill, T. M., et al. (2009). In vivo micro-CT analysis of bone remodeling in a rat calvarial defect model. *Phys. Med. Biol.* 54, 2147–2161. doi: 10.1088/0031-9155/54/7/020

Vandeghinste, B., Trachet, B., Renard, M., Casteleyn, C., Staelens, S., Loeys, B., et al. (2011). Replacing vascular corrosion casting by in vivo micro-CT imaging for building 3D cardiovascular models in mice. *Mol. Imaging Biol.* 13, 78–86. doi: 10.1007/s11307-010-0335-8

Varenika, V., Fu, Y., Maher, J. J., Gao, D., Kakar, S., Cabarrus, M. C., et al. (2013). Hepatic fibrosis: evaluation with semiquantitative contrast-enhanced CT. *Radiology* 266, 151–158. doi: 10.1148/radiol.12112452

Voelker, M. T., Fichtner, F., Kasper, M., Kamprad, M., Sack, U., Kaisers, U. X., et al. (2014). Characterization of a double-hit murine model of acute respiratory distress syndrome. *Clin. Exp. Pharmacol. Physiol.* 41, 844–853. doi: 10.1111/1440-1681.12283

Waarsing, J. H., Day, J. S., and Weinans, H. (2005). Longitudinal micro-CT scans to evaluate bone architecture. *J Musculoskelet. Neuronal Interact.* 5, 310–312.

Wang, C. L., Cohan, R. H., Ellis, J. H., Adusumilli, S., and Dunnick, N. R. (2007). Frequency, management, and outcome of extravasation of nonionic iodinated contrast medium in 69,657 intravenous injections. *Radiology* 243, 80–87. doi: 10.1148/radiol.2431060554

Wang, H., Zheng, L., Peng, C., Shen, M., Shi, X., and Zhang, G. (2013). Folic acid-modified dendrimer-entrapped gold nanoparticles as nanoprobes for targeted CT imaging of human lung adencarcinoma. *Biomaterials* 34, 470–480. doi: 10.1016/j.biomaterials.2012.09.054

Wetzel, A. W., Badea, C. T., Pomerantz, S. M., Mistry, N., Nave, D., and Johnson, G. A. (2007). "Measurement and modeling of 4D live mouse heart volumes from CT time series," in *Proceedings of the SPIE 6491*, Vol. 6491, *Videometrics IX*, eds J.-A. Beraldin, F. Remondino, and M. R. Shortis, San Jose, CA, 64910J-1.

Winter, P. M., Shukla, H. P., Caruthers, S. D., Scott, M. J., Fuhrhop, R. W., Robertson, J. D., et al. (2005). Molecular imaging of human thrombus with computed tomography. *Acad. Radiol.* 12(Suppl. 1), S9–S13. doi: 10.1016/j.acra.2005.02.016

Wolfe, T., Chatterjee, D., Lee, J., Grant, J. D., Bhattarai, S., Tailor, R., et al. (2015). Targeted gold nanoparticles enhance sensitization of prostate tumors to megavoltage radiation therapy in vivo. *Nanomedicine* 11, 1277–1283. doi: 10.1016/j.nano.2014.12.016

Wyss, C., Schaefer, S. C., Juillerat-Jeanneret, L., Lagopoulos, L., Lehr, H. A., Becker, C. D., et al. (2009). Molecular imaging by micro-CT: specific E-selectin imaging. *Eur. Radiol.* 19, 2487–2494. doi: 10.1007/s00330-009-1434-2

Xue, S. H., Wang, Y., Wang, M. X., Zhang, L., Du, X. X., Gu, H. C., et al. (2014). Iodinated oil-loaded, fluorescent mesoporous silica-coated iron oxide nanoparticles for magnetic resonance imaging/computed tomography/fluorescence trimodal imaging. *Int. J. Nanomed.* 9, 2527–2538. doi: 10.2147/IJN.S59754

Yao, W., Hadi, T., Jiang, Y., Lotz, J., Wronski, T. J., and Lane, N. E. (2005). Basic fibroblast growth factor improves trabecular bone connectivity and bone strength in the lumbar vertebral body of osteopenic rats. *Osteoporos. Int.* 16, 1939–1947. doi: 10.1007/s00198-005-1969-2

Yu, S. B., and Watson, A. D. (1999). Metal-Based X-ray contrast media. *Chem. Rev.* 99, 2353–2378. doi: 10.1021/cr980441p

Zheng, J., Jaffray, D., and Allen, C. (2009). Quantitative CT imaging of the spatial and temporal distribution of liposomes in a rabbit tumor model. *Mol. Pharm.* 6, 571–580. doi: 10.1021/mp800234r

Zheng, J., Perkins, G., Kirilova, A., Allen, C., and Jaffray, D. A. (2006). Multimodal contrast agent for combined computed tomography and magnetic resonance imaging applications. *Invest. Radiol.* 41, 339–348. doi: 10.1097/01.rli.0000186568.50265.64

Zhou, Y., Chen, H., Ambalavanan, N., Liu, G., Antony, V. B., Ding, Q., et al. (2015). Noninvasive imaging of experimental lung fibrosis. *Am. J. Respir. Cell Mol. Biol.* 53, 8–13. doi: 10.1165/rcmb.2015-0032TR

Zhu, J. Y., Zheng, L. F., Wen, S. H., Tang, Y. Q., Shen, M. W., Zhang, G. X., et al. (2014). Targeted cancer theranostics using alpha-tocopheryl succinate-conjugated multifunctional dendrimer-entrapped gold nanoparticles. *Biomaterials* 35, 7635–7646. doi: 10.1016/j.biomaterials.2014.05.046

Conflict of Interest Statement: The authors declare that the research was conducted in the absence of any commercial or financial relationships that could be construed as a potential conflict of interest.

12

Advancing Cardiovascular, Neurovascular, and Renal Magnetic Resonance Imaging in Small Rodents using Cryogenic Radiofrequency Coil Technology

Thoralf Niendorf[1,2]*, Andreas Pohlmann[1], Henning M. Reimann[1], Helmar Waiczies[3], Eva Peper[1], Till Huelnhagen[1], Erdmann Seeliger[4], Adrian Schreiber[5], Ralph Kettritz[5], Klaus Strobel[6], Min-Chi Ku[1] and Sonia Waiczies[1]

[1] Berlin Ultrahigh Field Facility, Max Delbrück Center for Molecular Medicine in the Helmholtz Association, Berlin, Germany, [2] German Centre for Cardiovascular Research, Berlin, Germany, [3] MRI.TOOLS GmbH, Berlin, Germany, [4] Center for Cardiovascular Research, Institute of Physiology, Charité—Universitätsmedizin Berlin, Berlin, Germany, [5] Clinic for Nephrology and Intensive Care Medicine, Charité Medical Faculty and Experimental and Clinical Research Center, Berlin, Germany, [6] Bruker BioSpin MRI GmbH, Ettlingen, Germany

Edited by:
Nicolau Beckmann,
Novartis Institutes for BioMedical
Research, Switzerland

Reviewed by:
Władysław Piotr Węglarz,
Institute of Nuclear Physics Polish
Academy of Sciences, Poland
Luc Darrasse,
Centre National de la Recherche
Scientifique, France

*Correspondence:
Thoralf Niendorf
thoralf.niendorf@mdc-berlin.de

Research in pathologies of the brain, heart and kidney have gained immensely from the plethora of studies that have helped shape new methods in magnetic resonance (MR) for characterizing preclinical disease models. Methodical probing into preclinical animal models by MR is invaluable since it allows a careful interpretation and extrapolation of data derived from these models to human disease. In this review we will focus on the applications of cryogenic radiofrequency (RF) coils in small animal MR as a means of boosting image quality (e.g., by supporting MR microscopy) and making data acquisition more efficient (e.g., by reducing measuring time); both being important constituents for thorough investigational studies on animal models of disease. This review attempts to make the (bio)medical imaging, molecular medicine, and pharmaceutical communities aware of this productive ferment and its outstanding significance for anatomical and functional MR in small rodents. The goal is to inspire a more intense interdisciplinary collaboration across the fields to further advance and progress non-invasive MR methods that ultimately support thorough (patho)physiological characterization of animal disease models. In this review, current and potential future applications for the RF coil technology in cardiovascular, neurovascular, and renal disease will be discussed.

Keywords: magnetic resonance, MRI, cardiovascular imaging, neurovascular imaging; renal imaging, MR technology, radio frequency coils, cryogenic

INTRODUCTION

For several decades animal models have served a wide span of applications in the life sciences. Transgenic systems have been invaluable for studying molecular signatures and specific cell populations as well as tools for non-invasive reporter gene imaging. Animal models that simulate human pathologies have also been indispensable for uncovering mechanisms behind major diseases as well as the identification of their respective treatments.

A thorough characterization of each animal model remains the crux of the matter. It ensures that the right conclusions are drawn from preclinical studies dealing with questions around pathogenesis and therapy as well as molecular studies that set the groundwork for future therapies and drug design. It is getting increasingly clear that most conditions and diseases, even those with an underlying genetic component, are multi-factorial and complex in nature suggesting that therapy should be equally intricate and versatile. It has been suggested that partial, but multiple, drug actions might be more efficient than a complete drug action at a single target in complex multifactorial disease. This calls for novel drug-design strategies that will depend not only on computational modeling for identifying correct multiple targets but also importantly on more-efficient and high-throughput *in vivo* testing. Further developments in non-invasive *in vivo* imaging in small rodents are necessary to guarantee this, as well as a swift and robust translation into clinical practice. For this to be achieved there is an absolute need for (i) anatomical and function imaging with a superb spatial and temporal resolution, (ii) high reproducibility in results, and (iii) longitudinal studies with sufficient statistical power.

Preclinical Magnetic Resonance Imaging (MRI) is conceptually appealing in the pursuit of basic and translational research as well as for explorations into cardiovascular, neurovascular, and renal disease. MRI has become increasingly important for small animal imaging at multiple levels of pre-clinical research. A growing number of reports manifest the advances for morphological and functional MRI of the heart, large blood vessels, CNS, and kidney. Notwithstanding its success and ubiquity, the relatively low sensitivity of conventional MRI constitutes an impediment for translational research and pre-clinical applications. Constraints common to standard room temperature RF MR detectors include contrast-to-noise-ratio (CNR) and spatial resolution but also acquisition time and signal-to-noise ratio (SNR), which are particular currencies spent for image quality.

In recent years, cryogenic RF coil technology that provides significant improvements in image quality has been made commercially available to small animal researchers. The cryogenic technology substantially increases SNR over standard room temperature RF-coils by considerably reducing thermal noise and signal losses in the RF receiver electronics. This facilitates the acquisition of high spatial resolution images within shorter scan times. The gain in SNR via cryogenic-cooling corresponds to the gain achieved by an equivalent increase in magnetic field strength, but without the extra challenges and costs—which could be prohibitive at extreme ultrahigh magnetic fields.

Recognizing the technical advancement in cryogenic RF coil technology this review attempts to make the (bio)medical imaging, molecular medicine, and pharmaceutical communities aware of this productive ferment and its outstanding significance for anatomical and functional MR in small rodents. The goal is to inspire collaborations across disciplinary boundaries and to attract basic scientists, translational researchers, clinician scientists, and new entrants into the field to advance the capabilities of non-invasive MR imaging through the RF coil

technology. In the sections that follow some of the potential applications for cryogenic RF coil technology are discussed. Neurovascular applications for cryogenic RF coil technology include morphological imaging and functional brain mapping in mice. The benefits of cryogenically-cooled RF coils in supporting MRI microscopy (defined by a spatial resolution <100 μm) *in vivo* are demonstrated; the morphological detail reveals brain pathology in animal models of neuroinflammatory diseases, which opens the opportunity to follow neuroinflammatory processes even during the early stages of disease progression. Examples of MR angiography are presented, especially within the context of neurovascular disease. Early and frontier applications of cryogenic RF coil technology in cardiovascular MRI are surveyed together with the opportunities for high spatial resolution cardiac chamber quantification and parametric mapping; all being facilitated by the traits of cryogenic RF coil technology. Last but not least, the sensitivity gain of cryogenic RF coil technology is put to good use for renal MR microscopy and *in vivo* MRI to support explorations into renal diseases with non-invasive techniques for probing renal perfusion, hypoxia and inflammation. A concluding section ventures a glance beyond the horizon and explores future directions. Of course, MRI of small rodents is an area of vigorous ongoing research, and many potentially valuable developments will receive only brief mention here.

TECHNICAL CONSIDERATIONS

State of the Art

To date, cryogenic RF coils have been developed by making use of either copper or high-temperature superconducting (HTS) material. In this review we limit ourselves primarily to copper cryogenic coils (CryoProbe, Bruker Biospin, Erlangen, Germany) since these are available to a broader spectrum of users. Pioneering HTS coils have been developed by specialized research groups and are not commercially available yet. Although complex to operate, these coils can achieve SNR gains of more than 10-fold as demonstrated in small excised samples at high field (Black et al., 1993) or in the living mouse at 1.5 T (Poirier-Quinot et al., 2008).

Image Quality and Signal-to-noise Ratio

Image quality describes the perceived or quantitatively measured degradation of an image in comparison to its "perfect" counterpart. In MRI this translates into how well the reconstructed image represents the characteristics of the RF signals originating from the excited MR nuclei. Image contrasts are the core information in the majority of MRI applications. Contrasts allow the delineation of morphological structures and pathological lesions (spatial contrast) or the detection of signal intensity changes over time in functional MRI (temporal contrast). Detrimental factors for MR image quality include artifacts and noise.

The SNR is a quantitative metric of image quality with regards to noise. From an MR image SNR is commonly calculated by dividing the mean signal intensity of a uniform region of interest covering the target region by the standard deviation of the noise commonly derived from the background free of signal or artifacts. While high SNRs (>100) allow high confidence in the MR data, low SNRs (<20) mean that the true image characteristics are increasingly masked by noise.

The SNR dependence on MR protocol parameters for a conventional 2D experiment is (McRobbie et al., 2006):

$$SNR \propto \frac{FOV_{\text{FE}} \cdot FOV_{\text{PE}} \cdot \Delta z \cdot F_{\text{sequence}} \cdot \sqrt{NA}}{\sqrt{BW \cdot N_{\text{FE}} \cdot N_{\text{PE}}}} \qquad (1)$$

where FOV is the field-of-view in frequency encoding (FE) and phase encoding (PE) direction, Δz is the slice thickness, F_{sequence} is the appropriate sequence dependent factor [including repetition time TR and echo time TE in relation to the relaxation times T_1 and $T_2^{(*)}$], NA is the number of signal averages, BW is the receiver bandwidth across the image and N is the acquisition matrix size in FE and PE direction. In practice, temporal signal averaging is the most commonly used approach to balance the competing needs for high spatial resolution, high spatial coverage, temporal resolution, and sufficient signal to noise. Yet, signal averaging comes at the cost of scan time when using standard gradient echo or spin echo imaging techniques, without the implementation of acceleration techniques such as parallel imaging or compressed sensing. The square root relation of SNR with the number of averages very quickly sets a limit at which more averages can no longer be justified with a substantial SNR gain due to the severe scan time penalty governed by the power of 2 of the number of averages.

Why Cooling the Radiofrequency Hardware Improves Image Quality

SNR of an MR image is closely linked to the quality of the acquired RF signals it is composed of. These RF signal measurements—like all analog electronic measurements—are degraded by noise, which reduces signal quality and hence image quality. RF coil efficiency relies on overcoming thermal noise induced by conductive samples (Hoult and Lauterbur, 1979). The noise in MR signal acquisitions originates predominantly from thermal (Brownian) motion of electrical charge carriers within the passive receiver electronics (e.g., coil, conductors, passive components) and within the sample itself. Particularly susceptible to noise are those parts of the electronics in which the RF signal is very small, i.e., from the RF coil until the preamplifier output. The contribution of a 50 Ohm preamplifier to the noise cannot be so easily described because of the reactive part of its impedance, though it can be evaluated by acquiring and comparing noise images at different temperatures e.g., at 77 and 293 K (Poirier-Quinot et al., 2008; Vaughan and Griffiths, 2012).

The concept of cooling RF coil hardware to reduce thermal noise was originally proposed in the 1970s by D. I. Hoult and R. E. Richards (Hoult and Richards, 1976), although the first actual application of cooled RF coils in room-temperature samples was introduced nearly a decade later (Styles et al., 1984). The temperature dependency of the SNR can be described with (Kovacs et al., 2005; Junge, 2012):

$$SNR \propto \frac{\omega_0 B_1}{\sqrt{R_S T_S + R_C T_C + (R_S + R_C) T_A}} \qquad (2)$$

where ω_0 is the Larmor angular frequency, B_1 is the effective RF field in the sample volume, R_S represents the so-called magnetic and electric loss in the sample (sample resistance), R_C is the resistive loss in the RF coil and $T_{S/C/A}$ is the temperature of the sample, coil, and the noise temperature of the preamplifier, respectively. Cooling reduces the coil noise $R_C T_C$ and preamplifier noise $(R_S + R_C)T_A$ and directly increases SNR. An additional benefit of cooling the receiver electronics is owed to the decrease of electrical resistances in the conductor (R_C) with decreasing temperatures. Reducing losses within the RF receive chain enhances the SNR.

However, SNR is also dependent on other factors such as frequency ω_0, RF coil geometry/quality (creating the effective B_1) and sample noise $R_S T_S$. Comparing the impacts of coil noise and sample noise on SNR in the context of RF coil size helps to answer the question whether—and under which circumstances—cooling the RF coil is worthwhile. As shown by Junge (2012), the coil and sample noise contributions to SNR at room temperature are of comparable magnitude for a single loop coil with a diameter of approximately 3.0 cm (at 1.5 T) or 1.4 cm (at 9.4 T). For larger RF coils sizes, as commonly used in human MRI, sample noise contributions dominate SNR. For small animal MRI the volumes of interest and RF coil sizes are typically in the range of 1–2 cm, rendering coil noise contributions comparable or larger than sample noise contributions. Although cooling the RF hardware will always reduce noise, the engineering and cost of cryogenic RF hardware starts to pay off only when the thermal noise originating from the receiver electronics is comparable or larger than the noise originating from the sample (patient, animal, object under investigation). It is for that reason that cryogenic RF coils have been developed primarily for nuclear magnetic resonance spectroscopy (NMR; see review Kovacs et al., 2005) using small samples of few millimeter diameter or few cubic-millimeter volume and more recently for small animal MRI.

The theoretical upper limit for the SNR improvement at a magnetic field strength of 9.4 T (f = 400 MHz) is an estimated factor of 2.8 for a transmission line resonator consisting of two planar split rings (with an inner diameter of 14 mm) that are placed on either side of a dielectric substrate, under the assumption of cooling the RF coil from room temperature down to 0 K (Junge, 2012). Cooling the preamplifier has a similar effect on SNR for small samples (Kovacs et al., 2005), but taking a typical preamplifier noise temperature of 15 K with a dominating sample noise ($R_S >> R_C$) at 310 K, the SNR equation shows that the noise contribution from the preamplifier is not that critical. In practice however the SNR gain achievable by a cryogenic RF coil is lower than the theoretical estimate. The RF hardware cannot be cooled down to 0 K. RF coil and preamplifier are typically operated at temperatures around −253°C (20 K) and −193°C (80 K), respectively. Notwithstanding these limitations, an SNR gain as high as 2.5 was reported for *in vivo* mouse brain MRI when comparing cryogenic RF hardware (400 MHz CryoProbe, Bruker Biospin MRI GmbH, Ettlingen, Germany) with a conventional room temperature RF coil setup of similar geometry (Baltes et al., 2009).

According to Hoult and Lauterbur (1979), sample resistance R_S increases quadratically with the Lamor frequency ω_0 for a well-designed RF coil. Thus, it may counterbalance the upper frequency term in the above Equation (2) toward higher frequencies. Higher SNR gains are expected at frequencies lower than 400 MHz and have been indeed reported at 200 MHz using the same cooled copper coil technology (Ratering et al., 2008). The gain becomes even higher when using the HTS coil technology at lower frequencies (Darrasse and Ginefri, 2003): SNR gains larger than 10-fold were achieved at 64 MHz in the living mouse brain (Poirier-Quinot et al., 2008). Thus, the cryogenic technology will be particularly valuable for preclinical studies when used in combination with clinical field strengths.

Cryogenic Radiofrequency Coil Hardware

The first commercial cryogenically cooled RF probe for NMR spectroscopy was installed in 1999 (Kovacs et al., 2005). It took almost 10 years for this technology to mature and to become commercially available for small animal MR scanners. The feasibility and benefit of cryogenically-cooled MRI RF probes was demonstrated for *in vivo* mouse brain imaging at 9.4 T (Baltes et al., 2009). This success built upon the pioneering explorations into cryogenic RF coil designs for biomedical MRI by researches such as Hurlston et al. (1999), Ginefri et al. (2007), Nouls et al. (2008) and the successful development of a prototype for 4.7 T (Ratering et al., 2008).

Modern cryogenic RF hardware employs high temperature superconducting (HTS) materials to dramatically reduce resistive losses (Black et al., 1993; Hurlston et al., 1999; Darrasse and Ginefri, 2003; Ginefri et al., 2007; Nouls et al., 2008; Junge, 2012; not commercially available yet). Cold helium gas has replaced liquid cryogens as cooling media. Simply speaking, Helium gas is compressed in one chamber and then chilled through expansion in another chamber in a closed-loop cooling system—comprised of the RF coil, a cryogenic cooling unit and a helium compressor. The waste heat produced during the gas compression is transferred from the helium compressor to a cold water system via a connected water chiller.

For a review of cryogenically cooled RF coil hardware, we will focus here on the range of commercially available cryogenic RF surface coils for preclinical MRI (CryoProbe™, Bruker Biospin MRI GmbH, Ettlingen, Germany). The RF coil head (CryoProbe; **Figure**   left) is installed at the center of the magnet bore. In this type, a set of torque rods (**Figure**   center) are fitted to the RF probe to allow its tuning and matching from the rear end of the MR system. The preamplifier and the interconnection between preamplifier and CryoProbe are also cryogenically cooled (**Figure**   right). Positioning of the mouse underneath the CryoProbe is facilitated by a dedicated animal cradle (**Figure**   top), which features a warm water heated floor, nose cone with tooth bar and anesthetic gas outlet, ear bars for head fixation, and spacers to adjust the z-axis position of the cradle, as well as a lever system to permit lifting the cradle closer to the CryoProbe once both are fully inserted and the mouse is located below the RF coil (**Figure**   bottom).

Since the introduction of the first cryogenic MRI RF coil the range of CryoProbes is steadily expanding. The initial mouse brain quadrature transmit/receive MRI CryoProbes (for

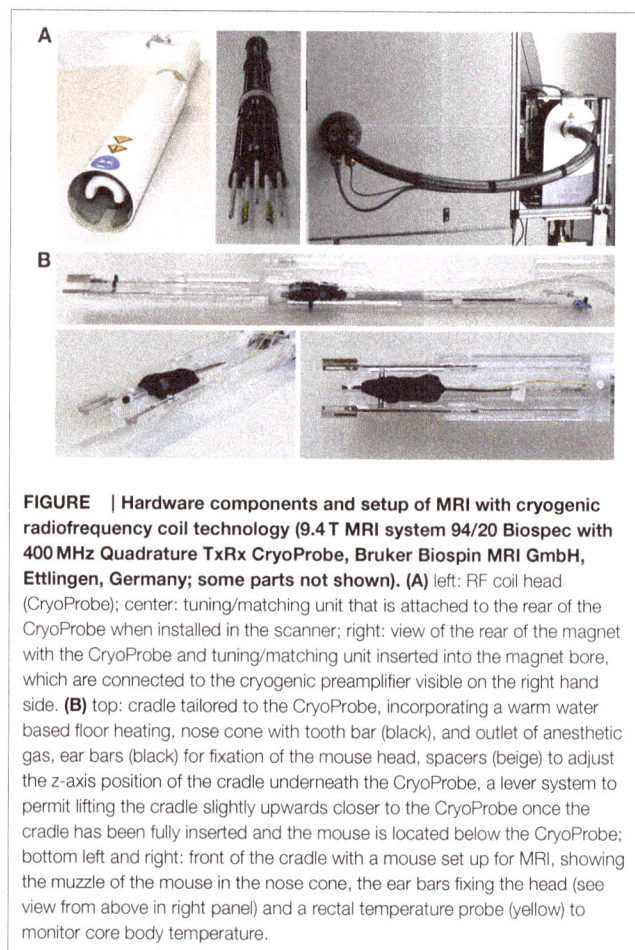

FIGURE | Hardware components and setup of MRI with cryogenic radiofrequency coil technology (9.4 T MRI system 94/20 Biospec with 400 MHz Quadrature TxRx CryoProbe, Bruker Biospin MRI GmbH, Ettlingen, Germany; some parts not shown). **(A)** left: RF coil head (CryoProbe); center: tuning/matching unit that is attached to the rear of the CryoProbe when installed in the scanner; right: view of the rear of the magnet with the CryoProbe and tuning/matching unit inserted into the magnet bore, which are connected to the cryogenic preamplifier visible on the right hand side. **(B)** top: cradle tailored to the CryoProbe, incorporating a warm water based floor heating, nose cone with tooth bar (black), and outlet of anesthetic gas, ear bars (black) for fixation of the mouse head, spacers (beige) to adjust the z-axis position of the cradle underneath the CryoProbe, a lever system to permit lifting the cradle slightly upwards closer to the CryoProbe once the cradle has been fully inserted and the mouse is located below the CryoProbe; bottom left and right: front of the cradle with a mouse set up for MRI, showing the muzzle of the mouse in the nose cone, the ear bars fixing the head (see view from above in right panel) and a rectal temperature probe (yellow) to monitor core body temperature.

4.7–15.2 T MR systems) are now-a-days complemented by four-channel array receive-only CryoProbes (for 7.0 and 9.4 T MR systems), four-channel array CryoProbes for rats, and mouse X-nuclei CryoProbes (for 9.4 T; e.g., ^{13}C, Sack et al., 2014). The latter are used in conjunction with a built-in room temperature ^{1}H RF coil for decoupling and acquisition of anatomical reference images. Finally, the receive-only CryoProbes allow for the use of a room temperature volume resonator for RF excitation, which improves transmission field (B_1^+) homogeneity.

Characteristics of Cryogenic RF Surface Coils—The Pros and Cons

Cryogenic cooling of the RF coil and preamplifier more than doubles the SNR compared with an equivalent RT coil setup. *In vivo* mouse studies revealed typical SNR gains of 2.5–2.8 in the brain (**Figure** ; Baltes et al., 2009, 2011; Junge, 2012), 3.0–5.0 in the heart (Wagenhaus et al., 2012), and 3.0–3.5 for ^{13}C spectroscopy in the brain (Sack et al., 2014). These examples of sensitivity enhancements obtained for 400 MHz (9.4 T) may only serve as a basic reference because the SNR gain depends on the frequency (see equation for SNR and Ratering et al., 2008) and the choice of RT coil against which the performance of the CryoProbe is benchmarked.

In practical terms, a 100% SNR gain by use of a CryoProbe is substantial enough to facilitate an improvement in spatial resolution from e.g., $(100 \times 100)\,\mu m^2$ to $(71 \times 71)\,\mu m^2$ by reducing the FOV. Maintaining the same FOV and acquisition time the spatial resolution can be improved to $(63 \times 63)\,\mu m^2$, as a result of increasing the matrix size (by 58%) combined with a reduction in the number of averages (by 36%). Alternatively an acquisition time reduction by 75% could be attained with this SNR gain via reducing the number of averages.

An SNR gain of 100% is equivalent to significantly increasing the magnet field strength, which is not only more cost intensive, but also comes along with challenges such as increased susceptibility artifacts, disadvantageous relaxation time changes, extra constraints for RF coil design at higher frequencies due to wave length shortening and adverse effects for physiological signals due to the interference with the magnetic field.

A surface coil design CryoProbe is essential to position the coil as close as possible to the object under investigation, to conform the coil geometry to the target anatomy, to keep coil size small and remain within the coil noise dominated regime. Although beneficial for signal sensitivity, an inherent limitation of surface coils is an inhomogeneous distribution in both the transmit RF field (B_1^+) and receive sensitivity profile (B_1^-). **Figure** demonstrates the depth dependence of SNR for a spin-echo imaging protocol. SNR is greatly enhanced by the CryoProbe, but only within a certain range of depth, here approximately 2–8 mm from the surface of the coil. The receive sensitivity profile of the surface RF coil reduces the ability to detect RF signals from locations very close to as well as far away from the RF coil. These variations might be a result of a transmit RF field inhomogeneity of the coil which then translates into a variation in flip angle across the field of view, thereby impacting on the signal intensity and T_1 image contrast. This applies to flip angles of excitation pulses as well as any other RF pulses, such as refocussing RF pulses with the exception of adiabatic pulses. Over a typical field of view of 6–8 mm (perpendicular to RF coil surface) the relative B_1 that is proportional to the flip angle can vary by up to a factor of 2 (**Figure** ; Baltes et al., 2009; Wagenhaus et al., 2012). In gradient-echo images this variability may often go unnoticed. However, in spin-echo images, large deviations from the 90° excitation pulses and the 180° refocusing pulses will eventually lead to inevitable signal losses. Transmit/receive surface coils like most of the CryoProbes require RF power adjustment on a coronal slice (rather than the standard axial slice) which must be carefully positioned to achieve sufficient RF power at larger depths while avoiding signal loss close to the RF coil in spin-echo acquisitions due to too much RF power. B_1^+ inhomogeneity can be largely avoided with the recently available receive-only CryoProbes, which make use of an additional RT volume resonator for RF transmission.

In conclusion, various factors play a role in determining the actual SNR gain, including magnet field strength, MR nucleus, distance to the RF coil, RF power adjustment as well as the MRI acquisition method. The typical improvement in SNR by

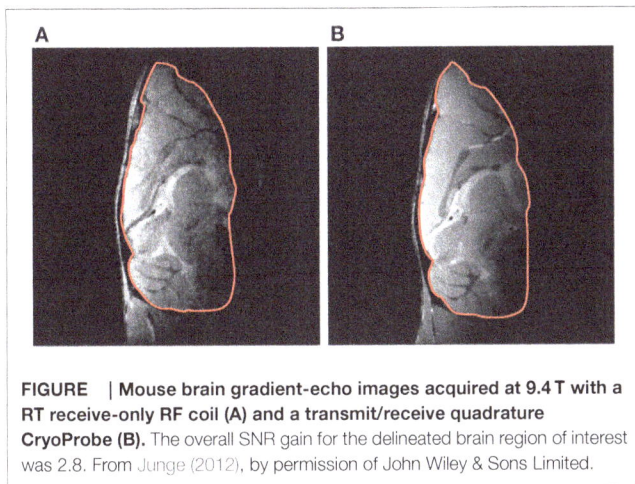

FIGURE | Mouse brain gradient-echo images acquired at 9.4 T with a RT receive-only RF coil (A) and a transmit/receive quadrature CryoProbe (B). The overall SNR gain for the delineated brain region of interest was 2.8. From Junge (2012), by permission of John Wiley & Sons Limited.

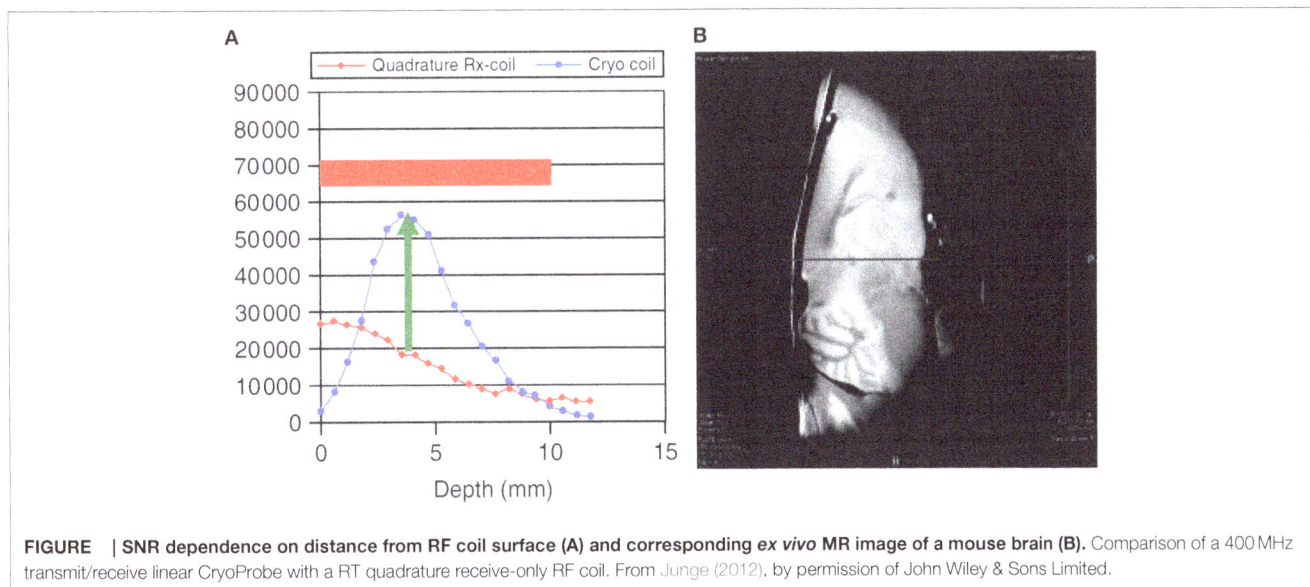

FIGURE | SNR dependence on distance from RF coil surface (A) and corresponding *ex vivo* MR image of a mouse brain (B). Comparison of a 400 MHz transmit/receive linear CryoProbe with a RT quadrature receive-only RF coil. From Junge (2012), by permission of John Wiley & Sons Limited.

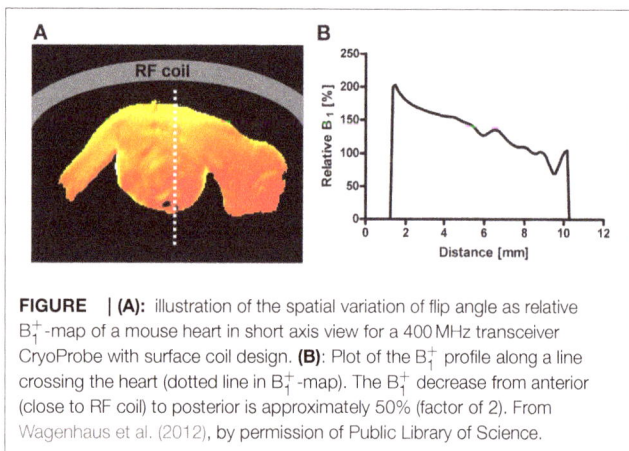

FIGURE | **(A):** illustration of the spatial variation of flip angle as relative B_1^+-map of a mouse heart in short axis view for a 400 MHz transceiver CryoProbe with surface coil design. **(B):** Plot of the B_1^+ profile along a line crossing the heart (dotted line in B_1^+-map). The B_1^+ decrease from anterior (close to RF coil) to posterior is approximately 50% (factor of 2). From Wagenhaus et al. (2012), by permission of Public Library of Science.

commercially-available CryoProbes can be expected to be a factor of 2–3, which can be translated into more than 60% higher spatial in-plane resolution or 75% shorter acquisition time.

NEUROVASCULAR APPLICATIONS

Animal Models of Multiple Sclerosis

The two key benefits of an SNR gain when using cryogenically-cooled coils—namely reduced scan time and/or increased image detail—are fundamental for studying dynamic pathological processes in animal models of disease. In several pathological conditions, especially those related to inflammation and vascular remodeling, an important challenge is to differentiate between hemodynamic alterations, inflammation, and degenerative processes during different stages of disease. Differentiating between pathological processes is essential in chronic neuroinflammatory conditions such as multiple sclerosis (MS) that include an inflammatory, demyelinating and neurodegenerative component. A differentiation between these processes is necessary to make the right therapeutic decision and follow the correct line of treatment for each individual patient (Sinnecker et al., 2012a,b, 2013; Wuerfel et al., 2012; Kuchling et al., 2014).

The histopathological hallmark of MS is the demyelinated plaque, which is associated with perivascular and parenchymal inflammatory cell infiltration and axonal injury (Kuhlmann et al., 2008). MS plaques can occur throughout the CNS; in periventricular and deep white matter, optic nerves and tracts, cerebellar peduncles, brainstem, spinal cord, and also in the gray matter (Sinnecker et al., 2012b). MRI is the most sensitive test to detect and demonstrate MS lesions (Milo and Miller, 2014): while active inflammation is associated with newly appearing, hyperintense MS lesions on T_2-weighted MRI and enhancement on T_1-weighted MRI after contrast agent (Barkhof et al., 1997; Brück et al., 1997), neurodegeneration is associated with hypointensities on T_1-weighted images and indicates severe tissue damage (Van Waesberghe et al., 1999).

An animal model that resembles MS pathology is the experimental autoimmune encephalomyelitis (EAE). EAE can be induced by immunizing different susceptible species of animals

with specific CNS antigen e.g., proteolipid protein (PLP) in SJL/J mice. The EAE model has been indispensable for understanding neuroinflammatory disease (Ransohoff, 2009) and for evaluating the effectiveness of nascent therapeutic approaches for MS (Ben Nun et al., 1981; Steinman and Zamvil, 2006; Ransohoff, 2012). Similarly to MS, lesions that are hyperintense on T_2-weighted MRI are present in EAE brains and correspond to inflammation, demyelination and neurodegeneration (Deboy et al., 2007). Also similar to MS, EAE lesions are distributed in time and space (Baxter, 2007), commonly in the brain stem, midbrain, cerebellum and periventricular area (especially in non-human primates) but also in spinal cord, corpus callosum and cerebral gray matter in small rodents (Verhoye et al., 1996; Hart et al., 1998; Boretius et al., 2006; Deboy et al., 2007; Wuerfel et al., 2007; Waiczies et al., 2012).

Brain MR microscopy is an invaluable tool to visualize succinct inflammatory patterns, even prior to neurological disease in the EAE. The main strengths of cryogenically-cooled coils to boost SNR and thereby provide high resolution MR microscopy and/or reduced scan time are best appreciated in animal models such as EAE that undergo highly dynamic disease profiles. Apart from the established hyperintense lesions on T_2-weighted images (commonly in the cerebellum), focal hypo-intense lesions were identified in the somatosensory cortex of EAE mice, when using high spatial resolution T_2^* and T_2 MRI in association with the CryoProbe (Waiczies et al., 2012). With the cryogenic system, an in plane resolution is as good as $(35 \times 35) \mu m^2$ and complete coverage of the brain could be achieved on both T_2^* and T_2-weighted imaging. With this capacity clear punctate lesions in cerebral gray matter could be revealed in association with intracortical vessels and distributing into the corpus callosum (Waiczies et al., 2012). Thanks to the spatial resolution facilitated by Cryoprobe technology the lesions that were revealed *in vivo* by MR histology could be clearly corroborated as inflammatory infiltrates with hematoxylin and eosin histology (**Figure**).

To gain a comprehensive and longitudinal view of brain inflammation, particularly during the early stages of EAE, MR methods that increase SNR are advantageous not only to increase detail via high resolved brain microscopic imaging but also to reduce scan time. Highly resolved MR images of the whole brain could be achieved in 11 min with the CryoProbe (**Figure** ; Waiczies et al., 2012). By reducing scan time, the number of measurements per individual animal can be increased during progression of disease. Repeated MR measurements are fundamental when making assessments regarding structural changes relevant to the pathology; even macroscopic changes (that do not require highly resolved MRI to be revealed) can be easily revealed. As a result of the reduced scan time and repeated measurements achievable by the CryoProbe, ventriculomegaly prior to neurological symptoms was revealed in the EAE (Lepore et al., 2013).

In the past few years animal models that simulate the neurodegenerative and demyelinating components of MS have been studied independently of the inflammatory component (Ransohoff, 2012). For instance transgenic models involving suicide genes that induce oligodendrogliopathy are powerful

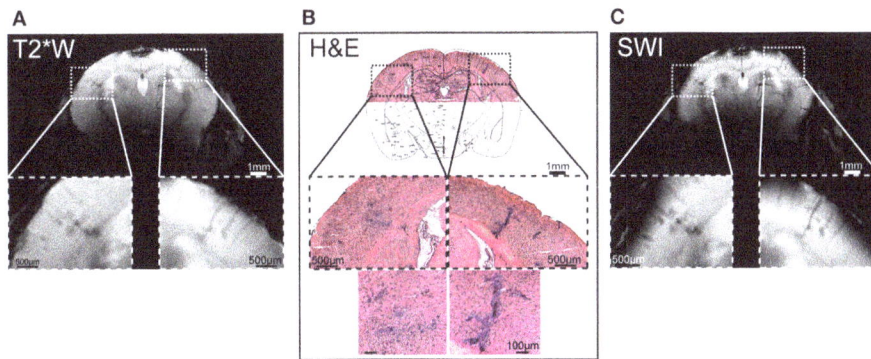

FIGURE | **Hypo-intense regions on microscopic MRI correspond to cellular infiltrates detected by histology. (A)** Coronal T_2^* weighted imaging (T_2^*W) using a multislice fast low angle shot (2D FLASH: TR/TE: 473/18 ms, FA 40°, matrix 512 × 512) sequence with an in plane resolution of (35 × 35) μm^2, 22 slices of 500 μm, acquisition time to image the whole mouse brain = 11 min. **(B)** Cellular infiltrates in cerebral cortex; the overview of the H&E histology is overlaid with a coronal slice (plate 41) from Paxinos and Franklin (2013), by permission of Elsevier. **(C)** Susceptibility weighted imaging (SWI) of T_2^*W scans using fully-automated post-processing by ParaVision 5.1 (Bruker, Ettlingen, Germany). From Waiczies et al. (2012), by permission of Public Library of Science.

tools for studying non-inflammatory demyelination and remyelination (Traka et al., 2010; Pohl et al., 2011). Using a cryogenically-cooled RF coil, pronounced T_2 hyperintensities were revealed in brain stem and cerebellar structures of this model (**Figure**); these changes were accompanied with a decreased magnetization transfer ratio (MTR; **Figure** ; Mueggler et al., 2012). MTR reflects the exchange of magnetization between pools of differently mobilized protons (Wolff and Balaban, 1989), commonly a rather freely mobile pool and a rather immobile pool associated with macromolecules, such as in axonal membranes or myelin (Alonso-Ortiz et al., 2015). MTR correlates significantly with the degree of myelination as shown in postmortem tissue of MS patients (Schmierer et al., 2004). The decline in MTR that was observed in the oligodendrogliopathy model with the aid of the CryoProbe (**Figure**) could be corroborated with evidence of white matter pathology upon histological analysis (**Figure** ; Mueggler et al., 2012).

Animal Models of Cerebral Amyloid Angiopathies

Neurodegenerative pathologies that involve cerebrovascular dysfunction include the cerebral amyloid angiopathies (CAA); these form a major part of the pathophysiology of Alzheimer's disease (AD; Biffi and Greenberg, 2011). Also in this field, transgenic systems and high resolution MR imaging are proving extremely valuable for investigating the role of vascular dysfunction and amyloid deposition in the pathophysiology and treatment of CAA and AD (Klohs et al., 2014). An important role for MR methods is for them to capture vascular remodeling as a result of hemodynamic alterations; this is important when studying the outcome of CAA on vascular integrity and function (Salat, 2014). The cerebral vascular tree can be assessed by different magnetic resonance angiography (MRA) techniques. The signal in time-of-flight (TOF)-MRA depends on the blood flow and is useful for determining changes in the architecture of major blood vessels as well as reduced blood flow in mouse

models of AD and CAA. When spatial resolution is limited, the tissue surrounding vessels also contributes to the MR signal. Originally TOF-MRA was limited to large cerebral vessels with high flow rates; small vessels suffer from both spin-saturation artifacts and partial volume effects and their edges are more difficult to visualize (Lin et al., 1997). The application of a cryogenically-cooled coil system to increase the resolution of TOF-MRA is a key to improve the detection of smaller vessel (**Figure**) in order to help identification of pathologies related to neurovascular disease. The enhanced spatial resolution per unit time introduced by the cryogenic system is key to start overcoming some of the partial volume effects that contribute to loss of small vessel visualization. Using a spatial resolution of $(150 \times 100 \times 100)\,\mu m^3$, flow disturbances at the level of the circle of Willis could be observed in the major arteries of aged animals containing the amyloid precursor protein (APP)23 transgene using TOF-MRA (Beckmann et al., 2003). Administration of superparamagnetic iron oxide (SPIO) particles in association with signal attenuations on three-dimensional (3D) gradient-echo MRI also revealed CAA-related microvascular lesions in different transgenic mouse models of AD including APP23 even at a spatial resolution of $(109 \times 133 \times 300)\,\mu m^3$ (Beckmann et al., 2011). Using a cryogenically-cooled coil system and a spatial resolution of $(60 \times 60 \times 61)\,\mu m^3$, contrast-enhanced (CE) micro (μ)MRA identified age-dependent and CAA-related remodeling of the cerebral microvasculature in arcAβ mice (Klohs et al., 2012). These transgenic mice express human APP and are characterized by strong CAA pathology (Merlini et al., 2011). Using longer san times, CE-μMRA was performed at even higher spatial resolutions of $(31 \times 31 \times 93)\,\mu m^3$ and vessels could be tracked far into the periphery (Figueiredo et al., 2012). Contrast enhanced (CE)-μMRI is expected to complement TOF-MRA (Klohs et al., 2012); after administration of the iron oxide contrast agent, hypointensities not discernable on the precontrast image become visible; these represent intact blood vessels (**Figure**). In this study, CE-μMRA in association with a CryoProbe revealed a reduction in the density of the

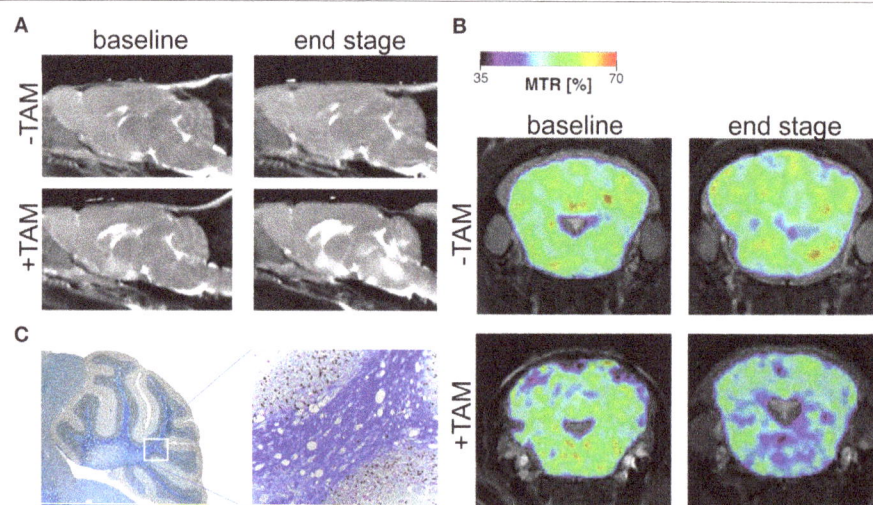

FIGURE | **MRI signature in a novel mouse model of genetically induced adult oligodendrocyte cell death. (A)** Parasagittal, quantitative T_2 maps at baseline (day 2), and end stage (day 41) oligodendrogliopathy following tamoxifen-induced ablation of oligodendrocytes (+TAM) and controls (−TAM). **(B)** MTR maps from representative animals before (−TAM) and after (+TAM) oligodendrocyte ablation at baseline (day 2) and end stage (day 41). MTR maps are color-coded for percentage and superimposed on T_2-weighted images (cerebellum and brainstem section at the level of −2.3 mm relative to Bregma). **(C)** Magnifications of Histological cerebellar sections from end stage diseased animal stained with Luxol-Nissl for myelin content. From Mueggler et al. (2012), by permission of Academic Press.

microvasculature in the arcAβ mouse during advanced disease state (Klohs et al., 2012).

Tumor Models

The summed-up advantages of the Cryoprobe are of significant benefit to visualize the pathology of tumor disease as well as assess the outcome of treatment options. One major drawback of standard clinical tumor imaging is associated with limitations in spatial resolution. This major limitation hinders an adequate delineation of tumor tissue from the surrounding healthy tissue prior to surgical tumor resection and results in the reported brain shift during navigated neurosurgical procedures (Reinges et al., 2004). A thorough delineation of tumor borders could be recently achieved in an animal model of high grade glioma by using a Cryoprobe for acquisition of MR images with an in-plane spatial resolution of 51 mm (Ku et al., 2013; Vinnakota et al., 2013). In these studies tumor MR microscopy was employed to determine the molecular mechanisms behind tumorgenesis as a precursor to therapeutic studies directed toward identified molecular targets.

Angiogenesis and neovascularization are histopathological hallmarks of cancer (Welti et al., 2013). Molecular determinants that pave these processes need to be targeted to overcome the current limitation of standard treatment regimen in reaching malignant gliomas (Agarwal et al., 2011). The tumor vasculature is functionally and structurally irregular and anti-angiogenic therapies aim to normalize this vascular irregularity (Jain, 2005). MR methods measuring perfusion, permeability, and vessel size has been a necessary tool, commonly requiring application of different contrast agents to monitor tumor neovascularization especially as a means of assessing antiangiogenic therapy response (Zwick et al., 2009; Knutsson et al., 2010). Recently,

vessel architectural imaging (VAI) was introduced and exploited to study tumor vessel caliber, hemodynamics, and relative oxygen saturation and used as a determinant of vessel type and function, especially for therapy response, in glioma patients (Emblem et al., 2013). Vessel size imaging (VSI) and DCE-MRI produce complementary information about the tumor vasculature but need to be performed separately due to the interaction between contrast agents regarding magnetization (Beaumont et al., 2009; Zwick et al., 2009). Recently, a cryogenically-cooled RF coil system was used to combine VSI and DCE-MRI in a glioma mouse model; a single shot gradient echo spin echo (GE-SE) sequence was combined with echo-planar imaging (EPI) and one contrast agent was used (Kording et al., 2014). The superior SNR of the cryogenically-cooled coil that made an increase in the receiver bandwidth possible, in combination with careful shimming routines, ascertained that segmentation and geometry between T_2 maps, ADC maps, GE and SE echo planar images (EPI) was not severely distorted (Kording et al., 2014). In this study the distribution of vessel size was shown to be larger in untreated glioma mice when compared to glioma mice treated with anti-VEGF antibody (bevacizumab) (Kording et al., 2014).

Blood Oxygenation Level Dependent (BOLD) Functional MRI

With the increase of SNR in small animal MRI it has become increasingly rewarding to advance upon investigations related to central nervous processing. Functional MRI (fMRI) in mice is a crucial tool to characterize transgenic mouse models of human cerebral pathologies and determine the outcome of therapies on the function of large-scale brain circuits. Functional

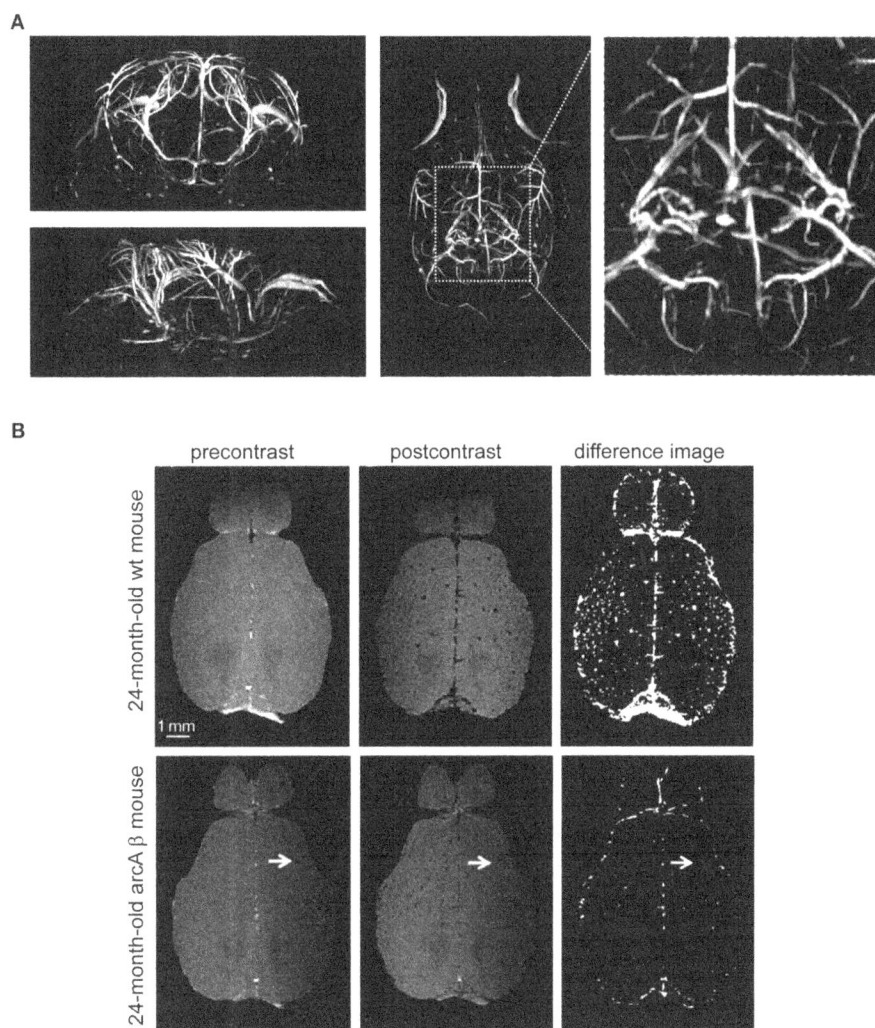

FIGURE | Visualization of vascular structures using cryogenically cooled RF coil technology to provide high resolution time-of-flight (TOF)-MRA and spin dephasing following intravascular iron oxide contrast agent. (A) High-resolution 3D TOF-MRA (axial and horizontal view) of the intracranial and extracranial vasculature of a 2-month-old wild type control mouse using a gradient echo sequence with flow compensation acquired at 9.4 T using the CryoProbe (TR = 30 ms, TE = 5.9 ms, FOV = (30 × 15 × 15) mm^3, 512 × 256 × 256, isotropic resolution = 59 μm^3. From Supplementary Data in Waiczies et al. (2012), by permission of Public Library of Science. **(B)** Contrast-enhanced cerebral MRA of a 24-month-old wt mouse and an age-matched arcAβ mouse before and after administration of a superparamagnetic iron oxide contrast agent. Images were acquired using a 3D FLASH sequence [TR = 150 ms, TE = 2.9 ms, FA = 20°, FOV = (15 × 12 × 2.2) mm^3, spatial resolution of (60 × 60 × 61) mm^3]. Difference images were obtained by subtraction of postcontrast image from precontrast image. The arrows point to focal hypointense areas that are present before administration of the contrast agent. Scale bar: 1 mm. From Klohs et al. (2012), by permission of Elsevier.

MRI takes advantage of neurovascular coupling as surrogate of neuronal activity. Established measuring techniques track local temporal changes in either blood flow, blood volume or blood oxygenation—all shown as positively correlated with firing rates of adjacent neuronal cell populations (Kim and Ogawa, 2012). Most common techniques in human fMRI make use of the blood oxygenation level-dependent (BOLD) effect. Due to different magnetic properties of oxygenated and deoxygenated hemoglobin temporal changes in local field homogeneity can be detected by T_2^* weighted MR techniques. Single shot gradient echo based echo planar imaging (GE-EPI) is commonly applied to meet the requirements on BOLD signal sensitivity and high temporal resolution.

To gain sufficient SNR at short acquisition times of 1–8 s comes at the cost of spatial resolution limits in mouse fMRI. At (ultra)high magnetic fields partial brain volumes are commonly acquired with in plane resolutions of about 190–260 microns and a slice thickness of 500 μm (Adamczak et al., 2010; Baltes et al., 2011; Bosshard et al., 2012; Nasrallah et al., 2014; Schroeter et al., 2014). At these voxel sizes GE-EPI is prone to severe image distortions induced by macroscopic magnetic field inhomogeneities, which increase with field strength. Mostly affected regions are air-tissue boundaries (interfaces of bone, tissue, and air). Gaining SNR by using systems with $B_0 \geq 11.7$ T further increases EPI image distortions (Adamczak et al., 2010). Improving upon SNR by utilizing a CryoProbe permits preserving MR signal in imperiled brain regions. The CryoProbe was shown to achieve a three-fold increase in SNR for GE-EPI at 9.4 T compared to a conventional RT surface coil (Baltes et al., 2011). Leveraging on the sensitivity gain of a cryogenically cooled RF coil permits increases in receiver bandwidth, which facilitates inter-echo time shortening in EPI. This results in an increase in the bandwidth along the phase encoding direction which allows for reduction in EPI image distortion (**Figure**).

Functional brain mapping surveys voxel-wise signal changes over time series of acquired image volumes. Signal and image consistency can be significantly impaired by physical (thermal noise, gradient heating) and physiological noise (cardiac, respiration, vascular oscillations). For mouse fMRI physiological noise is particularly relevant: due to the small body size inner organs like heart and lungs are in close proximity to the receiving RF head coil. Physiological noise (e.g., respiratory induced periodic changes in B_0 field homogeneity) gets amplified with higher field strengths. Temporal SNR (tSNR) considers physical and physiological fluctuations over time making it an important measure for fMRI data quality. Baltes and colleagues reported a 1 to 3-fold increase in tSNR with the CryoProbe over a conventional RT mouse head coil at 9.4 T (Baltes et al., 2011).

Somatosensory studies using the CryoProbe revealed most significant BOLD signal magnitudes in mouse fMRI with external stimuli (Bosshard et al., 2010, 2012, 2015; Baltes et al., 2011; Mueggler et al., 2011; Schroeter et al., 2014). Signal

intensity changes of up to 3.5% were observed in the primary somatosensory cortex for electro-stimulation (**Figures** , ; Bosshard et al., 2010, 2012; Baltes et al., 2011; Schroeter et al., 2014) and moderate noxious heat stimulation (Bosshard et al., 2015) of the murine paw under isoflurane anesthesia. In murine fMRI studies investigating somatosensation and pain commonly anesthesia is applied for ethical and practical reasons (Borsook and Becerra, 2011). Under these conditions BOLD magnitude strongly depends on the applied anesthetic protocol and control of physiological parameters (Schroeter et al., 2014). This makes it somewhat difficult to compare fMRI data obtained with a CryoProbe setup to other somatosensory mouse fMRI studies using conventional room temperature RF coils.

A direct comparison of maximum BOLD signal changes during electrostimulation of the murine forepaw using the CryoProbe compared to a conventional RF mouse head coil was conducted by Baltes et al. (2011). In this study scalp temperature was found to be an important factor influencing the BOLD signal magnitude. To ensure physiological temperatures at the surface of the CryoProbe it features a thermal shield, which can be adjusted in a certain temperature range. An internal heater generates a thermal gradient along the ceramic surface. The shield heating can be adjusted to result in the desired temperature at the scalp-coil interface. In anesthetized mice reduced scalp temperatures promote vasoconstrictive effects ascertained by reduced baseline perfusion (Baltes et al., 2011). Higher SNR

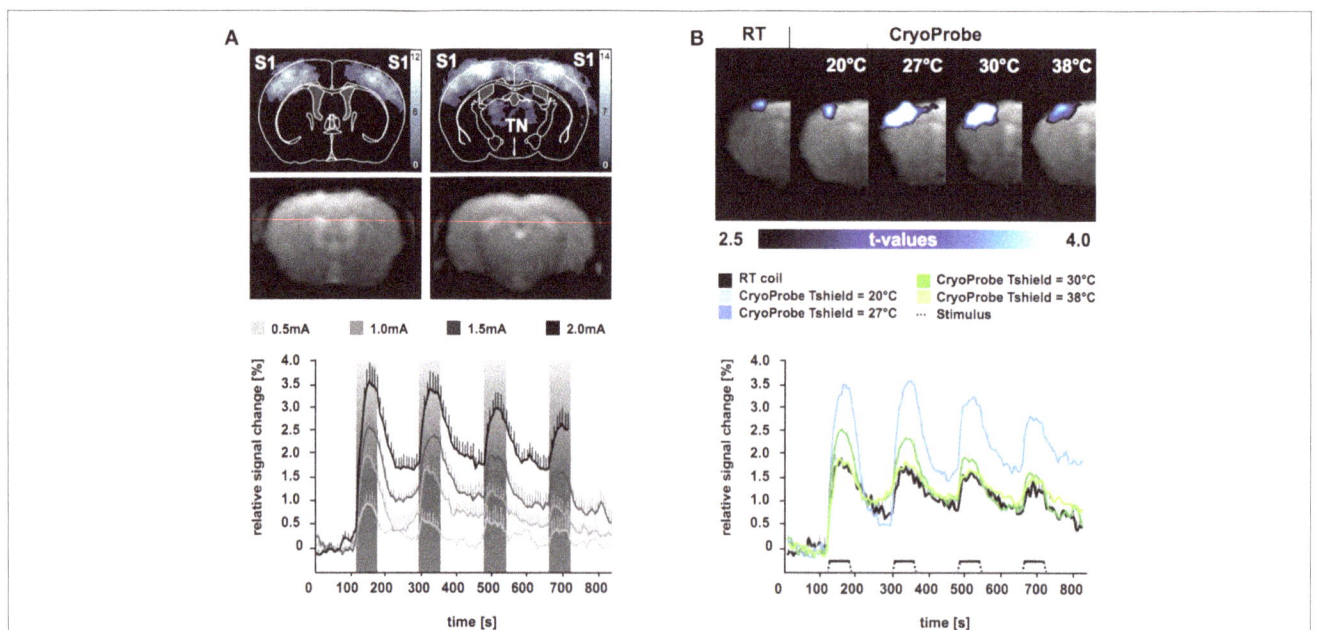

FIGURE | Blood oxygenation level-dependent (BOLD) fMRI significance maps (upper panel) and signal intensity time courses (lower panel) in mice for electrical stimulation of the forepaw during isoflurane anesthesia (1%) and mechanical ventilation. (A) Upper panel shows BOLD significance maps (upper row) for time series acquired using the CryoProbe revealing significant voxel clusters in primary somatosensory cortex (S1) and thalamic nuclei (TN) at 1.5 mA ($p < 0.0001$). Intensity corresponds to the number of animals displaying a significant BOLD signal. GE-EPI images (lower row) reveal only slight distortions. Lower panel shows signal intensity changes over time for significant voxel clusters in S1 during stimulation at 0.5, 1.0, 1.5, and 2.0 mA. Stimulus periods shaded in gray. From Bosshard et al. (2010), by permission of Wolters Kluwer Health, Inc. (B) Comparison of mouse fMRI data for significant voxel clusters in S1 acquired using a room temperature (RT) radiofrequency mouse head coil and the CryoCoil at different thermal shield temperatures. From Baltes et al. (2011), by permission of John Wiley & Sons Limited.

is expected to aid BOLD signal detection but should not alter the BOLD effect itself. At physiological temperatures (T_{scalp} of approx. 33.5°C) maximum BOLD magnitude was found to be similar for the CryoProbe and conventional RF mouse head coil during electrostimulation of the forepaw (**Figure**). Mild cerebral hypothermia (T_{shield} = 27°C) was shown to significantly boost BOLD signal magnitude whereas severe hypothermia (T_{shield} = 20°C) decreased BOLD signal intensity, most likely due to impairments in physiological processes. The temporal noise for baseline measurements was significantly reduced for the CryoProbe for all thermal shield temperatures up to factor 2 compared to conventional RF mouse head coil (Baltes et al., 2011). Therefore, the CryoProbe provides higher BOLD signal sensitivity and might be capable to detect smaller neurovascular changes. The possibility to adjust its surface temperature permits to sustain more physiological thermal conditions in anesthetized mice.

CARDIOVASCULAR APPLICATIONS

In Vivo Assessment of Cardiac Morphology and Function

Realizing that cardiovascular disease (CVD) is one of the leading causes of death (Heidenreich et al., 2011), research in pathologies related to heart function remain at the forefront of academia and pharmaceutical industry. For phenotyping of disease models (e.g., myocardial infarction or hypertension-induced myocardial injury/remodeling), as well as assessment of gender effects, evaluation of novel therapeutics and long-term follow-up studies non-invasive *in vivo* imaging of the heart is conceptually appealing. Cardiovascular magnetic resonance (CMR) is widely used in preclinical studies, the workhorse being an assessment of cardiac morphology and function. For a comprehensive and up-to-date review of CMR in small rodents please refer to Bakermans et al. (2015).

A highly reproducible quantitative assessment of cardiac morphology and function by CMR demands excellent spatial and temporal resolution. Both come at the cost of SNR loss, which can only be partially compensated for by increasing measurement time. Together with the small size of the mouse heart and its rapid motion (typical heart rates are 400–600 beats per minute) these SNR limitations pose serious challenges to CMR in mice. For cardiac chamber quantification and left ventricular function assessment an excellent delineation of myocardial borders, high ventricular blood-to-myocardium contrast and full coverage of the cardiac cycle with high temporal resolution are required. Furthermore, a complete coverage of the entire heart with a sufficiently high spatial resolution to facilitate reliable segmentation of the endo- and epicardial borders is crucial.

Current experimental CMR of mice uses dedicated birdcage volume RF coils or surface RF coil arrays with the geometry adjusted to the anatomy of the mice (Epstein, 2007; Heijman et al., 2007; Hiba et al., 2007; Young et al., 2009; Ratering et al., 2010; Schneider, 2011; Schneider et al., 2011) and affords images with a typical in-plane spatial resolution of 100–200 µm, heart coverage of 6–13 slices of 1.0 mm thickness and measurement

of 10–20 cardiac phases (Epstein, 2007; Heijman et al., 2007, 2008; Hiba et al., 2007; Sosnovik et al., 2007; Young et al., 2009; Ratering et al., 2010; Bovens et al., 2011; Schneider, 2011; Schneider et al., 2011). Although providing acceptable image quality for the quantitative assessment of the left ventricle (LV), further improvement in image quality is highly desirable, particularly for the assessment of the right ventricle (RV). To meet this goal, enhancements in the spatial resolution are essential, which in turn build upon SNR improvements.

An average gain in SNR of 3.6 in murine cardiac MRI was achieved when comparing a CryoProbe at 9.4 T with a conventional room temperature RF coil setup (receive-only four-element mouse heart surface array RF coil in combination with a volume resonator for transmission (Wagenhaus et al., 2012). The SNR gain ranged 3.0–5.0 within the myocardium and could be translated into higher spatial resolution imaging. The highly detailed anatomical images derived from the CryoProbe acquisitions provided significantly improved myocardial border sharpness vs. the RT-coil acquisitions as illustrated in **Figure** . Hard evidence for the benefit of the enhanced image quality was the improved reproducibility of the quantitative morphology and function assessment. Using the CryoProbe, intraobserver, and interobserver variability were smaller for almost all cardiac function parameters. For instance intraobserver variability in end-diastolic mass (EDM), end-diastolic volume (EDV), and end-systolic volume (ESV) were reduced on average by 59 and 66% for the left and right ventricle, respectively. The practical advantage is two-fold. An increased sensitivity will allow an earlier detection of pathological changes as well as a more thorough assessment of therapeutic effects. A smaller statistical variability within experimental groups allows for a significant reduction in animal group size.

Currently available cryogenic RF technology comes along with some challenges for performing CMR. The CryoProbe cannot easily be placed onto any anatomical region of interest since it must be installed inside the magnet bore. Instead, the animal is placed underneath the surface RF coil using a dedicated cradle. This set-up is tailored and well-suited for mouse brain MRI. To use it for CMR requires a special supine positioning of the mouse. Training and practice is necessary to position the heart correctly within the field of view of the CryoProbe. The supine position alters the shape of the RV (see short-axis view in **Figure** and long-axis view in Wagenhaus et al., 2012) but does not impact on the functional parameters (Wagenhaus et al., 2012). In some animals the supine position is accompanied by a difference in motion of the septum, which continues throughout diastole and results in blurring of the endocardial borders of the septum.

Inherent to surface coils is a decrease in signal-amplitude with increasing distance (as explained above). Hence the CryoProbe setup—just like the conventional RT surface RF coil setup—displays a spatial variation in SNR across the myocardial segments of a short axis view (**Figure**), which can be explained with the proximity to the surface coil. Inhomogeneity on the RF transmit side (B_1^+) is usually of little concern for gradient-echo based protocols such as the CINE FLASH commonly used for assessment of cardiac morphology and function (**Figure** ; Wagenhaus et al., 2012). Yet for techniques in which an exact

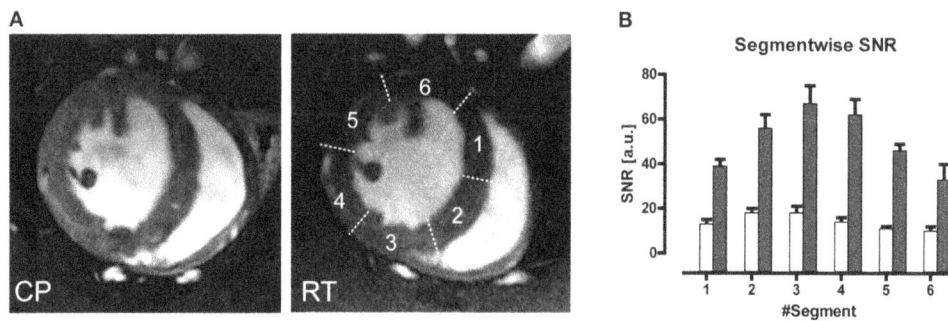

FIGURE | **(A)** Comparison of end-diastole short axis views acquired using a spatial resolution of $(69 \times 115 \times 800)\,\mu m^3$. Myocardial border delineation and depiction of anatomic details for left ventricular papillary muscles and right ventricular trabeculae is enhanced in the CryoProbe (CP) image compared to the room temperature (RT) coil image. **(B)** Bar plot of mean left ventricular myocardium SNR measured in images acquired with the CryoProbe (gray bars) or RT RF coil (white bars) in the different segments of a six-segment model. The segments were numbered clockwise, starting at the inferoseptal segment. The region closest to the coil (segment 3) showed the highest SNR, and SNR decreased with distance from the coil. From Wagenhaus et al. (2012), by permission of Public Library of Science.

flip angle is crucial—such as saturation based T_1-weighted gadolinium-enhanced first pass bolus perfusion studies (Utz et al., 2007, 2008) or inversion recovery prepared T_1-mapping for detection of fibrosis or characterization of myocardial tissue (Messroghli et al., 2003)—B_1^+ inhomogeneity may be an unfavorable characteristic of the CryoProbe. Such cardiac applications can benefit from using a volume resonator for transmission in conjunction with the state-of-the-art receive-only CryoProbe.

In conclusion, cryogenically cooled RF coils represent a valuable means of enhancing the image quality in *in-vivo* CMR of mice. They permit high spatial resolution CINE imaging of the mouse heart with excellent SNR, which measurably improves the reproducibility of quantitative cardiac morphology and function assessment. This is important since segmentation of the myocardium is challenging and prone to introduce significant data variability.

Ex Vivo MR Microscopy of the Rodent Heart

MR microscopy is a powerful tool to get an insight into the micro architecture of myocardial tissue and provides results similar to histology in a non-invasive matter. High spatial resolution and an appropriate organ coverage are both essential. Quantitative techniques like T_2^* mapping, diffusion tensor imaging (DTI) or quantitative susceptibility mapping (QSM) can complement the information provided from common MR contrasts and allow intersubject assessment. DTI or QSM require 3D datasets with high isotropic resolution. Combining the requirements of high resolution MR microscopy with large volume or whole heart spatial coverage already puts a strain on balancing SNR with scan time. T_2^* weighting and diffusion weighting, as needed for DTI or QSM, are also factors that inherently reduce SNR: Sufficient initial SNR is needed, to ensure adequate signal even at long TEs or for strong diffusion weighting. Thus, several features of quantitative myocardial MR microscopy constrain SNR and bring about the need for lengthy scan times to compensate for SNR losses. Even in *ex vivo* scans where acquisition time is by far not as limited as in *in vivo* scans, counteracting SNR

losses by averaging can easily result in days of acquisition time. Unfortunately, this condition is not feasible even in an *ex vivo* setting. Using a cryogenic RF probe helps to balance the competing constraints of high spatial resolution, high spatial coverage and sufficient T_2^* or diffusion weighting in acceptable acquisition times at ample signal to noise.

Figure shows examples for high resolution T_2^* weighted 3D MR microscopy of the fixed *ex vivo* rat heart at 9.4 T. These short and long axis views of the heart were derived from acquisitions using a conventional room temperature birdcage RF coil and a cryogenic surface RF coil (Huelnhagen et al., 2014; Peper et al., 2015). Signal magnitude and corresponding T_2^* maps derived from fitting the signal decay over 5 echo times are shown. Sub-millimeter structures, which can clearly be delineated in images obtained with the CryoProbe, are dominated by noise in the images acquired using the room temperature RF coil. With identical sequence and protocol settings and equal acquisition times approximately a five-fold mean SNR enhancement was achieved in this example when using the cryogenic RF probe. Attributing the SNR increase in this case solely to the fact that a cryogenic probe has been used would not be entirely appropriate since moving from a volume to a surface RF resonator usually goes along with an SNR gain at least in regions close to the RF coil. Notwithstanding this limitation it is fair to state that high SNR level images obtained with the cryogenic RF probe cannot be accomplished with the room temperature probe using the same imaging protocol and scan times. The SNR and signal uniformity implications of the limited field of view and B_1 gradient of the cryogenic surface RF coil can be recognized from the axial images. These non-uniformities can be corrected but might constitute a challenge for sample sizes not matching the coil geometry. If the sample size however, is in the range of the field of view specifications of the cryogenic RF surface coil, high resolution MR microscopy provides images that are comparable with histology, earning heart MR microscopy the moniker of cardiac MR histology. **Figure** illustrates an example of a fixed *ex-vivo* mouse heart scanned in 3D with an isotropic spatial resolution of $55\,\mu m^3$ using a cryogenic surface RF coil at 9.4 T (Peper et al., 2015).

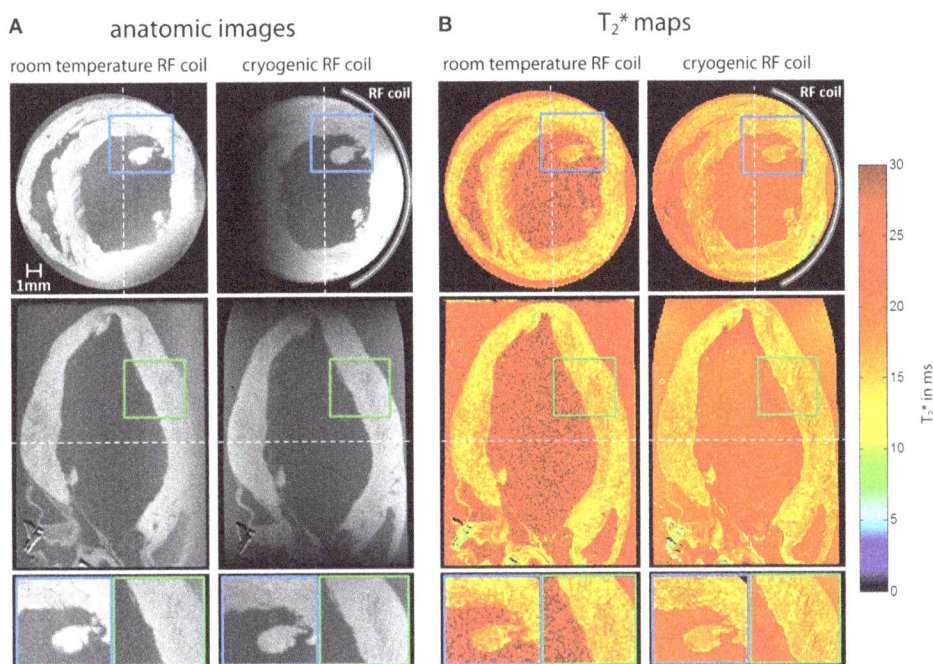

FIGURE | Axial (top) and coronal (center) views of high resolution T_2* weighted 3D MR microscopy images (A) and corresponding T_2* maps (B) of the fixed *ex vivo* rat heart acquired using a room temperature volume RF resonator and a cryogenic surface RF probe at 9.4 T [3D multi echo gradient echo technique, TR = 19 ms, TE = 2.14–13.54 ms, TE spacing 2.85 ms, spatial resolution = (94 × 94 × 94) μm³, FOV = (20 × 15 × 15) mm², acquisition time 12.7 h]. Bottom: Detail views of areas marked by colored rectangles. Dashed white lines mark the position of the slices. Data from Huelnhagen et al. (2014); Peper et al. (2015).

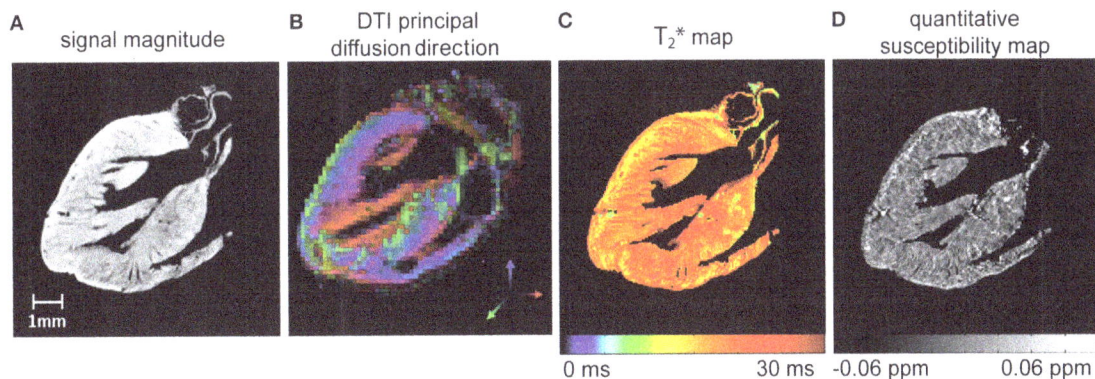

FIGURE | Sagittal slices of high resolution 3D MR microscopy images of the fixed *ex vivo* mouse heart acquired at 9.4 T using a cryogenic RF probe: (A) signal magnitude image, TE = 2.14 ms (B) principal diffusion direction derived from DTI (C) T_2* map and (D) quantitative susceptibility map. Acquisition parameters: 3D multi echo GRE: TR = 250 ms, TE = 2.14–44.96 ms, TE spacing 2.85 ms, spatial resolution = (55 × 55 × 55) μm³, FOV = (10 × 10 × 10) mm³, TA = 13.7 h; DTI-EPI: TR = 1000 ms, TE = 22.84 ms, spatial resolution = (156 × 156 × 156) μm³, FOV = (10 × 10 × 10) mm³, b = 2000 s/mm², 30 directions, TA = 17 h. Data from Peper et al. (2015).

Making use of the SNR gain of the cryogenic RF probe, despite the very high spatial resolution, an SNR of more than 60 was achieved for the first echo (TE = 2.14 ms). Even for long echo times SNR obtained with the cryogenic RF coil is appropriate to accommodate accurate T_2* mapping.

To summarize, MR microscopy of the heart with a high spatial coverage heavily benefits from using cryogenic RF resonators especially when contrast weighting is required, as in parametric mapping or diffusion weighted applications. The benefit is paramount during the characterization and phenotyping of animal models of cardiac disease as it provides a valuable means of getting a better understanding of myocardial microstructure and myocardial remodeling. The value of such improvements are in positive alignment with human MR studies at ultrahigh magnetic fields (Von Knobelsdorff-Brenkenhoff et al., 2010, 2013; Dieringer et al., 2011; Thalhammer et al., 2012; Winter et al.,

2012; Graessl et al., 2014) which strive for a relative spatial resolution (number of pixel per cardiac anatomy) approaching that of experimental MRI in small rodents with the ultimate goal to provide imaging means for diagnostics and for guiding treatment decisions in cardiovascular and metabolic diseases (Niendorf et al., 2010, 2013, 2015a).

RENAL APPLICATIONS

Ex Vivo MR Microscopy of the Rodent Kidney

Hurlston et al. (1999) ventured into an early exploration of ex vivo mouse kidney MR microscopy; their prototype HTS Helmholtz RF probe provided a seven-fold gain in SNR compared to a room temperature Helmholtz RF coil. Using the superconducting coil, the feasibility of renal MR microscopy was demonstrated at 9.4 T with 17 µm in-plane resolution in little more than an hour scan time (**Figure** ; 3D spin-echo, $(17 \times 17 \times 136)$ µm^3 spatial resolution).

The sensitivity gain of cryogenic RF coil technology can be put to good use for renal MR microscopy of glomeruli, the microscopic filtering units of the kidney. Glomerular size and number is thought to be linked to several renal and cardiovascular diseases (Hoy et al., 2008). While established techniques for measuring/counting glomeruli rely on extrapolations made from measurements/counts within small samples (Beeman et al., 2011), a total and direct quantification can be made by renal MR microscopy (Beeman et al., 2011; Heilmann et al., 2012). By exploiting the sensitivity boost of a CryoProbe, Heilmann et al. (2012) were able to quantify glomerular number and size in ferritin labeled rat kidneys ex vivo with a scan of less than 5 h duration. Automatic segmentation of 3D GRE images with $(35 \times 35 \times 35)$ µm^3 spatial resolution yielded glomerular diameters (mean $\pm$ SD = 109 ± 4.9 µm) and counts (mean $\pm$ SD = $32,785 \pm 3117$) with low intra-subject variability in one-seventh of the time required for traditional stereology.

In Vivo Structural and Functional Renal MRI

To date the potential for improving spatial resolution and increasing temporal resolution by use of a CryoProbe for in vivo renal MRI remains largely untapped. The boost in SNR can be expected to be similar to that reported for cardiac applications,

i.e., approximately three-fold (Wagenhaus et al., 2012). Organ size and depth of location within the thorax/abdomen are comparable. The same room temperature RF coils are typically used for both applications, commonly a four-element saddle-shaped receiver (RX) array in conjunction with a larger transmit (TX) volume resonator. In vivo MRI of a mouse kidney is perfectly feasible with a mouse CryoProbe (Xie et al., 2014; **Figure**). However, imaging of both kidneys simultaneously requires a much larger field of view than needed for a single kidney or the heart. The rat CryoProbe may be an attractive alternative as it provides a uniform signal intensity distribution over a larger field of view than the mouse CryoProbe (**Figure**). Objective signal and noise measurements will however still be required since these coils were not originally designed for matching the geometry of the mouse body and for optimized kidney imaging.

The combination of high speed acquisition with almost microscopic spatial resolution is of great interest also in other areas of functional renal MRI, such as T_2^* monitoring, as surrogate for renal blood oxygenation. Parametric mapping of T_2^* with sub-minute temporal resolution is essential for capturing the fast dynamic changes in renal hemodynamics and oxygenation during acute ischemic events or physiological test stimuli (Pohlmann et al., 2013b, 2014a). Comparison with renal MR microscopy images (Xie et al., 2012; Niendorf et al., 2015b) suggests that the limited spatial resolution of current in vivo protocols used for monitoring T_2^* masks some of the underlying intra-layer heterogeneity of renal structure and function. Higher spatial resolution for renal parametric MRI, which puts a strain on SNR, is therefore warranted especially in the mouse. Reduced oxygenation of intrarenal blood can lead to an additional loss of signal, which can be substantial in images acquired at larger echo times. Elucidating ischemia/reperfusion (I/R) injury, a consequence of kidney hypoperfusion or temporary interruption of blood flow—a common cause of acute kidney injury (AKI)—requires fast continuous T_2^*/T_2 mapping throughout baseline, ischemia, early reperfusion, and recovery (Pohlmann et al., 2013b) and hence benefits from scan acceleration using parallel imaging strategies. To this end, the SNR gain offered by a multi-channel receive cryogenic RF coil array is instrumental for compensating noise amplification inherent to parallel imaging (Niendorf and Sodickson, 2006a,b, 2008). The speed gain is of benefit in preclinical renal MRI studies where multiple parameters are assessed by multiple modalities including (i) quantitative physiological measurements such as renal perfusion pressure, renal blood flow, local cortical and medullary tissue pO_2 and blood flux and, (ii) comprehensive MRI protocols with tight spatio-temporal resolution constraints dictated by renal (patho)physiology and the interleaving with the quantitative physiological measurements (Pohlmann et al., 2014a). For all these reasons, cryogenic RF coil technology holds great potential for enabling non-invasive in vivo investigations into renal hemodynamics and oxygenation with MRI. Conventional methods for assessing renal hemodynamics and oxygenation such as fiber-optical pO_2 probes or ultrasonic flow probes provide quantitative physiological data, but are invasive and the

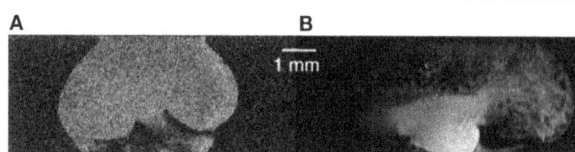

FIGURE | **Early proof-of-concept for renal MR microscopy at 9.4 T with 17 µm in-plane resolution. (A)** Room temperature Helmholtz RF coil. **(B)** High-temperature superconducting Helmholtz RF probe. From Hurlston et al. (1999) by permission of John Wiley & Sons Limited.

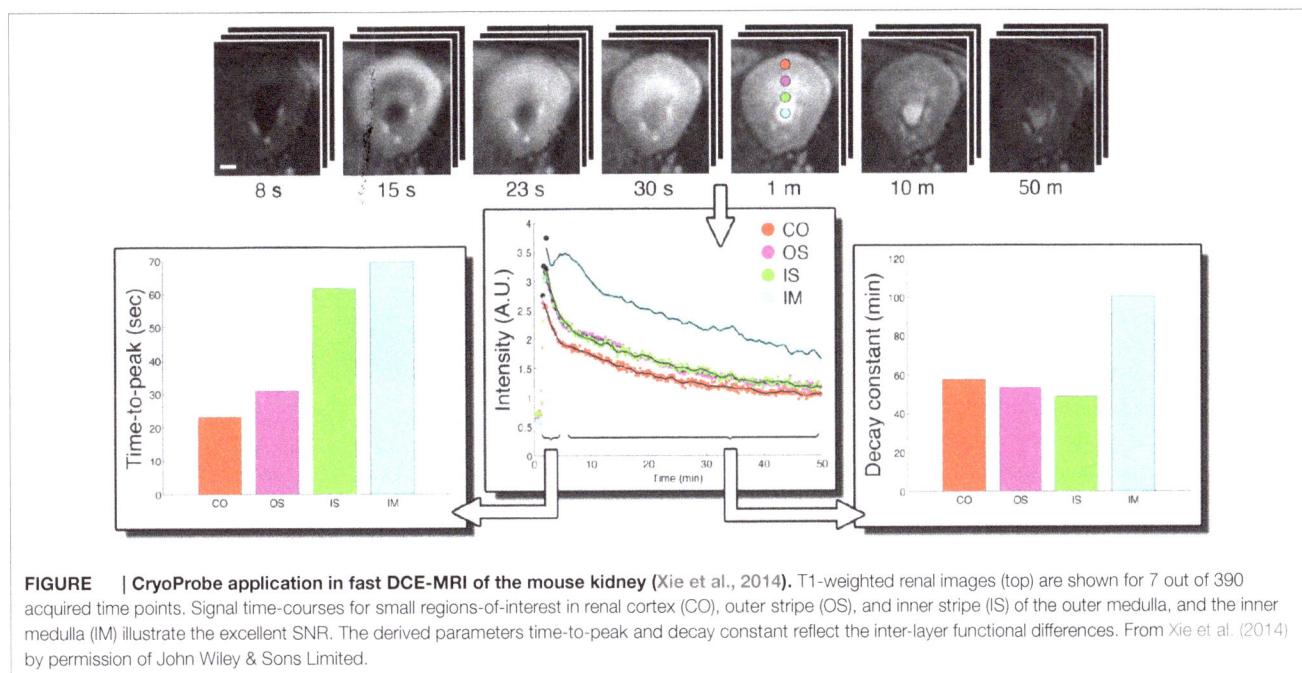

FIGURE | **CryoProbe application in fast DCE-MRI of the mouse kidney** (Xie et al., 2014). T1-weighted renal images (top) are shown for 7 out of 390 acquired time points. Signal time-courses for small regions-of-interest in renal cortex (CO), outer stripe (OS), and inner stripe (IS) of the outer medulla, and the inner medulla (IM) illustrate the excellent SNR. The derived parameters time-to-peak and decay constant reflect the inter-layer functional differences. From Xie et al. (2014) by permission of John Wiley & Sons Limited.

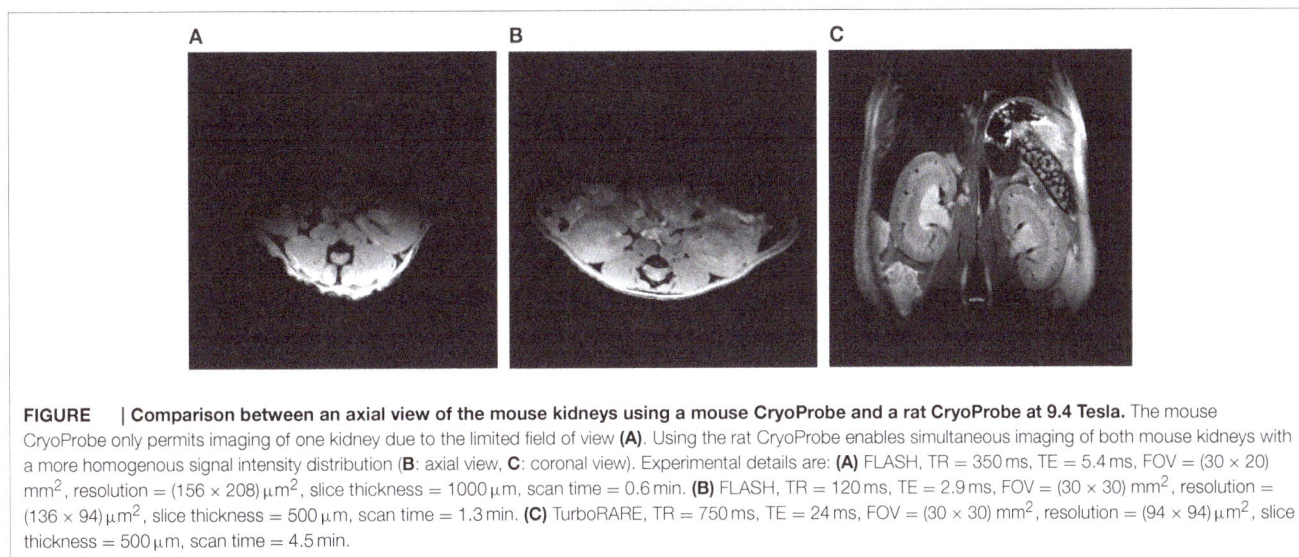

FIGURE | **Comparison between an axial view of the mouse kidneys using a mouse CryoProbe and a rat CryoProbe at 9.4 Tesla.** The mouse CryoProbe only permits imaging of one kidney due to the limited field of view (**A**). Using the rat CryoProbe enables simultaneous imaging of both mouse kidneys with a more homogenous signal intensity distribution (**B**: axial view, **C**: coronal view). Experimental details are: (**A**) FLASH, TR = 350 ms, TE = 5.4 ms, FOV = (30 × 20) mm^2, resolution = (156 × 208) μm^2, slice thickness = 1000 μm, scan time = 0.6 min. (**B**) FLASH, TR = 120 ms, TE = 2.9 ms, FOV = (30 × 30) mm^2, resolution = (136 × 94) μm^2, slice thickness = 500 μm, scan time = 1.3 min. (**C**) TurboRARE, TR = 750 ms, TE = 24 ms, FOV = (30 × 30) mm^2, resolution = (94 × 94) μm^2, slice thickness = 500 μm, scan time = 4.5 min.

fiber probes enable measurements in pin-point locations only (Arakelyan et al., 2013; Pohlmann et al., 2013a).

Assessing Renal Perfusion, Oxygenation, or Inflammatory Cell Infiltration Using Fluorine (^{19}F) MRI

Renal tissue hypoxia and inflammatory mechanisms play prominent roles in the pathophysiological chain of events that lead to acute kidney injury and promotes progression from acute injury to chronic kidney disease. Dependent on disease etiology, the contribution and impact of inflammatory mechanisms may vary (Chawla et al., 2014). Inflammatory processes, including early responses dominated by the innate immune system as well as later responses by the adaptive immune system, can support repair and restoration of renal functions but may also promote renal tissue injury and transition to chronic disease (Bonventre and Yang, 2011; Kinsey and Okusa, 2014; Molitoris, 2014).

Acute kidney injury can also trigger a systemic immune response that may lead to secondary dysfunction of organs such as heart, brain, and lung (Grams and Rabb, 2012). Alternatively, systemic immune diseases can have a crucial impact on the kidney e.g., antineutrophil cytoplasmic antibody (ANCA)-associated vasculitis often affects the kidneys leading to rapid-progressive glomerulonephritis (Schreiber and Choi, 2015).

Renal blood volume, blood oxygenation, and inflammatory cell migration can be assessed and monitored using cutting-edge ^{19}F MR techniques (Ruiz-Cabello et al., 2011; Hu et al., 2014). MRI of x-nuclei suffers from an inherently low SNR due to limited MR sensitivity (^{19}F ≈ ^{1}H) but also a low abundance of nuclei in the tissue of interest. Indeed, ^{19}F is virtually absent in the living tissues of rodents and the ^{19}F signal is created by injection of exogenous ^{19}F contrast agents. A commonly used variant of such ^{19}F agents is perfluorocarbon (PFC) (Ruiz-Cabello et al., 2011), which can be used to label inflammatory cells *in vivo* after systemic application (Waiczies et al., 2013) or track specific immune cells *in vivo* after *in vitro* labeling (Ahrens et al., 2005; Waiczies et al., 2011).

Systemic i.v. administration of ^{19}F nanoparticles (droplet emulsion) results in uptake and self-labeling by phagocytic immune cells e.g., macrophages, neutrophils or dendritic cells. Application of these nanoparticles to an ANCA-induced glomerulonephritis model demonstrated a significant ^{19}F MRI signal in the kidney (in contrast to kidneys of control animals that showed negligible signal). This method provides an *in vivo* depiction of renal inflammatory cell dynamics (**Figure** ; Pohlmann et al., 2014b).

Yet, the rather low spatial resolution of (0.94 × 0.94 × 1.88) mm^3 and required acquisition time of almost an hour leave a lot to be desired. Here the low SNR is a fundamental factor that is restricting the capabilities of ^{19}F MR in rodents. SNR negatively correlates to the detection limit for ^{19}F labeled cells. Applications in which harvested immune cells are labeled *in vitro* and re-applied to an animal have an even greater need for high sensitivity because in this case the number of labeled cells in the region of interest is much smaller (Waiczies et al., 2013).

Noteworthy for ^{19}F MRI, a gain in SNR of 3.0–3.5 for the ^{13}C CryoProbe (Sack et al., 2014) and 2.5 for the ^{1}H CryoProbe (Baltes et al., 2009) were reported at 9.4 T. Considering the close proximity of ^{19}F and ^{1}H frequency, an SNR gain of at least 2.5 will be expected for a ^{19}F CryoProbe at 9.4 T, a gain that would permit an enhanced spatio-temporal resolution of preclinical ^{19}F MRI and pave the way for better detection and more efficient tracking of cellular therapies such as dendritic cells that are used in a variety of cancers. With a technology that provides better detection of cells, even in far reaching organs, the best cell therapy solutions for pathologies such as recalcitrant cancers can be determined more efficiently and swiftly. These therapeutic solutions in combination with advanced clinical imaging technologies can ultimately be translated to the clinic and incorporated into personalized medicine.

OUTLOOK

The cryogenic RF coil technology has introduced significant advancements to small animal MR image acquisition in different areas of disease research. With the ever increasing clinical needs and research explorations looming over the MR horizon, further innovations in association with this technology are nevertheless likely to be expected. The opportunity of increasing sensitivity as well as spectral, spatial, and temporal resolution as a result of increased SNR with the cryogenic RF coil technology opens

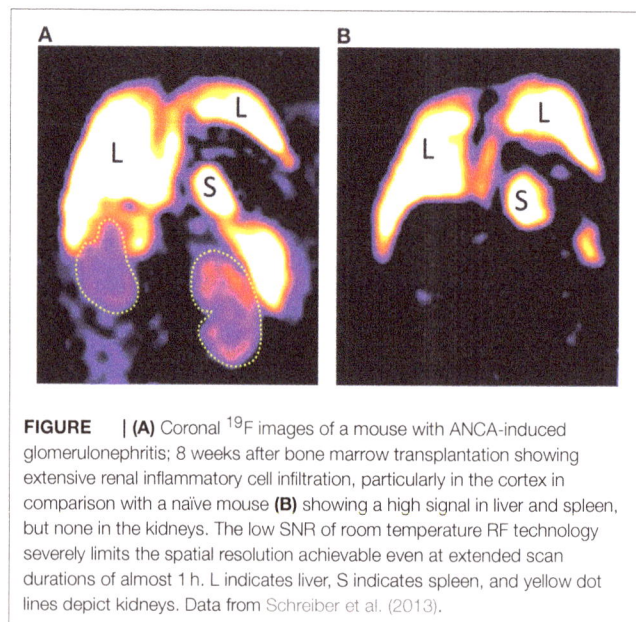

FIGURE | **(A)** Coronal ^{19}F images of a mouse with ANCA-induced glomerulonephritis; 8 weeks after bone marrow transplantation showing extensive renal inflammatory cell infiltration, particularly in the cortex in comparison with a naïve mouse **(B)** showing a high signal in liver and spleen, but none in the kidneys. The low SNR of room temperature RF technology severely limits the spatial resolution achievable even at extended scan durations of almost 1 h. L indicates liver, S indicates spleen, and yellow dot lines depict kidneys. Data from Schreiber et al. (2013).

up more prospects for advancing evolving MR techniques in spectroscopy (MRS), imaging (MRI), or spectroscopic imaging (MRSI). MR methods for studying the detection and distribution of metabolites containing proton (^{1}H) and x-nuclei e.g., carbon (^{13}C), oxygen (^{17}O), sodium (^{23}Na), and phosphorous (^{31}P) will benefit immensely from the introduction of cryogenically-cooled coils. In addition to the increased SNR, which is particularly favorable for nuclei with a relatively low biological abundance (e.g., ^{13}C, ^{23}Na, ^{31}P), better spectral resolutions are expected to reveal metabolites that have until now remained undetected, keeping in mind that resolution comes at a cost in SNR. Another evolving field that will benefit from cryogenically cooled RF coils is functional MRS (fMRS), which when used in conjunction with BOLD fMRI will be invaluable to study changes in resting and activation states in the brain. MRSI employing high-speed echo-planar encoding will also benefit from sensitivity gains to spatially map multiple tissue metabolite signals *in vivo*.

A gain in sensitivity and resolution that can be delivered by cryogenically cooled RF coils can be attained by increasing magnetic field (B$_0$) strengths, but the side effects and costs associated with higher B$_0$ are in such a case non-existent. Challenging adverse effects of higher B$_0$ (that can be eliminated with cryogenic RF coil cooling at lower fields) include saturation-related signal losses due to longer T1 relaxation times, shorter echo time acquisitions to compensate for sensitivity losses due to shorter T$_2$ relaxation times and line broadening or off-resonant effects due to B$_0$ susceptibility effects. For small animal imaging, cryogenically cooled RF coils would benefit from small cryogen-liquid free magnets systems with variable field operation and automatic field ramping. These MR systems can be operated at magnetic field strengths of 1.5, 3.0, or 7.0 T and hence provide opportunities for harmonizing basic with translational research. The installation and maintenance of such MR systems is affordable and thus ideal for preclinical research. Equipped with one cryogenically cooled RF coil such MR systems with cryogenic

Advancing Cardiovascular, Neurovascular, and Renal Magnetic Resonance Imaging in Small Rodents...

191

liquid-free magnets will be an invaluable technology for disease phenotyping, multi-modal imaging as well as for spanning of an assortment of x-nuclei for metabolic, molecular, and cellular imaging.

The benefits of the cryogenically-cooled RF coil technologies are in positive alignment with our human MR studies at ultrahigh B_0 fields, which strive for the spatial resolution used in experimental small animal MRI, but necessitate complex techniques (such as volume-selective higher-order B_0 shimming and phase correction strategies) to counterbalance the B_0 adverse effects. Considering the advantages of cryogenically cooled RF coils and the expected immense application for human studies a swift clinical translation is warranted. For starters, tremendous sensitivity gains will be expected when using smaller cryogenically cooled coils in association with higher B_0; the stronger magnetic coupling between small coil and sample is attributed to higher signal sensitivities and the smaller volume of tissue seen by smaller coils is attributed to lower noise. MR applications that will particularly benefit from cryogenically-cooled RF coil systems, particularly at UHF strengths, are diffusion weighted imaging (DWI) methods employing stronger diffusion-weighting (b-values > 2000 s/mm^{-2}) in order to demonstrate the biexponential decay of brain diffusion, and better differentiate between different water compartments, especially during ischaemic and other brain pathology (Norris and Niendorf, 1995; Dijkhuizen et al., 1996; Niendorf et al., 1996). Although higher b-values yield higher diffusion contrast, lower SNR is expected on heavily diffusion-weighted images, such that cryogenically-cooled coils will surely be invaluable for this application. Alternatively, the SNR gain inherent to cryogenically-cooled RF coils could be transferred into using a larger range of diffusion weighting, which would be of great benefit for *in vivo* explorations into the biophysics of water diffusion in tissue (Niendorf et al., 1994; Norris et al., 1994; Pyatigorskaya et al., 2014; Le Bihan and Iima, 2015) but also for the study of intracellular compartmentation of metabolites, with the implication feeding into neuroradiology, neurology and related clinical disciplines (Najac et al., 2014). Other foreseen human applications for cryogenically-cooled RF coils will include anatomic micro-imaging of the skin. Pioneering work undertaken with a HTS coil at 1.5 T recently demonstrated a subnanoliter spatial resolution (80 μm^3) for human skin MR microscopy (Laistler et al., 2015). Skin-sodium storage, as a physiologically important regulatory mechanism for blood pressure, volume regulation, and indeed survival, has recently been rediscovered. This prompted the development of MRI methods to assess sodium storage in humans with ^{23}Na-MRI at 3.0 Tesla (Kopp et al., 2012, 2013) and at 7.0 T; the latter facilitating a spatial resolution across the skin of as good as 1 mm in-plane (Linz et al., 2015). To this end, cryogenically cooled RF technology indeed represents a powerful research tool that can potentially help to unlock questions regarding Na$^+$ balance and Na$^+$ storage functions of skin with the ultimate goal to provide imaging means for diagnostics and for guiding treatment decisions in cardiovascular and metabolic diseases. It is however envisioned that the benefits of cryogenically-cooled coils for human application at ultrahigh fields will also go beyond skin microimaging of sub-nanoliter voxels. The significance of the cryogenic technology to advance upon current x-nuclei MR methods for metabolic probing (Linz et al., 2015) and pharmacological studies (Ji et al., 2015) is an area that will definitely receive considerable attention in the coming years.

AUTHOR CONTRIBUTIONS

TN, AP, and SW wrote the manuscript with help from HR, TH, and MK. HW, EP, ES, AS, RK, and KS contributed to data and intellectual feedback.

GRANT SPONSORS

This work was supported (in part, TH) by the DZHK (German Centre for Cardiovascular Research) and by the BMBF (German Ministry of Education and Research. HW received support by the German Federal Ministry of Education and Research (KMU-innovativ- Medizintechnik, MED-373-046). AP and HR were supported by the Helmholtz Alliance HGF/HMGU (Imaging and Curing Environmental Metabolic Diseases, HA-314).

ACKNOWLEDGMENTS

The authors wish to thank Leili Riazy (B.U.F.F., MDC) as well as Tim Wokrina and Daniel Marek (Bruker BioSpin).

REFERENCES

Adamczak, J. M., Farr, T. D., Seehafer, J. U., Kalthoff, D., and Hoehn, M. (2010). High field BOLD response to forepaw stimulation in the mouse. *Neuroimage* 51, 704–712. doi: 10.1016/j.neuroimage.2010.02.083

Agarwal, S., Sane, R., Oberoi, R., Ohlfest, J. R., and Elmquist, W. F. (2011). Delivery of molecularly targeted therapy to malignant glioma, a disease of the whole brain. *Expert Rev. Mol. Med.* 13:e17. doi: 10.1017/S1462399411001888

Ahrens, E. T., Flores, R., Xu, H., and Morel, P. A. (2005). *In vivo* imaging platform for tracking immunotherapeutic cells. *Nat. Biotechnol.* 23, 983–987. doi: 10.1038/nbt1121

Alonso-Ortiz, E., Levesque, I. R., and Pike, G. B. (2015). MRI-based myelin water imaging: a technical review. *Magn. Reson. Med.* 73, 70–81. doi: 10.1002/mrm.25198

Arakelyan, K., Cantow, K., Hentschel, J., Flemming, B., Pohlmann, A., Ladwig, M., et al. (2013). Early effects of an x-ray contrast medium on renal T(2) */T(2) MRI as compared to short-term hyperoxia, hypoxia and aortic occlusion in rats. *Acta Physiol.* 208, 202–213. doi: 10.1111/apha.12094

Bakermans, A. J., Abdurrachim, D., Moonen, R. P., Motaal, A. G., Prompers, J. J., Strijkers, G. J., et al. (2015). Small animal cardiovascular MR imaging and spectroscopy. *Prog. Nucl. Magn. Reson. Spectrosc.* 88–89, 1–47. doi: 10.1016/j.pnmrs.2015.03.001

Baltes, C., Bosshard, S., Mueggler, T., Ratering, D., and Rudin, M. (2011). Increased blood oxygen level−dependent (BOLD) sensitivity in the mouse somatosensory cortex during electrical forepaw stimulation using a cryogenic radiofrequency probe. *NMR Biomed.* 24, 439–446. doi: 10.1002/nbm.1613

Baltes, C., Radzwill, N., Bosshard, S., Marek, D., and Rudin, M. (2009). Micro MRI of the mouse brain using a novel 400 MHz cryogenic quadrature RF probe. *NMR Biomed.* 22, 834–842. doi: 10.1002/nbm.1396

Barkhof, F., Filippi, M., Miller, D. H., Scheltens, P., Campi, A., Polman, C. H., et al. (1997). Comparison of MRI criteria at first presentation to predict conversion to clinically definite multiple sclerosis. *Brain* 120, 2059–2069. doi: 10.1093/brain/120.11.2059

Baxter, A. G. (2007). The origin and application of experimental autoimmune encephalomyelitis. *Nat. Rev. Immunol.* 7, 904–912. doi: 10.1038/nri2190

Beaumont, M., Lemasson, B., Farion, R., Segebarth, C., Rémy, C., and Barbier, E. L. (2009). Characterization of tumor angiogenesis in rat brain using iron-based vessel size index MRI in combination with gadolinium-based dynamic contrast-enhanced MRI. *J. Cereb. Blood Flow Metab.* 29, 1714–1726. doi: 10.1038/jcbfm.2009.86

Beckmann, N., Gérard, C., Abramowski, D., Cannet, C., and Staufenbiel, M. (2011). Noninvasive magnetic resonance imaging detection of cerebral amyloid angiopathy-related microvascular alterations using superparamagnetic iron oxide particles in APP transgenic mouse models of Alzheimer's disease: application to passive Aβ immunotherapy. *J. Neurosci.* 31, 1023–1031. doi: 10.1523/JNEUROSCI.4936-10.2011

Beckmann, N., Schuler, A., Mueggler, T., Meyer, E. P., Wiederhold, K.-H., Staufenbiel, M., et al. (2003). Age-dependent cerebrovascular abnormalities and blood flow disturbances in APP23 mice modeling Alzheimer's disease. *J. Neurosci.* 23, 8453–8459. doi: 10.5167/uzh-182

Beeman, S. C., Zhang, M., Gubhaju, L., Wu, T., Bertram, J. F., Frakes, D. H., et al. (2011). Measuring glomerular number and size in perfused kidneys using MRI. *Am. J. Physiol. Renal Physiol.* 300, F1454–F1457. doi: 10.1152/ajprenal.00044.2011

Ben Nun, A., Wekerle, H., and Cohen, I. R. (1981). Vaccination against autoimmune encephalomyelitis with T-lymphocyte line cells reactive against myelin basic protein. *Nature* 292, 60–61. doi: 10.1038/292060a0

Biffi, A., and Greenberg, S. M. (2011). Cerebral amyloid angiopathy: a systematic review. *J. Clin. Neurol.* 7, 1–9. doi: 10.3988/jcn.2011.7.1.1

Black, R., Early, T., Roemer, P., Mueller, O., Mogro-Campero, A., Turner, L., et al. (1993). A high-temperature superconducting receiver for nuclear magnetic resonance microscopy. *Science* 259, 793–795. doi: 10.1126/science.8430331

Bonventre, J. V., and Yang, L. (2011). Cellular pathophysiology of ischemic acute kidney injury. *J. Clin. Invest.* 121, 4210. doi: 10.1172/JCI45161

Boretius, S., Schmelting, B., Watanabe, T., Merkler, D., Tammer, R., Czéh, B., et al. (2006). Monitoring of EAE onset and progression in the common marmoset monkey by sequential high-resolution 3D MRI. *NMR Biomed.* 19, 41–49. doi: 10.1002/nbm.999

Borsook, D., and Becerra, L. (2011). CNS animal fMRI in pain and analgesia. *Neurosci. Biobehav. Rev.* 35, 1125–1143. doi: 10.1016/j.neubiorev.2010.11.005

Bosshard, S. C., Baltes, C., Wyss, M. T., Mueggler, T., Weber, B., and Rudin, M. (2010). Assessment of brain responses to innocuous and noxious electrical forepaw stimulation in mice using BOLD fMRI. *Pain* 151, 655–663. doi: 10.1016/j.pain.2010.08.025

Bosshard, S. C., Grandjean, J., Schroeter, A., Baltes, C., Zeilhofer, H. U., and Rudin, M. (2012). Hyperalgesia by low doses of the local anesthetic lidocaine involves cannabinoid signaling: an fMRI study in mice. *Pain* 153, 1450–1458. doi: 10.1016/j.pain.2012.04.001

Bosshard, S. C., Stuker, F., Von Deuster, C., Schroeter, A., and Rudin, M. (2015). BOLD fMRI of C-fiber mediated nociceptive processing in mouse brain in response to thermal stimulation of the forepaws. *PLoS ONE* 10:e0126513. doi: 10.1371/journal.pone.0126513

Bovens, S. M., Te Boekhorst, B., Ouden, K. D., Van De Kolk, K. W., Nauerth, A., Nederhoff, M. G., et al. (2011). Evaluation of infarcted murine heart function: comparison of prospectively triggered with self–gated MRI. *NMR Biomed.* 24, 307–315. doi: 10.1002/nbm.1593

Brück, W., Bitsch, A., Kolenda, H., Brück, Y., Stiefel, M., and Lassmann, H. (1997). Inflammatory central nervous system demyelination: correlation of magnetic resonance imaging findings with lesion pathology. *Ann. Neurol.* 42, 783–793. doi: 10.1002/ana.410420515

Chawla, L. S., Eggers, P. W., Star, R. A., and Kimmel, P. L. (2014). Acute kidney injury and chronic kidney disease as interconnected syndromes. *N Engl. J. Med.* 371, 58–66. doi: 10.1056/NEJMra1214243

Darrasse, L., and Ginefri, J.-C. (2003). Perspectives with cryogenic RF probes in biomedical MRI. *Biochimie* 85, 915–937. doi: 10.1016/j.biochi.2003.09.016

Deboy, C. A., Zhang, J., Dike, S., Shats, I., Jones, M., Reich, D. S., et al. (2007). High resolution diffusion tensor imaging of axonal damage in focal inflammatory and demyelinating lesions in rat spinal cord. *Brain* 130, 2199–2210. doi: 10.1093/brain/awm122

Dieringer, M. A., Renz, W., Lindel, T., Seifert, F., Frauenrath, T., Von Knobelsdorff-Brenkenhoff, F., et al. (2011). Design and application of a four-channel transmit/receive surface coil for functional cardiac imaging at 7T. *J. Magn. Reson. Imaging* 33, 736–741. doi: 10.1002/jmri.22451

Dijkhuizen, R. M., Van Lookeren Campagne, M., Niendorf, T., Dreher, W., Van Der Toorn, A., Hoehn-Berlage, M., et al. (1996). Status of the neonatal rat brain after NMDA-induced excitotoxic injury as measured by MRI, MRS and metabolic imaging. *NMR Biomed.* 9, 84–92.

Emblem, K. E., Mouridsen, K., Bjornerud, A., Farrar, C. T., Jennings, D., Borra, R. J. H., et al. (2013). Vessel architectural imaging identifies cancer patient responders to anti-angiogenic therapy. *Nat. Med.* 19, 1178–1183. doi: 10.1038/nm.3289

Epstein, F. H. (2007). MR in mouse models of cardiac disease. *NMR Biomed.* 20, 238–255. doi: 10.1002/nbm.1152

Figueiredo, G., Brockmann, C., Boll, H., Heilmann, M., Schambach, S. J., Fiebig, T., et al. (2012). Comparison of digital subtraction angiography, micro-computed tomography angiography and magnetic resonance angiography in the assessment of the cerebrovascular system in live mice. *Clin. Neuroradiol.* 22, 21–28. doi: 10.1007/s00062-011-0113-2

Ginefri, J. C., Poirier-Quinot, M., Girard, O., and Darrasse, L. (2007). Technical aspects: development, manufacture and installation of a cryo-cooled HTS coil system for high-resolution *in-vivo* imaging of the mouse at 1.5 T. *Methods* 43, 54–67. doi: 10.1016/j.ymeth.2007.03.011

Graessl, A., Renz, W., Hezel, F., Dieringer, M. A., Winter, L., Oezerdem, C., et al. (2014). Modular 32-channel transceiver coil array for cardiac MRI at 7.0T. *Magn. Reson. Med.* 72, 276–290. doi: 10.1002/mrm.24903

Grams, M. E., and Rabb, H. (2012). The distant organ effects of acute kidney injury. *Kidney Int.* 81, 942–948. doi: 10.1038/ki.2011.241

Hart, B. A., Bauer, J., Muller, H. J., Melchers, B., Nicolay, K., Brok, H., et al. (1998). Histopathological characterization of magnetic resonance imaging-detectable brain white matter lesions in a primate model of multiple sclerosis: a correlative study in the experimental autoimmune encephalomyelitis model in common marmosets (Callithrix jacchus). *Am. J. Pathol.* 153, 649–663. doi: 10.1016/S0002-9440(10)65606-4

Heidenreich, P. A., Trogdon, J. G., Khavjou, O. A., Butler, J., Dracup, K., Ezekowitz, M. D., et al. (2011). Forecasting the future of cardiovascular disease in the United States a policy statement from the American heart association. *Circulation* 123, 933–944. doi: 10.1161/CIR.0b013e31820a55f5

Heijman, E., Aben, J. P., Penners, C., Niessen, P., Guillaume, R., Van Eys, G., et al. (2008). Evaluation of manual and automatic segmentation of the mouse heart from CINE MR images. *J. Magn. Reson. Imaging* 27, 86–93. doi: 10.1002/jmri.21236

Heijman, E., De Graaf, W., Niessen, P., Nauerth, A., Van Eys, G., De Graaf, L., et al. (2007). Comparison between prospective and retrospective triggering for mouse cardiac MRI. *NMR Biomed.* 20, 439–447. doi: 10.1002/nbm.1110

Heilmann, M., Neudecker, S., Wolf, I., Gubhaju, L., Sticht, C., Schock-Kusch, D., et al. (2012). Quantification of glomerular number and size distribution in normal rat kidneys using magnetic resonance imaging. *Nephrol. Dial. Transplant.* 27, 100–107. doi: 10.1093/ndt/gfr273

Hiba, B., Richard, N., Thibault, H., and Janier, M. (2007). Cardiac and respiratory self–gated cine MRI in the mouse: comparison between radial and rectilinear techniques at 7T. *Magn. Reson. Med.* 58, 745–753. doi: 10.1002/mrm.21355

Hoult, D. I., and Richards, R. (1976). The signal-to-noise ratio of the nuclear magnetic resonance experiment. *J. Magn. Reson.* 24, 71–85. doi: 10.1016/0022-2364(76)90233-X

Hoult, D. I., and Lauterbur, P. C. (1979). The sensitivity of the zeugmatographic experiment involving human samples. *J. Magn. Reson.* 34, 425–433. doi: 10.1016/0022-2364(79)90019-2

Hoy, W. E., Bertram, J. F., Denton, R. D., Zimanyi, M., Samuel, T., and Hughson, M. D. (2008). Nephron number, glomerular volume, renal disease and hypertension. *Curr. Opin. Nephrol. Hypertens.* 17, 258–265. doi: 10.1097/MNH.0b013e3282f9b1a5

Hu, L., Chen, J., Yang, X., Senpan, A., Allen, J. S., Yanaba, N., et al. (2014). Assessing intrarenal nonperfusion and vascular leakage in acute kidney injury with multinuclear 1H/19F MRI and perfluorocarbon nanoparticles. *Magn. Reson. Med.* 71, 2186–2196. doi: 10.1002/mrm.24851

Huelnhagen, T., Pohlmann, A., Hezel, F., Peper, E., Ku, M.-C., and Niendorf, T. (2014). Detailing myocardial microstructure in the *ex vivo* rat heart using high isotropic spatial resolution susceptibility weighted MRI and quantitative susceptibility mapping. *Proc. Intl. Soc. Magn. Reson. Med.* 22, 2437. doi: 10.13140/RG.2.1.1358.1522

Hurlston, S. E., Brey, W. W., Suddarth, S. A., and Johnson, G. A. (1999). A high-temperature superconducting Helmholtz probe for microscopy at 9.4 T. *Magn. Reson. Med.* 41, 1032–1038.

Jain, R. K. (2005). Normalization of tumor vasculature: an emerging concept in antiangiogenic therapy. *Science* 307, 58–62. doi: 10.1126/science.1104819

Ji, Y., Waiczies, H., Winter, L., Neumanova, P., Hofmann, D., Rieger, J., et al. (2015). Eight-channel transceiver RF coil array tailored for (1) H/(19) F MR of the human knee and fluorinated drugs at 7.0 T. *NMR Biomed.* 28, 726–737. doi: 10.1002/nbm.3300

Junge, S. (2012). "Cryogenic and superconducting coils for MRI," in *eMagRes - Encyclopedia of Magnetic Resonance*, eds J. T. Vaughan and J. R. Griffiths (Hoboken, NJ: John Wiley & Sons, Ltd.), 505–514. doi: 10.1002/9780470034590.emrstm1162

Kim, S.-G., and Ogawa, S. (2012). Biophysical and physiological origins of blood oxygenation level-dependent fMRI signals. *J. Cereb. Blood Flow Metab.* 32, 1188–1206. doi: 10.1038/jcbfm.2012.23

Kinsey, G. R., and Okusa, M. D. (2014). Expanding role of T cells in acute kidney injury. *Curr. Opin. Nephrol. Hypertens.* 23, 9. doi: 10.1097/01.mnh.0000436695.29173.de

Klohs, J., Baltes, C., Princz-Kranz, F., Ratering, D., Nitsch, R. M., Knuesel, I., et al. (2012). Contrast-enhanced magnetic resonance microangiography reveals remodeling of the cerebral microvasculature in transgenic ArcAβ mice. *J. Neurosci.* 32, 1705–1713. doi: 10.1523/JNEUROSCI.5626-11.2012

Klohs, J., Rudin, M., Shimshek, D. R., and Beckmann, N. (2014). Imaging of cerebrovascular pathology in animal models of Alzheimer's disease. *Front. Aging Neurosci.* 6:32. doi: 10.3389/fnagi.2014.00032

Knutsson, L., Ståhlberg, F., and Wirestam, R. (2010). Absolute quantification of perfusion using dynamic susceptibility contrast MRI: pitfalls and possibilities. *Magn. Reson. Mater. Physics Biol. Med.* 23, 1–21. doi: 10.1007/s10334-009-0190-2

Kopp, C., Linz, P., Dahlmann, A., Hammon, M., Jantsch, J., Muller, D. N., et al. (2013). 23Na magnetic resonance imaging-determined tissue sodium in healthy subjects and hypertensive patients. *Hypertension* 61, 635–640. doi: 10.1161/HYPERTENSIONAHA.111.00566

Kopp, C., Linz, P., Wachsmuth, L., Dahlmann, A., Horbach, T., Schofl, C., et al. (2012). (23)Na magnetic resonance imaging of tissue sodium. *Hypertension* 59, 167–172. doi: 10.1161/HYPERTENSIONAHA.111.183517

Kording, F., Weidensteiner, C., Zwick, S., Osterberg, N., Weyerbrock, A., Staszewski, O., et al. (2014). Simultaneous assessment of vessel size index, relative blood volume, and vessel permeability in a mouse brain tumor model using a combined spin echo gradient echo echo-planar imaging sequence and viable tumor analysis. *J. Magn. Reson. Imaging* 40, 1310–1318. doi: 10.1002/jmri.24513

Kovacs, H., Moskau, D., and Spraul, M. (2005). Cryogenically cooled probes—a leap in NMR technology. *Prog. Nucl. Magn. Reson. Spectrosc.* 46, 131–155. doi: 10.1016/j.pnmrs.2005.03.001

Ku, M.-C., Wolf, S. A., Respondek, D., Matyash, V., Pohlmann, A., Waiczies, S., et al. (2013). GDNF mediates glioblastoma-induced microglia attraction but not astrogliosis. *Acta Neuropathol.* 125, 609–620. doi: 10.1007/s00401-013-1079-8

Kuchling, J., Ramien, C., Bozin, I., Dörr, J., Harms, L., Rosche, B., et al. (2014). Identical lesion morphology in primary progressive and relapsing-remitting MS -an ultrahigh field MRI study. *Mult. Scler.* 20, 1866–1871. doi: 10.1177/1352458514531084

Kuhlmann, T., Lassmann, H., and Brück, W. (2008). Diagnosis of inflammatory demyelination in biopsy specimens: a practical approach. *Acta Neuropathol.* 115, 275–287. doi: 10.1007/s00401-007-0320-8

Laistler, E., Poirier-Quinot, M., Lambert, S. A., Dubuisson, R. M., Girard, O. M., Moser, E., et al. (2015). *In vivo* MR imaging of the human skin at subnanoliter resolution using a superconducting surface coil at 1.5 Tesla. *J. Magn. Reson. Imaging* 41, 496–504. doi: 10.1002/jmri.24549

Le Bihan, D., and Iima, M. (2015). Diffusion magnetic resonance imaging: what water tells us about biological tissues. *PLoS Biol.* 13:e1002203. doi: 10.1371/journal.pbio.1002246

Lepore, S., Waiczies, H., Hentschel, J., Ji, Y., Skodowski, J., Pohlmann, A., et al. (2013). Enlargement of cerebral ventricles as an early indicator of encephalomyelitis. *PLoS ONE* 8:e72841. doi: 10.1371/journal.pone.0072841

Lin, W., Abendschein, D. R., Celik, A., Dolan, R. P., Lauffer, R. B., Walovitch, R. C., et al. (1997). Intravascular contrast agent improves magnetic resonance angiography of carotid arteries in minipigs. *J. Magn. Reson. Imaging* 7, 963–971. doi: 10.1002/jmri.1880070605

Linz, P., Santoro, D., Renz, W., Rieger, J., Ruehle, A., Ruff, J., et al. (2015). Skin sodium measured with (2)(3)Na MRI at 7.0 T. *NMR Biomed.* 28, 54–62. doi: 10.1002/nbm.3224

McRobbie, D. W., Moore, E. A., Graves, M. J., and Prince, M. R. (2006). *MRI from Picture to Proton.* Cambridge: Cambridge University Press.

Merlini, M., Meyer, E., Ulmann-Schuler, A., and Nitsch, R. (2011). Vascular β-amyloid and early astrocyte alterations impair cerebrovascular function and cerebral metabolism in transgenic arcAβ mice. *Acta Neuropathol.* 122, 293–311. doi: 10.1007/s00401-011-0834-y

Messroghli, D. R., Niendorf, T., Schulz-Menger, J., Dietz, R., and Friedrich, M. G. (2003). T1 mapping in patients with acute myocardial infarction. *J. Cardiovasc. Magn. Reson.* 5, 353–359. doi: 10.1081/JCMR-120019418

Milo, R., and Miller, A. (2014). Revised diagnostic criteria of multiple sclerosis. *Autoimmun. Rev.* 13, 518–524. doi: 10.1016/j.autrev.2014.01.012

Molitoris, B. A. (2014). Therapeutic translation in acute kidney injury: the epithelial/endothelial axis. *J. Clin. Invest.* 124, 2355–2363. doi: 10.1172/JCI72269

Mueggler, T., Pohl, H., Baltes, C., Riethmacher, D., Suter, U., and Rudin, M. (2012). MRI signature in a novel mouse model of genetically induced adult oligodendrocyte cell death. *Neuroimage* 59, 1028–1036. doi: 10.1016/j.neuroimage.2011.09.001

Mueggler, T., Razoux, F., Russig, H., Buehler, A., Franklin, T. B., Baltes, C., et al. (2011). Mapping of CBV changes in 5-HT 1A terminal fields by functional MRI in the mouse brain. *Eur. Neuropsychopharmacol.* 21, 344–353. doi: 10.1016/j.euroneuro.2010.06.010

Najac, C., Branzoli, F., Ronen, I., and Valette, J. (2014). Brain intracellular metabolites are freely diffusing along cell fibers in grey and white matter, as measured by diffusion-weighted MR spectroscopy in the human brain at 7 T. *Brain Struct. Funct.* doi: 10.1007/s00429-014-0968-5. [Epub ahead of print].

Nasrallah, F. A., Tay, H.-C., and Chuang, K.-H. (2014). Detection of functional connectivity in the resting mouse brain. *Neuroimage* 86, 417–424. doi: 10.1016/j.neuroimage.2013.10.025

Niendorf, T., Dijkhuizen, R. M., Norris, D. G., Van Lookeren Campagne, M., and Nicolay, K. (1996). Biexponential diffusion attenuation in various states of brain tissue: implications for diffusion-weighted imaging. *Magn. Reson. Med.* 36, 847–857. doi: 10.1002/mrm.1910360607

Niendorf, T., Graessl, A., Thalhammer, C., Dieringer, M. A., Kraus, O., Santoro, D., et al. (2013). Progress and promises of human cardiac magnetic resonance at ultrahigh fields: a physics perspective. *J. Magn. Reson.* 229, 208–222. doi: 10.1016/j.jmr.2012.11.015

Niendorf, T., Norris, D. G., and Leibfritz, D. (1994). Detection of apparent restricted diffusion in healthy rat brain at short diffusion times. *Magn. Reson. Med.* 32, 672–677. doi: 10.1002/mrm.1910320520

Niendorf, T., Paul, K., Oezerdem, C., Graessl, A., Klix, S., Huelnhagen, T., et al. (2015a). W(h)ither human cardiac and body magnetic resonance at ultrahigh fields? Technical advances, practical considerations, applications, and clinical opportunities. *NMR Biomed.* doi: 10.1002/nbm.3268. [Epub ahead of print].

Niendorf, T., Pohlmann, A., Arakelyan, K., Flemming, B., Cantow, K., Hentschel, J., et al. (2015b). How bold is blood oxygenation level−dependent (BOLD) magnetic resonance imaging of the kidney? Opportunities, challenges and future directions. *Acta Physiol.* 213, 19–38. doi: 10.1111/apha.12393

Niendorf, T., and Sodickson, D. (2006a). Acceleration of cardiovascular MRI using parallel imaging: basic principles, practical considerations, clinical applications and future directions. *Rofo* 178, 15–30. doi: 10.1055/s-2005-858686

Niendorf, T., and Sodickson, D. K. (2006b). Parallel imaging in cardiovascular MRI: methods and applications. *NMR Biomed.* 19, 325–341. doi: 10.1002/nbm.1051

Niendorf, T., and Sodickson, D. K. (2008). Highly accelerated cardiovascular MR imaging using many channel technology: concepts and clinical applications. *Eur. Radiol.* 18, 87–102. doi: 10.1007/s00330-007-0692-0

Niendorf, T., Sodickson, D. K., Krombach, G. A., and Schulz-Menger, J. (2010). Toward cardiovascular MRI at 7 T: clinical needs, technical solutions and research promises. *Eur. Radiol.* 20, 2806–2816. doi: 10.1007/s00330-010-1902-8

Norris, D. G., and Niendorf, T. (1995). Interpretation of DW-NMR data: dependence on experimental conditions. *NMR Biomed.* 8, 280–288. doi: 10.1002/nbm.1940080703

Norris, D. G., Niendorf, T., and Leibfritz, D. (1994). Health and infarcted brain tissues studied at short diffusion times: the origins of apparent restriction and the reduction in apparent diffusion coefficient. *NMR Biomed.* 7, 304–310. doi: 10.1002/nbm.1940070703

Nouls, J. C., Izenson, M. G., Greeley, H. P., and Johnson, G. A. (2008). Design of a superconducting volume coil for magnetic resonance microscopy of the mouse brain. *J. Magn. Reson.* 191, 231–238. doi: 10.1016/j.jmr.2007.12.018

Paxinos, G., and Franklin, K. B. (2013). *Paxinos and Franklin's the Mouse Brain in Stereotaxic Coordinates.* Amsterdam: Elsevier.

Peper, E., Huelnhagen, T., Pohlmann, A., Ku, M.-C., and Niendorf, T. (2015). Comparison of high resolution T2* mapping and quantitative susceptibility mapping to investigate myocardial microstructure in the *ex vivo* rodent heart. *Proc. Intl. Soc. Mag. Reson. Med.* 23, 2609. doi: 10.13140/RG.2.1.1882.4400

Pohl, H. B., Porcheri, C., Mueggler, T., Bachmann, L. C., Martino, G., Riethmacher, D., et al. (2011). Genetically induced adult oligodendrocyte cell death is associated with poor myelin clearance, reduced remyelination, and axonal damage. *J. Neurosci.* 31, 1069–1080. doi: 10.1523/JNEUROSCI.5035-10.2011

Pohlmann, A., Arakelyan, K., Hentschel, J., Cantow, K., Flemming, B., Ladwig, M., et al. (2014a). Detailing the relation between renal T2* and renal tissue pO2 using an integrated approach of parametric magnetic resonance imaging and invasive physiological measurements. *Invest. Radiol.* 49, 547–560. doi: 10.1097/RLI.0000000000000054

Pohlmann, A., Cantow, K., Hentschel, J., Arakelyan, K., Ladwig, M., Flemming, B., et al. (2013a). Linking non-invasive parametric MRI with invasive physiological measurements (MR-PHYSIOL): towards a hybrid and integrated approach for investigation of acute kidney injury in rats. *Acta Physiol.* 207, 673–689. doi: 10.1111/apha.12065

Pohlmann, A., Hentschel, J., Fechner, M., Hoff, U., Bubalo, G., Arakelyan, K., et al. (2013b). High temporal resolution parametric MRI monitoring of the initial ischemia/reperfusion phase in experimental acute kidney injury. *PLoS ONE* 8:e57411. doi: 10.1371/journal.pone.0057411

Pohlmann, A., Schreiber, A., Ku, M.-C., Waiczies, H., Kox, S., Kettritz, R., et al. (2014b). Assessment of renal inflammatory cell infiltration in a murine ANCA-induced glomerulonephritis model by 19F-MRI. *Proc. Intl. Soc. Mag. Reson. Med.* 22, 2207. doi: 10.13140/RG.2.1.4143.4326

Poirier-Quinot, M., Ginefri, J.-C., Girard, O., Robert, P., and Darrasse, L. (2008). Performance of a miniature high-temperature superconducting (HTS) surface coil for *in vivo* microimaging of the mouse in a standard 1.5T clinical whole-body scanner. *Magnetic Resonance in Medicine* 60, 917–927. doi: 10.1002/mrm.21605

Pyatigorskaya, N., Le Bihan, D., Reynaud, O., and Ciobanu, L. (2014). Relationship between the diffusion time and the diffusion MRI signal observed at 17.2 Tesla in the healthy rat brain cortex. *Magn. Reson. Med.* 72, 492–500. doi: 10.1002/mrm.24921

Ransohoff, R. M. (2009). Immunology: in the beginning. *Nature* 462, 41–42. doi: 10.1038/462041a

Ransohoff, R. M. (2012). Animal models of multiple sclerosis: the good, the bad and the bottom line. *Nat. Neurosci.* 15, 1074–1077. doi: 10.1038/nn.3168

Ratering, D., Baltes, C., Dörries, C., and Rudin, M. (2010). Accelerated cardiovascular magnetic resonance of the mouse heart using self-gated parallel imaging strategies does not compromise accuracy of structural and functional measures. *J. Cardiovasc. Magn. Reson.* 12:43. doi: 10.1186/1532-429X-12-43

Ratering, D., Baltes, C., Nordmeyer–Massner, J., Marek, D., and Rudin, M. (2008). Performance of a 200–MHz cryogenic RF probe designed for MRI and MRS of the murine brain. *Magn. Reson. Med.* 59, 1440–1447. doi: 10.1002/mrm.21629

Reinges, M. H. T., Nguyen, H. H., Krings, T., Hütter, B. O., Rohde, V., and Gilsbach, J. M. (2004). Course of brain shift during microsurgical resection of supratentorial cerebral lesions: limits of conventional neuronavigation. *Acta Neurochir.* 146, 369–377. doi: 10.1007/s00701-003-0204-1

Ruiz-Cabello, J., Barnett, B. P., Bottomley, P. A., and Bulte, J. W. (2011). Fluorine (19F) MRS and MRI in biomedicine. *NMR Biomed.* 24, 114–129. doi: 10.1002/nbm.1570

Sack, M., Wetterling, F., Sartorius, A., Ende, G., and Weber–Fahr, W. (2014). Signal–to–noise ratio of a mouse brain 13C CryoProbe™ system in comparison with room temperature coils: spectroscopic phantom and *in vivo* results. *NMR Biomed.* 27, 709–715. doi: 10.1002/nbm.3110

Salat, D. H. (2014). Imaging small vessel-associated white matter changes in aging. *Neuroscience* 276, 174–186. doi: 10.1016/j.neuroscience.2013.11.041

Schmierer, K., Scaravilli, F., Altmann, D. R., Barker, G. J., and Miller, D. H. (2004). Magnetization transfer ratio and myelin in postmortem multiple sclerosis brain. *Ann. Neurol.* 56, 407–415. doi: 10.1002/ana.20202

Schneider, J. E. (2011). "Assessment of global cardiac function," in *In Vivo NMR Imaging*, eds L. Schröder and C. Faber (Heidelberg: Springer), 387–405. doi: 10.1007/978-1-61779-219-9_20

Schneider, J. E., Lanz, T., Barnes, H., Stork, L. A., Bohl, S., Lygate, C. A., et al. (2011). Accelerated cardiac magnetic resonance imaging in the mouse using an eight–channel array at 9.4 Tesla. *Magn. Reson. Med.* 65, 60–70. doi: 10.1002/mrm.22605

Schreiber, A., and Choi, M. (2015). The role of neutrophils in causing antineutrophil cytoplasmic autoantibody-associated vasculitis. *Curr. Opin. Hematol.* 22, 60–66. doi: 10.1097/MOH.0000000000000098

Schreiber, A., Kettritz, R., Ku, M.-C., Waiczies, H., Waiczies, S., Niendorf, T., et al. (2013). 19F-MRI for noninvasive visualization of renal inflammation in a murine ANCA-induced glomerulonephritis model. *J. Am. Soc. Nephrol.* 24:308A. doi: 10.13140/RG.2.1.1265.9923

Schroeter, A., Schlegel, F., Seuwen, A., Grandjean, J., and Rudin, M. (2014). Specificity of stimulus-evoked fMRI responses in the mouse: the influence of systemic physiological changes associated with innocuous stimulation under four different anesthetics. *Neuroimage* 94, 372–384. doi: 10.1016/j.neuroimage.2014.01.046

Sinnecker, T., Bozin, I., Dörr, J., Pfueller, C. F., Harms, L., Niendorf, T., et al. (2013). Periventricular venous density in multiple sclerosis is inversely associated with T2 lesion count: a 7 Tesla MRI study. *Mult. Scler.* 19, 316–325. doi: 10.1177/1352458512451941

Sinnecker, T., Dörr, J., Pfueller, C. F., Harms, L., Ruprecht, K., Jarius, S., et al. (2012a). Distinct lesion morphology at 7-T MRI differentiates neuromyelitis optica from multiple sclerosis. *Neurology* 79, 708–714. doi: 10.1212/WNL.0b013e3182648bc8

Sinnecker, T., Mittelstaedt, P., Dörr, J., Pfueller, C. F., Harms, L., Niendorf, T., et al. (2012b). Multiple sclerosis lesions and irreversible brain tissue damage: a comparative ultrahigh-field strength magnetic resonance imaging study. *Arch. Neurol.* 69, 739–745. doi: 10.1001/archneurol.2011.2450

Sosnovik, D. E., Dai, G., Nahrendorf, M., Rosen, B. R., and Seethamraju, R. (2007). Cardiac MRI in mice at 9.4 Tesla with a transmit–receive surface coil and a cardiac–tailored intensity–correction algorithm. *J. Magn. Reson. Imaging* 26, 279–287. doi: 10.1002/jmri.20966

Steinman, L., and Zamvil, S. S. (2006). How to successfully apply animal studies in experimental allergic encephalomyelitis to research on multiple sclerosis. *Ann. Neurol.* 60, 12–21. doi: 10.1002/ana.20913

Styles, P., Soffe, N. F., Scott, C. A., Cragg, D. A., Row, F., White, D. J., et al. (1984). A high-resolution NMR probe in which the coil and preamplifier are cooled with liquid helium. *J. Magn. Reson.* 213, 347–354. doi: 10.1016/j.jmr.2011.09.002

Thalhammer, C., Renz, W., Winter, L., Hezel, F., Rieger, J., Pfeiffer, H., et al. (2012). Two-dimensional sixteen channel transmit/receive coil array for cardiac MRI at 7.0 T: design, evaluation, and application. *J. Magn. Reson. Imaging* 36, 847–857. doi: 10.1002/jmri.23724

Traka, M., Arasi, K., Avila, R. L., Podojil, J. R., Christakos, A., Miller, S. D., et al. (2010). A genetic mouse model of adult-onset, pervasive central nervous system demyelination with robust remyelination. *Brain* 133, 3017–3029. doi: 10.1093/brain/awq247

Utz, W., Greiser, A., Niendorf, T., Dietz, R., and Schulz-Menger, J. (2008). Single- or dual-bolus approach for the assessment of myocardial perfusion reserve in quantitative MR perfusion imaging. *Magn. Reson. Med.* 59, 1373–1377. doi: 10.1002/mrm.21611

Utz, W., Niendorf, T., Wassmuth, R., Messroghli, D., Dietz, R., and Schulz-Menger, J. (2007). Contrast-dose relation in first-pass myocardial MR perfusion imaging. *J. Magn. Reson. Imaging* 25, 1131–1135. doi: 10.1002/jmri.20910

Van Waesberghe, J., Kamphorst, W., De Groot, C. J., Van Walderveen, M. A., Castelijns, J. A., Ravid, R., et al. (1999). Axonal loss in multiple sclerosis lesions: magnetic resonance imaging insights into substrates of disability. *Ann. Neurol.* 46, 747–754.

Vaughan, J. T., and Griffiths, J. R. (2012). *RF Coils for MRI*. Hoboken, NJ: John Wiley & Sons.

Verhoye, M. R., Gravenmade, E. J., Raman, E. R., Van Reempts, J., and Van Der Linden, A. (1996). *In vivo* noninvasive determination of abnormal water diffusion in the rat brain studied in an animal model for multiple sclerosis by diffusion- weighted NMR imaging. *Magn. Reson. Imaging* 14, 521–532. doi: 10.1016/0730-725X(96)00047-1

Vinnakota, K., Hu, F., Ku, M.-C., Georgieva, P. B., Szulzewsky, F., Pohlmann, A., et al. (2013). Toll-like receptor 2 mediates microglia/brain macrophage MT1-MMP expression and glioma expansion. *Neuro Oncol.* 15, 1457–1468. doi: 10.1093/neuonc/not115

Von Knobelsdorff-Brenkenhoff, F., Frauenrath, T., Prothmann, M., Dieringer, M. A., Hezel, F., Renz, W., et al. (2010). Cardiac chamber quantification using magnetic resonance imaging at 7 Tesla–a pilot study. *Eur. Radiol.* 20, 2844–2852. doi: 10.1007/s00330-010-1888-2

Von Knobelsdorff-Brenkenhoff, F., Tkachenko, V., Winter, L., Rieger, J., Thalhammer, C., Hezel, F., et al. (2013). Assessment of the right ventricle with cardiovascular magnetic resonance at 7 Tesla. *J. Cardiovasc. Magn. Reson.* 15:23. doi: 10.1186/1532-429x-15-23

Wagenhaus, B., Pohlmann, A., Dieringer, M. A., Els, A., Waiczies, H., Waiczies, S., et al. (2012). Functional and morphological cardiac magnetic resonance imaging of mice using a cryogenic quadrature radiofrequency coil. *PLoS ONE* 7:e42383. doi: 10.1371/journal.pone.0042383

Waiczies, H., Lepore, S., Drechsler, S., Qadri, F., Purfürst, B., Sydow, K., et al. (2013). Visualizing brain inflammation with a shingled-leg radio-frequency head probe for 19F/1H MRI. *Sci. Rep.* 3:1280. doi: 10.1038/srep01280

Waiczies, H., Lepore, S., Janitzek, N., Hagen, U., Seifert, F., Ittermann, B., et al. (2011). Perfluorocarbon particle size influences magnetic resonance signal and immunological properties of dendritic cells. *PLoS ONE* 6:e21981. doi: 10.1371/journal.pone.0021981

Waiczies, H., Millward, J. M., Lepore, S., Infante-Duarte, C., Pohlmann, A., Niendorf, T., et al. (2012). Identification of cellular infiltrates during early stages of brain inflammation with magnetic resonance microscopy. *PLoS ONE* 7:e32796. doi: 10.1371/journal.pone.0032796

Welti, J., Loges, S., Dimmeler, S., and Carmeliet, P. (2013). Recent molecular discoveries in angiogenesis and antiangiogenic therapies in cancer. *J. Clin. Invest.* 123, 3190–3200. doi: 10.1172/JCI70212

Winter, L., Kellman, P., Renz, W., Gräßl, A., Hezel, F., Thalhammer, C., et al. (2012). Comparison of three multichannel transmit/receive radiofrequency coil configurations for anatomic and functional cardiac MRI at 7.0T: implications for clinical imaging. *Eur. Radiol.* 22, 2211–2220. doi: 10.1007/s00330-012-2487-1

Wolff, S. D., and Balaban, R. S. (1989). Magnetization transfer contrast (MTC) and tissue water proton relaxation *in vivo*. *Magn. Reson. Med.* 10, 135–144. doi: 10.1002/mrm.1910100113

Wuerfel, J., Sinnecker, T., Ringelstein, E. B., Jarius, S., Schwindt, W., Niendorf, T., et al. (2012). Lesion morphology at 7 Tesla MRI differentiates Susac syndrome from multiple sclerosis. *Mult. Scler.* 18, 1592–1599. doi: 10.1177/1352458512441270

Wuerfel, J., Tysiak, E., Prozorovski, T., Smyth, M., Mueller, S., Schnorr, J., et al. (2007). Mouse model mimics multiple sclerosis in the clinico-radiological paradox. *Eur. J. Neurosci.* 26, 190–198. doi: 10.1111/j.1460-9568.2007.05644.x

Xie, L., Cianciolo, R. E., Hulette, B., Lee, H. W., Qi, Y., Cofer, G., et al. (2012). Magnetic resonance histology of age-related nephropathy in the Sprague Dawley rat. *Toxicol. Pathol.* 40, 764–778. doi: 10.1177/0192623312441408

Xie, L., Subashi, E., Qi, Y., Knepper, M. A., and Johnson, G. A. (2014). Four-dimensional MRI of renal function in the developing mouse. *NMR Biomed.* 27, 1094–1102. doi: 10.1002/nbm.3162

Young, A. A., Barnes, H., Davison, D., Neubauer, S., and Schneider, J. E. (2009). Fast left ventricular mass and volume assessment in mice with three-dimensional guide-point modeling. *J. Magn. Reson. Imaging* 30, 514–520. doi: 10.1002/jmri.21873

Zwick, S., Strecker, R., Kiselev, V., Gall, P., Huppert, J., Palmowski, M., et al. (2009). Assessment of vascular remodeling under antiangiogenic therapy using DCE-MRI and vessel size imaging. *J. Magn. Reson. Imaging* 29, 1125–1133. doi: 10.1002/jmri.21710

Conflict of Interest Statement: Sonia Waiczies received research grants from Novartis for a different project. Helmar Waiczies is employed by and Thoralf Niendorf is founder of MRI.TOOLS GmbH. Klaus Strobel is employed by Bruker BioSpin. No conflicts of interest were disclosed by the other authors.

13

Evolution of Contrast Agents for Ultrasound Imaging and Ultrasound-Mediated Drug Delivery

Vera Paefgen, Dennis Doleschel and Fabian Kiessling*

Institute for Experimental Molecular Imaging, RWTH Aachen University Hospital, Aachen, Germany

Edited by:
Nicolau Beckmann,
Novartis Institutes for BioMedical
Research, Switzerland

Reviewed by:
Ghanshyam Upadhyay,
City University of New York, USA
Claus Christian Glüer,
Christian-Albrechts-Universität zu Kiel,
Germany
Nathalie Lassau,
Gustave Roussy and IR4M UMR
8081, France

*Correspondence:
Fabian Kiessling,
Institute for Experimental Molecular
Imaging, RWTH Aachen University
Hospital, Pauwelsstrasse 30,
52074 Aachen, Germany
fkiessling@ukaachen.de

Ultrasound (US) is one of the most frequently used diagnostic methods. It is a non-invasive, comparably inexpensive imaging method with a broad spectrum of applications, which can be increased even more by using bubbles as contrast agents (CAs). There are various different types of bubbles: filled with different gases, composed of soft- or hard-shell materials, and ranging in size from nano- to micrometers. These intravascular CAs enable functional analyses, e.g., to acquire organ perfusion in real-time. Molecular analyses are achieved by coupling specific ligands to the bubbles' shell, which bind to marker molecules in the area of interest. Bubbles can also be loaded with or attached to drugs, peptides or genes and can be destroyed by US pulses to locally release the entrapped agent. Recent studies show that US CAs are also valuable tools in hyperthermia-induced ablation therapy of tumors, or can increase cellular uptake of locally released drugs by enhancing membrane permeability. This review summarizes important steps in the development of US CAs and introduces the current clinical applications of contrast-enhanced US. Additionally, an overview of the recent developments in US probe design for functional and molecular diagnosis as well as for drug delivery is given.

Keywords: ultrasound, contrast agent, microbubbles, nanobubbles, molecular imaging, drug delivery, theranostics

Introduction

Ultrasound (US) imaging enables cheap, non-invasive imaging in real-time with a high soft tissue contrast and without exposing the patient to radiation. This, together with its broad field of applications, explains the extensive use of clinical US imaging. Applications range from first-look examinations in abdomen or extremities to cardiac applications and endosonography, e.g., in the female genital tract. US regularly supplements x-ray mammography and it is used for the assessment of tissue vascularization and of vessel occlusion using Doppler. In many cases, additional CA are not needed to find the right diagnosis. For poorly vascularized tumors or regions with many small vessels with slow blood flow Doppler US is not sufficient. Hence CEUS is an option and was shown to improve cancer detection and tumor characterization, decreasing the number of

Abbreviations: BBB, blood-brain barrier; CA, contrast agent(s); CEUS, contrast-enhanced ultrasound; HIFU, high-intensity focused ultrasound; HS-MB, hard-shell microbubble(s); LOFU, low-intensity focused ultrasound; MB, microbubble(s); NB, nanobubble(s); PBCA, poly(n-butylcyanoacrylate); PEG, polyethylene glycol; PFC, perfluorocarbon(s); PLGA, poly(D,L-lactide-co-glycolide); PVA, poly(vinyl-alcohol); SS-MB, soft-shell microbubble(s); tPA, tissue plasminogen activator; US, ultrasound; USCA, ultrasound contrast agent(s); (U)SPIO, (ultrasmall) superparamagnetic iron oxide.

biopsies, or during surgery in brain cancer patients (Kitano et al., 2012; Uemura et al., 2013; Prada et al., 2014).

Application of CEUS started in the late 1960s after finding that the injection of agitated saline caused a detectable signal change during US examination (Gramiak and Shah, 1968). Contrast enhancement was caused by the compressible gas core of saline bubbles, enabling the bubble to backscatter the applied US wave. Those first saline bubbles were unstable due to the high surface tension. By injection of autologous blood at adequately rapid rates, the formation of more stable bubbles was described (Kremkau et al., 1970), nonetheless those bubbles still lacked sufficient lifetime and a defined size. It took more than 20 years to develop the first stable, commercially available and FDA-approved USCA (Feinstein et al., 1990), Albunex®, an albumin-coated and air-filled microsphere.

Since then, stability and biocompatibility of USCA have been continuously improved and bubbles have been modified to specifically target certain surface molecules expressed in pathological alterations. Apart from their support for imaging and diagnostics, micro- and NBs are object of increased interest for therapeutic applications. Recent studies used the disrupting effect of MB-enhanced US on the BBB in combination with transplantation of mesenchymal stem cells for treatment of brain ischemia, or used MBs as carriers of drugs, siRNA and mRNA (Dewitte et al., 2014; Gong et al., 2014). This broad field of different uses makes USCA attractive for research and beneficial for patients. Currently three different MB-based CA are clinically approved in the United States/North America and Europe, and a fourth is clinically used in Japan and South Korea, but the variety among the investigative CA is much broader and frequently produces new, promising progenies. Since examinations with those approved CA are common in the clinics, guidelines for CEUS imaging of the liver exist to guarantee proper and comparable examinations and an improvement for the patients' diagnosis and therapy (Claudon et al., 2013).

Diagnostics

Due to their broad applicability and low risks, many different types of USCA have been developed. To get started, an overview of the different possibilities to use bubbles of varying size, shell material, or gas cores will be presented, as well as their properties, applications, and advantages.

Microbubbles

The majority of USCA in use are MBs. As their name suggests, their diameters range between 1 and 10 µm. This size normally limits the application of MB to the intravascular system to assess functional parameters like vascularity, perfusion, blood flow velocity, angiogenicity, or to characterize vasculature molecularly by using targeted MB (Yuan and Rychak, 2013). Extravasation of MB to surrounding tissue is inhibited, preventing unspecific accumulation in the interstitial space and unwanted background signals. Micron-sized bubbles were found to cause proper backscattering of applied US pulses, not only with linear oscillations, but also with non-linear ones, which are not strongly

present in most tissues. Thus, MB can be detected with high sensitivity and a good contrast.

In this review we will introduce the main different shell materials, normally divided in soft- and hard-shell bubbles, will be introduced. Even though the included gas is responsible for the majority of the bubbles' acoustic properties, the shell adds a mechanical stiffness and reduces the compressibility of the gas. Therefore, the shell material provides multiple possibilities to tailor the MB to their specific application by changing visco-elastic properties (Hoff et al., 1996; Kiessling et al., 2014),

Nonetheless, the choice of gas is a factor that has to be considered. First experiments used air, but still suffered from poor stability and very short circulation times due to the high solubility of air in water. The same difficulties occurred in tests using a nitrogen filling, though a less gas-permeable coating slightly improved lifetime (Unger et al., 1994; Schutt et al., 2003). It was found that PFC were a good choice with their low solubility in water/blood and their good compatibility. With introduction of PFC it became possible to produce MB of a defined size with a lifetime of several minutes, long enough for diagnostic examinations in vivo. To rule out possible changes in bubble-size by air diffusing along the concentration gradient between blood and bubble, MB can be produced with a defined mixture of PFC and air, so that Laplace and arterial pressure are in equilibrium (Schutt et al., 1996). Another useful side effect of using PFC is the possible application of those USCA for MRI, since fluorine (19F) is NMR-detectable, even with a normal, slightly adjusted proton setup (Siemens TIM Trio 3T MRI scanner, transmit/receive 19F/1H dual-tune volume RF coil, a pre-amplifier), and does not cause background signals in patients (Rapoport et al., 2011). However, the amount of fluorine to detect is extremely small and requires a highly sensitive setup.

Hard-Shell Microbubbles

The group of HS-MBs mainly consists of gas bubbles with a coating of lower visco-elastical properties such as polymers or denatured proteins, as well as porous silica materials encapsulating gas. Generally, HS-MB show an increased circulation time in vivo and are the preferred type of CA for higher-intensity US applications where they provide a higher echogenicity than SS-MBs which might rupture.

Polymer-shelled microbubbles

The first polymers used for US applications were naturally occurring air-filled polymers. Gelatin was among the first biopolymers to be tested, but the production of adequately small MB turned out to be difficult and their circulation time was short (Carroll et al., 1980). Wheatley et al. (1990) pointed out the lack of appropriate CA for US diagnostics 20 years after the discovery of gas bubbles as a suitable system. They developed a setup for alginate-air MB, but again struggled with the needed maximal size of approximately 10 µm (Wheatley et al., 1990). Other approaches used agarose gel as shell material (D'Arrigo, 1981) with similar complications. For all natural polymers an increased risk of material contaminations was found, in addition to decreased reproducibility of size-defined bubbles and adequate in vivo stability to enable clinical examinations (Cohen et al.,

1996; Schutt et al., 2003). Until today, there are no clinically approved CA derived from those natural polymers, though a few groups still work with those materials due to their good compatibility (Huang et al., 2013). By switching to synthetic polymers, the risk of contamination could be decreased and many of them have proven their biocompatibility in other applications (Kelly et al., 2003). Modern polymer-shelled MB are normally made of synthetic polymers with a PFC/air-filling.

Cyanoacrylate polymers were first used as a shell material by Fritzsch et al. (1994). Under the name SHU 563 A, later on Sonovist®, (Schering AG, Berlin), those air-filled MB were shown to last more than 10 min *in vivo*, both in animals and in patients, to have a good biocompatibility and to be taken up by the reticuloendothelial system effectively. These properties made SHU 563 A an interesting tool for liver and spleen US examination (Bauer et al., 1999; Forsberg et al., 1999). Apart from Sonovist®, other cyanoacrylates are investigated for US applications as well. PBCA is a well-known biocompatible polymer and, as a gas-filled MB, tested for various diagnostic or therapeutic US-supporting applications. Synthesis of PBCA-MB includes intensive stirring during polymerization in presence of a detergent like Triton X-100 and hydrochloric acid (pH = 2). Olbrich et al. (2006) compared one- and two-step synthesis protocols and stirring intensity to vary size, shell thickness and the resulting properties of MB under acoustic pressure, as well as the MB survival time in plasma and serum. Factors that might interfere with MB stability were high injection rates and small needle diameters during MB injection, but when handled and stored correctly, PBCA-MB remained stable for multiple weeks (Fokong et al., 2011). Besides using PBCA-MB for drug delivery in therapeutic approaches, they can also be labeled with fluorophores or iron nanoparticles and thus be a useful tool for multimodal imaging with US and 2-photon-/fluorescence microscopy or MRI (Koczera et al., 2012; Lammers et al., 2015).

Poly(D,L-lactide-co-glycolide) is another commonly used material for MB synthesis. Here, bubbles are produced from a double emulsion of water, oil, and water, followed by evaporation of solvents. Compared to PLLA, PLGA has a faster degradation rate (Cui et al., 2005a). By varying factors like the molecular weight or adding capping structures to the polymers' ends, US scattering properties could be adjusted (Eisenbrey et al., 2008). Among the first animal experiments for PLGA-MB, myocardial contrast echocardiography was successfully done in dogs (Cui et al., 2005b). More recent approaches make use of PLGA-MB as delivery vectors, often in tumor treatment. Niu et al. (2012, 2013) used PLGA-MB to support identification of lymph nodes near tumor sides during surgery by delivering Sudan black, as well as the chemotherapeutic drug doxorubicin and iron particles, to make use of both US and MRI evaluation. PLGA-MB have been used as CA with sonosensitizer properties for tumor treatment as well, when coupled to hematoporphyrin that gets activated by US and is supposed to induce tumor necrosis (Zheng et al., 2012). Nonetheless there are currently no FDA-approved PLGA-MB for clinical applications.

Poly(vinyl-alcohol) is characterized by a good biocompatibility and its hydroxylic moiety which allows multiple chemical modifications (Cavalieri et al., 2005). Around 10 years ago several groups started working on PVA-MB. Similar to PBCA-MB, bubbles are synthesized during high stirring and in presence of hydrochloric acid, but due to its water soluble character, no detergent is needed, therefore the crosslinking occurs at the water/air interface (Cavalieri et al., 2006). By slight variations of temperature and pH value in the synthesis phase, the bubbles' diameter could be changed. PVA-MB were able to produce signal enhancements up to 20 dB in suspensions and have successfully been combined with SPIO nanoparticles to enable multimodal imaging (Grishenkov et al., 2009; Brismar et al., 2012).

Finally, MB can be produced by ink-jet printing using a polyperfluorooctyloxycaronyl-poly(lactic acid) copolymer. The printing method allows to specifically generate bubbles of a defined size and thus studies of swelling or shrinking processes (Böhmer et al., 2006, 2010).

Protein-shelled microbubbles

Though less resistant to US waves than polymer-coated MB, but with a longer history of use and development, the first commercially available USCA was the protein-shelled MB Albunex® (Molecular Biosystems, San Diego, CA, USA). On their way to develop a useful USCA for clinical applications, Keller et al. (1987) discovered that a 5% heat-denatured human albumin solution after sonication produces adequately stabilized, air-filled bubbles of mostly less than 10 μm in diameter. First animal experiments showed an enhanced contrast in 2D echocardiography after intravenous injection (Keller et al., 1987) and a behavior similar to erythrocytes to guarantee no interferences in coronary flow or hemodynamics caused by the CA during myocardial US examination (Keller et al., 1988, 1989). Still, Albunex® had a very limited lifetime *in vivo* due to its air-filled core, and the general principle of albumin-shelled MB was soon refined by replacing air with perfluoropropane. This was the beginning of the 'second generation' USCA Optison® (GE Healthcare, Buckinghamshire, UK). With a diameter of 2–5 μm, a shell thickness of approximately 15 nm, similar to its predecessor, but consisting of only 1% albumin, clinical trials proved a prolonged and better contrast enhancement compared to Albunex®, and a high preference of physicians for Optison® in left ventricular echocardiography (Cohen et al., 1998). Optison® under US application has been used for temporary disruption of the BBB, though side effects like vasoconstriction and hemorrhages might occur with sub-optimal US setting (Hynynen et al., 2001; Raymond et al., 2007). For echocardiography, application of Optison® was found to be generally safe in patients with different cardiologic problems, and potential induction of myocardial necrosis was ruled out (Borges et al., 2002; Wei et al., 2014). Nonetheless, in patients with an unstable cardiopulmonary status or an acute myocardial infarction, application is contraindicated (Dolan et al., 2009). Soltani et al. (2011) tested a mixture of tPA and the CA Optison® and the soft-shell MB SonoVue® (now Lumason®, Bracco, Milano, Italy) in a different setup. Using a catheter as a model of human vessels, they treated *in vitro* an acute ischemic stroke via intra-arterial sonothrombolysis, suggesting an effective treatment for some stroke patients (Soltani et al.,

2011). Optison® is FDA-approved for cardiac applications such as left ventricular opafication and endocardial border definition. Like polymer-shelled MB, it was shown by Korpanty et al. (2005) to use albumin-based MB, here in combination with dextrose, for molecular targeting. Avidin was incorporated in the shell, so that biotinylated antibodies could be bound functionally to the bubbles (Korpanty et al., 2005). Another more recent approach uses targeted poly-D,L-lactide/albumin hybrid MB for differential diagnosis in patients with chest pain to detect recent ischemia (Leng et al., 2014).

Soft-Shell Microbubbles

Soft-shell MB are commonly used for examinations using a low mechanical index (MI) since these MB are sensitively detectable by their non-linear oscillations. The better oscillation properties of SS-MB compared with HS-MB are due to the thinner, more flexible shells, which are held together not by covalent bonding, but hydrophobic interactions. Therefore, after slight shell disruptions, the shell seals itself to minimize surface tension (Borden et al., 2005; Brismar et al., 2012). If sealing is not possible due to the high acoustic pressure, the MB will split into several smaller bubbles instead of bursting like HS-MB (**Figure**). To achieve optimal contrast, the shells' characteristics should be considered and the acoustic power adjusted to the type of MB (Leong-Poi et al., 2002).

The most common shell materials for SS-MB are surfactant molecules or phospholipids, where the length of the acyl chain mainly influences the bubbles' acoustic dissolution and the monolayers' cohesiveness (Borden et al., 2005).

Phospholipid microbubbles

Several patents from Unger et al. (1994) describe early approaches for the synthesis of SS-MB and handling of gas-filled liposomes with a diameter of approximately 2 μm. Those liposomes were easy to produce by just adding the phospholipid of choice to water or buffer of the temperature slightly above the lipids' transition point from gel to a liquid crystalline state in which the liposomes form, cooling it back down and removing the liquid by negative pressure application (Unger, 1994). Dried liposomes, in presence of protectants such as trehalose, were found to have a greatly increased shelf life stability and to regain their shape and functionality when refilled with gas again (Crowe et al., 1985).

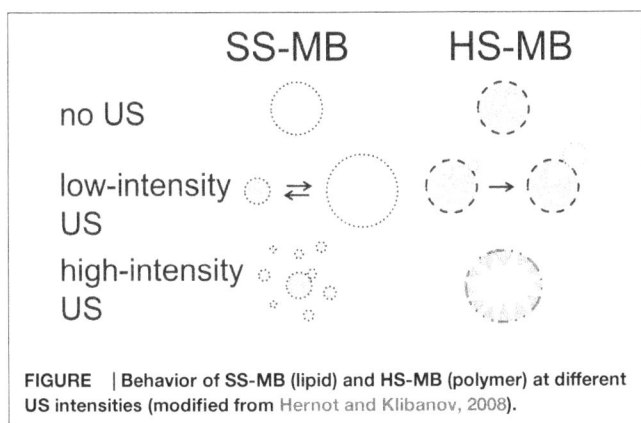

FIGURE | Behavior of SS-MB (lipid) and HS-MB (polymer) at different US intensities (modified from Hernot and Klibanov, 2008).

Upscaling production of lipid-layer MB, as well as the use of those bubbles for multimodal imaging via inclusion of paramagnetic particles such as gadolinium in the bubbles for MRI has been patented by D'Arrigo (1993), who also described the potential of MB for tumor treatment, even in the brain (D'Arrigo, 1993).

The first lipid-based USCA that made it to clinical trials and the clinics was Perflutren, sold as Definity® or Luminity® (Lantheus Medical Imaging, North Billerica, MA, USA). It contains perfluoropropane-filled MB in a shell made of three different saturated 16-carbon-long phospholipids. With an average size between only 1–2 μm they are smaller than most HS-MB (Unger et al., 2004). During the trial phase, a good compatibility was seen, as well as left ventricular cavity and myocardial enhancement (Fritz et al., 1997). Despite being developed and FDA approved primarily for echocardiography and cardiologic application, studies showed further clinical applications (Barr, 2013), such as their use to improve detection of tumors, e.g., in the liver. It takes a few minutes to examine a whole liver with US, but the MB lifetime of approximately 3.5 min after bolus injection was found to be sufficient. Compared to non-CEUS, the usage of Definity® showed a higher reliability in tumor- and nodule detection in the liver of rabbits, though the CA itself does not accumulate in the liver (Maruyama et al., 2005).

Similar to HS-MB, lipid-based MB have been found to be useful for therapeutic applications. Integration of lipophilic drugs in the shell, coupling to the outer side of the shell, or encapsulation of therapeutic agents have been shown and are under development for US-assisted and guided therapy, i.e., in cancer treatment. They have also been successfully tested for thrombolysis in combination with US and thrombolytic agents (Unger et al., 2004). More about therapeutical applications will be described later on (see Bubbles as Therapeutics).

Apart from Definity®/Luminity®, another SS-MB has clinical approval for cardiologic applications. SonoVue® (Bracco Imaging) gained FDA-approval in 2001 and, after a withdrawal, again in 2014, now under the name Lumason®. This sulfur hexafluoride filled phospholipid-MB are generally used for left ventricular opafication and endocardial border definition, but in some countries also have approval for general vessel diagnostic or imaging of microvascular structures in the breast or differentiation of lesions in the liver (Claudon et al., 2013; Appis et al., 2015). Apart from that, SonoVue® has also been tested in clinical trials for monitoring of uterine fibroid vascularization and improved ablation (Henri et al., 2014; Jiang et al., 2014).

Surfactant-stabilized microbubbles

Hilmann et al. (1985) already suggested the usage of surfactant-stabilized gaseous MB for US diagnostics, but it was not before the mid-90s that this method found its way into more clinically-related *in vitro* research. Among the first surfactant-stabilized MB were those derived from a mixture of the non-ionic surfactants Span60 (sorbitan monostearat) and Tween80 (polyoxyethylene sorbitan monooleate) in different molar ratios, but also other members of the Span/Tween family. MBs of a diameter below the maximum of 10 μm were obtainable and for certain mixtures a shelf time of several weeks and a high echogenicity in B-mode

US imaging were shown (Singhal et al., 1993; Wheatley et al., 1994). Still, those MB that succeeded in clinical trials were of different materials. Imagent® (IMCOR Pharmaceuticals Inc., San Diego, CA, USA) MB of approximately 5 μm in diameter, filled with a mixture of air and PFCs, were first tested for renal and liver perfusion studies in rabbits, later for myocardial perfusion and detection of general blood flow abnormalities using Doppler US. It showed promising contrast and compatibility with almost no adverse side effects in first clinical trials (Taylor et al., 1996; Sirlin et al., 1997; Pelura, 1998). Nonetheless other CA from this family dominated and still dominate, both in research and in the clinics. One of them, Levovist® (Schering AG, Berlin, Germany) or SHU-508, was developed in the late 1980s and has been tested and used for several applications since then. Consisting of a saccharide- and palmitic acid-containing shell and air-filled in early versions, it was first tested for examinations of the left ventricle in dogs. A huge advantage was the mean size below 6 μm and the described transpulmonary circulation, making intravenous injections possible and injections directly into the left heart chamber superfluous, (Smith et al., 1989). Clinical trials on echocardiography in patients showed good contrast enhancement and only minor adverse side effects (Schlief et al., 1991). In patients with liver metastases Levovist® greatly enhanced the visualization of blood flow in the tumors, which led to a better differentiation between cancer, hemangiomas and fatty lesions (Ernst et al., 1997). Similarly, more recent studies investigated the advantages of CEUS using Levovist® for differentiation between benign and malignant tumors in several organs, such as spleen, breast, and ovaries. A clear differentiation between malignant and benign tumors was possible, which led to the conclusion that CEUS with Levovist® can help to avoid unnecessary biopsies and surgeries (Ota and Ono, 2004; Wu et al., 2015).

The other main player in the field of surfactant-stabilized MB is Echogen® (Sonus Pharmaceuticals, Bothel, WA, USA) with a core of dodecafluorpentane. First described by Cotter et al. (1994) it quickly became an object of interest (Kronzon et al., 1994). Dodecafluorpentane has a boiling point of approximately 29°C, so it can be injected intravenously as nano-sized, non-echogenic liquid droplets, and immediately transit to echogenic bubbles of 1–2 μm (Forsberg et al., 1994). In direct comparison with Albunex® for echocardiography, the dodecafluorpentane-based CA was found to lead to better results regarding enhancement duration, endocardial border delineation and diagnostic confidence (Grayburn et al., 1998). However, among the surfactant-stabilized MB, Levovist® was the more common, especially since it received approval for clinical applications and in Europe and Canada, whereas Sonus Pharmaceuticals stated withdrawal of their application for FDA approval in 2000 (Correas et al., 2014). By now, Levovist® is not approved anymore for clinical use either. A list of USCA which have/had clinical approval is given in **Table** .

Nanobubbles

Due to their size, MB are unable to leave the vasculature, even in solid tumors, which often have leaky vasculature and a poor lymphatic drainage. This leads to extravasation and retention of macromolecules, also known as the EPR effect (enhanced permeability and retention). To extravasate to the tumor itself, bubbles need to be smaller than 400–800 nm in diameter, therefore referred to as NBs. It has been shown that even bubbles of this dimension were able to produce an enhanced backscatter after US application (Oeffinger and Wheatley, 2004). Additionally, high accumulation of NB in tumors was described, also referred to as passive targeting (Yin et al., 2012). Enhancement of more than 20 dB could be detected for several minutes in vitro, using NB of approximately 500 nm in size and being composed of a Span60/Tween80 shell and octafluoropropane as a gaseous core. However, similar to experiments with MB derived from Span60/Tween80, some adverse side effects such as tachycardia were seen in patients due to the limited biocompatibility of the material. Using the highly compatible polyoxyethylene-40-stearate as a substitute for Tween80 to create a "parents suspension" with MB and separation of NB populations by centrifugation led to the development of biocompatible NB of 400-600 nm size. Extravasation into the tumor tissue and contrast enhancement for several minutes was seen using power Doppler (Xing et al., 2010). In different approaches, PLGA and PBCA instead of surfactants have been used to develop biocompatible NB between 150–450 nm (300–500 nm, respectively) in diameter that have been labeled with antibodies binding to HLA-G or TAG-72 to specifically bind to tumors deriving from trophoblastic or epithelial tissue (Xu et al., 2010; Zhang et al., 2014).

Regarding in vivo lifetime of NB, results from different studies vary between a few minutes to more than 1 h of contrast enhancement (du Toit et al., 2011; Yin et al., 2012). The size of NB, their material composition and additional coatings or added ligands strongly influence the circulation time and their uptake by the reticuloendothelial system, so that for each NB formulation this factor needs to be determined individually.

If exclusively imaging is wanted, MB still are the first choice due to their higher gaseous content and better oscillation. Nonetheless, accumulation of PFC-containing nanodroplets in the tumor interstitium and US-induced fusion of droplets into MB has been reported (Rapoport et al., 2011). Additionally injection of a nanoparticle emulsion with a generally poor acoustic reflectivity strongly enhances US-contrast when bound in great numbers to specific target sites (Lanza et al., 2000). However, NB are of high interest for therapeutic approaches such as thermal sensitizers in tumors that undergo radiofrequency treatment (Perera et al., 2014). When filled with or coupled to drugs, generally for cancer treatment, the passive targeting to the tumor and the EPR effect might be used for more specific drug delivery and enhanced therapeutic success. Additionally, several groups are also working on the development of targeted, drug-, nucleic acid-filled, or drug-free NBs, directed against different tumor markers.

The current state of the art and preclinical studies with NB will be described later on.

TABLE | Ultrasound contrast agent that have/had been clinically approved.

Name	First approved for clinical use	Shell material	Gas	Application (examples)	Producer/distributor	Countries
Optison	1998	Cross-linked serum albumin	Octafluoropropane	Left ventricular opafication	GE healthcare, Buckinghamshire, UK	US, Europe
Sonazoid	2007	Phospholipid	Perfluorobutane	Myocardial perfusion, liver imaging	GE healthcare, Buckinghamshire, UK/ Daiichi Saniko, Tokyo, JP	Japan, South Korea
Lumason/SonoVue	2001/2014	Phospholipid	Sulphurhexafluoride	Left ventricular opafication, microvascular enhancement (liver and breast lesion detection)	Bracco diagnostics, Milano, Italy	US, Europe, China
Definity/Luminity	2001/2006	Phospholipid	Octafluoropropane	Echocardiography, liver/kidney imaging (Canada)	Lantheus medical Imaging, North Billerica, MA	North America, Europe (approval filed)
Imagent/Imavist	2002, withdrawn	Phospholipid	Perfluorohexane, Nitrogen	Echocardiography, heart perfusion, tumor/blood flow anomalies	Schering AG, Berlin, DE	US
Echovist	1991, withdrawn	Galactose microparticles	Air	Right heart imaging	Schering AG, Berlin, DE	Germany, UK
Levovist	1995, withdrawn	Galactose microparticles, palmitic acid	Air	Whole heart imaging, doppler imaging	Schering AG, Berlin, DE	Canada, Europe, China, Japan
Albunex	1993, withdrawn	Sonicated serum albumin	air	Transpulmonary imaging	Molecular Biosystems Inc., San Diego, CA, USA	Japan, US

Silica Shells

With a size between 0.2–2 μm, silica hard-shell particles cannot be placed uniformly in the groups of MB or NB, nor can they be called bubbles, but they are an interesting and new USCA as well. Their rise started around 2009 when Lin et al. (2009) showed their first experiments with gas-filled silica shells *in vitro*. A high MI is required to rupture the shells, releasing the gas of the porous particles and thus produce an US-detectable signal (Lin et al., 2009). Synthesis of silica shells is more complicated compared to other USCA, as it requires templates, generally polystyrene particles, which have to be removed by suitable solvents and replaced by PFCs afterward. After evaluation of possible cytotoxic or hemolytic effects of clinically reasonable concentrations, silica shells were injected in rat testicles and detected with US at varying MI (Hu et al., 2011a). A clearly visible contrast enhancement was seen up to 20 min after injection. In a murine cancer model silica micro- and nano-shells were injected intraperitoneally and imaged using a MI of 1.9 which destroyed the shells and led to detectable "Loss of correlation" signals, when the air sucked out of the particle shell. After image processing steps for motion correction and threshold-, median- and high-pass filter application the high background signals could be subtracted and the accumulation of silica shells in the tumor could be reliably detected (Ta et al., 2012). Liberman et al. (2012, 2014) suggested the usage of silica micro-shells for labeling breast tumors. In their study, the shells were shown to stay in place and being detectable after a local injection for more than 1 day, providing an alternative to guiding wires which are clinical standard. Additionally, those silica particles were found to be promising sonosensitizers in US-mediated ablation therapies in *ex vivo* and some first *in vivo* experiments (Liberman et al., 2012, 2014), whereas another approach combined silica-coated shells

with PFC-filling and additionally an included chemotherapeutic drug. With a USCA like that, imaging, ablation and drug delivery would be possible at the same time, but further development is needed here (Ma et al., 2014).

Similar to bubble CA, researchers work on modifications of silica shells for specific targeting. A first attempt of micron-sized shells with a functionalization involved the addition of an amino ($-NH_2$) group (Hu et al., 2011b). In their publication they also describe a simple way to control the shells' diameter and thickness by variation of tetraethylorthosilicate content. Another approach to modify silica particles involves conjugation of hollow silica nano-sized spheres to Gd-DTPA and cycloRGD. This construct has been tested successfully in a murine tumor model for targeted tumor imaging with MRI and US, but animals have only been observed for 8 h after injection and long-term studies will be needed for a proper evaluation (An et al., 2014).

Biodistribution and Degradation

For the development of new CA, often clinically approved or as biocompatible considered biomaterials are chosen. Parallel to the investigation of the material's behavior in its bubble/particle shape under US application, *in vitro* toxicity and stability tests under physiological conditions need to be done. Here, first experiments with the CA in presence of blood can be made to rule out potential hemolytic effects of MB under US application (Dalecki, 2005), or a low stability when confronted with blood. For the gaseous filling, it has been shown that PFC as not-naturally in living organisms existing gases, are biologically inert and completely excreted by exhalation within less than 1 day without undergoing modification (Hutter et al., 1999;

Hvattum et al., 2001; Toft et al., 2006). Clearance of the shell material happens via the reticuloendothelial system, namely liver and spleen, where macrophages engulf what is left after the gaseous content left the shell by diffusion. Renal clearance has not been reported for clinically approved USCA, which makes CEUS a suitable diagnostic tool also in patients with renal insufficiency, without the need for other examinations and before CA application. Temporary pain in the kidney area after CA injection is most likely caused by the MBs' accumulation in the small renal vessels, though an effect on blood circulation and function could not be found (Cokkinos et al., 2013; Liu et al., 2013). To the best of our knowledge, a broad comparison study of the exact degradation and clearance processes of the most common USCA has not been done so far, most likely because severe side effects rarely occur and long term impairments have not been described.

Not only degassed, empty shells and fragments, but also intact MB can be taken up by Kupffer cells in the liver, and similar observations have been made for other macrophage populations and neutrophils outside of the liver as well (Kindberg et al., 2003) for Sonazoid® (GE Healthcare, Buckinghamshire, UK). The general tendency to enhance signal in the liver after injection is best known for Levovist®, but also Sonazoid® and Optison®, and enables detection of liver and spleen anomalies, whereas SonoVue® and Imavist® (Alliance Pharmaceuticals Corp., Chippenham, UK) show little to no uptake by Kupffer cells (Albrecht et al., 2000; Wilson et al., 2000). Due to an accumulation of these CA in the smaller vessels of the liver and a reduced blood flow velocity, both blood pool CA can be used for differentiation of benign and malign liver lesions anyway (Maruyama et al., 2004; von Herbay et al., 2004; Quaia, 2006; Yanagisawa et al., 2007). Shell composition, size and surface properties are responsible for their circulation time and uptake by phagocytes, and no general behavior for phospholipid- or protein-based bubbles can be predicted. So even between materials from the same shell material 'family', differences can be seen, most likely due to activation of the complement-system by slightly different surface structures (Chen and Borden, 2011; Kiessling et al., 2012). For unbound bubbles, clearance via the reticuloendothelial system normally happens within the first 10 min after injection (Yuan and Rychak, 2013). To reduce the fast uptake, addition of PEG to the outer surface can help to prolong circulation time and further improve the general biocompatibility (Ryan et al., 2008; Chen and Borden, 2011). For polymer-coated MB, currently not clinically approved, renal excretion after shell breakdown (Palmowski et al., 2008) has been described and for some nanoparticles, excretion by the renal and hepatic system by feces has been shown, though leftovers were still detectable in animals after 3 months (Chen et al., 2013).

Micro- and NB were applied in patients with impaired organ function without mentionable side effects (Albrecht et al., 2004). SonoVue® has been tested in patients with chronic obstructive pulmonary disease without showing more than temporary light impairments like headaches, rushes, or dizziness (Bokor et al., 2001). The theoretical risk of MB injections in patients with coronary diseases is known and premature ventricular contractions have been documented, especially at higher MI and mostly after continuous injection instead of a bolus injection. Adverse effects though are rare and generally mild and temporary, and unlike other imaging modalities, USCA have been safely applied to patients with renal diseases, kidney failure or a generally very bad health condition without an increase in side effects. In at least three cases, however, patients died after SonoVue® injection, but it is uncertain if the CA injections caused the events (van der Wouw et al., 2000; ter Haar, 2009; Wei et al., 2014).

Active and Passive Targeting

As mentioned before, the EPR effect enables the accumulation of NB in the tissue of tumors, without any specific modifications or targeting molecules. This type of contrast enhancement or drug accumulation in the tissue is therefore referred to as passive targeting (Yin et al., 2012). However, also MB can be used up to a certain point for passive targeting. The chemical composition of the shell affects its behavior in the body, causing accumulations in tissues or attachment to cells. For example, Lindner et al. (2000a) were able to show binding of albumin- and lipid-shelled MB to activated leukocytes adherent to the venular wall without further specific targeting moieties in an inflammation model. Binding was mediated by β2-integrin and the complement system (Lindner et al., 2000a). The same group also demonstrated that incorporation of phosphatidylserine in the lipid shell enables binding to activated leukocytes in inflammation (Lindner et al., 2000b).

Active targeting requires specific surface modification. Since MB are limited to the vascular compartment, their targets need to be expressed on the luminal side of endothelial cells in pathological environments (**Figure**). Therefore, the first approaches toward targeted MB aimed for thrombosis diagnostics and investigated the blood clot dissolving properties of US application. Unger et al. (1998, 2000) used for their first in vitro system the shortest functional peptide sequence of fibrinogen, known to bind to glycoprotein IIb/IIIa on platelets, and linked it to a lipid-shell bubble. In a binding assay, they observed both binding and signal enhancement. Their first in vivo studies in a dog model showed similarly promising results (Unger et al., 1998, 2000). Other early approaches involved targeting the intercellular adhesion molecule 1 (ICAM-1) for the detection of atherogenesis. Villanueva et al. (1998) used an anti-ICAM-1 antibody covalently bound to a lipid-shell bubble, showing a 40-times higher adhesion of labeled bubbles to interleukin-1β-activated ICAM-1 overexpressing endothelial cells in an in vitro flow system, compared to untreated endothelial cells. For a first in vivo approach, a rat model of heterotopic heart transplant rejection was chosen. Both successful binding and a strong US contrast enhancement were demonstrated in the transplanted organ undergoing acute rejection (Weller et al., 2003).

A marker of angiogenesis in tumors is integrin $\alpha_V\beta_3$ expressed by proliferating and activated endothelial cells. To specifically

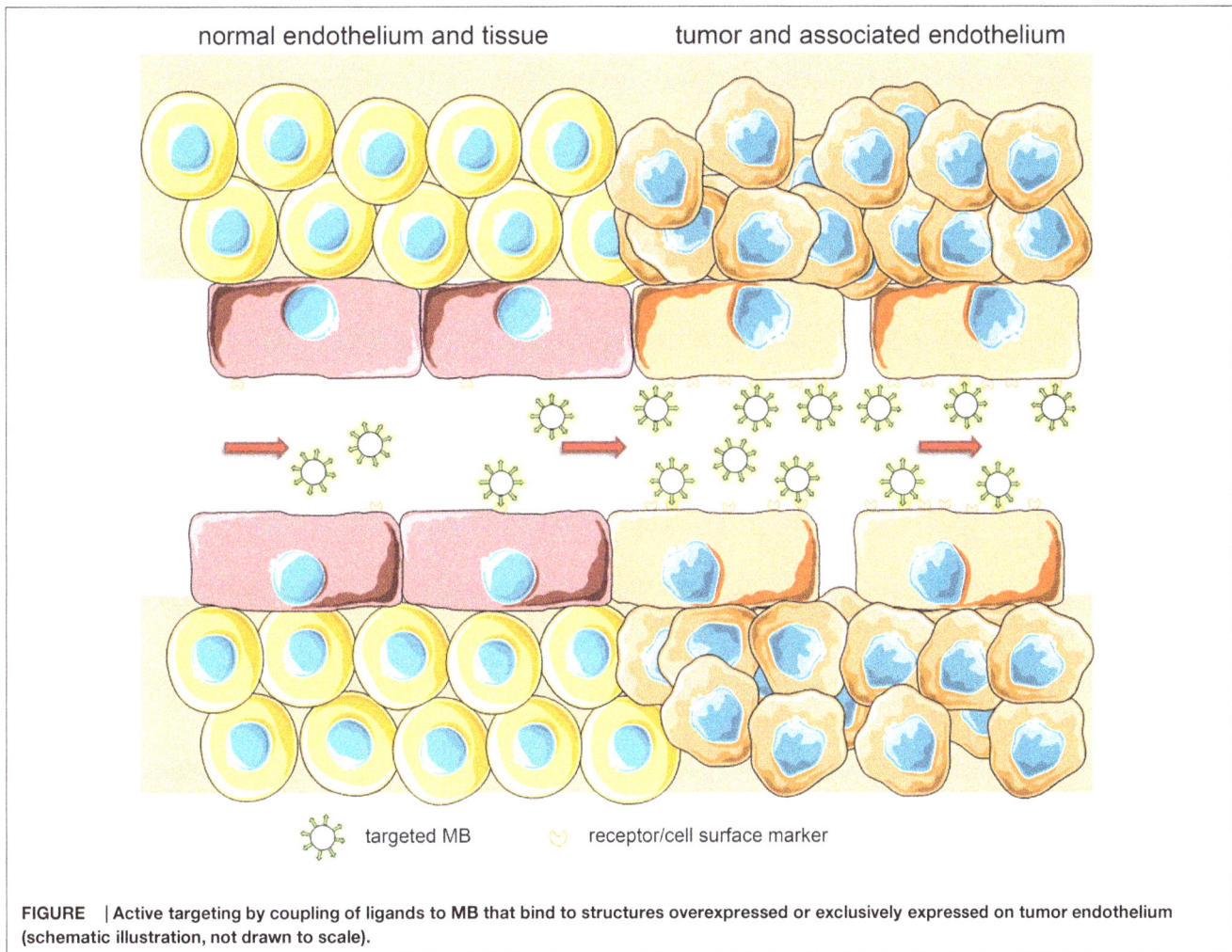

FIGURE | Active targeting by coupling of ligands to MB that bind to structures overexpressed or exclusively expressed on tumor endothelium (schematic illustration, not drawn to scale).

target tumors, antibodies binding to the α_V-integrin subunit were linked to MB and injected in mice that underwent local growth factor treatment to induce neovascularization at the injection site, and thus endothelial activation. A significantly greater amount of MB was found in this area, as well as a higher acoustic activity (Leong-Poi, 2002). Short peptide sequences like RGD can be used instead of α_V-integrin-antibodies. In a murine Met-1 breast cancer model, Ellegala et al. (2003) were able to show similar results with MB linked to the integrin-recognition peptide sequence RGD, and suggested $\alpha_V\beta_3$-targeted MB for early tumor angiogenesis detection. Similar to $\alpha_V\beta_3$, the vascular endothelial growth factor receptor 2 (VEGFR2) is commonly expressed on activated, proliferating endothelial cells, which makes it another target of interest for the detection of tumor angiogenesis. VEGFR2 was successfully targeted with lipid-shell MB in tumor models (Willmann et al., 2008). However, in a murine model α_V and VEGFR2 performed poorly as markers for evaluation of early response to treatment. In this study, endoglin was found to be a more suitable target molecule (Leguerney et al., 2015).

Alternatively, Fokong et al. (2013) linked the peptide sequence IELLQAR to PBCA-MB and achieved a strong contrast

enhancement in a murine breast cancer model due to the MB binding to E-selectin, a marker of vascular inflammation and early angiogenesis. Despite many positive pre-clinical studies, evaluation in patients still has to be done. Here, it has to be considered that the recognition motif to the MB which leads to immunogenic responses in patients.

Active targeting has also been tested for NB. The principle is the same, but contrary to MB, NB can also target receptors and other molecules outside the endothelium due to their possible extravasation to the tumor tissue (**Figure**). Functional coupling of an antibody, in this case directed against the TAG-72 antigen overexpressed on several epithelial tumors, to polymer-coated NB and successful binding of those to cancer cells *in vitro* has been shown by Xu et al. (2010). The usefulness of such an approach for tumor treatment has also been demonstrated *in vivo* using HLA-G as a target for antibody-coupled polymer-NB (Zhang et al., 2014). The combination of HIFU and the local release of chemotherapeutics after bubble disruption was shown to strongly enhance apoptosis of tumor cells. Recently Jiang et al. (2015) presented a promising new construct for tumor imaging, improving the idea and the *in vitro* model of Liu et al. (2007). Their lipid-based NB were coupled to

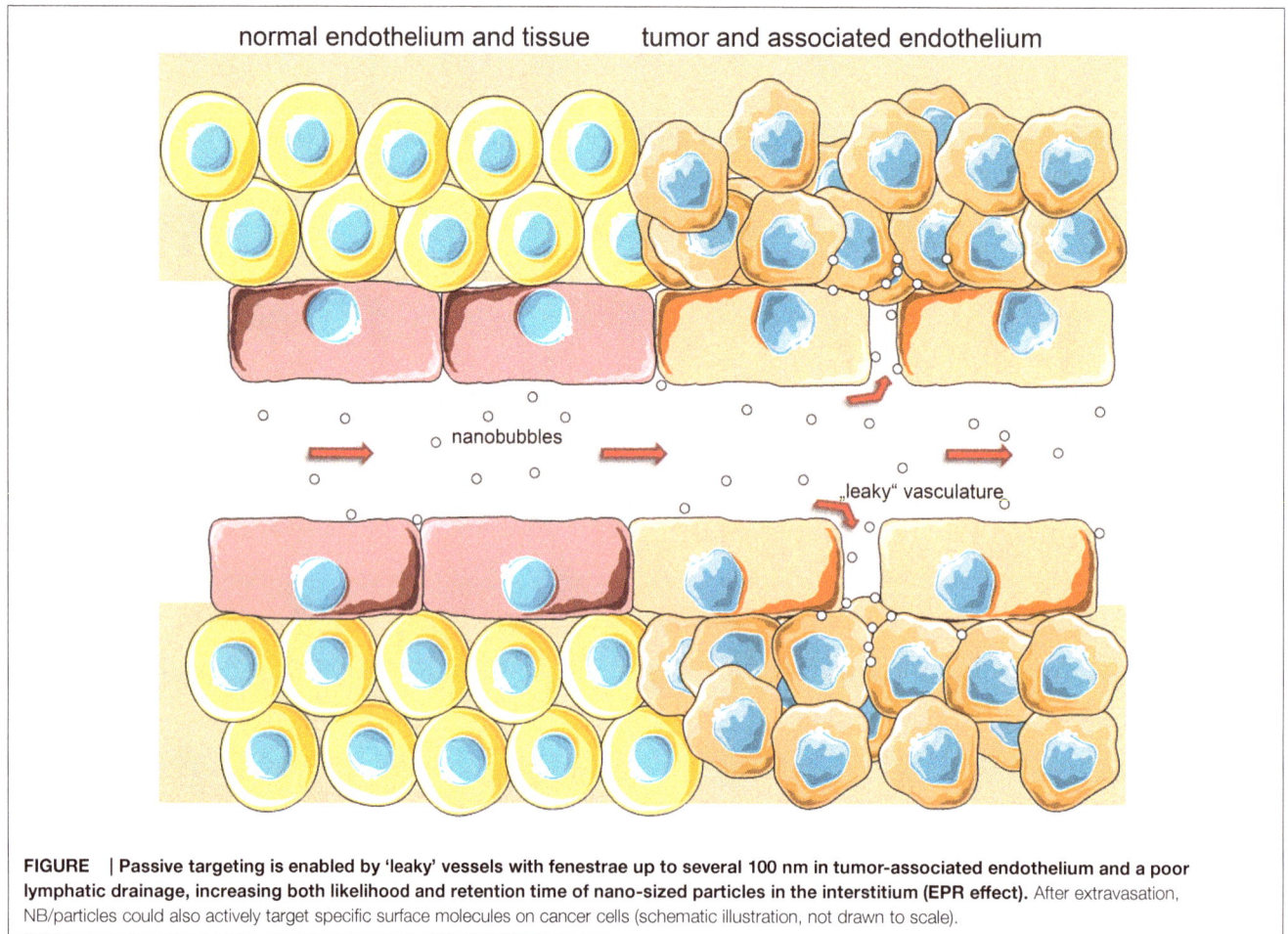

FIGURE | Passive targeting is enabled by 'leaky' vessels with fenestrae up to several 100 nm in tumor-associated endothelium and a poor lymphatic drainage, increasing both likelihood and retention time of nano-sized particles in the interstitium (EPR effect). After extravasation, NB/particles could also actively target specific surface molecules on cancer cells (schematic illustration, not drawn to scale).

Herceptin® (Roche, Basel, CH), also known as trastuzumab, a therapeutic monoclonal antibody binding to Her-2, which is overexpressed in many breast tumors. They found a significant increase in NB-binding to the tumor in xenograft-models which are known to overexpress Her-2, but only little accumulation in tumor xenografts with low Her-2 expression. Targeted NB in Her-2 overexpressing tumors also had an increased washout half-time, enabling longer observation times. Additionally, their bubble-construct was found to be of a low cytotoxicity (Jiang et al., 2015). To this date, this might be the approach being the closest to clinical studies. Herceptin® has also been conjugated to mesoporous silica nanoparticles and showed tumor-specific toxicity *in vitro,* suggesting further development of silica particles in the field of targeted imaging and drug delivery (Milgroom et al., 2014).

Bubbles as Therapeutics

The basic idea behind using MB for therapeutic purposes is their ability to enhance vibration-effects generated by US pulses. Already Tachibana and Tachibana (1995) observed that US-mediated thrombolysis is more effective in the presence of bubbles, resulting from acoustic cavitation of the sonicated

bubbles. Then, Molina et al. (2006) could demonstrate in a clinical study on stroke patients that the rate of complete arterial recanalization after sonification was significantly higher in the group that received MB and tPA, compared to only tPA. Similar results were found in a sonothrombolysis trial with transcranial US (Molina et al., 2009). Thus, the application of MB to enhance US-mediated thrombolysis has the potential for improving therapy of acute stroke patients (Tsivgoulis et al., 2010). Recent results from Petit et al. (2015). support the claim of strong synergistic effects when US, MB, and tPA are combined due to an enhanced clot lysis and degradation of fibrin.

Another application area for USCA as therapeutics is HIFU-based tumor ablation. In the non-contrast-enhanced setting, this is facilitated by thermal and mechanical effects in the target tissue arising from absorption of high-frequency US waves and the internal conversion into heat and vibration, including acoustic cavitation and radiation forces (Saha et al., 2014). The group of Jiang et al. (2014) could demonstrate in a clinical study that the additional administration of MB (SonoVue®) to patients prior to HIFU ablation increased the HIFU-mediated tumor ablation significantly more than solely HIFU, even at lower sonification power and less sonification time. The mechanism of the bubble-enhanced HIFU-mediated tissue ablation is suspected to be a result of the violent bubble collapse, which may cause mechanical injury in the target tissue (Farny et al., 2010).

A further application area for USCA as therapeutics is sonoporation. LOFU pulses mediate temporal permeabilization of cell membranes and enable drug delivery across biological barriers like blood vessels or even the BBB (Kiessling et al., 2012). Without bubbles, the low-intensity acoustic US-field promotes inertial cavitation, resulting in gas bubble creation, leading to streaming and radiation forces to the tissue. The addition of MB decreases the energy required to create cavitation and increases the effectiveness of cell membrane permeation and of cell transfections (Delalande et al., 2013).

Microbubbles might also be used for gene therapy. Here, the transport of genes or nucleic acids to and their introduction into cells is facilitated by CEUS. Wang et al. (2008) showed that in presence of MB the efficacy of cell transfection was 1–2 orders of magnitude higher than with plasmid DNA alone. However, the efficacy of US-mediated gene transfer is low in comparison to electroporation or viral transfection. Thus, the group around Sun intends to design MB, which are better suited for gene delivery than the commercially available Definity®. They increased the

lipid-shell acyl-chain length to enhance the bubble stability or charged the spheres' shell positively in order to improve DNA-binding affinity. Using the designed MB for gene transfection, the group observed significantly enhanced transfection effectiveness by stronger transgene expression compared to gene transfection with Definity®. Still, transfection efficacy is not comparable to viral transfection, but since US-mediated transfection using MB contains less risks regarding immunotoxicity and possible oncogenic effects and provides a better spatial and temporal control of the process, work in this field will be continued (Sun et al., 2014). Dewitte et al. (2014) also used a combination of lipid MB and nucleic acids for transfections. In their setup, mRNA coding for cancer antigens was bound to the lipid bubbles. Application of US led to transfection of murine dendritic cells ex vivo. These were later on injected, similar to a vaccination, into lymph nodes near the tumors of nude mice. The matured antigen-presenting dendritic cells then lead to a strong reduction of tumor mass, in some cases even complete remission and long-term immunity to tumors expressing this antigen (Dewitte et al., 2014). Similar to transfection studies with MB, Yin et al. (2014) used NB to transfect cells in vitro and in vivo with siRNA to enhance apoptosis in tumors

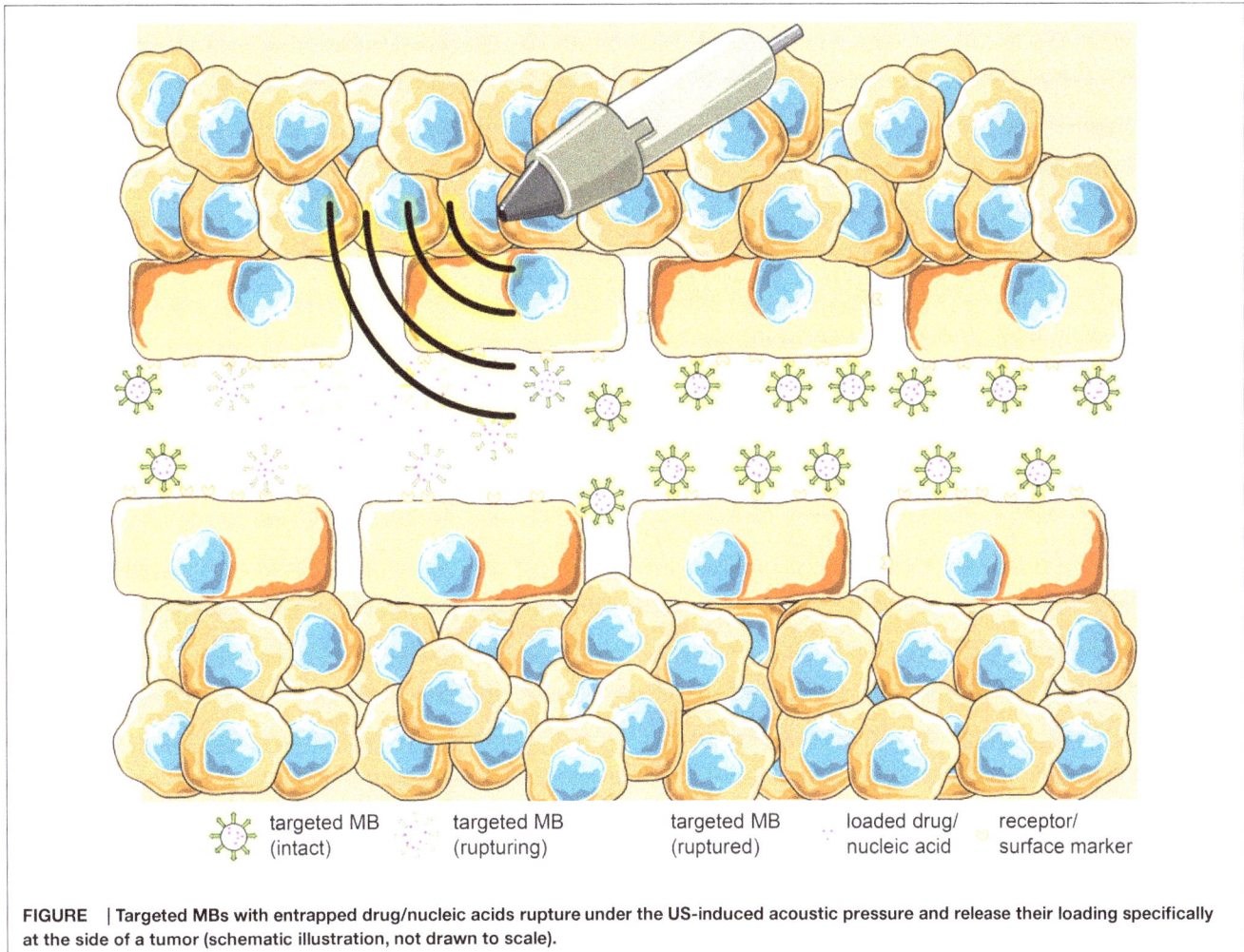

targeted MB (intact) targeted MB (rupturing) targeted MB (ruptured) loaded drug/ nucleic acid receptor/ surface marker

FIGURE | Targeted MBs with entrapped drug/nucleic acids rupture under the US-induced acoustic pressure and release their loading specifically at the side of a tumor (schematic illustration, not drawn to scale).

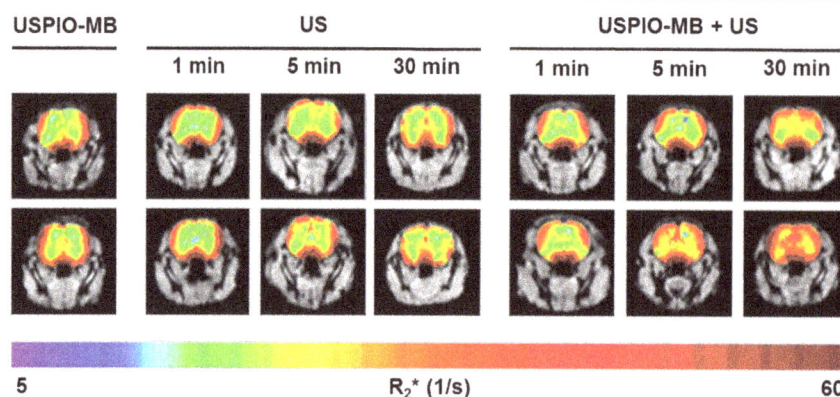

FIGURE | **Effect of US only (US) and USPIO-labeled MB with US (USPIO-MB+US) on the BBB.** T_2*-weighted MRI images were taken before and after US/USPIO-MB+US application, R_2* values of each measurement were color-coded and overlayed. The most striking difference can be seen after US application for 30 min, comparing pre- and post-scan in both groups (from: Lammers et al., 2015, ©2014 WILEY-VCH Verlag GmbH & Co. KGaA, Weinheim).

after NB injection and US treatment with promising first results.

The second application field for bubble-enhanced sonoporation is US-mediated drug release (**Figure**). Using drug-loaded MB, it is possible to spatiotemporally apply LOFU pulses at certain organs to increase the membrane permeability, and at the same time increase the energy to promote bubble collapse and particle release (Tzu-Yin et al., 2013). This way, the group around Kiessling and co-workers used USPIO containing PBCA-MB (USPIO-MB) as a proof of principle approach to demonstrate drug delivery across the BBB in mice (**Figure**). For the experiment, mice were scanned by MRI before and after injection of USPIO-MB and successive US treatment in the head region using destructive pulses. In comparison to control groups, the USPIO brain incorporation was significantly increased in the group receiving US treatment. Drug delivery across the BBB was additionally confirmed by histology, and significantly enhanced FITC-dextran extravasation and deposition within the brain was detected in animals receiving USPIO-MB and sonification. The temporal and spatial BBB-opening offers a new perspective to treat gliomas, but also neurodegenerative disorders like Alzheimer or Parkinson's disease, where macromolecular drugs or growth factors have to be locally accumulated (Lammers et al., 2015). However, also outside of the brain US-supported drug delivery is promising. In an animal model of incomplete tumor resection, cetuximab-loaded MB and US stimulation had stronger therapeutic effects on the remaining tumor mass than cetuximab-only treated animals, which was confirmed by *in vivo* fluorescence and bioluminescence, as well as caliper measurements (Sorace et al., 2014). Co-delivery of paclitaxel and siRNA to inhibit anti-apoptotic protein production also showed very promising results in a murine HepG2 tumor model. Here, tumor growth was strongly inhibited in animals which received NB with paclitaxel entrapped in and siRNA-containing micelles attached to the shell, additionally to US application. Furthermore those animals showed longer survival (Yin et al., 2014). Despite those promising results further animal studies need to be done before similar setups can go into clinical trials.

Besides being or delivering the therapeutic agents themselves, MB were shown to be highly useful in monitoring of oncological therapies. Shortly after chemotherapy started, Lassau et al. (2005, 2006). could show changes in tumor vascularity or increasing necrosis in patients with metastatic melanoma and gastrointestinal stroma tumors after injection of Levovist® and SonoVue®. Using standardized dynamic CEUS measurements, the group was even able to predict the outcome of antiangiogenic tumor therapy by evaluating the "area under the perfusion curve." Among several criteria, this one was found to be highly correlated to therapy response and freedom from progression (Lassau et al., 2014). Differentiation of responders and non-responders at early points in time is needed to plan if the therapy will be continued or if an alternative has to be considered.

Conclusion

In this review we presented the historical development of CAs for US imaging from the early steps to the current state of the art. MBs are established CA for clinical vascular analysis and liver diagnosis, but also other applications. A broad variety of materials and sizes generates the basis for those multiple diagnostic and therapeutic applications. Currently, there are three clinically approved CAs, but with many on-going pre-clinical studies and promising first results, more clinical trials can be expected to start within the next years. The combination of US CAs for diagnostics and therapy in one single injection therefore holds a great potential for the future and might be a valuable tool for treatment of widespread and deadly diseases like cancer or cardiovascular diseases. But also for neurodegenerative diseases USCA might play a growing role in treatment. A temporary increase in vessel permeability could enhance drug delivery to the brain or other tumors while reducing systemic side effects due to the mostly local delivery. USCA might also gain more importance in non-invasive ablation therapies.

When functional analysis or tissue vascularization does not suffice, the application of molecularly-targeted CA would be complementary, both in diagnosis and targeted drug delivery. For targeted MB and NB, the pre-clinically common biotin-streptavidin linking method needs a similarly strong and easy alternative to avoid immune reactions. Additionally, more targets with a sufficiently strong binding to the ligand are required, otherwise the shear stress in vessels might inhibit successful binding of the CAs and thus impair the contrast enhancement. Another point that might need refinement is the CA's circulation time. So far even PEGylated bubbles with PFC have a very limited lifetime, limiting the time frame for examination. But with no described long term impairments after injection, rare side effects and a valuable role in diagnostics, sonothrombolysis, monitoring of treatment, specific and targeted substance delivery vesicles or sonosensitizers, the technology of CA and US in combination is –with some specific adjustments- the swiss army knife among CAs and imaging modalities.

Acknowledgments

This work was supported by the German Ministry for Education and Research/Bundesministerium für Bildung und Forschung (BMBF), project numbers 0315415C and 0316042F, as well as by the German Research Foundation/Deutsche Forschungsgemeinschaft (DFG), project KI 1072/15-1.

References

Albrecht, T., Blomley, M., Bolondi, L., Claudon, M., Correas, J.-M., Cosgrove, D., et al. (2004). Guidelines for the use of contrast agents in ultrasound: january 2004. *Ultraschall. Medizin.* 25, 249–256. doi: 10.1055/s-2004-813245

Albrecht, T., Blomley, M. J., Heckemann, R. A., Cosgrove, D. O., Jayaram, V., Butler-Barnes, J., et al. (2000). Stimulated acoustic emissions with the ultrasound contrast medium Levovist: a clinically useful contrast effect with liver-specific properties. *Rofo* 172, 61–67. doi: 10.1055/s-2000-11101

An, L., Hu, H., Du, J., Wei, J., Wang, L., Yang, H., et al. (2014). Paramagnetic hollow silica nanospheres for in vivo targeted ultrasound and magnetic resonance imaging. *Biomaterials* 35, 5381–5392. doi: 10.1016/j.biomaterials.2014.03.030

Appis, A. W., Tracy, M. J., and Feinstein, S. B. (2015). Update on the safety and efficacy of commercial ultrasound contrast agents in cardiac applications. *Echo Res. Pract.* 2, R55–R62. doi: 10.1530/ERP-15-0018

Barr, R. G. (2013). Off-label use of ultrasound contrast agents for abdominal imaging in the United States. *J. Ultrasound Med.* 32, 7–12.

Bauer, A., Blomley, M., Leen, E., Cosgrove, D., and Schlief, R. (1999). Liver-specific imaging with SHU 563A: diagnostic potential of a new class of ultrasound contrast media. *Eur. Radiol.* 9, S349–S352. doi: 10.1007/PL00014072

Böhmer, M. R., Schroeders, R., Steenbakkers, J. A. M., de Winter, S. H. P. M., Duineveld, P. A., Lub, J., et al. (2006). Preparation of monodisperse polymer particles and capsules by ink-jet printing. Colloids Surfaces A Physicochem. *Eng. Asp.* 289, 96–104. doi: 10.1016/j.colsurfa.2006.04.011

Böhmer, M. R., Steenbakkers, J. A. M., and Chlon, C. (2010). Monodisperse polymeric particles prepared by ink-jet printing: double emulsions, hydrogels and polymer mixtures. *Colloids Surfaces B Biointerfaces* 79, 47–52. doi: 10.1016/j.colsurfb.2010.03.021

Bokor, D., Chambers, J. B., Rees, P. J., Mant, T. G., Luzzani, F., and Spinazzi, A. (2001). *Clinical Safety of SonoVue, a New Contrast Agent for Ultrasound Imaging, in Healthy Volunteers and in Patients with Chronic Obstructive Pulmonary Disease.* Available at: http://www.mendeley.com/research/clinical-safety-sonovue-new-contrast-agent-ultrasound-imaging-healthy-volunteers-patients-chronic-ob-1 doi: 10.1097/00004424-200102000-00006

Borden, M. A., Kruse, D. E., Caskey, C. F., Zhao, S., Dayton, P. A., and Ferrara, K. W. (2005). Influence of lipid shell physicochemical properties on ultrasound-induced microbubble destruction. *IEEE Trans. Ultrason. Ferroelectr. Freq. Control* 52, 1992–2002. doi: 10.1109/TUFFC.2005.1561668

Borges, A. C., Walde, T., Reibis, R. K., Grohmann, A., Ziebig, R., Rutsch, W., et al. (2002). Does contrast echocardiography with optison induce myocardial necrosis in humans? *J. Am. Soc. Echocardiogr.* 15, 1080–1086. doi: 10.1067/mje.2002.121833

Brismar, T. B., Grishenkov, D., Gustafsson, B., Härmark, J., Barrefelt, Å., Kothapalli, S. V. V. N., et al. (2012). Magnetite nanoparticles can be coupled to microbubbles to support multimodal imaging. *Biomacromolecules* 13, 1390–1399. doi: 10.1021/bm300099f

Carroll, B. A., Turner, R. J., Tickner, E. G., Boyle, D. B., and Young, S. W. (1980). Gelatin encapsulated nitrogen microbubbles as ultrasonic contrast agents. *Invest. Radiol.* 15, 260–266. doi: 10.1097/00004424-198005000-1980 05013

Cavalieri, F., El Hamassi, A., Chiessi, E., and Paradossi, G. (2005). Stable polymeric microballoons as multifunctional device for biomedical uses: synthesis and characterization. *Langmuir* 21, 8758–8764. doi: 10.1021/la050287j

Cavalieri, F., El Hamassi, A., Chiessi, E., Paradossi, G., Villa, R., and Zaffaroni, N. (2006). Ligands tethering to biocompatible ultrasound active polymeric microbubbles surface. *Macromol. Symp.* 234, 94–101. doi: 10.1002/masy.200650213

Chen, C. C., and Borden, M. A. (2011). The role of poly(ethylene glycol) brush architecture in complement activation on targeted microbubble surfaces. *Biomaterials* 32, 6579–6587. doi: 10.1016/j.biomaterials.2011.05.027

Chen, Y., Chen, H., and Shi, J. (2013). In vivo bio-safety evaluations and diagnostic/therapeutic applications of chemically designed mesoporous silica nanoparticles. *Adv. Mater.* 25, 3144–3176. doi: 10.1002/adma.2012 05292

Claudon, M., Dietrich, C. F., Choi, B. I., Cosgrove, D. O., Kudo, M., Nolsøe, C. P., et al. (2013). Guidelines and good clinical practice recommendations for contrast enhanced ultrasound (CEUS) in the Liver - Update 2012. A WFUMB-EFSUMB Initiative in Cooperation with Representatives of AFSUMB, AIUM, ASUM, FLAUS and ICUS. *Ultrasound Med. Biol.* 39, 187–210. doi: 10.1016/j.ultrasmedbio.2012.09.002

Cohen, J. L., Cheirif, J., Segar, D. S., Gillam, L. D., Gottdiener, J. S., Hausnerova, E., et al. (1998). Improved left ventricular endocardial border delineation and opacification with OPTISON (FS069), a new echocardiographic contrast agent: results of a phase III multicenter trial. *J. Am. Coll. Cardiol.* 32, 746–752. doi: 10.1016/S0735-1097(98)00311-318

Cohen, S., Andrianov, A. K., Wheatley, M., Allcock, H. R., and Langer, R. S. (1996). Gas-filled polymeric microbubbles for ultrasound imaging. US. Paten 54 87390.

Cokkinos, D. D., Antypa, E. G., Skilakaki, M., Kriketou, D., Tavernaraki, E., and Piperopoulos, P. N. (2013). Contrast enhanced ultrasound of the kidneys: what is it capable of? *Biomed. Res. Int.* 2013, 1–13. doi: 10.1155/2013/595873

Correas, J.-M., Bridal, L., Lesavre, A., Méjean, A., Claudon, M., and Hélénon, O. (2014). Ultrasound contrast agents: properties, principles of action, tolerance, and artifacts. *Eur. Radiol.* 11, 1316–1328. doi: 10.1007/s0033001 00940

Cotter, B., Kwan, O. L., Kimura, B., Leese, P., Quay, S., Worah, D., et al. (1994). Evaluation of the efficacy, safety and pharmacokinetics of QW3600 (Echogen) in man. *Circulation* 90:555.

Crowe, L. M., Crowe, J. H., Rudolph, A., Womersley, C., and Appel, L. (1985). Preservation of freeze-dried liposomes by Trehalose. *Arch. Biochem. Biophys.* 242, 240–247. doi: 10.1016/0003-9861(85)90498-9

Cui, W., Bei, J., Wang, S., Zhi, G., Zhao, Y., and Zhou, X. (2005a). "In vitro and in vivo evaluation of poly(L-lactide-co-glycolide) (PLGA) microbubbles as a contrast agent," in *Proceedings of the 8. Arab International Conference on Polymer Science and Technology*, Sharm Elshiekh.

Cui, W., Bei, J., Wang, S., Zhi, G., Zhao, Y., Zhou, X., et al. (2005b). Preparation and evaluation of poly(L-lactide-co-glycolide) (PLGA) microbubbles as a contrast agent for myocardial contrast echocardiography. *J. Biomed. Mater. Res. Part B Appl. Biomater.* 73, 171–178. doi: 10.1002/jbm.b.30189

Dalecki, D. (2005). "Biological effects of microbubble-based ultrasound contrast agents," in *Contrast Media in Ultrasonography - Basic Principles and Clinical Applications*, eds A. L. Baert, L. W. Bragy, H.-P. Heilmann, M. Molls, and K. Sartor (Heidelberg: Springer-Verlag), 77–87.

D'Arrigo, J. S. (1981). Aromatic proteinaceous surfactants stabilize long-lived gas microbubbles from natural sources. *J. Chem. Phys.* 75, 962. doi: 10.1063/1.442096

D'Arrigo, J. S. (1993). Method for teh production of medical-grad lipid-coated microbubbles, paramagnetic labeling of such microbubbles and therapeutic use of microbubbles. US. Patent No 5215680.

Delalande, A., Kotopoulis, S., Postema, M., Midoux, P., and Pichon, C. (2013). Sonoporation: mechanistic insights and ongoing challenges for gene transfer. *Gene* 525, 191–199. doi: 10.1016/j.gene.2013.03.095

Dewitte, H., Van Lint, S., Heirman, C., Thielemans, K., De Smedt, S. C., Breckpot, K., et al. (2014). The potential of antigen and TriMix sonoporation using mRNA-loaded microbubbles for ultrasound-triggered cancer immunotherapy. *J. Control. Release Submitted* 194, 28–36. doi: 10.1016/j.jconrel.2014.08.011

Dolan, M. S., Gala, S. S., Dodla, S., Abdelmoneim, S. S., Xie, F., Cloutier, D., et al. (2009). Safety and efficacy of commercially available ultrasound contrast agents for rest and stress echocardiography a multicenter experience. *J. Am. Coll. Cardiol.* 53, 32–38. doi: 10.1016/j.jacc.2008.08.066

du Toit, L. C., Govender, T., Pillay, V., Choonara, Y. E., and Kodama, T. (2011). Investigating the effect of polymeric approaches on circulation time and physical properties of nanobubbles. *Pharm. Res.* 28, 494–504. doi: 10.1007/s11095-010-0247-y

Eisenbrey, J. R., Burstein, O. M., and Wheatley, M. A. (2008). Effect of molecular weight and end capping on poly(lactic- co -glycolic acid) ultrasound contrast agents. *Polym. Eng. Sci.* 48, 1785–1792. doi: 10.1002/pen.21146

Ellegala, D. B., Leong-Poi, H., Carpenter, J. E., Klibanov, A. L., Kaul, S., Shaffrey, M. E., et al. (2003). Imaging tumor angiogenesis with contrast ultrasound and microbubbles targeted to alpha(v)beta3. *Circulation* 108, 336–341. doi: 10.1161/01.CIR.0000080326.15367.0C

Ernst, H., Nusko, G., Hahn, E. G., and Heyder, N. (1997). Color Doppler endosonography of esophageal varices: signal enhancement after intravenous injection of the ultrasound contrast agent Levovist. *Endoscopy* 29, S42–S43. doi: 10.1055/s-2007-1004290

Farny, C. H., Glynn Holt, R., and Roy, R. A. (2010). The correlation between bubble-enhanced HIFU heating and cavitation power. *IEEE Trans. Biomed. Eng.* 57, 175–184. doi: 10.1109/TBME.2009.2028133

Feinstein, S. B., Cheirif, J., Ten Cate, F. J., Silverman, P. R., Heidenreich, P. A., Dick, C., et al. (1990). Safety and efficacy of a new transpulmonary ultrasound contrast agent: initial multicenter clinical results. *J. Am. Coll. Cardiol.* 16, 316–324. doi: 10.1016/0735-1097(90)90580-I

Fokong, S., Fragoso, A., Rix, A., Curaj, A., Wu, Z., Lederle, W., et al. (2013). Ultrasound molecular imaging of E-selectin in tumor vessels using poly n-butyl cyanoacrylate microbubbles covalently coupled to a short targeting peptide. *Investig. Radiol.* 48, 843–850. doi: 10.1097/RLI.0b013e31829d03ec

Fokong, S., Siepmann, M., Liu, Z., Schmitz, G., Kiessling, F., and Gätjens, J. (2011). Advanced characterization and refinement of poly N-butyl cyanoacrylate microbubbles for ultrasound imaging. *Ultrasound Med. Biol.* 37, 1622–1634. doi: 10.1016/j.ultrasmedbio.2011.07.001

Forsberg, F., Goldberg, B. B., Liu, J. B., Merton, D. A., Rawool, N. M., and Shi, W. T. (1999). Tissue-specific US contrast agent for evaluation of hepatic and splenic parenchyma. *Radiology* 210, 125–132. doi: 10.1148/radiology.210.1.r99ja11125

Forsberg, F., Liu, J.-B., Merton, D. A., Rawool, N. M., and Goldberg, B. B. (1994). "In vivo evaluation of a new ultrasound contrast agent," in *Proceedings of the IEEE Ultrasonics Symposium*, Vol. 3 (Cannes: IEEE), 1555–1558. doi: 10.1109/ultsym.1994.401888

Fritz, T. A., Unger, E. C., Sutherland, D. G., and Sahn, D. (1997). Phase I clinical trials of MRX-115. *Invest. Radiol.* 32, 735–740. doi: 10.1097/00004424-199712000-199712003

Fritzsch, T., Hauff, P., Heldmann, F., Lüders, F., Uhlendorf, V., and Weitschies, W. (1994). Preliminary results with a new liver specific ultrasound contrast agent. *Ultrasound. Med. Biol.* 20, S137.

Gong, Z., Ran, H., Wu, S., Zhu, J., and Zheng, J. (2014). Ultrasound-microbubble transplantation of bone marrow stromal cells improves neurological function after forebrain ischemia in adult mice. *Cell Biochem. Biophys.* 70, 499–504. doi: 10.1007/s12013-014-9947-y

Gramiak, R., and Shah, P. M. (1968). Echocardiography of the Aortic Root. *Invest. Radiol.* 3, 301–388. doi: 10.1097/00004424-196809000-00011

Grayburn, P. A., Weiss, J. L., Hack, T. C., Klodas, E., Raichlen, J. S., Vannan, M. A., et al. (1998). Phase III multicenter trial comparing the efficacy of 2% dodecafluoropentane emulsion (EchoGen) and sonicated 5% human albumin (Albunex) as ultrasound contrast agents in patients with suboptimal echocardiograms. *J. Am. Coll. Cardiol.* 32, 230–236. doi: 10.1016/S0735-1097(98)00219-218

Grishenkov, D., Pecorari, C., Brismar, T. B., and Paradossi, G. (2009). Characterization of acoustic properties of pva-shelled ultrasound contrast agents: linear properties (Part I). *Ultrasound. Med. Biol.* 35, 1127–1138. doi: 10.1016/j.ultrasmedbio.2009.02.002

Henri, M., Florence, E., Aurore, B., Denis, H., Frederic, P., Francois, T., et al. (2014). Contribution of contrast-enhanced ultrasound with Sonovue to describe the microvascularization of uterine fibroid tumors before and after uterine artery embolization. *Eur. J. Obstet. Gynecol. Reprod. Biol.* 181, 104–110. doi: 10.1016/j.ejogrb.2014.07.030

Hernot, S., and Klibanov, A. L. (2008). Microbubbles in ultrasound-triggered drug and gene delivery. *Adv. Drug Deliv. Rev.* 60, 1153–1166. doi: 10.1016/j.addr.2008.03.005

Hilmann, J., Hoffmann, R. R., Muetzel, W., and Zimmermann, I. (1985). Carrier liquid solutions for the production of gas microbubbles, preparation thereof, and use thereof as contrast medium for ultrasonic diagnostics. *Ultrasound Med. Biol.* US Patent 4466442: 11, II.

Hoff, L., Sontum, P. C., and Hoff, B. (1996). Acoustic properties of shell-encapsulated, gas-filled ultrasound contrast agents. *Proc. IEEE Ultrason. Symp.* 2, 1441–1444. doi: 10.1109/ULTSYM.1996.584337

Hu, H., Zhou, H., Du, J., Wang, Z., An, L., Yang, H., et al. (2011a). Biocompatiable hollow silica microspheres as novel ultrasound contrast agents for in vivo imaging. *J. Mater. Chem.* 21, 6576. doi: 10.1039/c0jm03915b

Hu, H., Zhou, H., Liang, J., An, L., Dai, A., Li, X., et al. (2011b). Facile synthesis of amino-functionalized hollow silica microspheres and their potential application for ultrasound imaging. *J. Colloid Interface Sci.* 358, 392–398. doi: 10.1016/j.jcis.2011.03.051

Huang, K. S., Lin, Y. S., Chang, W. R., Wang, Y. L., and Yang, C. H. (2013). A facile fabrication of alginate microbubbles using a gas foaming reaction. *Molecules* 18, 9594–9602. doi: 10.3390/molecules18089594

Hutter, J. C., Luu, H. M., Mehlhaff, P. M., Killam, A. L., and Dittrich, H. C. (1999). Physiologically based pharmacokinetic model for fluorocarbon elimination after the administration of an octafluoropropane-albumin microsphere sonographic contrast agent. *J. Ultrasound Med.* 18, 1–11.

Hvattum, E., Normann, P. T., Oulie, I., Uran, S., Ringstad, O., and Skotland, T. (2001). Determination of perfluorobutane in rat blood by automatic headspace capillary gas chromatography and selected ion monitoring mass spectrometry. *J. Pharm. Biomed. Anal.* 24, 487–494. doi: 10.1016/S0731-7085(00)00432-5

Hynynen, K., McDannold, N., Vykhodtseva, N., and Jolesz, F. A. (2001). Noninvasive MR imaging-guided focal opening of the blood-brain barrier in rabbits. *Radiology* 220, 640–646. doi: 10.1148/radiol.2202001804

Jiang, N., Xie, B., Zhang, X., He, M., Li, K., Bai, J., et al. (2014). Enhancing ablation effects of a microbubble-enhancing contrast agent ("sonovue") in the treatment of uterine fibroids with high-intensity focused ultrasound: a randomized controlled trial. *Cardiovasc. Intervent. Radiol.* 37, 1321–1328. doi: 10.1007/s00270-013-0803-z

Jiang, Q., Hao, S., Xiao, X., Yao, J., Ou, B., Zhao, Z., et al. (2015). Production and characterization of a novel long-acting Herceptin-targeted nanobubble contrast agent specific for Her-2-positive breast cancers. *Breast Cancer.* doi: 10.1007/s12282-014-0581-588 [Epub ahead of print].

Keller, M. W., Feinstein, S. B., and Watson, D. D. (1987). Successful left ventricular opacification following peripheral venous injection of sonicated contrast agent: an experimental evaluation. *Am. Heart J.* 114, 570–575. doi: 10.1016/0002-8703(87)90754-X

Keller, M. W., Glasheen, W., Teja, K., Gear, A., and Kaul, S. (1988). Myocardial contrast echocardiography without significant hemodynamic effects or reactive hyperemia: a major advantage in the imaging of regional myocardial perfusion. *J. Am. Coll. Cardiol.* 12, 1039–1047. doi: 10.1016/0735-1097(88)9047 4-90473

Keller, M. W., Segal, S. S., Kaul, S., and Duling, B. (1989). The behavior of sonicated albumin microbubbles within the microcirculation: a basis for their use during myocardial contrast echocardiography. *Circ. Res.* 65, 458–467. doi: 10.1161/01.RES.65.2.458

Kelly, C. M., DeMerlis, C. C., Schoneker, D. R., and Borzelleca, J. F. (2003). Subchronic toxicity study in rats and genotoxicity tests with polyvinyl alcohol. *Food Chem. Toxicol.* 41, 719–727. doi: 10.1016/S0278-6915(03)0 0003-6

Kiessling, F., Fokong, S., Koczera, P., Lederle, W., and Lammers, T. (2012). Ultrasound microbubbles for molecular diagnosis, therapy, and theranostics. *J. Nucl. Med.* 53, 345–348. doi: 10.2967/jnumed.111.099754

Kiessling, F., Mertens, M. E., Grimm, J., and Lammers, T. (2014). Nanoparticles for imaging: top or flop? *Radiology* 273, 10–28. doi: 10.1148/radiol.141 31520

Kindberg, G. M., Tolleshaug, H., Roos, N., and Skotland, T. (2003). Hepatic clearance of Sonazoid perfluorobutane microbubbles by Kupffer cells does not reduce the ability of liver to phagocytose or degrade albumin microspheres. *Cell Tissue Res.* 312, 49–54. doi: 10.1007/s00441-003-0698-690

Kitano, M., Kudo, M., Yamao, K., Takagi, T., Sakamoto, H., Komaki, T., et al. (2012). Characterization of small solid tumors in the pancreas: the value of contrast-enhanced harmonic endoscopic ultrasonography. *Am. J. Gastroenterol.* 107, 303–310. doi: 10.1038/ajg.2011.354

Koczera, P., Wu, Z., Fokong, S., Theek, B., Appold, L., Jorge, S., et al. (2012). Fluorescently labeled microbubbles for facilitating translational molecular ultrasound studies. *Drug Deliv. Transl. Res.* 2, 56–64. doi: 10.1007/s13346-011-0056-59

Korpanty, G., Grayburn, P. A., Shohet, R. V, and Brekken, R. A. (2005). Targeting vascular endothelium with avidin microbubbles. *Ultrasound Med. Biol.* 31, 1279–1283. doi: 10.1016/j.ultrasmedbio.2005.06.001

Kremkau, F. W., Gramiak, R., Carstensen, E. L., Shah, P. M., and Kramer, D. H. (1970). Ultrasonic detection of cavitation at catheter tips. *Am. J. Roentgenol.* 110, 177–183. doi: 10.2214/ajr.110.1.177

Kronzon, I., Goodkin, G. M., Culliford, A., Scholes, J. V., Boctor, F., Freedberg, R. S., et al. (1994). Right atrial and right ventricular obstruction by recurrent stromomyoma. *J. Am. Soc. Echocardiogr.* 7, 528–533. doi: 10.1016/S0894-7317(14)80010-80012

Lammers, T., Koczera, P., Fokong, S., Gremse, F., Ehling, J., Vogt, M., et al. (2015). Theranostic USPIO-loaded microbubbles for mediating and monitoring blood-brain barrier permeation. *Adv. Funct. Mater.* 25, 36–43. doi: 10.1002/adfm.201401199

Lanza, G. M., Abendschein, D. R., Hall, C. S., Scott, M. J., Scherrer, D. E., Houseman, A., et al. (2000). In vivo molecular imaging of stretch-induced tissue factor in carotid arteries with ligand-targeted nanoparticles. *J. Am. Soc. Echocardiogr.* 13, 608–614. doi: 10.1067/mje.2000.105840

Lassau, N., Bonastre, J., Kind, M., Vilgrain, V., Lacroix, J., Cuinet, M., et al. (2014). Validation of dynamic contrast-enhanced ultrasound in predicting outcomes of antiangiogenic therapy for solid tumors: the french multicenter support for innovative and expensive techniques study. *Invest. Radiol.* 49, 794–800. doi: 10.1097/RLI.0000000000000085

Lassau, N., Lamuraglia, M., Chami, L., Leclère, J., Bonvalot, S., Terrier, P., et al. (2006). Gastrointestinal stromal tumors treated with imatinib: monitoring response with contrast-enhanced sonography. *Am. J. Roentgenol.* 187, 1267–1273. doi: 10.2214/AJR.05.1192

Lassau, N., Lamuraglia, M., Vanel, D., Le Cesne, A., Chami, L., Jaziri, S., et al. (2005). Doppler US with perfusion software and contrast medium injection in the early evaluation of isolated limb perfusion of limb sarcomas: prospective study of 49 cases. *Ann. Oncol.* 16, 1054–1060. doi: 10.1093/annonc/m di214

Leguerney, I., Scoazec, J.-Y., Gadot, N., Robin, N., Pénault-Llorca, F., Victorin, S., et al. (2015). Molecular ultrasound imaging using contrast agents targeting endoglin, vascular endothelial growth factor receptor 2 and integrin. *Ultrasound Med. Biol.* 41, 197–207. doi: 10.1016/j.ultrasmedbio.2014.06.014

Leng, X., Wang, J., Carson, A., Chen, X., Fu, H., Ottoboni, S., et al. (2014). Ultrasound detection of myocardial ischemic memory using an e-selectin targeting Peptide amenable to human application. *Mol. Imag.* 16, 1–9.

Leong-Poi, H. (2002). Noninvasive assessment of angiogenesis by ultrasound and microbubbles targeted to alphav-integrins. *Circulation* 107, 455–460. doi: 10.1161/01.CIR.0000044916.05919.8B

Leong-Poi, H., Song, J., Rim, S. J., Christiansen, J., Kaul, S., and Lindner, J. R. (2002). Influence of microbubble shell properties on ultrasound signal: Implications for low-power perfusion imaging. *J. Am. Soc. Echocardiogr.* 15, 1269–1276. doi: 10.1067/mje.2002.124516

Liberman, A., Martinez, H. P., Ta, C. N., Barback, C. V., Mattrey, R. F., Kono, Y., et al. (2012). Hollow silica and silica-boron nano/microparticles for contrast-enhanced ultrasound to detect small tumors. *Biomaterials* 33, 5124–5129. doi: 10.1016/j.biomaterials.2012.03.066

Liberman, A., Wu, Z., Barback, C. V., Viveros, R. D., Wang, J., Ellies, L. G., et al. (2014). Hollow iron-silica nanoshells for enhanced high intensity focused ultrasound. *J. Surg. Res.* 190, 391–398. doi: 10.1016/j.jss.2014. 05.009

Lin, P.-L., Eckersley, R. J., and Hall, E. A. H. (2009). Ultrabubble: a laminated ultrasound contrast agent with narrow size range. *Adv. Mater.* 21, 3949–3952. doi: 10.1002/adma.200901096

Lindner, J. R., Coggins, M. P., Kaul, S., Klibanov, A. L., Brandenburger, G. H., and Ley, K. (2000a). Microbubble persistence in the microcirculation during ischemia/reperfusion and inflammation is caused by integrin- and complement-mediated adherence to activated leukocytes. *Circulation* 101, 668–675. doi: 10.1161/01.CIR.101.6.668

Lindner, J. R., Song, J., Xu, F., Klibanov, A. L., Singbartl, K., Ley, K., et al. (2000b). Noninvasive ultrasound imaging of inflammation using microbubbles targeted to activated leukocytes. *Circulation* 102, 2745–2750. doi: 10.1161/01.CIR.102.22.2745

Liu, J., Li, J., Rosol, T. J., Pan, X., and Voorhees, J. L. (2007). Biodegradable nanoparticles for targeted ultrasound imaging of breast cancer cells in vitro. *Phys. Med. Biol.* 52, 4739–4747. doi: 10.1088/0031-9155/52/16/002

Liu, Y. N., Khangura, J., Xie, A., Belcik, J. T., Qi, Y., Davidson, B. P., et al. (2013). Renal retention of lipid microbubbles: a potential mechanism for flank discomfort during ultrasound contrast administration. *J. Am. Soc. Echocardiogr.* 26, 1474–1481. doi: 10.1016/j.echo.2013.08.004

Ma, M., Xu, H., Chen, H., Jia, X., Zhang, K., Wang, Q., et al. (2014). A drug-perfluorocarbon nanoemulsion with an ultrathin silica coating for the synergistic effect of chemotherapy and ablation by high-intensity focused ultrasound. *Adv. Mater.* 26, 7378–7385. doi: 10.1002/adma.2014 02969

Maruyama, H., Matsutani, S., Saisho, H., Mine, Y., Kamiyama, N., Hirata, T., et al. (2005). Real-time blood-pool images of contrast enhanced ultrasound with Definity in the detection of tumour nodules in the liver. *Br. J. Radiol.* 78, 512–518. doi: 10.1259/bjr/59648297

Maruyama, H., Matsutani, S., Saisho, H., Mine, Y., Yuki, H., and Miyata, K. (2004). Different behaviors of microbubbles in the liver: time-related quantitative analysis of two ultrasound contrast agents, Levovist and Definity. *Ultrasound Med. Biol.* 30, 1035–1040. doi: 10.1016/j.ultrasmedbio.2004.06.008

Milgroom, A., Intrator, M., Madhavan, K., Mazzaro, L., Shandas, R., Liu, B., et al. (2014). Mesoporous silica nanoparticles as a breast-cancer targeting ultrasound contrast agent. *Colloids Surf. B Biointerfaces* 116, 652–657. doi: 10.1016/j.colsurfb.2013.10.038

Molina, C. A., Barreto, A. D., Tsivgoulis, G., Sierzenski, P., Malkoff, M. D., Rubiera, M., et al. (2009). Transcranial ultrasound in clinical sonothrombolysis (TUCSON) trial. *Ann. Neurol.* 66, 28–38. doi: 10.1002/ana.21723

Molina, C. A., Ribo, M., Rubiera, M., Montaner, J., Santamarina, E., Delgado-Mederos, R., et al. (2006). Microbubble administration accelerates clot lysis during continuous 2-MHz ultrasound monitoring in stroke patients treated with intravenous tissue plasminogen activator. *Stroke* 37, 425–429. doi: 10.1161/01.STR.0000199064.94588.39

Niu, C., Wang, Z., Lu, G., Krupka, T. M., Sun, Y., You, Y., et al. (2013). Doxorubicin loaded superparamagnetic PLGA-iron oxide multifunctional microbubbles for dual-mode US/MR imaging and therapy of metastasis in lymph nodes. *Biomaterials* 34, 2307–2317. doi: 10.1016/j.biomaterials.2012. 12.003

Niu, C., Wang, Z., Zuo, G., Krupka, T. M., Ran, H., Zhang, P., et al. (2012). Poly(Lactide-co-glycolide) ultrasonographic microbubbles carrying Sudan black for preoperative and intraoperative localization of lymph nodes. *Clin. Breast Cancer* 12, 199–206. doi: 10.1016/j.clbc.2012.01.005

Oeffinger, B. E., and Wheatley, M. A. (2004). Development and characterization of a nano-scale contrast agent. *Ultrasonics* 42, 343–347. doi: 10.1016/j.ultras.2003.11.011

Olbrich, C., Hauff, P., Scholle, F., Schmidt, W., Bakowsky, U., Briel, A., et al. (2006). The in vitro stability of air-filled polybutylcyanoacrylate microparticles. *Biomaterials* 27, 3549–3559. doi: 10.1016/j.biomaterials.2006.02.034

Ota, T., and Ono, S. (2004). Intrapancreatic accessory spleen: diagnosis using contrast enhanced ultrasound. *Br. J. Radiol.* 77, 148–149. doi: 10.1259/bjr/56352047

Palmowski, M., Morgenstern, B., Hauff, P., Reinhardt, M., Huppert, J., Maurer, M., et al. (2008). Pharmacodynamics of streptavidin-coated cyanoacrylate microbubbles designed for molecular ultrasound imaging. *Investig. Radiol.* 43, 162–169. doi: 10.1097/RLI.0b013e31815a251b

Pelura, T. J. (1998). Clinical experience with AF0150 (Imagent US), a new ultrasound contrast agent. *Acad. Radiol.* 5, S69–S71. doi: 10.1016/S1076-6332(98)80064-80060

Perera, R. H., Solorio, L., Wu, H., Gangolli, M., Silverman, E., Hernandez, C., et al. (2014). Nanobubble ultrasound contrast agents for enhanced delivery of thermal sensitizer to tumors undergoing radiofrequency ablation. *Pharm. Res.* 31, 1407–1417. doi: 10.1007/s11095-013-1100-x

Petit, B., Yan, F., Bussat, P., Bohren, Y., Gaud, E., Fontana, P., et al. (2015). Fibrin degradation during sonothrombolysis – Effect of ultrasound, microbubbles and tissue plasminogen activator. *J. Drug Deliv. Sci. Technol.* 25, 29–35. doi: 10.1016/j.jddst.2014.12.001

Prada, F., Perin, A., Martegani, A., Aiani, L., Solbiati, L., Lamperti, M., et al. (2014). Intraoperative contrast-enhanced ultrasound for brain tumor surgery. *Neurosurgery* 74, 542–552. doi: 10.1227/NEU.0000000000000301

Quaia, E. (2006). "Contrast media in ultrasonography," in *Basic Principles and Clinical Applications*, eds A. L. Baert, L. W. Brady, H.-P. Heilmann, M. Molls, and K. Sartor (Berlin: Springer-Verlag), 9–11.

Rapoport, N., Nam, K. H., Gupta, R., Gao, Z., Mohan, P., Payne, A., et al. (2011). Ultrasound-mediated tumor imaging and nanotherapy using drug loaded, block copolymer stabilized perfluorocarbon nanoemulsions. *J. Control. Release* 153, 4–15. doi: 10.1016/j.jconrel.2011.01.022

Raymond, S. B., Skoch, J., Hynynen, K., and Bacskai, B. J. (2007). Multiphoton imaging of ultrasound/Optison mediated cerebrovascular effects in vivo. *J. Cereb. Blood Flow Metab.* 27, 393–403. doi: 10.1038/sj.jcbfm.9600336

Ryan, S. M., Mantovani, G., Wang, X., Haddleton, D. M., and Brayden, D. J. (2008). Advances in PEGylation of important biotech molecules: delivery aspects. *Expert Opin. Drug Deliv.* 5, 371–383. doi: 10.1517/17425247.5.4.371

Saha, S., Bhanja, P., Partanem, A., Zhang, W., Liu, L., Tomé, W., et al. (2014). Low intensity focused ultrasound (LOFU) modulates unfolded protein response and sensitizes prostate cancer to 17AAG. *Oncoscience* 1, 434–445.

Schlief, R., Schürmann, R., and Niendorf, H. P. (1991). Blood-pool enhancement with SH U 508 a: results of phase II clinical trials. *Investig. Radiol.* 26, S188–S189. doi: 10.1097/00004424-199111001-00064

Schutt, E. G., Klein, D. H., Mattrey, R. M., and Riess, J. G. (2003). Injectable microbubbles as contrast agents for diagnostic ultrasound imaging: the key role of perfluorochemicals. *Angew. Chemie Int. Ed.* 42, 3218–3235. doi: 10.1002/anie.200200550

Schutt, E. G., Pelura, T. J., and Hopkins, R. M. (1996). Osmotically stabilized microbubble sonographic contrast agents. *Acad. Radiol.* 3(Suppl. 2), S188–S190. doi: 10.1016/S1076-6332(96)80530-80537

Singhal, S., Moser, C. C., and Wheatley, M. A. (1993). Surfactant-stabilized microbubbles as ultrasound contrast agents: stability study of span-60 and tween-80 mixtures using a langmuir trough. *Langmuir* 9, 2426–2429. doi: 10.1021/la00033a027

Sirlin, C. B., Girard, M. S., Steinbach, G. C., Baker, K. G., Broderdorf, S. K., Hall, L. A., et al. (1997). Effect of ultrasound transmit power on liver enhancement with Imagent US, a PFC-stabilized microbubble contrast agent. *Int. J. Imaging Syst. Technol.* 8, 82–88. doi: 10.1002/(SICI)1098-1098(1997)8:1<82::AID-IMA10>3.0.CO 2-N

Smith, M. D., Elion, J. L., McClure, R. R., Kwan, O. L., and DeMaria, A. N. (1989). Left heart opacification with peripheral venous injection of a new saccharide echo contrast agent in dogs. *J. Am. Coll. Cardiol.* 13, 1622–1628. doi: 10.1016/0735-1097(89)90357-90354

Soltani, A., Singhal, R., Obtera, M., Roy, R. A., Clark, W. M., and Hansmann, D. R. (2011). Potentiating intra-arterial sonothrombolysis for acute ischemic stroke by the addition of the ultrasound contrast agents (Optison & SonoVue). *J. Thromb. Thrombolysis* 31, 71–84. doi: 10.1007/s11239-010-0483-483

Sorace, A. G., Korb, M., Warram, J. M., Umphrey, H., Zinn, K. R., Rosenthal, E., et al. (2014). Ultrasound-stimulated drug delivery for treatment of residual disease after incomplete resection of head and neck cancer. *Ultrasound Med. Biol.* 40, 755–764. doi: 10.1016/j.ultrasmedbio.2013.11.002

Sun, R. R., Noble, M. L., Sun, S. S., Song, S., and Miao, C. H. (2014). Development of therapeutic microbubbles for enhancing ultrasound-mediated gene delivery. *J. Control. Release Off. J. Control. Release Soc.* 182, 111–120. doi: 10.1016/j.jconrel.2014.03.002

Ta, C. N., Liberman, A., Martinez, H. P., Barback, C. V., Mattrey, R. F., Blair, S. L., et al. (2012). Integrated processing of contrast pulse sequencing ultrasound imaging for enhanced active contrast of hollow gas filled silica nanoshells and microshells. *J. Vac. Sci. Technol. B Microelectron. Nanom. Struct.* 30, 02C104. doi: 10.1116/1.3694835

Tachibana, K., and Tachibana, S. (1995). Albumin microbubble echo-contrast material as an enhancer for ultrasound accelerated thrombolysis. *Circulation* 92, 1148–1150. doi: 10.1161/01.CIR.92.5.1148

Taylor, G. A., Ecklund, K., and Dunning, P. S. (1996). Renal cortical perfusion in rabbits: visualization with color amplitude imaging and an experimental microbubble-based US contrast agent. *Radiology* 201, 125–129. doi: 10.1148/radiology.201.1.8816532

ter Haar, G. (2009). Safety and bio-effects of ultrasound contrast agents. *Med. Biol. Eng. Comput.* 47, 893–900. doi: 10.1007/s11517-009-0507-3

Toft, K. G., Hustvedt, S. O., Hals, P.-A., Oulie, I., Uran, S., Landmark, K., et al. (2006). Disposition of perfluorobutane in rats after intravenous injection of SonazoidTM. *Ultrasound Med. Biol.* 32, 107–114. doi: 10.1016/j.ultrasmedbio.2005.09.008

Tsivgoulis, G., Eggers, J., Ribo, M., Perren, F., Saqqur, M., Rubiera, M., et al. (2010). Safety and efficacy of ultrasound-enhanced thrombolysis: a comprehensive review and meta-analysis of randomized and nonrandomized studies. *Stroke* 41, 280–287. doi: 10.1161/STROKEAHA.109.563304

Tzu-Yin, W., Wilson, K. E., Machtaler, S., and Willmann, J. K. (2013). Ultrasound and microbubble guided drug delivery: mechanistic understanding and clinical implications. *Curr. Pharm. Biotechnol.* 14, 743–752.

Uemura, H., Sano, F., Nomiya, A., Yamamoto, T., Nakamura, M., Miyoshi, Y., et al. (2013). Usefulness of perflubutane microbubble-enhanced ultrasound in imaging and detection of prostate cancer: phase II multicenter clinical trial. *World J. Urol.* 31, 1123–1128. doi: 10.1007/s00345-012-0833-831

Unger, E., Fritz, T., Shen, D.-K., Lund, P., Sahn, D., Ramasswami, R., et al. (1994). Gas-filled lipid bilayers as Imaging Contrast Agents. *J. Liposome Res.* 4, 861–874. doi: 10.3109/08982109409018605

Unger, E., McCreery, T. P., Sweitzer, R. H., Shen, D., and Wu, G. (1998). In vitro studies of a new thrombus-specific ultrasound contrast agent. *Am. J. Cardiol.* 81, 58G–61G. doi: 10.1016/S0002-9149(98)00055-1

Unger, E., Metzger, P., Krupinski, E., Baker, M., Hulett, R., Gabaeff, D., et al. (2000). The use of a thrombus-specific ultrasound contrast agent to detect thrombus in arteriovenous fistulae. *Invest. Radiol.* 35, 86–89. doi: 10.1097/00004424-200001000-200001010

Unger, E. C. (1994). Gas filled liposomes and their use as ultrasonic contrast agents. US. Patent 5305757.

Unger, E. C., Porter, T., Culp, W., Labell, R., Matsunaga, T., and Zutshi, R. (2004). Therapeutic applications of lipid-coated microbubbles. *Adv. Drug Deliv. Rev.* 56, 1291–1314. doi: 10.1016/j.addr.2003.12.006

van der Wouw, P. A., Brauns, A. C., Bailey, S. E., Powers, J. E., and Wilde, A. A. (2000). Premature ventricular contractions during triggered imaging with ultrasound contrast. *J. Am. Soc. Echocardiogr.* 13, 288–294. doi: 10.1067/mje.2000.103865

Villanueva, F. S., Jankowski, R. J., Klibanov, A. L., Pina, M. L., Alber, S. M., Watkins, S. C., et al. (1998). Microbubbles targeted to intercellular adhesion molecule-1 bind to activated coronary artery endothelial cells. *Circulation* 98, 1–5. doi: 10.1161/01.CIR.98.1.1

von Herbay, A., Vogt, C., Willers, R., and Häussinger, D. (2004). Real-time imaging with the sonographic contrast agent SonoVue: differentiation between benign and malignant hepatic lesions. *J. Ultrasound. Med.* 23, 1557–1568.

Wang, J.-F., Wang, J.-B., Chen, H., Zhang, C.-M., Liu, L., Pan, S.-H., et al. (2008). Ultrasound-mediated microbubble destruction enhances gene transfection in pancreatic cancer cells. *Adv. Ther.* 25, 412–421. doi: 10.1007/s12325-008-0051-59

Wei, K., Shah, S., Jaber, W. A., and DeMaria, A. (2014). An observational study of the occurrence of serious adverse reactions among patients who receive optison in routine medical practice. *J. Am. Soc. Echocardiogr.* 27, 1006–1010. doi: 10.1016/j.echo.2014.04.020

Weller, G. E. R., Lu, E., Csikari, M. M., Klibanov, A. L., Fischer, D., Wagner, W. R., et al. (2003). Ultrasound imaging of acute cardiac transplant rejection with microbubbles targeted to intercellular adhesion molecule-1. *Circulation* 108, 218–224. doi: 10.1161/01.CIR.0000080287.74762.60

Wheatley, M. A., Peng, S., Singhal, S., and Goldberg, B. B. (1994). Surfactant-stabilized microbubble mixtures, process for preparing and methods of using the same. US. Patent 5352436.

Wheatley, M., Schrope, B., and Shen, P. (1990). Contrast agents for diagnostic ultrasound: development and evaluation of polymer-coated microbubbles. *Biomaterials* 11, 713–717. doi: 10.1016/0142-9612(90)90033-M

Willmann, J. K., Paulmurugan, R., Chen, K., Gheysens, O., Rodriguez-Porcel, M., Lutz, A. M., et al. (2008). US imaging of tumor angiogenesis with microbubbles targeted to vascular endothelial growth factor receptor type 2 in mice. *Radiology* 246, 508–518. doi: 10.1148/radiol.2462070536

Wilson, S. R., Burns, P. N., Muradali, D., Wilson, J. A., and Lai, X. (2000). Harmonic hepatic US with microbubble contrast agent: initial experience showing improved characterization of hemangioma, hepatocellular carcinoma, and metastasis. *Radiology* 215, 153–161. doi: 10.1148/radiology.215.1.r00ap08153

Wu, Y., Peng, H., and Zhao, X. (2015). Diagnostic performance of contrast-enhanced ultrasound for ovarian cancer: a meta-analysis. *Ultrasound Med. Biol.* 41, 967–974. doi: 10.1016/j.ultrasmedbio.2014.11.018

Xing, Z., Wang, J., Ke, H., Zhao, B., Yue, X., Dai, Z., et al. (2010). The fabrication of novel nanobubble ultrasound contrast agent for potential tumor imaging. *Nanotechnology* 21, 145607. doi: 10.1088/0957-4484/21/14/145607

Xu, J. S., Huang, J., Qin, R., Hinkle, G. H., Povoski, S. P., Martin, E. W., et al. (2010). Synthesizing and binding dual-mode poly (lactic-co-glycolic acid) (PLGA) nanobubbles for cancer targeting and imaging. *Biomaterials* 31, 1716–1722. doi: 10.1016/j.biomaterials.2009.11.052

Yanagisawa, K., Moriyasu, F., Miyahara, T., Yuki, M., and Iijima, H. (2007). Phagocytosis of ultrasound contrast agent microbubbles by Kupffer cells. *Ultrasound Med. Biol.* 33, 318–325. doi: 10.1016/j.ultrasmedbio.2006.08.008

Yin, T., Wang, P., Li, J., Wang, Y., Zheng, B., Zheng, R., et al. (2014). Tumor-penetrating codelivery of siRNA and paclitaxel with ultrasound-responsive nanobubbles hetero-assembled from polymeric micelles and liposomes. *Biomaterials* 35, 5932–5943. doi: 10.1016/j.biomaterials.2014.03.072

Yin, T., Wang, P., Zheng, R., Zheng, B., Cheng, D., Zhang, X., et al. (2012). Nanobubbles for enhanced ultrasound imaging of tumors. *Int. J. Nanomedicine* 7, 895–904. doi: 10.2147/IJN.S28830

Yuan, B., and Rychak, J. (2013). Tumor functional and molecular imaging utilizing ultrasound and ultrasound-mediated optical techniques. *Am. J. Pathol.* 182, 305–311. doi: 10.1016/j.ajpath.2012.07.036

Zhang, X., Zheng, Y., Wang, Z., Huang, S., Chen, Y., Jiang, W., et al. (2014). Methotrexate-loaded PLGA nanobubbles for ultrasound imaging and Synergistic Targeted therapy of residual tumor during HIFU ablation. *Biomaterials* 35, 5148–5161. doi: 10.1016/j.biomaterials.2014.02.036

Zheng, Y., Zhang, Y., Ao, M., Zhang, P., Zhang, H., Li, P., et al. (2012). Hematoporphyrin encapsulated PLGA microbubble for contrast enhanced ultrasound imaging and sonodynamic therapy. *J. Microencapsul.* 29, 437–444. doi: 10.3109/02652048.2012.655333

Conflict of Interest Statement: The reviewer Claus Christian Glüer declares that, despite having collaborated with the author Fabian Kiessling, the review process was handled objectively. The authors declare that the research was conducted in the absence of any commercial or financial relationships that could be construed as a potential conflict of interest.

Permissions

The contributors of this book come from diverse backgrounds, making this book a truly international effort. This book will bring forth new frontiers with its revolutionizing research information and detailed analysis of the nascent developments around the world.

We would like to thank all the contributing authors for lending their expertise to make the book truly unique. They have played a crucial role in the development of this book. Without their invaluable contributions this book wouldn't have been possible. They have made vital efforts to compile up to date information on the varied aspects of this subject to make this book a valuable addition to the collection of many professionals and students.

This book was conceptualized with the vision of imparting up-to-date information and advanced data in this field. To ensure the same, a matchless editorial board was set up. Every individual on the board went through rigorous rounds of assessment to prove their worth. After which they invested a large part of their time researching and compiling the most relevant data for our readers.

The editorial board has been involved in producing this book since its inception. They have spent rigorous hours researching and exploring the diverse topics which have resulted in the successful publishing of this book. They have passed on their knowledge of decades through this book. To expedite this challenging task, the publisher supported the team at every step. A small team of assistant editors was also appointed to further simplify the editing procedure and attain best results for the readers.

Apart from the editorial board, the designing team has also invested a significant amount of their time in understanding the subject and creating the most relevant covers. They scrutinized every image to scout for the most suitable representation of the subject and create an appropriate cover for the book.

The publishing team has been an ardent support to the editorial, designing and production team. Their endless efforts to recruit the best for this project, has resulted in the accomplishment of this book. They are a veteran in the field of academics and their pool of knowledge is as vast as their experience in printing. Their expertise and guidance has proved useful at every step. Their uncompromising quality standards have made this book an exceptional effort. Their encouragement from time to time has been an inspiration for everyone.

The publisher and the editorial board hope that this book will prove to be a valuable piece of knowledge for researchers, students, practitioners and scholars across the globe.

List of Contributors

Bridget M. Seitz, Gregory D. Fink and Stephanie W. Watts
Department of Pharmacology and Toxicology, Michigan State University, East Lansing, MI, USA

Teresa Krieger-Burke
In Vivo Facility, Michigan State University, East Lansing, MI, USA

Lieven D. Declercq, Alfons Verbruggen and Guy Bormans
Laboratory for Radiopharmacy, Department of Pharmaceutical and Pharmacological Sciences, KU Leuven, Leuven, Belgium

Rik Vandenberghe
Laboratory for Cognitive Neurology, Department of Neurosciences, KU Leuven, Leuven, Belgium

Koen Van Laere
Nuclear Medicine and Molecular Imaging, Department of Imaging and Pathology, KU Leuven, Leuven, Belgium

Jinghai J. Xu
Merck and Co., Kenilworth, NJ, USA

Yvonne W. S. Jauw and Josée M. Zijlstra
Department of Hematology, VU University Medical Center, Amsterdam, Netherlands

C. Willemien Menke-van der Houven van Oordt
Department of Medical Oncology, VU University Medical Center, Amsterdam, Netherlands

Otto S. Hoekstra, Danielle J. Vugts, Marc C. Huisman and Guus A. M. S. van Dongen
Department of Radiology and Nuclear Medicine, VU University Medical Center, Amsterdam, Netherlands

N. Harry Hendrikse
Department of Radiology and Nuclear Medicine, VU University Medical Center, Amsterdam, Netherlands
Department of Clinical Pharmacology and Pharmacy, VU University Medical Center, Amsterdam, Netherlands

Xiaobo Fan
Center of Clinical Laboratory Medicine of Zhongda Hospital, Southeast University, Nanjing, China
Medical School, Southeast University, Nanjing, China

Juxiang Fan and Xiyong Wang
Medical School, Southeast University, Nanjing, China

Pengpeng Wu and Guoqiu Wu
Center of Clinical Laboratory Medicine of Zhongda Hospital, Southeast University, Nanjing, China

Pasquina Marzola and Federico Boschi
Department of Computer Science, University of Verona, Verona, Italy

Francesco Moneta
Preclinical Imaging Division – Bruker BioSpin, Bruker Italia s.r.l, Milano, Italy

Andrea Sbarbati and Carlo Zancanaro
Department of Neurosciences, Biomedicine and Movement Sciences, University of Verona, Verona, Italy

Alicia Arranz
Department of Cell Biology and Immunology, Center for Molecular Biology "Severo Ochoa", Spanish National Research Council, Madrid, Spain

Jorge Ripoll
Department of Bioengineering and Aerospace Engineering, Universidad Carlos III of Madrid, Madrid, Spain
Experimental Medicine and Surgery Unit, Instituto de Investigación Sanitaria del Hospital Gregorio Marañón, Madrid, Spain

Arnoldo Santos
Centro Nacional de Investigaciones Cardiovasculares Carlos III, Madrid, Spain
CIBER de Enfermedades Respiratorias (CIBERES), Madrid, Spain
Madrid-MIT M+Visión Consortium, Madrid, Spain
Department of Anesthesia, Massachusetts General Hospital, Harvard Medical School, Boston, MA, USA

Leticia Fernández-Friera and Beatriz López-Melgar
Centro Nacional de Investigaciones Cardiovasculares Carlos III, Madrid, Spain
Hospital Universitario HM Monteprincipe, Madrid, Spain

María Villalba
Centro Nacional de Investigaciones Cardiovasculares Carlos III, Madrid, Spain

Samuel España
Centro Nacional de Investigaciones Cardiovasculares
Carlos III, Madrid, Spain
CIBER de Enfermedades Respiratorias (CIBERES),
Madrid, Spain
Madrid-MIT M+Visión Consortium, Madrid, Spain

Jesús Mateo
Centro Nacional de Investigaciones Cardiovasculares
Carlos III, Madrid, Spain
CIBER de Enfermedades Respiratorias (CIBERES),
Madrid, Spain

Ruben A. Mota
Centro Nacional de Investigaciones Cardiovasculares
Carlos III, Madrid, Spain
Charles River, Barcelona, Spain

Jesús Jiménez-Borreguero
Centro Nacional de Investigaciones Cardiovasculares
Carlos III, Madrid, Spain
Cardiac Imaging Department, Hospital de La Princesa,
Madrid, Spain

Jesús Ruiz-Cabello
Centro Nacional de Investigaciones Cardiovasculares
Carlos III, Madrid, Spain
CIBER de Enfermedades Respiratorias (CIBERES),
Madrid, Spain
Universidad Complutense de Madrid, Madrid, Spain

**Bart H. A. Lammertink, Clemens Bos, Roel Deckers,
Chrit T. W. Moonen and Jean-Michel Escoffre**
Image Guided Therapy, Imaging Division, University
Medical Center Utrecht, Utrecht, Netherlands

Gert Storm
Department of Pharmaceutical Sciences, Faculty of
Science, Utrecht University, Utrecht, Netherlands
Targeted Therapeutics, MIRA Institute for Biomedical
Technology and Technical Medicine, University of
Twente, Enschede, Netherlands

**Elisabeth Jonckers, Disha Shah, Julie Hamaide,
Marleen Verhoye and Annemie Van der Linden**
Bio-Imaging Lab, Department of Biomedical Sciences,
University of Antwerp, Antwerp, Belgium

Jeffrey R. Ashton
Department of Biomedical Engineering, Duke
University, Durham, NC, USA
Department of Radiology, Center for In Vivo
Microscopy, Duke University Medical Center, Durham,
NC, USA

Jennifer L. West
Department of Biomedical Engineering, Duke
University, Durham, NC, USA

Cristian T. Badea
Department of Radiology, Center for In Vivo
Microscopy, Duke University Medical Center, Durham,
NC, USA

Thoralf Niendorf
Berlin Ultrahigh Field Facility, Max Delbrück Center
for Molecular Medicine in the Helmholtz Association,
Berlin, Germany

German Centre for Cardiovascular Research, Berlin,
Germany

**Andreas Pohlmann, Henning M. Reimann, Eva Peper,
Till Huelnhagen, Min-Chi Ku and Sonia Waiczies**
Berlin Ultrahigh Field Facility, Max Delbrück Center
for Molecular Medicine in the Helmholtz Association,
Berlin, Germany

Helmar Waiczies
MRI.TOOLS GmbH, Berlin, Germany

Erdmann Seeliger
Center for Cardiovascular Research, Institute of
Physiology, Charité—Universitätsmedizin Berlin,
Berlin, Germany

Adrian Schreiber and Ralph Kettritz
Clinic for Nephrology and Intensive Care Medicine,
Charité Medical Faculty and Experimental and Clinical
Research Center, Berlin, Germany

Klaus Strobel
Bruker BioSpin MRI GmbH, Ettlingen, Germany

Vera Paefgen, Dennis Doleschel and Fabian Kiessling
Institute for Experimental Molecular Imaging, RWTH
Aachen University Hospital, Aachen, Germany

Index

www.ingramcontent.com/pod-product-compliance
Lightning Source LLC
Chambersburg PA
CBHW080634200326

41458CB00013B/4627